Hemodynamic Rounds

Hemodynamic Rounds

Interpretation of Cardiac Pathophysiology from
Pressure Waveform Analysis

Fourth Edition

Edited by

Morton J. Kern
University of California
USA

Michael J. Lim
St. Louis University Health Sciences Center
USA

James A. Goldstein
William Beaumont Hospital
USA

WILEY Blackwell

Registered Office(s)
John Wiley & Sons, Inc., 111 River Street, Hoboken, NJ 07030, USA
John Wiley & Sons Ltd, The Atrium, Southern Gate, Chichester, West Sussex, PO19 8SQ, UK

Editorial Office
9600 Garsington Road, Oxford, OX4 2DQ, UK

For details of our global editorial offices, customer services, and more information about Wiley products visit us at www.wiley.com.

Wiley also publishes its books in a variety of electronic formats and by print-on-demand. Some content that appears in standard print versions of this book may not be available in other formats.

Library of Congress Cataloging-in-Publication Data
Names: Kern, Morton J., editor. | Lim, Michael J., editor. | Goldstein, James A., editor.
Title: Hemodynamic rounds : interpretation of cardiac pathophysiology from pressure waveform analysis / edited by Morton J. Kern, Michael J. Lim, James A. Goldstein.
Description: Fourth edition. | Hoboken, NJ : Wiley, 2018. | Includes bibliographical references and index. |
Identifiers: LCCN 2017055956 (print) | LCCN 2017056803 (ebook) | ISBN 9781119095637 (pdf) | ISBN 9781119095644 (epub) | ISBN 9781119095613 (paperback)
Subjects: | MESH: Hemodynamics–physiology | Coronary Circulation–physiology | Coronary Disease–physiopathology | Case Reports
Classification: LCC RC670.5.H45 (ebook) | LCC RC670.5.H45 (print) | NLM WG 106 | DDC 616.1/0754–dc23
LC record available at https://lccn.loc.gov/2017055956

Cover design: Wiley
Cover image: Courtesy of Morton J. Kern

Set in 10/12pt Warnock by SPi Global, Pondicherry, India

10 9 8 7 6 5 4 3 2 1

MJK—I thank Margaret and Anna Rose, the continuing systole of my life, and my deepest appreciation to my fellows-in-training, for without them there would be no point in these exercises.

MJL—To Amy, Parker, and Taylor, the essential pieces to my life.

JAG—To my wife Cindy, who keeps life fun while I am working.

Contents

List of Contributors

Robin Abdelmalik, MD,
Former Cardiology Fellow, University California,
Irvine, CA, USA

Frank V. Aguirre, MD,
Interventional Cardiologist, Prarire Cardiovascular
Associates Spramfield, IL, USA

Steven Appleby, MD,
Interventional Cardiologist, Long Beach Memorial
Medical Center, CA, USA

Elie Azrak, MD,
Interventional Cardiologist, Cardiology Consultants,
St. Louis, MO, USA

Richard G. Bach, MD,
Associate Professor of Medicine, Cardiovascular
Division, Washington University, School of Medicine;
Director, Cardiac Intensive Care Unit, Barnes-Jewish
Hospital, St. Louis, MO, USA

James Bergin, MD,
Interventional Cardiologist, Cardiovascular Division,
University of Virginia Health System, Charlottesville,
VA, USA

Jeff Ciaramita, MD,
Former fellow in Cardiology, St. Louis University,
St. Louis, MO, USA

Larry S. Dean, MD,
Interventional Cardiologist, Professor of Medicine,
Director, UW Regional Heart Center, Division of
Cardiology, University of Washington, Seattle, WA, USA

Ubeydullah Deligonul, MD,
Interventional Cardiologist, Cardiovascular
Consultants, St. Louis, MO, USA

Thomas J. Donohue, MD,
Chief of Cardiology, St. Raphael's Hospital, New Havern,
CT, USA

Ziad Elghoul, MD,
Interventional Cardiologist, Division of Cardiology,
University of Louisville, Louisville, KY, USA

Ted Feldman, MD,
Interventional Cardiologist, University of Chicago,
Chicago, IL, USA

Krystof J. Godlewski, MD,
Interventional Cardiologist, University of Louisville,
Louisville, KY, USA

Steven L. Goldberg, MD,
Clinical Associate Professor, Director, Cardiac
Catheterization Laboratory, Division of Cardiology,
University of Washington, Seattle, WA, USA

James A. Goldstein, MD,
Director, Cardiovascular Research, William Beaumont
Hospital, MI, USA

Marco Guerrero, MD,
Former fellow in Cardiology, St. Louis University,
St. Louis, MO, USA

Ivan D. Hanson, M.D.
Interventional Cardiologist, Department of
Cardiovascular Medicine, Beaumont Health System,
Royal Oak, MI, USA

Stuart T. Higano, MD,
Interventional Cardiologist, Cardiovascular
Consultants, St. Louis, MO, USA

Ziyad M. Hijazi, MD, FSCAI,
Director, Congenital & Structural Heart Disease,
Professor of Pediatrics & Internal Medicine,
Sidra Medical and Research Center, Doha,
Qatar

Ralf J. Holzer, MD, MSc.
Assistant Director, Cardiac Catheterization &
Interventional Therapy, Assistant Professor of
Pediatrics, Cardiology Division, The Ohio State
University, The Heart Center, Columbus Children's
Hospital, Columbus, OH, USA

John Kern, MD,
Department of Cardiothoracic Surgery, University of Virginia Health System, Cardiovascular Division, Charlottesville, VA, USA

Morton J. Kern, MD, MFSCAI, FAHA, FACC,
Chief of Medicine, Veterans Administration Long Beach Health Care System, Professor of Medicine, University of California, Irvine, CA, USA

Douglas L. Kosmicki, MD,
Former fellow in Cardiology, University of Utah, Salt Lake City, UT, USA

Eric V. Krieger, MD,
Interventional Cardiologist, Cardiology Fellow, Division of Cardiology, University of Washington, Seattle, WA, USA

Abhay Laddu, MD,
Former Resident Internal Medicine, St. Louis University, St. Louis, MO, USA

Massoud A. Leesar, MD,
Interventional Cardiologist, University of Cincinatti, Cincinatti, OH, USA

Michael J. Lim, MD,
Chief of Cardiology, St. Louis University, St. Louis, MO, USA

D. Scott Lim, MD,
Interventional Cardiologist, University of Colorado, Danver, CO, USA

Crystal Medina, MD MPH,
Cardiovascular Disease Fellow, 2nd year, University of California, Irvine, CA, USA

Andrew D. Michaels, MD,
Interventional Cardiologist, University of Utah, Salt Lake City, UT, USA

Leslie Miller, MD,
Heart Failure Transplant Cardiologist, University of South Florida, Tampa, FL, USA

Gary S. Mintz, MD,
Professor of Medicine, Division of Cardiology, Columbia University, New York, NY, USA

Glenn T. Morris, MD,
Interventional Cardiologist, University of Louisville, Louisville, KY, USA

Robert H. Neumayr, MD,
Interventional Cardiology, St. Louis University, St. Louis, MO, USA

Michael Ragosta, MD,
Director, Cardiac Catheterization Laboratories, University of Virginia Health System, Cardiovascular Division, Charlottesville, VA, USA

Syed T. Reza, MD,
Interventional Cardiology, Division of Cardiology, University of Louisville, Louisville, KY, USA

Tariq S. Siddiqui, MD,
Interventional Cardiologist, Division of Cardiology, University of Louisville, Louisville, KY, USA

Paul Sorajja, MD,
Director, Center for Valve and Structural Heart Disease, Minneapolis Heart Institute, Abbott Northwestern Hospital, Minneapolis, MN, USA

Douglas K. Stewart, MD,
Professor, University of Washington Medical Center, Director, Interventional Cardiology Fellowship, Division of Cardiology, University of Washington, Seattle, WA, USA

George A. Stouffer, MD,
Interventional Cardiologist, University of Virginia, Charlottesville, VA, USA

Justin A. Strote, MD,
Interventional Cardiologist, Division of Cardiology, University of Washington, Seattle, WA, USA

Williams M. Suh, MD,
Interventional Cardiologist, University California Irvine, Orange, CA, USA

Naeem K. Tahirkheli, MD,
Former fellow in Cardiology, Mayo Clinic Rochester, MN, USA

J. David Talley, MD,
Interventional Cardiologist, University of Louisville, Louisville, KY, USA

Joshua W. Todd, MD,
Former fellow, Division of Cardiology, University of North Carolina, Chapel Hill, NC, USA

Zoltan Turi, MD,
Professor of Medicine, Co-Director Structural Heart Program, Hackensack University Medical Center, Hackensack, NJ, USA

Preface to the Fourth Edition

Although superseded by modern echocardiography, invasive hemodynamic data continue to be an integral part of cardiology training and comprise validation for much of the pathophysiology obtained from clinical examination, echocardiography, and new imaging modalities. With the advances in imaging technology, the continued reliance on the graphics of hemodynamics has been in decline. However, hemodynamics remain useful for diagnosis and treatment of the multitude of cardiovascular conditions. In the care of the cardiac patient, a critical integration of clinical symptoms, anatomical disorders, and the physiologic underpinnings of these disorders often leads to the best diagnosis and treatment. The understanding of hemodynamic waveforms and the insights provided into the patient's pathophysiology remain the cornerstone for this text.

The first edition of *Hemodynamic Rounds* emphasized the interpretation of hemodynamic waveforms for clinical decision-making as presented from a series of cases published in *Catheterization and Cardiovascular Diagnosis*, now known as *Catheterization and Cardiovascular Interventions*. The case-based format limited itself to description of individual hemodynamic tracings, but was not presented in a formalized textbook fashion. The subsequent two editions of *Hemodynamic Rounds* extended this work, enlarged it, and reorganized it into new sections, providing a more logical approach to the study of pressure waveforms and the associated pathology.

This fourth edition further expands a more thematic approach to the understanding of pathophysiologic waveforms. Since the last edition new procedures such as TAVR (transaortic valve replacement) have provided unique insights into intraprocedural hemodynamics as guides or warning signs of impending complications. The text has been divided into six major parts, logically arranging the previously material and adding new and dynamic tracings, incorporating some of the latest publications on novel hemodynamic topics as they continue to evolve and move into our modern practice.

Part One describes normal and pathophysiologic hemodynamic waveforms and is organized according to the study of pressure wave measurement systems, artifacts, and normal waveforms. The hemodynamics of the tricuspid valve, the mitral valve, and left-sided V waves are reviewed. Left ventricular end diastolic pressure, simultaneous right and left heart pressures, and effects of nitroglycerin and pulsus alternans are also discussed.

Parts Two, Three, and Four cover valvular, constrictive, and restrictive physiology and structural heart disease hemodynamics, respectively. In Part Three, constrictive, restrictive, and tamponade physiologic waveforms are described in detail. Among the topics in valvular heart disease in Part Two, hypertrophic obstructive cardiomyopathy is included in an expanded presentation on the history of the TASH methodology and its outcomes. More uncommon hemodynamics are provided again in Part Five, which covers several topics including coronary and renal hemodynamic assessment along with congenital heart disease, and a unique chapter on left ventricular support devices and "extra" hearts, both transplanted and mechanical. The material on coronary hemodynamics has been expanded given a decade of new studies demonstrating better outcomes using interventions guided by FFR (fractional flow reserve) and the emergence of basal indices to assess coronary stenoses. Of course, after two decades of study and publications, coronary hemodynamics can be used for better decision-making during coronary angiography in daily practice.

The concluding Part Six on clinical-pathophysiologic correlations is dedicated to a discussion of crucial clinical and bedside correlations of hemodynamics, describing the anatomic and pathophysiologic presentations of dyspnea, edema and anasarca, syncope, hypotension, and low cardiac output in four distinct blocks, presenting correlative findings between anatomy, hemodynamics, and clinical manifestations.

It is the hope of the authors that this work will be of lasting value to students, trainees, practicing physicians, and all related health-care personnel dealing with the important subject of cardiac hemodynamics. We thank Dr. Frank Hildner, first editor and founder of *Catheterization and Cardiovascular Interventions*, formerly *Catheterization and Cardiovascular Diagnosis*, for his encouragement and involvement with this work, without which this book would never have been published.

Morton J. Kern, MD
Michael J. Lim, MD
James A. Goldstein, MD

Introduction

Morton J. Kern and James A. Goldstein[1]

Historical Review

On February 28, 1733, the president of the Council of the Royal Society, Sir Hans Sloane, requested that Stephen Hales, one of the counselors, present his information on the mechanics of blood circulation from a previous presentation of a series of hemodynamic experiments reported in his book *Haemastaticks* [1]. Hales took his place in medical history next to William Harvey in studies of the human and animal circulation. *De Motu Cordis* [2] and *Haemastaticks* stimulated scientists' interest in the newly developed principles and mathematical computations of fluid mechanics as applied to circulatory physiologic events. The simple measurement of blood pressure now became a subject of great scientific concern.

From such basic interests, experimental physiologists at Oxford University in the 1800s, investigating the physiology of the circulation, began estimating the output of ventricular contraction and velocity of blood flow in the aorta, based on relatively primitive measurements of cardiovascular structures. These data remain valid today and correspond to those currently accepted and obtained by modern quantitative techniques. Cardiologists interested in hemodynamics should continue to emulate Stephen Hales, who relied on direct measurements and observations repeatedly checked and applied on simple but confirmed computations. Hales's numerous original achievements in hemodynamics are remarkable even by today's standards and include the first direct and accurate measurement of blood pressure in different animals (see Figure I.1) under different physiologic conditions such as hemorrhage and respiration; cardiac output estimated by left ventricular systolic stroke volume measured from the diastolic volume after death of the animal; calculations of pressure measured on the internal surface of the left ventricular at the beginning of systole; and

determination of blood flow velocity in the aorta approximating 0.5 m/sec. Hales introduced the concept of the wind castle or capacitance effect in the transformation of pulsatile flow in large vessels to continuous flow in smaller vessels. He also made the first direct measurement of venous blood pressure and correct interpretation of venous return on cardiac output in relation to contraction and respiration. Since recording equipment documenting Hales's observations was unavailable, understanding the unique collection of data depends on interpreting descriptive material.

Our current appreciation of hemodynamics, hopefully enhanced in this book, comes to us from a small group of modern physiologists active in the 1920s, among whom Dr. Carl Wiggers, from Western Reserve University in Ohio, emerges as a major figure. Advances in hemodynamic research arose from the development of recording instruments with fidelity, able to capture and reproduce the waveforms of rapidly changing pressures during the various phases of cardiac contractions. Importantly, Dr. Wiggers and colleagues also employed the newly developed electrocardiogram to obtain simultaneous pressure waveforms and electrical activity and, thus, establish the fundamental electrical–mechanical intervals. These relationships are the benchmark against which the observations of the pressure tracings of classical diseased conditions can be compared [4]. Almost a hundred years separate Wiggers and other originators of clinical cardiovascular physiology from today's cardiologists.

From the time Claude Bernard (1840) coined the phrase "cardiac catheterization" [5], laboratories of that type and name had been examining human physiology, ultimately incorporating radiologically determined anatomic information during the development of cardiac angiography in the 1960s. In 1929, Werner Forssman performed the first documented human

---

1 With special acknowledgments to Frank Hildner, MD for his contribution.

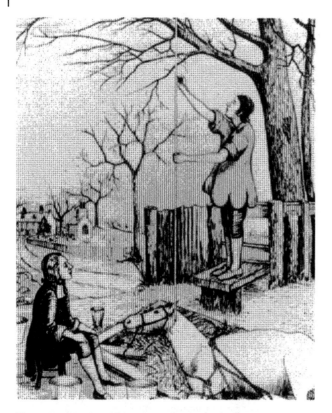

Figure I.1 Drawing depicting Dr. Stephen Hales (seated) directing and observing the measurement of arterial pressure in a sedated horse circa 1730. *Source:* Lyon 1987 [3]. Reproduced with permission of John Wiley & Sons.

cardiac catheterization—on himself [6]—changing the nature of the work from exclusively animal to human subjects. In the late 1930s, Cournand and Ranges [7] used the new right-heart catheterization technique to investigate pulmonary physiology. World War II expanded the scope and direction of their work to include hemorrhagic shock and drug effects on the circulation. However, in those days the most serious problems patients presented related to congenital and rheumatic heart disease. Accordingly, laboratories around the world began publishing data on the hemodynamics and physiology of atrial septal defects [8], ventricular septal defects [9], stenotic and insufficient mitral and aortic valves, and ventricular function. The beginning of invasive cardiology had now evolved into a distinct field of study that would produce valuable diagnostic and therapeutic results.

Without doubt, the most crucial development needed for the advancement of the field was the cathode ray tube, a direct result of the war. Before the image intensifier [10, 11], cardiac fluoroscopy utilized high-dose radiation and required physicians to accommodate their eyes to a green fluorescent screen by wearing red goggles for 15–20 minutes before starting. Indeed, the faintly glowing image in a completely dark room frequently failed to reveal even the position of the catheter [12]. Without the additional light provided by the image intensifier, "angiocardiography" was nothing more than a simple flat-plate radiograph, or perhaps a sequence of cut films obtained on the newly developed serial film changer [13]. Cineangiography was developed in the late 1950s through the persistent efforts of Janker (1954) [14] and Sones (1958) [15]. Advanced radiographic imaging spurred the development of catheter invasive techniques, permitting the investigation of heretofore unapproachable anatomical sites, clinical conditions, and disease entities. The findings in turn resulted in more effective and novel cardiac surgical techniques.

After the basic mechanics of congenital anomalies and rheumatic abnormalities were confirmed, expanded study was undertaken of conditions related to occlusive coronary artery disease such as myocardial infarction, left ventricular aneurysms, mitral chordal, and septal rupture. The concepts of systolic and diastolic myocardial mechanical function, hypertrophic obstructive and nonobstructive cardiomyopathy, electrophysiologic relations, and other previously unappreciated conditions came under scrutiny. The result was a new body of knowledge leading to the development and use of remarkable noninvasive techniques, including phonocardiographs, ballistocardiographs, exercise stress testing, radionuclide imaging, and echocardiography. While echocardiography and other important imaging techniques have superseded invasive approaches to some diagnoses, the acquisition and interpretation of hemodynamics remain critical to a proper understanding and appreciation of all cardiovascular conditions and situations.

Approach to Hemodynamic Waveform Interpretation

In the first edition of *Hemodynamic Rounds*, each chapter had been published in the journal *Catheterization and Cardiovascular Diagnosis*, now known as *Catheterization and Cardiovascular Interventions*, in a case-based format. The material was intended to provide both novice and advanced cardiologists with classical and, at times, unique pressure tracings to emphasize the value of careful waveform observation as it relates to different cardiac pathophysiologies. This fourth edition of the book carries this format forward and expands and updates the discussions to those areas where new information has been acquired, such as transaortic valve replacement (TAVR) procedures.

High-quality hemodynamic data are required for accurate hemodynamic determinations. As in the days of Stephen Hales, some hemodynamic data are extraordinarily simple, such as using a sphygmomanometer for indirect assessment of systemic arterial pressure. Some hemodynamic data are complex, requiring placement of multiple and specialized catheters within various locations and heart chambers to determine valvular gradients, myocardial contraction, relaxation, compliance, impedance, and work [16–18]. Percutaneous coronary and structural heart interventions prompted the development of the study of human coronary hemodynamics, now available easily to all on a daily basis. For coronary stenosis assessment, intracoronary pressure and flow measures are indispensable for accurate diagnosis beyond angiography alone. Intravascular ultrasound and optical coherence tomographic imaging catheters provide unique complementary anatomic information only dreamed about by the founders of our field.

As with all laboratory data, the significance of various hemodynamic findings should be placed in context of the ancillary historical, clinical, echocardiographic, roentgenographic, and electrocardiographic data. Acting on isolated laboratory values is dangerous and continues to be the nemesis of all technical innovations in medicine.

Methodologies Involved in Hemodynamic Data Collection

Each laboratory, and preferably all physicians, should establish protocols for right- and left-heart catheterization. A uniform and consistent approach to data collection insures complete, accurate, and reliable data for the majority of clinical problems. The standardized routine also obviates easily overlooked data collection steps being missed. Further, time is saved during procedure setup and data recording. The technical staff do not have to rethink what will happen for the unique and personal hemodynamic protocol of each different operator. Right-heart catheterization, sometimes performed sequentially with left-heart catheterization, may often be combined with it simultaneously to provide the most complete data. In most academic laboratories, a combined methodology is preferred.

The methodology for performing right-heart catheterization has been reviewed previously [19], but the indications have changed [19,20]. In general, routine right-heart catheterization is not indicated, but certainly should be liberally employed when patient care demands it. Shanes *et al.* [21] and Barron *et al.* [22], though arriving at opposite opinions, agree that right-heart catheterization is critical to evaluate patients with previous congenital heart disease, valvular heart disease, left- or right-heart failure, cardiomyopathy, or any unexplained significant clinical historical or physical findings.

Left-heart hemodynamic measurements most often use a single pressure transducer which screens for LV–aortic gradients. For accuracy, simultaneous left ventricular (LV) and central aortic pressure can easily be obtained using a dual-lumen pigtail catheter with two transducers. Measurements of cardiac work, calculation of flow resistance, valve areas, and shunt calculations require accurate hemodynamic data, arterial and venous blood oxygen saturations, and cardiac output determinations.

If hemodynamic information is considered important, the operators should take the time to obtain reliable and unequivocal pressure waveforms, separating artifact from true pathology. To achieve this goal, operators must be familiar with the equipment producing the waveforms and the sources of error found in recording techniques, tubing, transducers, and catheters. A complete description of the mechanics, techniques, pitfalls, and errors of hemodynamic data recording is provided in the *Cardiac Catheterization Handbook*, sixth edition, 2015 [23].

Initiating the Study of Pressure Waveforms

Pressure waveforms may be confusing for both the cardiovascular fellow-in-training and the clinician trying to understand the results of the procedure. After an intense training period in which the components of all pressure waves found in cardiovascular structures are reviewed and discussed, the young physician must be encouraged to continue practicing pattern recognition, deductive analysis, and a systematic approach to understanding the full meaning of the complete pressure data obtained. This systematic waveform interpretation includes consideration of the following key points:

1) Identify the cardiac rhythm. Most cardiac events can be identified by their timing from within the R–R cycle. Hemodynamic data obtained during arrhythmias may be confusing, since the various irregular contraction sequences distort pressure waves.
2) Determine the pressure scale on which the waveform is recorded and verify the pressure per division to be certain there is no recording artifact. Also, note the recording speed to assess the appropriate cardiac rhythm and timing of events occurring within one cardiac cycle. The comparison of waveforms for the chamber of interest should be made against known waveforms of normal physiology. The type of artifacts due to catheter fling or over- or underdamping will be discussed in the initial chapters.
3) Interpret the waveforms in conjunction with the clinical presentation and suspected diseased conditions

of the patient. A large V wave does not always represent valvular regurgitation. The equilibration of right and left ventricular diastolic pressures may be hypovolemia rather than pericardial constriction. Consider alternative clinical and physiologic explanations.

The examination, consideration of possible mechanisms, and clinical interpretation of the various waveform phenomena form the rationale for this book. We hope that this approach will enhance accuracy and lead to the best decisions for your patients' clinical care.

References

1 Hales S (ed.). *Statical Essays: Containing Haemastaticks*. New York: Hafner, 1964.

2 Harvey W (ed.). *Movement of the Heart and Blood in Animals*. Springfield, IL: Charles C Thomas, 1962.

3 Lyons AS, Petrucelli RJ II (eds.). *Medicine: An Illustrated History*. New York: Harry N. Abrams, 1987.

4 Wiggers CJ (ed.). *The Pressure Pulses in the Cardiovascular System*. New York: Longmans, Green, 1928.

5 Grmek MD. *Catalogue des manuscrits de Claude Bernard*. Paris: Masson, 1967.

6 Forssman W. Die Sondierung des rechten Herzens. *Klin Wochenschr* 8:2085–2087, 1929.

7 Cournand A, Ranges HA. Catheterization of the right auricle in man. *Proc Soc Exp Bioi Med* 46:462, 1941.

8 Brannon ES, Weens HS, Warren JV. Atrial septal defect: Study of hemodynamics by the technique of right heart catheterization. *Am J Med Sci* 210:480, 1945.

9 Baldwin E de F, Moore LV, Noble RP. The demonstration of ventricular septal defect by means of right heart catheterization. *Am Heart J* 32:152, 1944.

10 Sturm RE, Morgan RH. Screen intensification systems and their limitations. *Am J Roentgenol* 62:617, 1949.

11 Moon RJ. Amplifying and intensifying fluoroscopic images by means of scanning X-ray tube. *Science* 112:339, 1950.

12 Zimmerman HA. Presentation at the Twenty-Second Annual Scientific Session of the American Heart Association, Atlantic City, NJ, June 4, 1949.

13 Sanchez-Perez JM, Carter RA. Time factors in cerebral angiography and an automatic seriograph. *Am J Roentgenol* 62:509–518, 1949.

14 Janker R. *Roentgenotogische Funktionsdiagnostic Wupper*. Garandit, Elberfeld, 1954.

15 Sones FM Jr. Cinecardioangiography. *Pediatr Clin North Am* 5:945, 1958.

16 Moscucci M (ed.). *Grossman and Baim's Cardiac Catheterization, Angiography, and Intervention*, 8th ed. Wolters/Kluwer/Lippincott Williams, Wilkins, Philadelphia, PA, 2014.

17 Pepine CJ, Hill JA, Lambert CR (eds). *Diagnostic and Therapeutic Cardiac Catheterization*. Williams & Wilkins, Baltimore, MD, 1989.

18 Miller G (ed.). *Invasive Investigation of the Heart*. Blackwell Scientific, London, 1989.

19 Green DG, Society for Cardiac Angiography Officers and Trustees. Right heart catheterization and temporary pacemaker insertion during coronary arteriography for suspected coronary artery disease. *Cathet Cardiovasc Diagn* 10:429–430, 1984.

20 Samet P. The complete cardiac catheterization. *Cathet Cardiovasc Diagn* 10:431–432, 1984.

21 Shanes JG, Stein MA, Dierenfeldt BJ, Kondos GT. The value of routine right heart catheterization in patients undergoing coronary arteriography. *Am Heart J* 113:1261–1263, 1987.

22 Barron JT, Ruggie N, Uretz E, Messer JV. Findings on routine right heart catheterization in patients with suspected coronary artery disease. *Am Heart J* 115:1193, 1988.

23 Kern MJ. (ed.) *The Cardiac Catheterization Handbook*, 6th ed. Elsevier, Philadephia, PA, 2011.

Part One

Normal Waveforms

1

Principles of Normal Physiology and Pathophysiology

James A. Goldstein and Morton J. Kern

Pathophysiologic derangements of cardiac anatomic components and mechanics manifest as "cardinal" cardiovascular symptoms, most of which are reflected in distinct hemodynamic disturbances. These symptomatic–hemodynamic constellations include (i) dyspnea, reflecting pulmonary venous congestion; (ii) fatigue, attributable to inadequate cardiac output; (iii) syncope, resulting from transient profound hypotension; and (iv) peripheral edema, related to systemic venous congestion. Chest pain typically suggesting ischemia does not usually result directly from primary hemodynamic derangements, does not lend itself to this anatomic–pathophysiologic hemodynamic approach, and will not be addressed in these discussions.

It is important to emphasize that these symptom groups in isolation are nonspecific. Identical complaints reflecting disparate pathophysiologic processes can occur due to a variety of mechanisms. For example, dyspnea is an expected symptomatic manifestation of pulmonary venous hypertension attributable to a spectrum of left-heart derangements, the underlying mechanisms of which vary greatly (e.g., mitral stenosis, mitral regurgitation, left ventricular cardiomyopathy, etc.). The treatments and prognoses also vary greatly. Dyspnea is also commonly of pulmonary origin, with circumstances in which the heart may be completely normal or impacted only as an innocent bystander (e.g., cor pulmonale).

Similarly, peripheral edema and ascites reflect systemic venous congestion resulting from a spectrum of right-heart failure mechanisms (e.g., tricuspid valve disease, right ventricular cardiomyopathy, pericardial disorders, etc.). However, edema may also develop under conditions with normal systemic venous pressures, as may occur in patients with cirrhotic liver disease, nephrotic syndrome, inferior vena cava (IVC) compression, and so on. Thus, for cardiovascular assessment, symptoms and signs must be characterized according to the underlying anatomic–pathophysiologic mechanisms.

To establish an anatomic–pathophysiologic differential diagnosis, first consider the anatomic cardiac components (myocardium, valves, arteries, pericardium, and conduction tissue) that may be involved and then focus on the fundamental mechanisms that impact each anatomic component, finally asking how such anatomic–pathophysiologic derangements and hemodynamic perturbations are reflected in the symptoms, physical signs, and invasive waveforms.

Cardiac Mechanical Function and Hemodynamics

Hemodynamic assessment is an integral part of the anatomic–physiologic approach to circulatory pathophysiology, employing bedside examination with confirmatory or complementary invasive and noninvasive (echo-Doppler data) hemodynamic information.

The purpose of the cardiovascular system is to generate cardiac output to perfuse the body. However, although perfusion is the heart's "bottom line," perfusion depends on pressure to drive the blood through the tissues. Organ perfusion is determined by arterial driving pressure modulated by vascular bed resistances. The regulation of the circulation (pressure and flow) can be understood by the application of Ohm's law–related resistance to pressure and flow. In classical physics applied to an electrical circuit, Ohm's law is expressed as:

$$\Delta V = I \times R$$

where ΔV is the driving voltage potential difference across the circuit, I is the current flow, and R is the circuit resistance. Thus, circuit output or current flow is a function of the "driving" voltage divided by circuit resistance, or $I = \Delta V/R$. Translating Ohm's law to the cardiac circulation, blood pressure (dV) = cardiac output

Hemodynamic Rounds: Interpretation of Cardiac Pathophysiology from Pressure Waveform Analysis, Fourth Edition.
Edited by Morton J. Kern, Michael J. Lim, and James A. Goldstein.
© 2018 John Wiley & Sons Ltd. Published 2018 by John Wiley & Sons Ltd.

(I) × systemic vascular resistance (R) and can be applied to the systemic circulation or to individual organ beds.

The key components of blood pressure can be further considered. Thus, cardiac output (CO) = heart rate (HR) × stroke volume (SV). Furthermore, SV is a function of three cardiac mechanisms: preload, afterload, and contractility. Systemic vascular resistance is determined by total blood volume and vascular tone (a function of intrinsic vessel contraction or relaxation interacting with systemic and local neuro-hormonal influences, metabolic factors, other vasomotor mediators, etc.).

Fundamentals of Hemodynamic Waveforms: The Wiggers Diagram

All pressure waves of the cardiac cycle can be understood by reviewing and knowing how electrical and mechanical activity of the heart's contraction and relaxation are related. Every electrical activity is followed normally by a mechanical function (either contraction or relaxation), resulting in a pressure wave. The timing of mechanical events can be obtained by looking at the electrocardiogram (ECG) and corresponding pressure tracing (Figure 1.1) [1].

The ECG P wave is responsible for atrial contraction, the QRS for ventricular activation, and the T wave for ventricular relaxation. The periods between electrical activation reflect impulse transmission times to different areas of the heart. These time delays permit the mechanical functions to be in synchrony and generate efficient cardiac output and pressure. When the normal sequence of contraction and relaxation of the heart muscle is disturbed by arrhythmia, cardiac function is inefficient or ineffective, as demonstrated on the various pressure waveforms associated with the arrhythmia.

The cardiac cycle begins with the P wave. This is the electrical signal for atrial contraction. The atrial pressure wave (A wave; Figure 1.1, #1) follows the P wave by 30–50 msec. Following the A wave peak, the atrium relaxes and pressure falls, generating the X descent (point b). The next event is the depolarization of the ventricles with the QRS (point b). The left ventricular (LV) pressure after the A wave is called the end-diastolic pressure (LVEDP). It can be denoted by a vertical line dropped from the R wave to the intersection of the LV pressure (point b). About 15–30 msec after the QRS, the ventricles contract and the LV (and right ventricular, RV) pressure increases rapidly. This period of rise in LV pressure without change in LV volume is called the isovolumetric contraction period (interval b–c). When LV pressure rises above the pressure in the aorta, the aortic valve opens and blood is ejected into the circulation (point c). This point is the beginning of systole. Some hemodynamicists include isovolumetric contraction as part of systole.

About 200–250 msec after the QRS, at the T wave, repolarization starts and the heart begins relaxing. By the end of the T wave (point e), the LV contraction has ended and LV relaxation produces a fall in the LV (and aortic pressure). When the LV pressure falls below the aortic pressure, the aortic valve closes (point e). Systole concludes and diastole begins. After aortic valve closure, the ventricular pressure continues to fall. When the LV pressure falls below the left atrial (LA) pressure, the mitral valve opens and the LA empties into the LV (point f). The period from aortic valve closure to mitral valve opening is call the isovolumetric relaxation period (interval e–f). Diastole is the period from mitral valve opening to mitral valve closing.

Observing the atrial pressure wave across the cardiac cycle, it should be noted that after the A wave, pressure slowly rises across systole, continuing to increase until the end of systole when the pressure and volume of the LA are nearly maximal, producing a ventricular filling wave (V wave). The V wave (point f, #4) peak is followed by a rapid fall when the mitral valve opens. This V wave pressure descent is labeled the Y descent and usually parallels LV pressure. After the V wave, the LV is filled by the small pressure gradient assisting blood flow from the atria into the ventricles over the diastolic period (called diastasis), until the cycle begins again with atrial pressure building, until again atrial activation and contraction

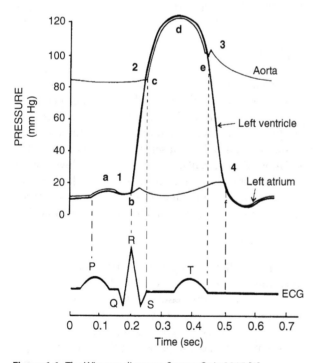

Figure 1.1 The Wiggers diagram. *Source:* Opie 2015 [1]. Reproduced with permission of Elsevier.

generate the A wave, ejecting atrial blood into the LV. The peaks and descents of the atrial pressure waves are changed by pathologic conditions and are used to support the diagnosis of these pathologies, as will be seen in the examples dealing with heart failure, constrictive physiology, and RV infarction.

Valve Hemodynamics

To appreciate hemodynamic valve dysfunction, consider when cardiac pressure normally opens and closes the valves. The aortic and pulmonary valves open in systole, when ventricular pressure exceeds aortic pressure (and RV exceeds pulmonary artery or PA pressure). Stenosis of these valves produces systolic pressure gradients and characteristic high-velocity heart murmurs. The mitral and tricuspid valves are closed in systole when LV pressure is greater than atrial pressure. A mitral or tricuspid regurgitant valve that fails to close is characterized by a low-velocity systolic murmur with a rumbling quality. Conversely, incompetent aortic valves fail to seal and let blood continue to rush backward into the LV in diastole. The blood rushes into the LV with a diastolic murmur. At the beginning of diastole, LA pressure is at its highest. If the mitral valve is stenotic, the high LA pressure emptying into the LV produces a diastolic rumble. When reviewing the cardiac hemodynamics, we can always refer to the Wiggers diagram for what the expected normal hemodynamic responses should be.

Systolic and Diastolic Performance

The hemodynamic evaluation of the circulation may be considered as two sides of a single coin of cardiac function: (i) systolic function, the ability of the heart to pump, generate pressure, and perfuse the body; and (ii) diastolic performance, the ability of the chambers to fill at physiologic pressures with the preload necessary to generate SV.

Systolic Function

Systolic function reflects the ability of the ventricle to contract and generate output or stroke work, a function determined by its loading conditions, including both preload (determined by venous return and end-diastolic volume), afterload (related to aortic impedance and wall stress), and the contractile state (the force generated at any given end-diastolic volume).

The Frank–Starling mechanism established the relationship between end-diastolic volume (preload) and ventricular performance (stroke volume, cardiac output, and/or stroke work), wherein isovolumetric force at any given contractile state is a function of the degree of end-diastolic fiber stretch (also known as a force–length relationship; Figure 1.2). Thus, the normal LV functions are on the ascending limb of this force–length relationship. Afterload, the impedance during ejection, is defined as the force per unit area acting upon myocardial fibers, a force resulting in wall stress, which is expressed by the Law of Laplace (Wall stress = Radius/2 x Thickness). Afterload is influenced by changes in ventricular volume and wall thickness, as well as aortic pressure or aortic impedance.

Frank–Starling and Ventricular Waveforms

Ventricular waveforms reflect both systolic and diastolic function and include the effects of chamber preload, contractility, and afterload. The upstroke of RV or LV pressure (+ dP/dt) is influenced by preload and contractility, but is a poor measure of either. A brisk upstroke suggests reasonable function versus a sluggish or delayed pressure rise of depressed performance. The peak amplitude reflects both contractility and afterload.

In diastole, ventricular relaxation (- dP/dt) is an active energy-requiring process and reflects intrinsic aspects of myocardial contractility as the ventricle actively "relaxes." The pressure wave of the downstroke relaxation phase is an active process requiring adenosine triphosphate (ATP) and closely mirrors systolic function. The pressure downstroke can also be used to assess cardiac dysfunction. A slurred or retarded negative dP/dt (also known as tau, a LV relaxation measurement) may indicate cardiomyopathy and adversely influenced diastolic properties.

Arterial Waveforms

Arterial waveforms reflect the ejection of blood from the LV (and therefore its preload, contractility, and afterload), together with the intrinsic resistance and compliance of the pulmonary or systemic circuit. Filling pressures in the ventricles reflect diastolic properties, influenced by intrinsic chamber factors (e.g., pressure overload hypertrophy, volume overload, ischemia, infiltration, inflammation), as well as extrinsic effects from the pericardium or contralateral ventricle through diastolic ventricular interactions. The arterial waveform reflects dynamic interactions between SV and the capacitance (distensibility) of the peripheral arterial tree (which determines the rate at which the ejected volume of blood flows from the proximal arterial compartment into the peripheral tissues). The first peak of the arterial pressure waveform is the percussion wave, which reflects

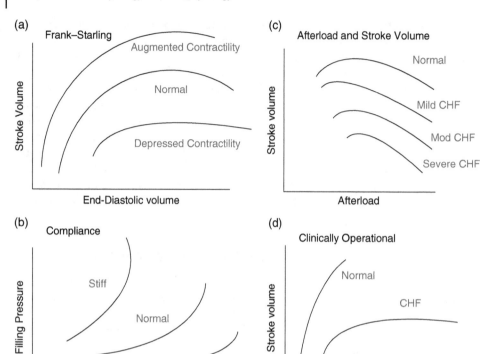

Figure 1.2 Family of cardiac function curves illustrating and combining principles of systolic function, diastolic compliance, effects of excess afterload, and a symphysis pertinent to clinical day-to-day life. (a) Classic Frank–Starling relationship of true end-diastolic volume output. (b) Compliance curves illustrating rapid rise in pressure attributable to impaired ventricular compliance. (c) Adverse effects of increasing afterload on ventricular stroke volume, particularly deleterious under conditions of depressed LV systolic function. (d) "Clinically operational" graph illustrating hemodynamic impact of mechanical abnormalities on patients who normally generate optimal stroke volume with low filling pressures, compared to dysfunctional ventricles (from both systolic and diastolic abnormalities) in which despite high filling pressures stroke volume is low.

the impulse of the LV stroke modulated by the reflected pressure from the vascular tree (and therefore its compliance); therefore, the arterial upstroke to its peak reflects LV preload, contractility, and afterload (both that imposed by the aortic valve and the stroke volume ratio or SVR). A secondary tidal wave follows, reflecting primarily the returning pulse wave from the upper body (peripheral tone), which then smoothly falls to the dichrotic notch (incisura) which corresponds to aortic valve closure. The subsequent decline in aortic pressure represents pure diastolic runoff. In early diastole, a small positive wave may be seen, the dichrotic wave, most likely an effect of reflected pulse from the lower body.

Pulse Amplification

As the pulse wave travels distally through the arterial circulation, the waveform may increase, a phenomenon termed peripheral amplification [2]. Amplification is characterized by a taller systolic peak, delayed dichrotic notch, lower end-diastolic pressure, and later pulse arrival. The systolic peak is steeper going to the periphery, attributable to summated reflected waves which develop as the narrowing and branching of blood vessels reflect some of the pulse back toward the aortic valve (Figure 1.3). As the resistance of the branching arterial tree increases, the more of the pressure wave is reflected. The more resistant the tree (i.e., the more atheromatous, hypertrophic, and calcified the arteries), the greater the magnitude of reflection. This is particularly relevant in those with stiff, noncompliant vessels (e.g., the elderly or hypertensive patients), in whom the pulse wave velocity is rapid and reflected waves from both upper and lower body return quickly during late systole, causing a more prominent tidal wave, which may even exceed the percussion wave. This condition may explain the absence of pulsus parvus et tardus in very elderly aortic stenosis patients in whom the carotid pulse is preserved and reflects an exaggerated peripheral amplification from noncompliant vessels). However, there is little change in mean arterial pressure (MAP) because there is little change in the resistance to flow from aorta to radial

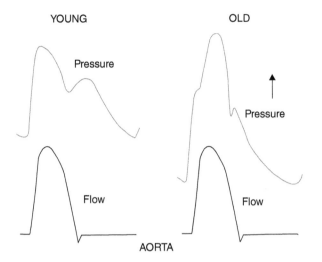

YOUNG   OLD

Pressure

Pressure

Flow   Flow

AORTA

Figure 1.3 Arterial pressure wave reflection comparing manifestations in young versus elderly patients. The pressure wave reflection arises from the junction of conduit and low-resistance arteries with high-resistance arteries. Given that there are firmer junctions in the lower versus upper body, most reflection returning from the periphery comes from the lower body up into the proximal thoracic aorta. This reflected wave injects stroke volume, giving rise to the peak systolic pressure in the contour of the tidal wave. In older patients with nondistensible vasculature, the augmented reflected wave results in higher peak systolic pressure for any given stroke volume. *Source:* O'Rourke 2006 [2]. Reproduced with permission of Elsevier.

artery; rather, MAP changes more dramatically at the arteriolar level.

Aortic diastolic pressure reflects the aggregate resistance of the systemic arterial tree back upon the aortic valve. Noncompliant vessels similarly cause this pressure to be raised. In contrast, the soft vasoplegic (dilated or relaxed) vessels of a septic patient will offer little resistance, and the diastolic pressure will be lower. A regurgitant aortic valve will also cause this pressure to be lower than normal, because the pressure wave travels all the way through to the ventricle manifested as the regurgitant jet.

Pulse pressure is the difference between peak systolic and end-diastolic aortic pressures. A widened pulse pressure suggests aortic regurgitation, because in diastole the arterial pressure drops to fill the left ventricle though the regurgitating aortic valve, and at the same time forward runoff is great, since peripheral resistance is also reduced. In contrast, a narrow pulse pressure may occur in conditions such as cardiac tamponade, or any other low-output state (e.g., severe cardiogenic shock, massive pulmonary embolism or tension pneumothorax).

Pressure–Volume Loops

In aggregate, the relationships between preload, afterload, and contractility are illustrated in ventricular pressure–volume (PV) loops which plot the changes of these variables over a cardiac cycle [3]. Each PV loop (Figure 1.4) represents one cardiac cycle. Beginning at end diastole (point a), LV volume has received the atrial contribution and is maximal. Isovolumic contraction (a to b) increases LV pressure with no change in volume. At the end of isovolumic contraction, LV pressure exceeds aortic pressure, the aortic valve opens, and blood is ejected from the LV into the aorta (point b). Over the systolic ejection phase, LV volume decreases and, as ventricular repolarization occurs, LV ejection ceases and relaxation begins. When LV pressure falls below aortic pressure, the aortic valve closes, a point also known as the end-systolic pressure–volume (ESPV) point (c). Isovolumic relaxation occurs until LV pressure decreases below the atrial pressure, opening the mitral valve (point d).

The stroke volume is represented by the width of the PV loop, the difference between end-systolic and end-diastolic volumes. The area within the loop represents stroke work. Load-independent LV contractility, also known as Emax, is defined as the maximal slope of the ESPV points under various loading conditions, and the line of these points is the ESPV relationship (ESPVR). Effective arterial elastance (Ea), a measure of LV afterload, is defined as the ratio of end-systolic pressure to stroke volume. Under steady-state conditions, optimal LV contractile efficiency occurs when the ratio of Ea:Emax approaches 1.

The PV loop describes contractile function, relaxation properties, SV, cardiac work, and myocardial oxygen consumption. Hemodynamic alterations and interventions change the PV relationship in predictable ways and comparisons of various hemodynamic interventions can be made more precisely by examining the PV loop (Figures 1.5 and 1.6).

Acute changes in cardiac function such as might occur with acute myocardial infarction (AMI) are also easily demonstrated. In AMI, LV contractility (Emax) is reduced; LV pressure, SV, and LV stroke work may be unchanged or reduced, and LVEDP is increased. In cardiogenic shock, Emax is severely reduced, LV afterload (Ea) may be increased, LVEDV and LVEDP are increased, and SV is reduced, findings easily seen to display reduced LV contractile function, acute diastolic dysfunction, elevated LVEDV and LVEDP, and increased LV work (oxygen demand). In more severe cases of myocardial infarction that evolve into cardiogenic shock, LV contractile function is more severely reduced, with associated significant increases in end-diastolic pressure and volume. The LV impairment results in a markedly reduced SV, with an increased myocardial oxygen demand.

The most common applications of PV loops characterize only left ventricular hemodynamics. For research into right ventricular function or extracardiac problems,

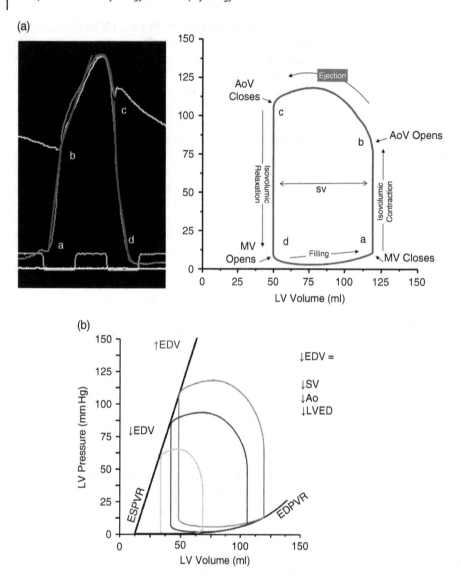

Figure 1.4 (a) The pressure–volume (PV) loop characterizes the changes in pressure flow over the course of one cardiac cycle. Left panel, the left ventricular (LV) and aortic pressure as measured during cardiac catheterization. Right panel, the PV loop derived from the hemodynamics of LV pressure and volume. Point a, LV end-diastolic pressure is followed by isovolumetric contraction ending at point b, the aortic valve (AoV) opening. Ejection continues until the repolarization of the LV produces a fall in LV ejection. LV pressure falls pasts point c, aortic valve closure, and continues to fall along the line of isovolumetric relaxation to point d, mitral valve (MV) opening. Changes in the shape of the PV loop demonstrate changes in contractility and cardiac output (stroke volume, SV). Load-independent LV contractility, also known as Emax, is defined as the maximal slope of the end-systolic pressure–volume (ESPV) point under various loading conditions, known as the ESPV relationship (ESPVR). Effective arterial elastance (Ea) is a measure of LV afterload and is defined as the ratio of end-systolic pressure and stroke volume. (b) The effect of changes in LV preload. Increasing the left ventricular end-diastolic pressure (LVEDP) along the line of the end-diastolic pressure–volume relationship (EDPVR). As volume is increased, LVEDP, SV, and aortic pressure increase. (*See insert for color representation of the figure.*)

the standard PV loops become complex and affected by additional factors, altering the PV loop configuration and interpretation.

Left Ventricular Rotational Mechanics: Systolic Twist and Diastolic Suction

Due to the spiral architecture of its myofibers, the LV twists or rotates from apex to base in a systolic "wringing" motion, generating the SV pathway through the LV outflow tract, an action that contributes significantly to LV systolic performance [4]. The LV twist also stores potential energy during the systolic phase. During subsequent isovolumic relaxation (an active ATP requiring process to re-sequester Ca++ into the sarcoplasmic reticulum), the "untwisting" or recoil of stored energy contributes to the diastolic "suction" that opens the mitral valve and accelerates atrial emptying along the LV inflow path. These important mechanics may be deranged under a wide variety of pathologic conditions,

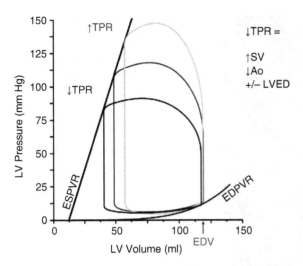

Figure 1.5 The effect of increasing afterload or total peripheral vascular resistance (TPR) decreases SV, increases aortic pressure, and minimally modifies LVEDP. (*See insert for color representation of the figure.*)

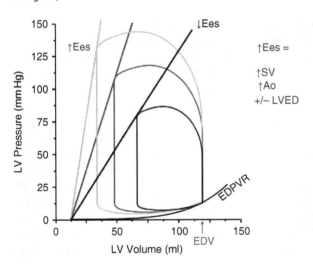

Figure 1.6 The effect of increasing contractility: the increasing slope of the line of end-systolic elastance (Ees) increases SV and aortic pressure, with minimal effect on LVEDP. (*See insert for color representation of the figure.*)

may be evident in hemodynamic traces, and contribute to clinical hemodynamic compromise.

Diastolic Performance and Cardiac Compliance

Diastolic function is the ability of a chamber to obtain its necessary preload at physiological filling pressures to generate CO under a variety of physiologic conditions, both at rest and during stress (exercise and metabolic stress such as infection, surgery, etc.). Diastole is not a passive process and is fundamentally influenced by various active factors. Diastole can be considered in four phases: isovolumic relaxation, early filling, diastasis, and atrial contraction. Isovolumic relaxation (lusitropic function) is a bit of

a misnomer, for this is an active ATP-requiring process that untwists the LV, rapidly reducing ventricular pressure and through suction opening the mitral valve and initiating the rapid early filling phase. The majority of LV filling occurs here, through ventricular suction; this is followed by equilibration of LA and LV pressures and temporary cessation of flow (diastasis). Finally, active atrial contraction contributes the booster pump function, which delivers additional ventricular preload. This booster optimizes ventricular filling at a lower mean atrial pressure, and the end-diastolic "kick" elevates ventricular end-diastolic pressure (EDP) as the atria actively relax (X descent), thereby facilitating ventricular–atrial pressure reversal which initiates AV valve closure; in aggregate, these effects optimize LV preload while concomitantly minimizing the effects of ventricular diastolic pressure on the back tributaries of filling; that is, the lungs. These diastolic patterns are best illustrated not by invasive catheter interrogation, but rather by Doppler echocardiography under physiologic conditions. LV inflow velocity across the mitral valve is most rapid early, reflected as a predominant E wave on the transmitral Doppler echocardiogram. In normal anatomy, the preload contributed by atrial contraction is relatively small (in contrast to when the ventricle is stiff or the AV valve is obstructed), and therefore the velocity imparted by atrial contraction (the transmitral inflow A wave) is relatively low, thus the normal E/A wave ratio is greater than 1 but less than 2.

Functional preload is the amount of blood actually distending the cardiac chamber. This volume is reflected in filling pressure according to chamber compliance, the relationship between diastolic pressure and volume in any anatomic chamber (ventricle, atrium, pericardium, cranium, etc.). Cardiac chamber diastolic pressure is determined by the volume of blood in the chamber and its distensibility (compliance). In normal anatomy, optimal filling occurs at low filling pressures (Figures 1.2 and 1.7).

During diastole, the LV, left atrium, and pulmonary veins form a "common chamber," which is continuous with the pulmonary capillary bed; in the right heart a similar relationship exists. Diastolic dysfunction is defined as a functional abnormality of diastolic relaxation, filling, or distensibility, in which filling is limited by abnormal chamber stiffness (hypertrophy, ischemia, fibrosis, infiltration, extrinsic pericardial resistance). Increased stiffness dictates that at any given level of chamber filling, the filling pressure is disproportionately elevated (Figure 1.7). Diastolic dysfunction may occur in association with chamber dilation and related systolic dysfunction (e.g., ischemic cardiomyopathy), or with a small stiff chamber with an intact ejection fraction (e.g., hypertensive cardiomyopathy). Figure 1.2a is the classic Frank–Starling curve wherein end-diastolic volume (true preload) generates output (SV) dependent on the inotropic state. Pure diastolic pressure–volume relationships are illustrated in

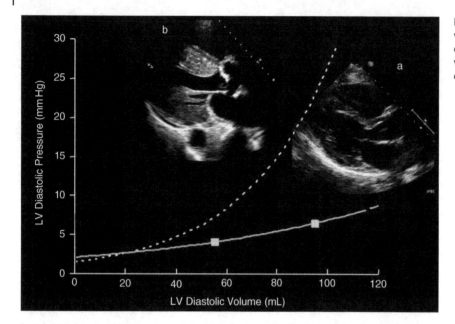

Figure 1.7 Left ventricular pressure–volume relationships demonstrating compliance curves in a normal LV (b) versus a thick stiff LV (a). (*See insert for color representation of the figure.*)

Figure 1.2b, wherein chamber compliance determines the actual distending pressure (and thus back pressure) for any given level of true preload (Figure 1.2c). What matters clinically is the diastolic pressure needed to generate a given SV. The compliant and contractile ventricle can accommodate a dramatically increased preload (i.e., stress or exercise) and generate high output at low filling pressures. In contrast, both types of heart failure, those with stiff hearts and preserved ejection fraction (HFPEF) and those with dilated hearts and reduced ejection fraction (HFREF), suffer elevated filling pressure and low output syndromes. Finally, consideration of these principles must also take into account the profound influence of excess afterload on ventricular performance (Figure 1.2c), which has disproportionate effects on SV in those with depressed ejection fraction (EF).

Differentiation of Cardiac Preload and Filling Pressures: Left Ventricular End-Diastolic Pressure Does Not Necessarily Reflect Left Ventricular Filling

Cardiac performance is optimal when SV is generated at low filling pressures. However, diastolic pressure generated by any given degree of filling (true preload) is a function of the compliance of the chamber, and therefore filling pressure reasonably reflects preload *only* if chamber compliance is normal.

Thus, impaired compliance attributable to intrinsic factors (hypertrophy, infiltration or ischemia, or primary pressure and volume overload) or extrinsic constraint (pericardial disease or ventricular interactions) distorts the relationship between filling pressure and true preload. This distortion may confound clinical and invasive

hemodynamic assessment. Measurement of intracardiac filling pressures (for example, LVEDP) is used for two basic purposes: (i) to determine whether preload is adequate to generate SV (i.e., whether the patient is volume depleted); and (ii) to determine whether there is elevated pressure exerting adverse "backward" congestive effects.

With respect to assessing true preload in a patient with clinical low-output hypoperfusion, pulmonary capillary wedge pressure (PCWP) or LVEDP is a convenient surrogate for left-heart preload, although under noncompliant conditions (e.g., severe LV hypertrophy or cardiac tamponade) LV preload may be markedly reduced, but intracardiac pressures may be strikingly elevated. In fact, in some cases patients may be in pulmonary edema despite an LV with small cavity and intact contractility (e.g., restrictive cardiomyopathy). Conversely, chronic volume overload lesion such as aortic regurgitation may result in dramatically increased chamber volumes, but in those who are well compensated, intracardiac pressures are relatively normal as the chamber and pericardium dilate and become more compliant.

Cardiac Mechanics, Atrial Waveforms, and the Venous Circulations

A critical relationship exists among cardiac mechanics and atrial waveforms, the physiology of the venous circulations, and the dynamic effects of intrathoracic pressure (ITP) and respiratory motion on cardiovascular physiology, permitting a better interpretation of the waveforms to reflect pathophysiology.

Atrial Waveforms

Analysis of the atrial waveforms (Figure 1.8) yields insight into cardiac chamber and pericardial compliance. The atrial waveforms are constituted by two positive waves (A and V peaks) and two collapsing waves (X and Y descents). The atrial A wave is generated by atrial systole following the P wave on ECG. Atrial mechanics behave in a manner similar to that of ventricular muscle. The strength of atrial contraction is reflected in the rapidity of the A wave upstroke and peak amplitude. The X descent follows the A wave and is generated by two events: the initial decline in pressure reflecting active atrial relaxation, with a latter descent component reflecting pericardial emptying during ventricular systole (also called systolic intrapericardial depressurization, a condition that is exaggerated when pericardial space is compromised). The X descent's second component is affected by the pericardial space and changes when the ventricles are maximally emptied, therefore pericardial volume and intrapericardial pressure (IPP) are at their nadir.

During ventricular systole, venous return results in atrial filling and pressure which peak with the V wave, whose height reflects the atrial pressure–volume compliance characteristics. The subsequent diastolic Y descent represents atrial emptying and depressurization. The steepness of the Y descent is influenced by the volume and pressure in the atrium just prior to atrioventricular (AV) valve opening (height of the V wave) and resistance to atrial emptying (AV valve resistance and ventricular–pericardial compliance).

Venous Circulations and Respiratory Oscillations

Venous return to both atria is inversely proportional to the instantaneous atrial pressure, which is itself dependent on compliance. The lowest return occurs when each pressure is highest. Under physiologic conditions, venous return to both atria is biphasic, with a systolic peak determined by atrial relaxation (corresponding to

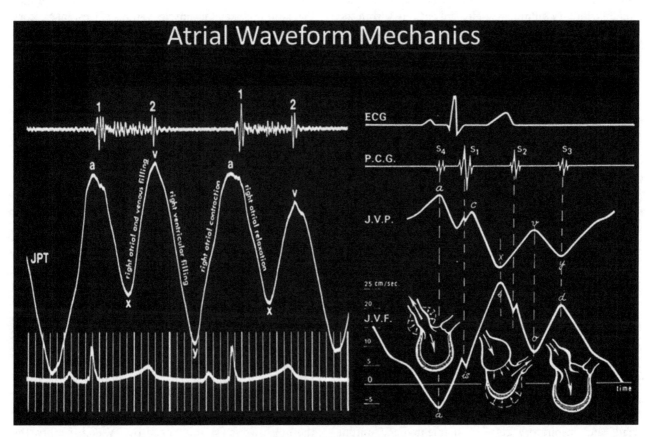

Figure 1.8 Atrial mechanical cycle. The upstroke and amplitude of the A wave reflect atrial contraction and the initial portion of the extra set reflects atrial relaxation, with the latter portion due to systolic intrapericardial pressurization. From the downslope of the latter portion of the extra set to the height of the V wave represents the peak period of atrial venous return filling (or regurgitant filling if the atrioventricular valve is incompetent), and therefore is a reflection of atrial compliance. The widest set reflects ventricular relaxation, opening of the AV valve, and subsequent atrial emptying. *Source:* Kalmanson 1971 [5]. Reproduced with permission of Oxford University Press.

the X descent of the atrial and jugular venous pressure [JVP] waveforms) and a diastolic peak determined by tricuspid valve (TV) resistance and RV compliance (corresponding to the Y descent of the atrial and JVP waveforms). It is essential to consider the relationship of IPP to atrial pressures and flows. Normal IPP is subatmospheric, and both approximates and varies with pleural pressure, decreasing dramatically during inspiration. IPP also tracks right atrial (RA) pressure and shows fluctuations that are associated with the cardiac cycle. In general, IPP increases when cardiac volumes are increased (peak ventricular filling, the V wave) and is lowest at peak ventricular emptying (the later portion of the X descent). It follows that inspiratory decrement in pleural pressure normally reduces pericardial, RA, RV, wedge, and systemic arterial pressures slightly. However, IPP decreases somewhat more than RA pressure, thereby augmenting right-heart filling and output.

Under physiologic conditions, respiratory oscillations exert complex effects on cardiac filling and dynamics since the respiratory effects on the right and the left heart are disparate, owing to differences in the venous return systems and the intrapleural space. The left heart and its tributary pulmonary veins are entirely within the intrathoracic space. In contrast, although both right-heart chambers are intrathoracic, the tributary systemic venous system is extrapleural. Normally, inspiration-induced decrements in ITP (from expiratory 5 to end-inspiratory 25–30 mm Hg) are transmitted through the pericardium to the cardiac chambers. In the right heart, these decrements in ITP enhance the filling gradient from the extrathoracic systemic veins to the right atrium, thereby increasing the caval–right atrial gradient and augmenting venous return flow by 50–60%, increasing right-heart filling and output.

In contrast, the left heart and its tributary pulmonary veins are entirely intrathoracic. Therefore, since pleural pressure changes are evenly distributed to the left heart and pulmonary veins, the pressure gradient from the pulmonary veins to the left ventricle shows minimal change with respiration. However, left-heart filling, stroke volume, and aortic systolic pressure normally decrease with inspiration (up to 10–12 mm Hg). The mechanisms responsible for this normal inspiratory oscillation in aortic pressure include variable ventricular volumes as each ventricle competes for its part of the entire cardiac volume constrained by the pericardium. This competition leads to leftward septal displacement due to augmented right-heart filling, increased LV "afterload," and inspiratory delay of augmented RV output through the lungs. This physiologic respiratory blood pressure oscillation phenomenon has somewhat confusingly been termed paradoxical pulse, but is normal when <10–12 mm Hg. The moniker pulsus paradoxus was

bestowed by W. Kussmaul in 1898, describing the findings of cardiac tamponade in a patient who was tachycardic by auscultation but manifested "paradoxical" phasic dropout of radial pulse on palpation. Paradoxical pulse >12–15 mm Hg is abnormal and may reflect cardiac tamponade and other conditions of enhanced ventricular interaction with intact inspiratory venous return.

Hemodynamics and Exercise/Stress

Cardiac output increases to meet peripheral demands during exercise or metabolic stress (e.g., infection, surgery). Under physiologic conditions, increased CO is mediated by neuro-hormonal stimulated tachycardia together with increased stroke volume achieved by augmented increased contractility, as well as by peripheral vasodilation (primarily of skeletal muscle). The increased heart rate is associated with enhanced contractility (the systolic "force–frequency relationship"). In addition, no increase in CO can be achieved without a proportional increase in venous return to both sides of the heart. During exercise, venous return is enhanced by the pumping action of skeletal muscle, venous valves, inspiratory suction induced by enhanced respiratory effort which augments right-heart filling, and ventricular suction during diastole. The LV "suction" effect related to active relaxation and "untwisting" further facilitates an increased diastolic filling rate during exercise by rapidly and markedly decreasing LV pressure during early diastole. Normal LV distensibility allows increased end-diastolic volume with minimal change in mean filling pressure. These mechanisms are frequently deranged in various pathologic conditions.

Ventricular Interactions

The right and left hearts are connected "in series" across the lungs. The right heart is designed to pump blood through the lungs to deliver oxygenated preload to the left heart. (This observation was first appreciated by Sir William Harvey, who stated that "The purpose of the right heart is to pump blood through the lungs, not to nourish them" [6]). Optimal in-series performance is essential to maintain adequate CO at rest and increased CO under conditions of exercise or stress. This requires (i) adequate RV preload (inflow; i.e., systemic venous return); and (ii) optimal pulmonary blood flow through the lungs, which is influenced by RV contractility, the pulmonary valve, and pulmonary vascular resistance (pre-, intra-, and postcapillary). It therefore follows that derangements of any component may lead to in-series failure, which may be subcategorized as "forward failure" due to primary derangements of RV preload and contractility, or RV afterload proximal to the pulmonary venous circulation, or "backward failure," in which the primary inciting pathophysiologic mechanism is elevated pulmonary capillary pressure attributable to distal downstream elevation of LA pressure, leading to elevated pulmonary vascular resistance.

Impairment of RV forward failure may result from primary impaired contractility (e.g., acute RV infarction or nonischemic cardiomyopathy), increased RV afterload, or both. RV afterload excess may result from obstruction at any site along the RV flow path (pulmonic stenosis, pulmonary emboli, or pulmonary hypertension of any cause). In the absence of pure obstruction, right-heart afterload failure is due to pulmonary hypertension, which may be differentiated based on anatomic–pathophysiologic hemodynamic considerations as precapillary, intracapillary (pulmonary), or postcapillary (Figure 1.9). Precapillary pulmonary hypertension reflects primary abnormalities of the pulmonary arterial

bed resulting from thromboembolic disease, primary pulmonary hypertension, or occasionally extrinsic mass obstruction of the major pulmonary arteries from mediastinal tumors. Primary intrapulmonary processes include the broad range of primary obstructive or restrictive lung diseases.

Acute RV Failure
Acute increases in afterload or acute ischemia may induce abrupt RV failure. Acutely increased pulmonary resistance imposed by massive and submassive acute pulmonary emboli commonly precipitate RV forward failure. In this setting, it is important to emphasize that the RV (a volume pump by design) is acutely ill equipped and therefore unable to adjust to abrupt increases in afterload imposed by abrupt increments in pulmonary vascular resistance. Acute RV failure is also commonly seen in patients with acute inferior ST elevation myocardial infarction, 50% of whom manifest with concomitant RV infarction. Acute ischemic depression of RV

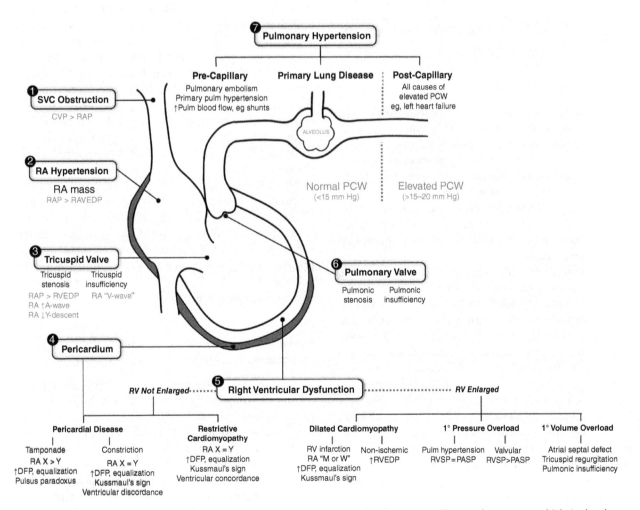

Figure 1.9 Post-capillary pulmonary hypertension is attributable to increased pulmonary capillary wedge pressure which, in the absence of pulmonary veno-occlusive disease, reflects elevated left atrial pressure.

contractility diminishes transpulmonary delivery of LV preload, leading to decreased cardiac output despite intact LV contractility. Biventricular diastolic dysfunction contributes to hemodynamic compromise in 25% of cases overall. Abrupt RV dilatation within the noncompliant pericardium elevates intrapericardial pressure, the resultant constraint further impairing RV and LV compliance and filling, and therefore forward output.

Chronic RV Failure

Under chronic conditions, the RV can hypertrophy to an extent in response to increased afterload (but not as well or as long as the more muscular LV), thus RV forward (and backward) failure ensues. This is the case in any patient with significant pulmonary hypertension, regardless of the cause. It is now well recognized that depressed RV systolic function is common in patients with dilated LV cardiomyopathies (either as part of the intrinsic depression of contractility in nonischemic patients, or in those with ischemic cardiomyopathy largely a result of pulmonary venous congestion leading to pulmonary hypertension. Regardless of the clinical congestive heart failure setting, chronic depression of RV output contributes to morbidity and mortality.

Backward Heart Failure

Elevated pulmonary capillary pressure leads to elevated pulmonary vascular resistance and ultimately pulmonary congestion. Such "post-capillary pulmonary hypertension" is attributable to increased pulmonary capillary wedge pressure which, in the absence of pulmonary veno-occlusive disease, reflects elevated LA pressure (Figure 1.9). Pathologic LA pressure increases are attributable to mitral valve disease or LV impairment (pressure overload, volume overload, or cardiomyopathy), or rarely LA myxomas.

Resting elevations of PCWP, particularly >25 mm Hg, lead to pulmonary hypertension that is tripartite in its "protective" pathophysiology, including vasoconstriction together with thickening of the pulmonary capillaries, pulmonary arteriolar intimal thickening, and medial hypertrophy. It is important to note that these protective mechanisms, including increased capillary lymphatic drainage, are designed to keep the lungs dry, but at the cost of reduced CO. These adaptive mechanisms may allow chronic resting elevations of PCWP even >25 mm Hg to be tolerated without resting dyspnea, rales or congestion seen on chest radiogram. A regurgitant mitral valve exerts disproportionate back pressure for any given mean elevation of PCWP (and thus greater magnitudes of pulmonary hypertension), a phenomenon undoubtedly attributable to the systolic pulsation of blood deep into the pulmonary venous system.

Parallel Ventricular Interactions: Septal-Mediated Diastolic Ventricular Interactions

Pressure or volume overload of one ventricle influences the compliance and filling of the contralateral ventricle by septal-mediated diastolic interactions. The normal pericardium more tightly constrains the ventricles and therefore enhances such interactions. Even in the absence of the pericardium, pressure or volume overload of one ventricle influences the compliance and filling of the contralateral ventricle. The pericardium envelopes the cardiac chambers and under physiological conditions exerts mechanical effects that enhance normal ventricular interactions, balancing left and right cardiac outputs. Because the pericardium is noncompliant, conditions that cause intrapericardial crowding (e.g., blood or masses) elevate intrapericardial pressure, which may be the mediator of adverse cardiac compressive effects.

Elevated IPP may result from primary disease of the pericardium itself (tamponade or constriction) or from abrupt chamber dilatation (e.g., right ventricular infarction [RVI] or abrupt RV dilation after major pulmonary embolus). Acute RV dilatation within the noncompliant pericardium elevates IPP, the resultant constraint further intensifying septal-mediated diastolic ventricular interactions and thereby impairing both RV and LV compliance and filling (Figure 1.10). These effects contribute to the pattern of equalized diastolic pressures and RV "dip-and-plateau" characteristic of both conditions. In patients with acute RVI, ischemic right ventricular free wall (RVFW) dysfunction diminishes transpulmonary delivery of LV preload, leading to decreased cardiac output despite intact LV contractility. Biventricular diastolic dysfunction contributes to hemodynamic compromise. The ischemic RV is stiff and dilated early in diastole, which impedes inflow, leading to rapid diastolic pressure elevation. Acute RV dilatation and elevated diastolic pressure shift the interventricular septum toward the volume-deprived left ventricle, further impairing LV compliance and filling.

Septal-Mediated Systolic Ventricular Interactions

Under conditions of acute ischemic RVFW dysfunction, RV performance is dependent on LV-septal contractile contributions transmitted via systolic ventricular interactions, mediated by the septum through both paradoxical septal motion and primary septal contributions. In early isovolumic systole, unopposed LV-septal pressure generation creates a left-to-right transseptal pressure gradient, resulting in early systolic septal bulging into the RV cavity. This paradoxical motion not only contributes to early generation of RV systolic pressure,

Figure 1.10 Pericardial mediated diastolic interactions. Under normal conditions, the interventricular septum is concave left to right, reflecting greater LV versus RV stiffness. RV dilatation and diastolic pressure elevation shift the septum right to left, altering LV filling and compliance. Abrupt RV dilatation (e.g., acute pulmonary embolus or RV infarction) also occurs across the pericardium, increasing pericardial pressure and exacerbating this adverse diastolic interaction. *Source:* Haddad 2008 [6]. Reproduced with permission of Wolters Kluwer Health, Inc.

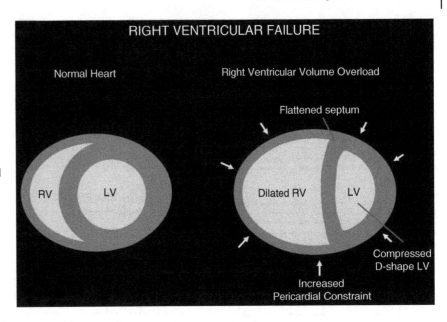

but also helps stretch the dyskinetic RVFW, a prerequisite to providing a stable buttress upon which later LV-septal thickening and shortening can generate peak RV pressure and effective pulmonary flow.

Fundamentals of Right-Heart Hemodynamics

Hemodynamics of Abnormal Cardiac Rhythms

One of the most common pitfalls in the interpretation of hemodynamic data is the failure to appreciate abnormalities in cardiac rhythms, which often account for the alteration and, at times, misinterpretation of pressure waveforms [8, 9]. Let us examine the right-heart hemodynamics in a patient undergoing evaluation for shortness of breath. The right atrial pressure (Figure 1.11, left and middle) demonstrates an alteration in the phasic waveform. At left, the V wave or S wave suggests tricuspid regurgitation. However, this waveform is significantly different during the measurements made only a few minutes later (Figure 1.11, middle). How has the physiology been affected?

Examining the ECG, a paced rhythm is responsible for the initially regurgitant wave in the right atrial pressure. The peak of the pressure wave corresponds to the QRS (the tracing lines align the specific wave or segment of the ECG to the pressure wave). As the rhythm changes to a sinus mechanism (Figure 1.11, center of middle panel), the normal right atrial waveform is restored and the regurgitant waveform is eliminated. The changing rhythm also affects the determination of maximal pulmonary artery pressures (Figure 1.11, right). During pacing, the pulmonary artery pressure has a larger respiratory variation and is higher than pressures obtained during normal sinus rhythm.

Observe the right-heart hemodynamics obtained in a patient undergoing evaluation for ischemia-induced ventricular dysrhythmia and congestive heart failure (Figure 1.12). The mean right atrial pressure (Figure 1.12, top left) is 9 mm Hg with large V waves. Why is the right atrial waveform different between the left and right panels of Figure 1.12? Consider the ECG. When sinus rhythm

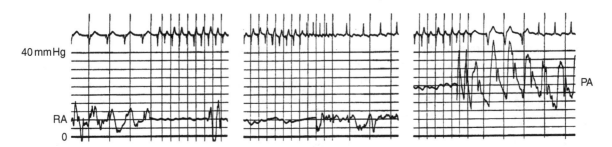

Figure 1.11 (Left) Right atrial (RA) pressure (0–40 mmHg scale) during alterations in cardiac rhythm (middle). (Far right) Change in pulmonary artery (PA) pressure.

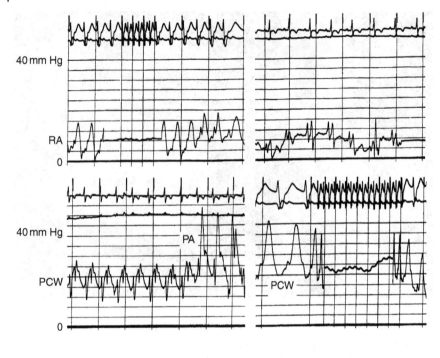

Figure 1.12 Right-heart hemodynamics during changes in cardiac rhythm. (Top left and right) RA, right atrial; (bottom left and right) PCWP, pulmonary capillary wedge pressure; PA, pulmonary artery.

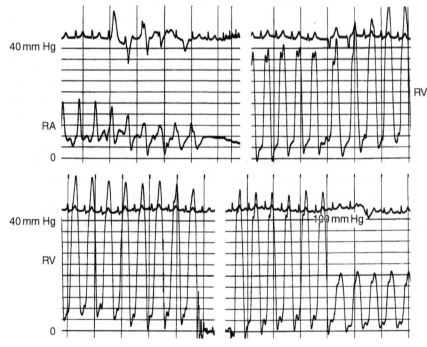

Figure 1.13 (Top right) Right atrial (RA) and (top left and lower right) right ventricular (RV) pressures (0–40 mm Hg scale) during alterations in cardiac rhythm. (Lower right) RV pressure scale change from 0–40 mm Hg to 0–100 mm Hg (far right).

is restored (note the P waves), the V wave is attenuated and a normal right atrial pressure waveform can be seen, with a reduction in right atrial pressure to a mean value of 7 mm Hg (Figure 1.12, top right). A similar response can be appreciated in the pulmonary capillary wedge pressure (Figure 1.12, lower left). During sinus rhythm, PCWP averages 18 mm Hg, with a V wave up to 24 mm Hg. However, during ventricular tachycardia, the mean PCWP markedly increases to 24 mm Hg, with V waves

up to 40 mm Hg (Figure 1.12, lower right). Interpretation of the hemodynamic waveform is thus critically dependent on the particular cardiac rhythm which reflects the physiologic responses generating the cardiac pressure (Figures 1.13 and 1.14).

The influence of cardiac rhythm on right-heart hemodynamics can be appreciated in a 39-year-old man with congestive heart failure and cardiomyopathy undergoes hemodynamic evaluation (Figure 1.13). Examine the

Figure 1.14 Right atrial (RA) pressure (0–40 mm Hg scale) in a patient after myocardial infarction. See text for details.

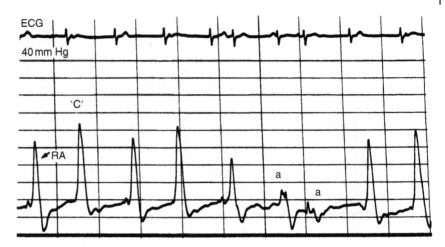

right atrial waveform at the top right (Figure 1.13). Note the alteration of the V wave configuration. How does one explain the large pointed waveforms at the left side in contrast to the smaller, broader waveforms demonstrated at the right? While considering the possibilities, examine the differences in right ventricular pressures obtained during this study (Figure 1.13, upper right and lower left panels). Compare the effects on the cardiac rhythm of the generation of right ventricular pressure.

The right atrial pressure V waves (Figure 1.13, top left) occur during junctional rhythm with atrial superimposition on the QRS and third-degree heart block. As the atrial time delay permits normal sinus mechanisms to intervene, the waveform changes into a sinus-type rhythm with a larger A wave and a small V wave. Note the decrease in mean right atrial pressure from 10–12 mm Hg to < 8 mm Hg when sinus rhythm is in play.

The evaluation of right ventricular pressure is also interesting, in that the accelerated junctional rhythm during complete heart block has a lower peak systolic pressure of approximately 38 mm Hg (Figure 1.13, top right, right side). When the rhythm changes, the peak systolic right ventricular pressure increases to approximately 50 mm Hg and the initiation of the atrial wave can be seen as a deflection on the QRS (Figure 1.13, mid-portion at upper right). As the sinus mechanism contributes to the filling of the ventricle and precedes QRS activation of ventricular contraction, the systolic pressure increases and remains in excess of 50 mm Hg. The rhythm changes explain the wide variations in right atrial and ventricular pressure waveforms, and should be important functional clues in the evaluation of hemodynamics for such individuals.

Consider the right atrial pressure wave obtained in a 66-year-old man following myocardial infarction (Figure 1.14). Cardiac rhythm disturbances were noted on the resting electrocardiogram on day 3. The right

atrial pressure wave was recorded using a fluid-filled catheter. Examine the pressure waves and consider the following: What is the etiology of the large, spiked waves (C)? Is the tricuspid valve normal? What accounts for the C spike variation from 16 to 24 mm Hg? What is responsible for the change in waveform on beats #6 and 7?

These large, spiked waves are C waves or (giant) cannon waves. This occurs when atrial contraction falls out of sequence with normal ventricular systole and the atria contract against a tricuspid valve closed by the increased right ventricular pressure during ejection. The size of the C wave is dependent on the timing of atrial contraction relative to ventricular filling (and the position of the tricuspid valve). When the atrial contraction precedes ventricular contraction in its normal synchronous mode, normal A waves are generated (beats #6 and 7). When atrial synchrony is lost, the cannon waves return. These cannon waves can be observed on bedside physical examination in the jugular venous pulse and should be differentiated from systolic tricuspid regurgitant waves (to be identified below). Iatrogenic induced (pacemaker) or spontaneous abnormalities of conduction also can produce similar types of cannon waves of atrial activity out of synchrony with ventricular contraction.

Large spiked pressure waves appeared in the right atrial tracing of a 78-year-old woman with a ventricular pacemaker (Figure 1.15). Examine the rhythm first. The pressure tracing demonstrates brief, sharp peaked waves, less prominent than the atrial contraction waves of the previous tracing. The dyssynchronous ventricular pacemaker timing relative to atrial dissociated contraction appears to be responsible. Note the wider C-type wave of beat #3 with the P wave falling on the QRS. The high-pressure spike of very narrow width also suggests artifact from catheter impaction, but the timing sequence also is highly consistent with "cannon"-type waves.

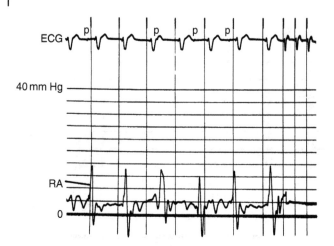

Figure 1.15 Right atrial (RA) pressure (0–40 mm Hg scale) in a patient with compensated heart failure. See text for details.

Vena Caval Pressure Waveforms in Tricuspid Regurgitation

Tricuspid regurgitation often produces distinct waveforms in the right atrial pressure [10–13]. Sometimes, transmission of the regurgitant wave can be detected beyond the vena cava (i.e., transmitted to the jugular veins) [14]. However, it is uncommon to observe changing waveforms in the inferior vena cava compared to those in the right atrium. For purposes of demonstration, we recorded the inferior vena caval pressure and compared the waveforms to those of the right atrial and ventricular pressures in a patient with modest tricuspid regurgitation (Figure 1.16).

A 61-year-old woman had tricuspid regurgitation of unknown etiology which was associated with mild pulmonary hypertension and dyspnea. Coronary arteriography was normal. Left ventriculography demonstrated mild global hypokinesis with an ejection fraction of 55%.

Aortic pressure was 125/70 mm Hg, left ventricular pressure was 125/12 mm Hg, and pulmonary capillary wedge pressure was 20 mm Hg with normal A and V wave configurations. The effects of tricuspid regurgitation on the right atrium and inferior vena cava were assessed by measuring two pressures simultaneously, one from each of the two lumens of a balloon-tipped pulmonary artery catheter. The systolic wave of regurgitation could be appreciated in both the right atrium and inferior vena cava. The right atrial pressure was measured with the tip of the balloon-tipped catheter looped within the right atrium (Figure 1.16, upper left). The inferior vena cava pressure was measured approximately 10 cm below the inferior border of the right atrium. The pressure wave fidelity between the two systems was demonstrated to be equivalent by comparing the right ventricular and right atrial pressures measured with the same transducers on advancement of the catheter into the right ventricular apex (Figure 1.16, top right).

The waveform of the inferior vena cava is slower in upstroke and downstroke, with reduced velocity. The blunted waveform is due, in part, to the considerably higher capacity and compliance of the vena cava compared to those of the right atrium. It is also important to note that the right atrial pressure mean, as expected, is lower than that of the vena cava, with a 2–4 mm Hg pressure gradient required for maintenance of normal blood flow. The pressure gradient between the inferior vena cava and right atrium occurs predominantly during the end of atrial diastole (Figure 1.16, top left).

The severity of tricuspid regurgitation can be appreciated when comparing the right ventricular and right atrial pressures (Figure 1.16, top right), showing the regurgitant S wave and large V wave of tricuspid regurgitation. Tricuspid regurgitation is, by waveform characteristics, most severe during the ventricular couplet

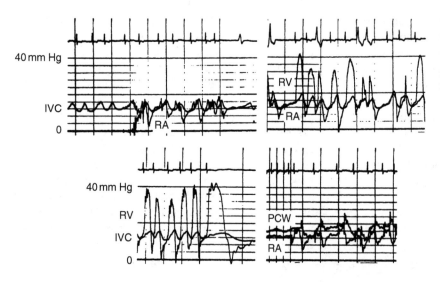

Figure 1.16 (Top left) Right atrial (RA) and inferior vena cava (IVC) pressures in a patient with tricuspid regurgitation. (Top right) RA and RV pressures. (Lower left) RV and IVC pressures. (Lower right) Pulmonary capillary wedge (PCW) and RA pressures.

appearing in the mid portion of this tracing, in which the pressure during systole is achieved for both beats. When comparing the vena cava and right ventricular pressures (Figure 1.16, lower left), the delay in waveform and transmission of the vena cava can be appreciated. Of interest is that the differences between the mean pulmonary capillary wedge (16 mm Hg) and mean right atrial pressures (12 mm Hg; Figure 1.16, lower right) demonstrate the larger Y descent in right atrial pressure (Figure 1.16, upper left) which drives the inferior vena cava flow. Inferior vena cava flow in most cases parallels that of superior vena cava flow and thus large V waves in the jugular vein on clinical examination can reflect either significant tricuspid regurgitation or functional regurgitation during cardiac arrhythmias [14].

The jugular pulse closely reflects events in right atrial pressure and also parallels changes observed in the vena cava [15, 16]. However, one must remember that the change in pressure within the right atrium is reflected principally by a change in volume for the venous system. It is thought that the pulse wave transmission from the right atrium to the jugular veins has the least disparity for pressure waves which are positive and are thought to be conducted more rapidly compared to negative pressure waves [17]. The venous pulse A and C waves have an average delay from right atrial pressures of approximately 60 msec, the V wave 80 msec, the Y trough 90 msec, and the X trough 110 msec [17]. It requires 60 msec for the right atrial A wave to reach the right ventricle and cause a positive defection in this chamber. These delays should be considered when examining the jugular venous pulse, as well as inferior vena caval pressure waves as a reflection of right atrial pressure [11].

Jugular vein pulsations may occur from an induced artifact of transmitted carotid arterial pressure waves. This artifact can be recognized by an irregular pulsation often obscuring the X descent. The irregular wave shows a carotid-like contour, with the dichrotic notch recognized in the middle of the X descent [11]. Tavel [14] notes that tricuspid insufficiency often produces a prominent V wave, beginning early and tending to obliterate the X descent. In severe tricuspid regurgitation, the V wave corresponds and begins with the C wave and shows a broad plateau terminating in a steep Y descent. This wave has been termed the regurgitant or S wave. In the setting of atrial fibrillation, nearly complete obliteration of the X descent is required before making the diagnosis of tricuspid insufficiency from a venous pulse wave. In patients with normal sinus rhythm, changes in the venous pulse suggesting tricuspid regurgitation may demonstrate only slight decrease in the X descent equal to or above the level of the Y trough. In some patients, a separate systolic wave may appear on the V wave ascent and may be an obscured clue to the presence of tricuspid

regurgitation [13]. In addition, in tricuspid regurgitation there may be a relatively normal venous pulse wave; hence the diagnostic accuracy of the waveform is helpful, in that a normal curve cannot be used to exclude tricuspid disease. The characteristic pulse waves may be absent at rest but brought on by inspiratory maneuvers or increasing heart rate [13].

Normal Tricuspid Valve Function

Simultaneous right ventricular and right atrial pressure waves using fluid-filled transducer systems were measured in a 40-year-old woman with a history of dyspnea and chronic obstructive pulmonary disease (COPD; Figure 1.17). Identical matching of the right atrial and right ventricular diastolic pressures is the norm. The A wave (atrial contraction) of the right atrial pressure corresponds to the A wave of the right ventricle. The V wave corresponds to the passive increase in right atrial pressure from venous return along with the rapid rise in right ventricle pressure during RV systole. The V wave peak precedes the tricuspid valve opening. Note that pressure immediately after the A wave, called the X descent, falls and does not begin to increase until late in systole. As right ventricular pressure falls below right atrial pressure, the tricuspid valve opens, releasing atrial pressure (the Y descent of the V wave). Not shown on this tracing is a C wave of ventricular contraction apparent on some beats as a "notch" immediately after an A wave or the initial upstroke of ventricular pressure.

The higher ejection velocity and faster development of the right ventricular pressure cause more oscillation of

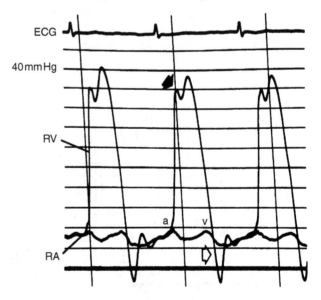

Figure 1.17 Simultaneous right ventricular (RV) and right atrial (RA) pressures measured through two fluid-filled catheters (0–40 mm Hg scale). See text for details.

the transducer system than those of the right atrial pressure, and therefore a high-frequency "ringing" is observed as a notch on the upstroke before the systolic peak of the right ventricle (Figure 1.17, black arrow) and a rapid dip (negative overshoot) in early diastole (open arrow). This common artifact using fluid-filled systems is important to consider when assessing tricuspid and pulmonary gradients.

Atrial Pressure X and Y Troughs

Compare the typical hemodynamic normal example (Figure 1.17) of tricuspid valve function to right and left atrial pressure waveforms in a 62-year-old man with aortic stenosis (Figure 1.18). These pressures were measured continuously on pullback of a fluid-filled transseptal Brockenbrough catheter. The mean left atrial pressure is elevated approximately 22 mm Hg with striking A and V waves. There are two principal negative or downward motions of the right (and left) atrial pressure waves. The X trough results from movement of the tricuspid (or mitral) valve away from the atrium when intrapericardial pressure is decreasing immediately after ventricular contraction begins and left ventricular volume falls. The Y trough occurs with opening of the tricuspid valve [18]. There is a reciprocal relationship between pressure and right atrial or venous flow. Flow is virtually absent at times of peak positive A and V waves [15, 19]. The left atrial V wave is giant (i.e., twice the mean pressure) and occurs, in this particular patient, in the absence of mitral regurgitation. The V wave reflects the pressure–volume relationship (also known as compliance of the atrium) and will be discussed in the review of the V wave below. A noncompliant or stiff ventricle often is associated with large A and V waves. The differences between left and right atrial pressures are easily appreciated during the

pullback from left to right atrium (Figure 1.18). The left atrial V waves are generally greater than V waves on the right atrial pressure where the A wave predominates. The C waves, again, are not evident. Also note that atrial arrhythmias may significantly alter the waveforms (Figure 1.18, first right atrial beat after *, a1).

Systolic Regurgitant Right Atrial Waves

In contrast to large cannon-type waves, positive systolic pressure waves on the right atrial tracing may also be due to an incompetent or occasionally a stenotic tricuspid valve. A 50-year-old woman with atrial fibrillation and a history of rheumatic fever has increasing pedal edema and dyspnea. Simultaneous right ventricular and right atrial pressures were measured with two fluid-filled catheters (Figure 1.19). The right atrial pressure matches the right ventricular pressure in diastole, and rises across the systolic period of right ventricular ejection, which is the most common pressure wave pattern of tricuspid regurgitation [12]. As anticipated in atrial fibrillation, the right atrial and ventricular A waves are absent. A prominent Y descent occurs after the point of the maximal right atrial pressure (V wave) and falls sharply with the drop in right ventricular pressure. Although the slope of the atrial pressure during right ventricular ejection is generally proportional to the severity of tricuspid regurgitation [Figure 1.15], the compliance or pressure–volume relationship of the atrium will determine the size and character of the pressure wave. Note that the diastolic pressures of the right atrial and right ventricular tracings are nearly identical throughout the majority of diastole. If the catheters are zeroed, calibrated properly, and the resonant features and sensitivity of the two fluid-filled systems are matched, small diastolic gradients of tricuspid stenosis can be reliably determined.

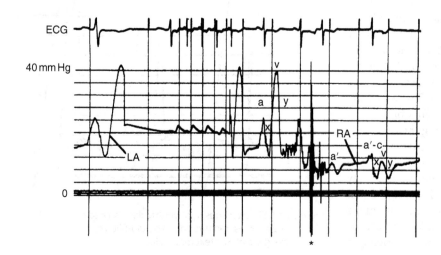

Figure 1.18 Continuous pressure recording from left atrium (LA) to right atrium (RA) on pullback (*) across the intra-atrial septum, demonstrating phasic waveforms A and V and X and Y descents, respectively, for the two atria. See text for details.

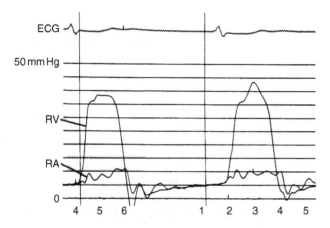

Figure 1.19 Right atrial (RA) pressure (0–40 mm Hg scale) with a varying murmur along the right sternal border. See text for details. *Source:* Lingamneni 1979 [12]. Reproduced with permission of John Wiley & Sons.

Pulsatile Venous Waves

A 39-year-old woman with severe ascites and dyspnea at rest has large V waves during jugular vein examination and a pulsatile liver. The simultaneous right ventricular and right atrial pressures (Figure 1.20) show the marked and more striking upslope of right atrial pressure during right ventricular ejection with a V or S (systolic) wave to 32 mm Hg. The more rapid rise of right atrial pressure indicates severe tricuspid regurgitation (compared with Figure 1.19). Early diastolic right ventricular pressure drop is associated with an early right atrial–right ventricular pressure gradient which equilibrates before the first one-third of diastole following a rapid decline, reflecting mostly high flow and not necessarily significant tricuspid valvular stenosis. The faster heart rate (compared with the previous patient in Figure 1.19) may also contribute to the early right atrial–right ventricular diastolic gradient. The regurgitant S wave, occurring slightly earlier than the V wave, is very prominent on physical examination and can be seen in the neck and even transmitted down to the femoral vein (Figure 1.20, lower panel). The marked regurgitant waves seen on the lower panel are measured in the femoral vein. Femoral vein pressure may be as high as 40 mm Hg. Thus, on puncture of the femoral vein, a "venous" pressure pulse may be observed. The timing of the V wave is coincident with the electrocardiographic T wave, but may be easily confused with an arterial pulse of low amplitude.

Tricuspid Valve Dysfunction: Right Atrial–Right Ventricular Gradients

Right atrial and right ventricular pressures were measured in a 49-year-old woman with increasing abdominal girth, dyspnea at rest and exercise, and systolic and

diastolic murmurs that varied markedly with respiration (Figure 1.21). The right atrial pressure (upper panel) demonstrated a prominent regurgitant wave with fusion of A and V waves, an absent X trough, and a marked Y descent. Is there truly an A wave? No, the rhythm is atrial fibrillation. Also observe absent A waves on the right ventricular tracing (lower panel). The C wave of ventricular contraction can now be seen (arrow, lower panel). Because of the resonant qualities of some fluid-filled systems, the pressure waveform with a blunted A wave and X descent (Figure 1.22) may occasionally be confused with the "M" configuration of constrictive or restrictive physiology [10, 20]. The broad and wide upsloping right atrial pressure of tricuspid regurgitation is importantly associated with a persistent gradient of approximately 4 mm Hg across the tricuspid valve throughout diastole. Compare this pressure tracing to that seen on Figure 1.21, in which a diastolic right ventricular–right atrial pressure diastolic gradient is not present. These small pressure gradients are always significant in tricuspid valve disease [10].

A 66-year-old white female had severe tricuspid regurgitation in 1985 and underwent a procedure with a symptom-free period until five years later. A marked increase in abdominal girth and severe lower-extremity edema were the predominant complaints, along with mild paroxysmal nocturnal dyspnea and orthopnea. There was no chest pain. High-flow velocities across the tricuspid valve were demonstrated by echocardiography. Moderate left ventricular dysfunction was also present. The hemodynamic tracings of the right-heart pressures were measured with fluid-filled transducers through two catheters (Figure 1.23). The left-hand panel of Figure 1.23 demonstrates the elevated and matched right atrial pressures. The rhythm was atrial bigeminy. Note the loss of distinct right atrial A and V waves. When simultaneous right ventricular and right atrial pressures are measured (Figure 1.23, right-hand panel), a significant right atrial–right ventricular diastolic gradient can be seen. The tricuspid valve, five years after bioprosthetic valve implantation, had a mean gradient of 11 mm Hg with a cardiac output of 6.4 L/min, which yielded a valve area of 1.5 cm^2. Importantly, matching of the two pressure transducers eliminated artifactual differences contributing to this gradient. As one can see, in significant tricuspid stenosis the gradient persists throughout diastole during both long and short cycles (compared to Figure 1.21). Repeat tricuspid valve replacement was subsequently performed.

Pressure Wave Artifacts

If the measurement of blood pressure were automatically available without having to attend to transducer flushing, pressure line, and manifold connections, and erroneous settings on the recorders or kinks in catheters, the study of

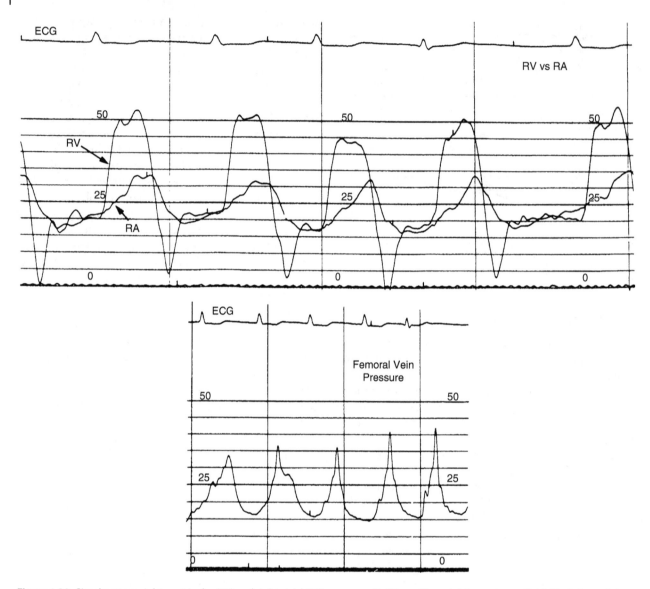

Figure 1.20 Simultaneous right ventricular (RV) and right atrial (RA) pressures (0–50 mm Hg scale) through two fluid-filled channels in a patient with pulsatile neck veins. See text for details.

hemodynamics would be as routine and reliable as that of electrocardiography. However, as with any recording system that requires specially trained personnel and multiple combinations of different connector types, the mechanical and electrical artifacts of both fluid-filled tubes and high-fidelity recording instruments produce pressure wave artifacts that must be recognized as the major flaw in accurate hemodynamic data interpretation [21].

In the measurement of right atrial pressure, the most common artifacts include failure to match the zero positions or transducer gain sensitivity of the two fluid-filled systems. When tricuspid valve disease is suspected, precise calibration and equisensitivity of transducers are critical, because small gradients may have large clinical importance.

An increase in right atrial mean pressure during inspiration is a common indication (Kussmaul's sign) of physiologic abnormalities of atrial filling, especially prevalent in patients with constrictive or restrictive physiology. However, how does one explain the inspiratory increases in right atrial pressure in a 46-year-old woman with atypical chest pain without suspected pericardial disease? To the unknowing observer, this increase in right atrial mean pressure would be consistent with pathophysiology of constrictive pericarditis, but the mean right atrial pressure is only 4 mm Hg (Figure 1.24, top). It would be unusual for an asymptomatic, untreated person with significant constrictive physiology to have a low mean right atrial pressure. Whenever a suspected potentially erroneous physiologic event occurs during mean

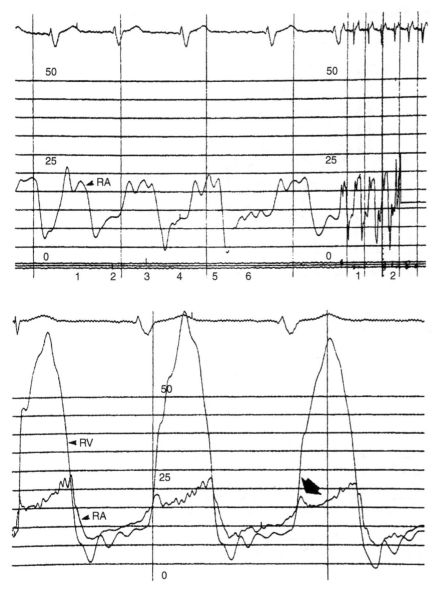

Figure 1.21 Simultaneous right ventricular (RV) and right atrial (RA) pressures (0–50 mm Hg scale) through two fluid-filled channels in a patient with prominent waves in neck veins and varying murmurs. See text for details.

pressure recording, observe the phasic waveform generating this response. As can be seen on the lower panel of Figure 1.24, the phasic right atrial waveform is displayed during inspiration. The initial several beats demonstrate the normal fall in right atrial pressure with an increasing Y descent and then the catheter accidentally enters the right ventricle. The artifact of measuring right ventricular pressure during mean right atrial waveform recording is the explanation for an abnormal increase in right atrial mean pressure during inspiration in this patient, in whom pericardial disease was not present.

Another common and disturbing artifact of fluid-filled pressure systems, especially in measuring right atrial and other right-heart pressures, is that of excessive catheter "fling" of an underdamped pressure (catheter, tubing, and transducer) system. This artifact is very common when using balloon-tipped pulmonary artery flotation catheters. The left side of Figures 1.25a and 1.25b shows right-heart pressures recorded prior to pressure system manipulation to reduce the underdamped signal. Interpretation of waveforms and other details of these pressure tracings cannot be discerned from the rapid high-frequency "ringing" artifact of the underdamped system. To improve hemodynamic recordings while continuously measuring pressure, a 50% saline and contrast solution was instilled through the catheter. The right-hand panel shows the distinct and strikingly elevated waveforms of a patient with congestive heart failure. The

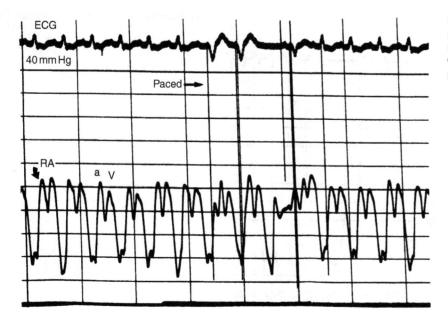

Figure 1.22 Right atrial (RA) pressure in a patient with dyspnea at rest (0–40 mm Hg scale). See text for details. *Source:* Grossman 1986 [10]. Reproduced with permission of Wolters Kluwer Health, Inc.

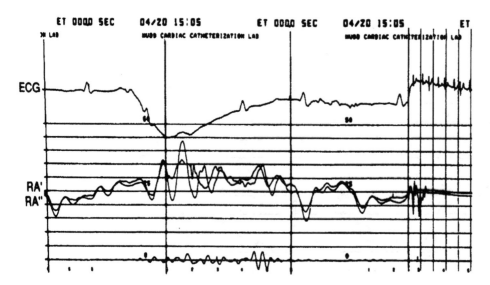

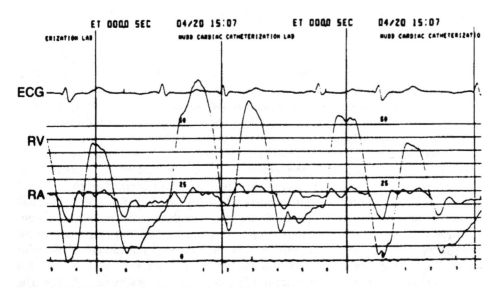

Figure 1.23 Right ventricular (RV) and right atrial (RA) pressures (0–50 mm Hg scale) measured in a patient with severe ascites and peripheral edema. Left panel shows two matching fluid-filled transducers prior to crossing the tricuspid valve (0–50 mm Hg scale). See text for details.

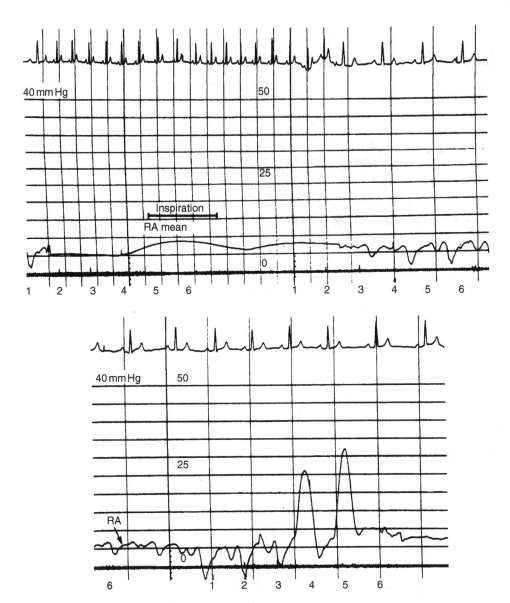

Figure 1.24 Right atrial (RA) mean pressure during inspiration: Kussmaul's sign? See text for details.

small A and large V waves with the prominent Y descent are evident [22]. In the same patient, the catheter was flushed with saline and passed to the pulmonary artery, which also demonstrated a marked high-frequency ringing artifact. Contrast media was again instilled which correctly damped the pressure waveform, providing accurate identification of pulmonary artery pressures (Figure 1.25b, right-hand panel).

Whenever the damping characteristics of the fluid-filled systems are not satisfactory, maneuvers to improve the resonant characteristics should be conducted to achieve satisfactory pressure responses. Accurate determination of waveforms will aid in the determination of diseased conditions using pressure patterns.

Pressure Wave Artifacts

If the measurement of blood pressure were automatically available without having to attend to transducer flushing, pressure line, and manifold connections, as well as erroneous settings on the recorders or kinks in catheters, the study of hemodynamics would be as routine and reliable as that of electrocardiography. However, as with any recording system that requires specially trained personnel and multiple combinations of different connector types, the mechanical and electrical artifacts of both fluid-filled tubes and high-fidelity recording instruments produce pressure wave artifacts that must be recognized as the major flaw in accurate hemodynamic data interpretation

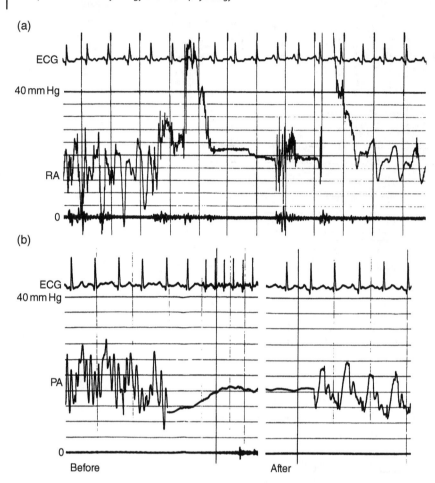

(a)

(b)

Figure 1.25 (a) Right atrial (RA) pressure and (b) pulmonary artery pressure (G–40 mm Hg scale) with high-frequency artifact. Left panels are before and right panels after pressure system manipulation.

Pressure System Resonance: The Under- and Overdamped Waveform

Probably the most common pressure wave artifacts of fluid-filled systems are the exaggerated ringing of underdamping and overly damped "rounded" waveforms. An underdamped pressure tracing is one in which the pressure wave is rapidly reflected within the system and produces an oscillating sinusoidal distortion of the pressure waveform [23]. This underdamped tracing is also called ringing, as in continued bounding of sound waves in a bell with a characteristic demonstration of the physics of reflected waves [24]. Commonly, an air bubble in the pressure line will be small enough to be rapidly accelerated and decelerated, moving the fluid column back and forth, resulting in ringing of the pressure tracing. The effect of a bubble in the pressure line connected to a 7 F pigtail catheter and fluid-filled transducer used to measure left ventricular pressure is illustrated in Figure 1.26, left panel. The bubble causes a high spike on the left ventricular upstroke and a large negative overshoot wave on the left ventricular pressure downstroke. When the pres-

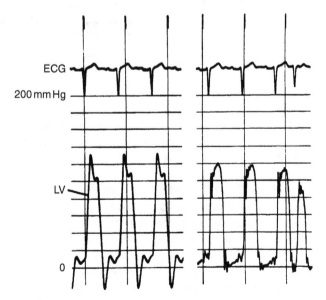

Figure 1.26 Left ventricular (LV) pressure with 7F pigtail catheter using fluid-filled transducers. Left panel demonstrates "ringing" artifact. See text for details.

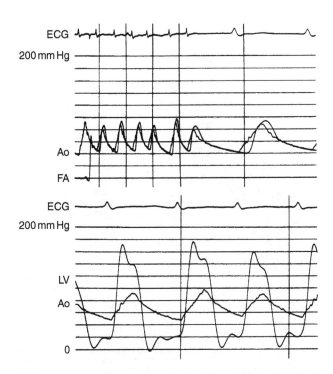

Figure 1.27 Overdamped left ventricle. (Top) Central and femoral (FA) pressures. (Bottom) Left ventricular (LV) and aortic (Ao) pressures in a patient with aortic stenosis. Note delay and unusual waveform in left ventricular pressure. See text for details.

sure line and transducer are properly flushed, the left ventricular pressure (Figure 1.26, right panel) shows an excellent and normal waveform, which should be expected with modern fluid-filled systems.

An overdamped waveform reduces the impact of the pressure wave, rounding the contours and delaying the upstroke and downstroke of the pressure wave. An example of pressure overdamping will be described later and is depicted in Figure 1.27.

A Hemodynamic Data Collection Method

Hemodynamic studies require accurate data collection techniques. For complex cases, one must record simultaneous pressure waveforms, working with multiple transducers. Below are the steps commonly used to minimize artifactual pressure recordings.

Step 1

Check the transducer connections to the recorder. This step is one of the greatest points of confusion and frustration in hemodynamic studies. It is not uncommon that the cables connecting the transducers to the table and the hemodynamic recorder are unplugged and

uncoiled, and scattered over the catheter table and floor. Numbering, labeling, and color-coding all cables and their inputs make reconnection easy and quick. In addition to clear labeling of the cables, an attachment device for the coiled cables to the tableside, such as Velcro strips or other tape, is also very helpful.

On the sterile field, it is also worth numbering and color-coding the transducers and tubing so that communications for recording the waveforms from the operators to the control room can proceed smoothly. For example, "zeroing transducer number 1; pressure is up on number 1; number 1 is a femoral artery pressure." Clear communications are always helpful and this is the best method to reduce frustration, save time, and decrease confusion during hemodynamic measurements.

Step 2

Set up the transducers on the sterile field or on the injector device. A small rack with transducer mounting brackets is placed opposite the operators and set at the patient's mid-chest level. Transducers are connected electrically to the catheter table sockets, sending the signals to the recorder. The transducers are flushed with saline through plastic tubing to be connected to the catheters on the sterile field. The transducers are flushed to ensure that bubbles are eliminated. All connections to stopcocks and tubing should be flushed and tightened. If possible, the shortest and stiffest tubing should be used to produce the best pressure transmission pathway.

Step 3

After flushing, the tableside transducers are zeroed at the mid-chest level of the patient. The transducers are opened to atmosphere; the recording technologist zeroes the signals on the hemodynamic recorder. The transducers are then closed. It may be necessary to reflush the transducers to be sure that they are free of air bubbles. Any remaining bubbles may produce underdamped pressure waveforms. This setup applies for multiple transducers and will provide accurate hemodynamic measurements for all cases.

Technical Note

The ACIST power injection system (Eden Prairie, MN) has a pressure transducer mounted on a built-in bracket with rubber-padded backing through which the pressure is transmitted to an electrical sensor. Although the transducer on the ACIST device is accurate, because of the mechanical plate interface, the signal is delayed by about 50–100 msec relative to the ECG. The computer-measured left ventricular end-diastolic pressure may be inaccurate, since the timing mark of the R wave from

(a)

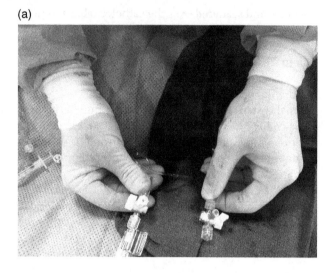

(c)

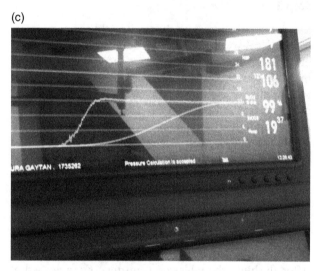

(b)

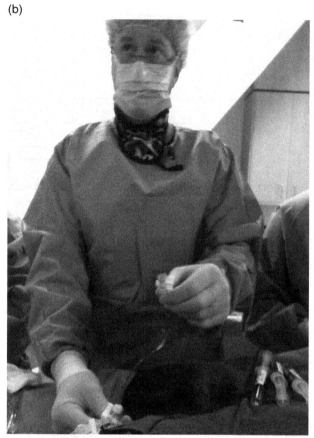

Figure 1.28 (a) The transducer (left) is connected to a fluid-filled tube (right) and a stopcock, which is open to the air. (b) Lifting either the tubing as shown here or the transducer changes the pressure, but once zero is set with the position of the tubing, there is no need to adjust the transducer. Connect the tubing to the catheter and you are ready to measure. (c) A hemodynamic monitor showing the effect of first raising the tubing. The blue line goes up and then raising the transducer to the same level will produce the same effect.

the ECG is out of synchrony with the pressure wave (Figures 1.28, 1.29, and 1.30). For all simultaneous two-pressure hemodynamic studies, or any study in which high accuracy is desired, two tableside-mounted transducers may be preferred.

Step 4

Continuously review the pressure waveforms during acquisition. The waveforms should make sense for the catheter location, cardiac rhythm, and clinical situation. The pressure waveform should be timed correctly with the ECG and should be of an appropriate scale. For example, does an arterial pressure of 60/40 with a heart rate of 80 bpm make sense in a perfectly comfortable, awake patient who is talking to you? First, check the patient. Then, check the scale factors on the recorder,

then the connections and tubing again, and whether or not the pressure transducer is connected to the left-sided or right-sided catheter. Errors like this are a common source of confusion among inexperienced personnel. Unusual waveforms should correlate to pathophysiology. If not, suspect some error in the recording technique, such as a loose connection, an air bubble, a clot in the line, a damped or kinked pressure tube or catheter, or a wrong recording scale. These checkpoints are necessary to record good-quality hemodynamics.

Technical Note on Using Simultaneous Right- and Left-Heart Hemodynamics

Usually, right-heart hemodynamics are performed in conjunction with left-heart hemodynamics to obtain a complete assessment of myocardial, pulmonary, and valvular

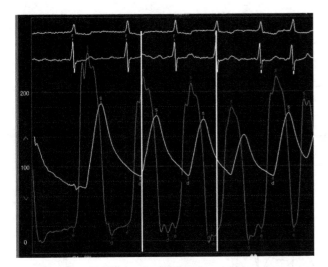

Figure 1.29 Left ventricular and aortic pressures measured from table-side transducers. The vertical yellow lines indicate left ventricular end diastolic pressure (LVEDP) and timing to ECG. Note the delay in aortic pressure due to pressure transmission from the femoral arterial sheath-side arm. The computer has placed "d" on aortic diastolic pressures and "e" on LVEDP. The "e" position varies, but is mostly close to the true LVEDP. Scale 0–200 mm Hg. (*See insert for color representation of the figure.*)

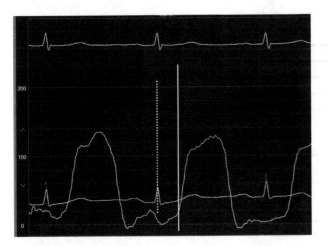

Figure 1.30 Left ventricular pressure recorded with an ACIST transducer, demonstrating delay in pressure relative to ECG. The R wave precedes the LVEDP by almost 100 msec. Manual selection of LVEDP is required. (*See insert for color representation of the figure.*)

function. Normally, when performing simultaneous right- and left-heart hemodynamics, a right-heart catheter is positioned in the pulmonary artery in the standard manner. After cardiac output is obtained, a pigtail catheter is positioned in the LV and LV hemodynamics and simultaneous wedge pressures are acquired to gauge mitral valve function. On pullback of the right-heart catheter, simultaneous RV and LV pressures are measured, especially useful in patients suspected of having constrictive or restrictive physiology. Finally, to evaluate aortic valve disease use a dual-lumen pigtail catheter or pressure wire and multipurpose catheter. Right- and left-heart catheterizations

performed in this manner will provide a complete hemodynamic assessment in 95% of cases and provide an accurate understanding of aortic, mitral, tricuspid, and pulmonary valve disease with minimal extra maneuvers. These protocols have been described elsewhere [23]. Improving the precision, organization, clarity, and operational protocols will produce better hemodynamic data.

Case of a Transiently Wide Pulse Pressure: Artifact or Episodic Aortic Insufficiency?

A continuous hemodynamic tracing was recorded during 7 F left ventricular catheter pullback after ventriculography (Figure 1.31a). The pullback was easily and smoothly, but slowly, performed. The operator noted a wide pulse pressure which appeared to diminish over the next several beats. Should the operator reload for aortography to demonstrate transient aortic insufficiency? To a new student of hemodynamics, this mystifying physiology of waxing aortic insufficiency might require more study. However, a slow pigtail catheter pullback from the left ventricle might be incomplete, leaving a portion of the uncoiled pigtail in the left ventricle with several side holes still transmitting the lower left ventricular diastolic pressure falsely, reducing aortic diastolic pressure. This phenomenon is demonstrated again with simultaneous femoral arterial and pigtail catheter pressures (Figures 1.31b, c). The changing diastolic pressure is due to catheter movement, with a different number of pigtail catheter side holes moving across the aortic valve.

With complete catheter removal, two systemic pressures match without the diastolic pressure artifact (Figure 1.31c, right side). This artifact can be easily recognized by the unusual diastolic waveform, with a late diastolic shoulder and rapid dip differentiating it from a wide pulse pressure of valvular insufficiency.

Case of a Late-Rising Central Aortic Pressure: Artifact or Pathology?

The most proximally measured aortic pressure wave rises before the pressure waves measured more distally. This constant physiologic requirement may be disturbed only by pressure waveform artifacts. Consider the hemodynamic data obtained in a 72-year-old man with aortic stenosis (Figure 1.27). Because of mild peripheral vascular disease, simultaneous pressures were initially obtained with a 6 F femoral arterial sheath and a 5 F pigtail catheter with fluid-filled transducers. The pressures measured before crossing the aortic valve demonstrated a good correspondence with two notable features: a slightly reduced femoral pressure overshoot consistent with mild peripheral vascular

(a)

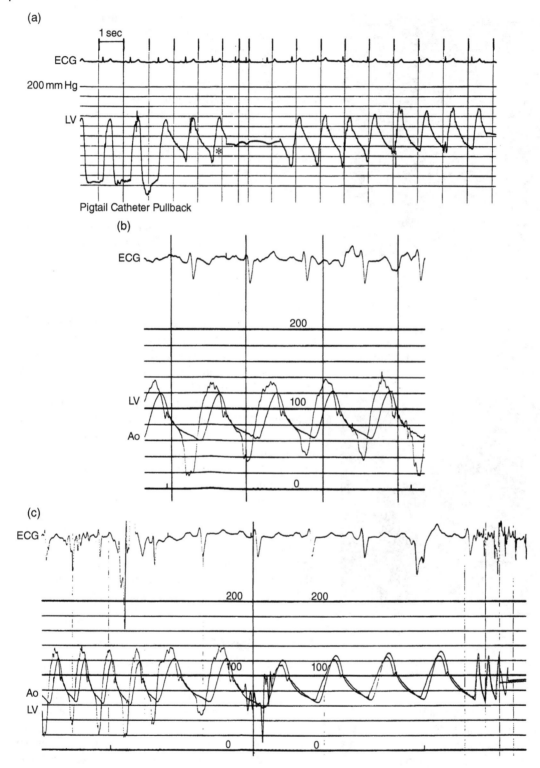

Pigtail Catheter Pullback

(b)

(c)

Figure 1.31 (a) Left ventricular (LV) catheter pullback with transient aortic insufficiency. Note unusual diastolic waveform. See text for details. (b, c) LV and simultaneous aortic (Ao) pressures. See text for details.

disease and a slow central aortic pressure upstroke consistent with aortic stenosis. These pressure waveforms are acceptable for routine clinical use. Crossing the heavily calcified valve in the enlarged aortic root was accomplished with the pigtail catheter and a 0.038″ straight guidewire. Mild difficulty in advancing the pigtail catheter over the valve and into the left ventricle was encountered.

Figure 1.32 (Upper panel) Catheter pullback from subclavian artery to aorta. Note gradient and waveform change. (Lower panel) Two central aortic pressures. P1 is in the aorta at the level of the left subclavian origin. Where Is P2? See text for details.

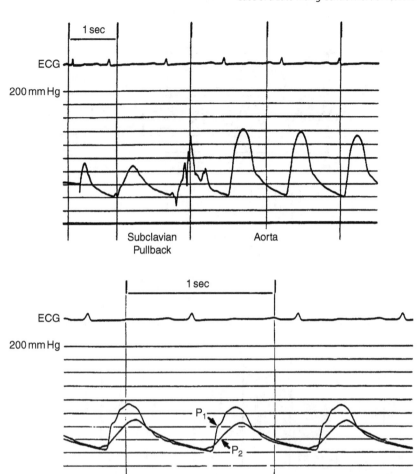

Examine the simultaneous left ventricular and aortic pressures (Figure 1.27, lower panel). Why does left ventricular pressure rise after aortic pressure? The LV pressure is overly damped with a rounded contour. A delay in pressure transmission is caused by an LV catheter kink in crossing the valve that could not be eliminated by vigorous flushing. Pressure overdamping can be caused by inadequate flushing, leaving an air bubble or blood in the line, reducing the fidelity of pressure transmission. This problem may be exaggerated in small-diameter tubes and catheters. Increasing the fluid viscosity with contrast media would also produce the damped and delayed tracing. This artifact was eliminated by changing catheters, in this case to a 7 F or 8 F sheath with a 6 F or 7 F pigtail. A second arterial puncture or the transseptal approach as discussed elsewhere [25] would be an alternative solution. In Figure 1.27 (top panel), why is the central aortic (Ao) pressure different from the femoral pressure (FA)? The presence of peripheral vascular disease creates a gradient measurement between the central aortic pressure measured by a second small pigtail catheter placed in the ascending aorta and the original femoral artery catheter.

Another example of a late rising proximal aortic pressure is shown in Figure 1.32 (lower panel). P1 and P2 are pressure tracings from two fluid-filled catheters located in the thoracic aorta. P1 has a brisk upstroke with an anachrotic shoulder and dichrotic notch. P2 is an earlier rising tracing with a considerably slower upslope and attenuated resonant waveform characteristics. What conditions produced this pattern and from which locations are these pressures obtained? P1 is in the descending aorta below the left subclavian artery origin. P2 is inadvertently just beyond the ostial portion of the left subclavian artery, which had a significant narrowing, producing a 30–40 mm Hg systolic gradient, slow upstroke, and loss of the anachrotic shoulder and dichrotic notch. On pullback from the subclavian artery to the aorta, the systolic gradient and changing waveform are evident (Figure 1.32, upper panel). Subclavian stenosis and coarctation are the two conditions that can cause this pressure with catheters in the central aorta.

In the consideration of aortic coarctation (Figure 1.33A, top panel), one pressure waveform should be delayed with a slightly slower upstroke, but

(a)

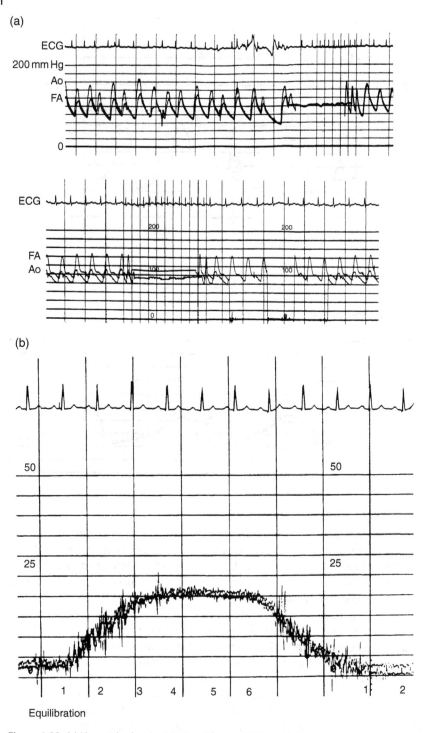

(b)

Equilibration

Figure 1.33 (a) Unmatched central (Ao) and femoral (FA) arterial pressures despite matched zero points. Is this consistant with coarctation? (b) Demonstration of equisensitivity and calibration of three fluid-filled transducers.

this pressure waveform will occur with the most distal pressure (e.g., not with P2 but with P1), since the delay in pulse transmission usually occurs in the aorta below the subclavian takeoff narrowing, not in the subclavian artery as shown on Figure 1.32.

Transducer Disequilibration

Differences in transducer signal response to the same pressure can cause false readings, artifactual gradients, and erroneous clinical decisions. Precision in measurement requires equisensitive amplifier settings and matched transducer gain settings. Matching of peripheral with central aortic pressure to assess the aortic valve gradient requires properly flushed transducers with equisensitive pressure responses. Although most transducers are highly reliable, an occasionally defective product or loose connection may produce a disparity in pressures expected to be equivalent. Examine the femoral artery sheath and central aortic pressures in Figure 1.33a. The pressure differences were not attributable to a loose pressure connection, overdamped or unflushed tubing, or unmatched amplifier settings. The aortic pressure transducer was faulty and subsequently replaced, permitting matching of the pressures similar to that shown in Figure 1.27. One way to quickly check the equisensitivity of pressure transducers is shown in Figure 1.33b. Hold all manifolds (in this example three manifolds are connected to three transducers) at the same level, then raise and lower the manifolds together, observing the equivalency of pressure responses. A separation of one of the transducer tracings indicates a faulty calibration or defective transducer.

Key Points

1) The most common pressure wave artifact of a fluid-filled system is exaggerated "ringing" of underdamping.
2) Recording artifacts such as mislabeled pressure scale and unlabeled time lines can affect data quality.

3) Slow pigtail catheter pullback (leaving side holes in LV) from the left ventricle can falsely reduce aortic diastolic pressure.
4) The most common pressure wave artifact of a fluid-filled system is exaggerated "ringing" of underdamping.
5) Recording artifacts such as mislabeled pressure scale and unlabeled time lines can affect data quality.
6) Slow pigtail catheter pullback (leaving side holes in LV) from the left ventricle can falsely reduce aortic diastolic pressure.
7) A very common mistake in interpretation of hemodynamic data is not recognizing cardiac dysrrhythmias.
8) During clinical examination, the presence of a large V wave in the jugular vein reflects either significant tricuspid regurgitation or functional regurgitation during cardiac arrhythmias.
9) The prominent V wave of tricuspid insufficiency begins early and tends to obliterate the X descent.
10) The left atrial V waves are generally greater than the V waves of right atrial pressure where the A wave predominates.
11) Large, spiked C waves, called cannon waves, are present when atrial contraction falls out of sequence with normal ventricular systole, resulting in atrial contraction against a closed tricuspid valve.
12) In general, the slope of the right atrial pressure during right ventricle ejection is proportional to the severity of tricuspid regurgitation.

References

1 Opie LH and Bers DM. Mechanisms of cardiac contraction and relaxation. In Mann D, Zipes, D, Libby P, Bonow R (eds), *Braunwald's Heart Disease*, 10th ed. Philadelphia, PA: Elsevier Saunders, 2015, pp. 429–453.

2 O'Rourke MF, Hashimoto J. Mechanical factors in arterial aging: A clinical perspective. *J Am Coll Cardiol* 50(1):1–13, 2007.

3 Burkhoff D, Sayer G, Doshi D, Uriel N. Hemodynamics of mechanical circulatory support. *J Am Coll Cardiol* 66:2663–74, 2015.

4 Bertini M, Sengupta PP, Nucifera G, Delgado V, Ng A, Marsan N, Shanks M, Van Bommel R, Schalij MJ, Narula J, Bax JJ. Role of left ventricular twist mechanics in the assessment of cardiac syssynchrony in heart failure. *J Am Coll Cardiol Img* 2:785–956, 2009

5 Kalmanson D, Veyrat C, Chiche P. Atrial versus ventricular contribution in determining systolic venous return: A new approach to an old riddle. *Cardiovasc Res* 5:293, 1971.

6 Harvey W (ed.). *Movement of the Heart and Blood in Animals*. Springfield, IL: Charles C Thomas, 1962.

7 Haddad F, Doyle R, Murphy DJ, Hunt SA. Right ventricular function in cardiovascular disease, Part I. *Circulation* 117:1717–1731, 2008.

8 Kern MJ (ed.) *Hemodynamic Rounds: Interpretation of Pathophysiology from Pressure Waveform Analysis*. New York: Wiley-Liss, 1993, pp. 1–6.

9 Kern MJ, Deligonul U, Donohue T, Caracciolo E, Feldman T. Hemodynamic data. In Kern MJ (ed.), *The Cardiac Catheterization Handbook*, 2nd ed. St. Louis: Mosby–Year Book, 1995, pp. 108–207.

10 Grossman W. Profiles in valvular heart disease. In *Cardiac Catheterization and Angiography*. Philadelphia: Lea & Febiger, 1986, p. 378.

11 Tavel ME. Normal sounds and pulses: Relationships and intervals between the various events. In *Clinical Phonocardiography and External Pulse Recording*,

2nd ed. Chicago, IL: Year Book Medical Publishers, 1972, pp. 35–58.

12 Lingamneni R, Cha SD, Maranhao V, Gooch AS, Goldberg H. Tricuspid regurgitation: Clinical and angiographic assessment. *Cathet Cardiovasc Diagn* 5:7–17, 1979.

13 Mueller O, Shillingford J. Tricuspid incompetence. *Br Heart J* 16:195–204, 1954.

14 Tavel ME (ed.). The jugular pulse tracing: Its clinical application. In *Clinical Phonocardiography and External Pulse Recording*, 2nd ed. Chicago, IL: Year Book Medical Publishers, 1972, pp. 207–226.

15 Morgan BC, Abel FL, Mullins GL, Guntheroth WG. Flow patterns in cavae, pulmonary artery, pulmonary vein and aorta in intact dogs. *Am J Physiol* 210:903–909, 1966.

16 Brecher GA, Hubay CA. Pulmonary blood flow and venous return during spontaneous respiration. *Circ Res* 3:210–214, 1955.

17 Brecher GA, Hubay CA. Pulmonary blood flow and venous return during spontaneous respiration. *Circ Res* 3:210–214, 1955.

18 Willems J, Roelandt J, Kesteloot H. The jugular venous pulse tracing. In *Proceedings of the Fifth European Congress of Cardiology*, September 1968, p. 433.

19 Brecher GA. Cardiac variations in venous return studied with a new bristle flow meter. *Am J Physiol* 176:423–430, 1954.

20 Tyberg JV, Taichman GC, Sith ER, Douglas NWS, Smiseth OA, Keon WJ. The relationship between pericardial pressure and right atrial pressure: An intraoperative study. *Circulation* 73:428–432, 1986.

21 Boltwood CM Jr, Carey JS, Feld G, Shah PM. Pericardial constraint in chronic heart failure. *Am Heart J* 113:847–849, 1987.

22 Kern MJ, Aguirre F, Donohue T. Hemodynamic rounds: Interpretation of cardiac pathophysiology from pressure waveform analysis: Pressure wave artifacts. *Cathet Cardiovasc Diagn* 27:147–154, 1992.

23 Nichols WW, O'Rourke MF. Measuring principles of arterial waves. In Nichols WW, O'Rourke MF, Vlachopoulos C (eds), *McDonald's Blood Flow in Arteries: Theoretical, Experimental and Clinical Practices*, 3rd ed. Philadelphia, PA: Lea & Febiger, 1990, pp. 143–161.

24 Kern MJ. Catheter selection for the stenotic aortic valve. *Cathet Cardiovasc Diagn* 17:190–191, 1989.

25 Kern MI, Deligonul U. Hemodynamic rounds: Interpretation of cardiac pathophysiology from pressure waveform analysis. I. The stenotic aortic valve. *Cathet Cardiovasc Diagn* 21:112–120, 1990.

2

Left Atrial Hemodynamics

Morton J. Kern

The hemodynamic waveforms obtained with pulmonary capillary wedge pressure tracings in the cardiac catheterization laboratory or during monitoring in the intensive care unit are probably among the most important and practical clinical hemodynamic data. These waveforms indicate filling pressure of the left ventricle, function of the mitral valve, and resistance of the pulmonary circuit. Normally, V waves on the pulmonary capillary wedge tracing reflect left atrial filling during ventricular systole and atrial emptying immediately after ventricular systole and ventricular relaxation. The morphology and magnitude of the V wave are determined principally by the pressure–volume relationship of the left atrium. Large V waves may be due to valvular mitral regurgitation or stenosis, or a number of other nonvalvular conditions in which the pressure–volume relationship of the atrial chamber is altered (e.g., high atrial volume due to ventricular septal defect or elevated atrial pressure needed to compensate for decreased ventricular compliance in the setting of diastolic dysfunction) [1, 2, 3]. The accurate interpretation of the V wave has clinical importance in a variety of common circumstances and has been the subject of numerous experimental and clinical studies characterizing factors of relevance.

Normal A and V Wave Patterns

Before discussing abnormal pulmonary capillary wedge waveforms, we should review briefly the normal atrial waveforms (Figure 2.1). The following definitions for atrial or pulmonary capillary wedge waveforms will be used. The A wave is the first positive wave due to contraction of the atria (after the P wave on the electrocardiogram or ECG). The second positive wave appearing on the downslope of the A wave is the C wave, which is due to ventricular contraction. The C wave is not always obvious on the pressure tracing. The third positive wave,

the V wave, is due to atrial filling occurring at the end of ventricular systole. The peak of the V wave usually corresponds to the electrocardiographic T wave. The negative slopes of the A and V waves are termed the X and Y descents. The X descent may be broken into X and X′, divided by the presence of a C wave. The Y descent occurs on the downslope of the V wave. The lowest pressures of the X and Y descents are called troughs, and these points of pressure measurements are thought to be better correlated with left ventricular (LV) end-diastolic pressure under pathologic conditions than is the mean pulmonary capillary wedge pressure [4]. The left ventricular end-diastolic pressure is obtained after atrial contraction, which usually produces a visible deformity of the left ventricular pressure (see Figure 2.1, LV A wave). The left ventricular end-diastolic pressure is measured immediately after the A wave of the LV pressure tracing and corresponds to the peak R wave of the QRS complex on the ECG (on Figure 2.1, follow the ventricular time line at the first R wave down to its crossing point on the LV pressure).

The tracings on Figure 2.1 were obtained in a 59-year-old woman 10 days after an inferior myocardial infarction. The left ventricular pressure A wave (of approximately 22 mm Hg) usually exceeds the pulmonary capillary wedge pressure A waves (of about 18 mm Hg). These particular pulmonary capillary wedge waveforms are elevated, but normal in morphology and timing. The normal delay in pressure transmission from the atria to the pulmonary capillaries of approximately 140 msec is also demonstrated on this tracing (see small arrows on beat #3, Figure 2.1). The peaks of both the A and V waves are similarly delayed. When measured directly, the true left atrial V wave peak, as we will see, should occur within the downslope of the left ventricular tracing. In contrast to the right atrial pressure waves, the left-sided V wave is usually greater than the A wave.

Hemodynamic Rounds: Interpretation of Cardiac Pathophysiology from Pressure Waveform Analysis, Fourth Edition.
Edited by Morton J. Kern, Michael J. Lim, and James A. Goldstein.
© 2018 John Wiley & Sons Ltd. Published 2018 by John Wiley & Sons Ltd.

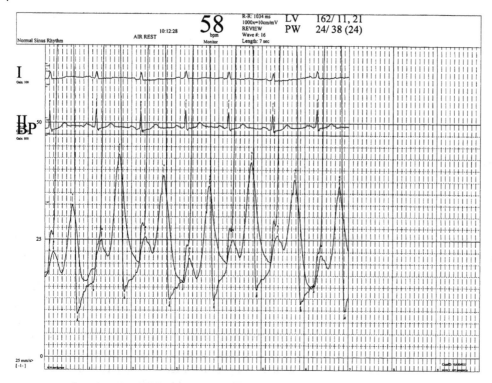

Figure 2.1 Simultaneous left ventricular (LV) and pulmonary capillary wedge (PCW) pressure tracing (0–40 mm Hg scale) in a patient after myocardial infarction.

Correspondence of Pulmonary Capillary Wedge and Left Ventricular End-Diastolic Pressures

The pulmonary capillary wedge pressure is a reliable indicator of left atrial and ventricular end-diastolic pressure in most circumstances. Simultaneous pulmonary capillary wedge pressures (using an 8F balloon-tipped catheter) and left atrial pressure (obtained from the transseptal approach using a Brockenbrough catheter) were measured during assessment of severe aortic stenosis (Figure 2.2). The pulmonary capillary wedge pressure is nearly identical in magnitude and duration to the left atrial pressure. The largest discrepancy between left

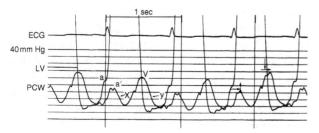

Figure 2.2 Simultaneous left atrial (LA) and pulmonary capillary wedge (PCW) pressures measured with fluid-filled catheters. See text for details (A' and V' are PCW waveforms).

atrial and pulmonary capillary wedge A and V wave pressures is usually ≤ 5 mm Hg [5]. In over 700 cardiac catheterizations, left atrial pressures obtained by transseptal and pulmonary artery diastolic pressures were nearly identical [6]. Simultaneous measurements of left atrial and pulmonary capillary wedge pressures at the time of surgery were also concordant in 90% of cases by < 1 mm Hg difference with a 95% confidence limit for a 2 mm Hg difference between left atrial and pulmonary capillary wedge pressures [5, 6]. The timing delay of the pulmonary capillary wedge pressure relative to left atrial pressure ranges from 140 to 200 msec.

However, the pulmonary capillary wedge pressure may not accurately reflect left ventricular end-diastolic pressure in the presence of obstructive airway disease and conditions altering intrathoracic pressures, such as assisted mechanical ventilation with positive end expiratory pressure [3, 5, 6]. Both the pulmonary capillary wedge and left atrial pressures may be disparate to the left ventricular end-diastolic pressure in patients with low left ventricular compliance (e.g., acute myocardial infarction, hypertension, hypertrophic or congestive cardiomyopathy) or with valvular mitral stenosis or regurgitation, or other conditions in which atrial flow characteristics are highly abnormal [5].

Obtaining an accurate pulmonary capillary wedge pressure may be difficult in patients with pulmonary hypertension, dilated right ventricle, severe tricuspid regurgitation, or anatomic deformations due to acquired (postoperative or calcified cardiac annulus) or congenital anomalies. When using a balloon-tipped catheter, an accurate pulmonary capillary wedge pressure is verified by clear A and V waves, as described above. Confirmation of catheter position by a small 1–2 cc injection of contrast may produce a characteristic angiographic "fern" pattern, but this is an antiquated and time-consuming maneuver. Besides pressure damping, clearing the catheter after this "test" may cause the catheter tip to migrate. Confirming an arterial oxygen saturation (>90%) value from the pulmonary capillary wedge location is difficult with an inflated balloon, since venous blood trapped by the balloon often mixes with oxygenated pulmonary capillary blood. If the pulmonary capillary wedge is in question, obtain a pressure tracing with the balloon deflated. A satisfactory oxygen saturation (>95%) may then be obtained. If this is not possible, consider using a stiff, large-diameter end-holed catheter, such as a Multipurpose, Cournand, or Goodale–Lubin catheter, or perform a transseptal puncture with left atrial cannulation.

A 63-year-old patient with significant mitral regurgitation following mitral commissurtomy eight years earlier underwent hemodynamic study for progressive fatigue. Simultaneous left atrial, pulmonary capillary wedge, and left ventricular pressures were obtained after transseptal catheterization (Figure 2.3). Atrial fibrillation is the underlying rhythm. The differences between left atrial and pulmonary capillary wedge pressure are evident on the upper-left panel of Figure 2.3, showing the higher left atrial pressure and lower pulmonary capillary wedge pressure with its characteristic phase delay and slower V wave downslope. In this patient, use of this pulmonary capillary wedge pressure would have introduced an error with regard to the presence of mitral stenosis. After flushing and rechecking zero levels of the pulmonary capillary wedge tracing (Figure 2.3, lower panel), the severity of the regurgitant valvular lesion can be better appreciated. The upper-right-hand panel of Figure 2.3 shows the left atrial pressure superimposed on the left ventricular pressure. The C and V waves evident on the left atrial pressure (compare with Figure 2.4) are less distinct than seen on the pulmonary capillary wedge pressure. From the shape of the V wave, severe mitral regurgitation would be anticipated. The bottom panel of Figure 2.3 shows the delay in the pulmonary capillary wedge and artifactual gradient of the pulmonary capillary wedge and left ventricular pressures when tracings are used without appropriate phase shifting. In patients with suspected mitral stenosis, a properly obtained and confirmed, time-adjusted pulmonary capillary wedge pressure accurately reflects left atrial pressure. In most cases, transseptal left-heart catheterization to measure

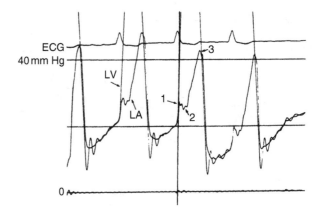

Figure 2.3 Simultaneous left atrial (LA) and left ventricular (LV) pressure tracings (0–40 mm Hg scale) in a patient with new onset of fatigue.

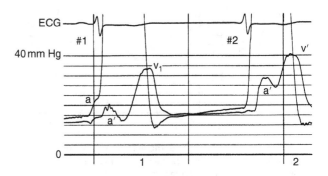

Figure 2.4 Simultaneous left atrial (LA) and left ventricular (LV) pressure tracings (0–40 mm Hg scale) in a patient with a new systolic murmur.

left atrial pressure is not necessary [7]. However, when a diastolic mitral valve gradient is a critical measurement, the left atrial pressure should be measured directly.

In summary, the left-sided V wave is dependent on the left atrial and ventricular pressure–volume filling relationship. The cardiac rhythm and timing of atrial systole also influence the V wave. The morphology of the V wave can reflect the severity of mitral regurgitation with stenosis, but valve areas in this setting may be better assessed by a pressure half-time method.

Factors Influencing the Size of the V Wave

The compliance of the ventricle and atrium is the major determinant of changes in the atrial and ventricular pressure waves. Figure 2.5 illustrates a hypothetical left atrial pressure–volume (P–V) relationship. Four principal factors acting on the P–V relationship influence the morphology of the V wave: (i) the volume of blood entering the atrium during ventricular systole; (ii) the rate of

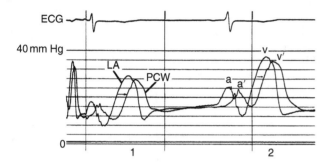

Figure 2.5 Pressure–volume relationship determining the morphology and magnitude of atrial pressure waves.

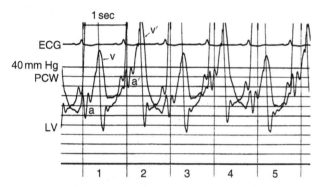

Figure 2.6 Simultaneous left ventricular (LV) and pulmonary capillary wedge (PCW) pressure tracings (0–40 mm Hg scale) in a patient with congestive heart failure.

forward flow into the atrium; (iii) systemic afterload (influencing emptying); and (iv) left ventricular contractile force (affecting left ventricular end-diastolic volume and pressure). In a highly compliant left atrium (such as that occurring with P–V curve B, Figure 2.5), a known increase in volume ("x" ml moving up the curve from points b to c) will produce a small change in pressure (Y$_1$, mm Hg), generating a small V wave. In contrast, when atrial compliance is reduced—that is, the atria become stiffer—a new compliance (P–V) curve is formed. The same volume of blood entering the left atrium on P–V curve A and moving from points b to c will produce a much larger increase in pressure (Y$_2$, mm Hg) and a large V wave. A change in the shape or location of the P–V curve can occur due to alteration in atrial chamber properties (i.e., postoperative or rheumatic inflammation), fluid mechanics (e.g., regurgitation), as well as alteration of atrial or ventricular musculature (e.g., ischemia). In a poorly compliant, stiff left ventricle, which occurs in a patient with a myocardial infarction (Figure 2.6), the atrial contraction and its contribution to left ventricular filling increase left ventricular end-diastolic pressure well above the mean left atrial pressure and pulmonary capillary wedge pressure. In patients with myocardial infarction, the mean pulmonary capillary wedge pressure often correlates better with the pressure before the A wave at

the beginning of atrial systole [8]. Haskell *et al.* [4] indicate that in patients with large left-sided V waves due to mitral regurgitation, the trough of the X descent is the best predictor of left ventricular end-diastolic pressure. In contrast, if the V wave is small, the mean pulmonary capillary wedge pressure or direct left atrial pressure is still the more accurate estimate of left ventricular end-diastolic pressure despite concurrent mitral regurgitation.

The Large V Wave and Mitral Regurgitation

It is known that the height of the V wave does not accurately reflect the degree of mitral regurgitation. Pichard *et al.* [9], Fuchs *et al.* [10], and others [11, 12] have shown that a large V wave in the pulmonary capillary wedge pressure tracings is neither sensitive nor specific for severe mitral regurgitation. The use of the X trough [4], the ratio of the QT to QV interval, and the downslope of the V wave [12] have been proposed as reliable signs of significant mitral regurgitation, but the sensitivity and specificity of these signs remain poor. The size of the V wave is determined by the position on the atrial compliance curve during the filling period rather than the degree of filling that is occurring. Severe mitral regurgitation in a very large and compliant atrium will produce little or no change in atrial pressure and, hence, little or no change in the pulmonary capillary wedge V wave. Giant V waves may be eliminated after changing ventricular afterload with nitroprusside [13]. Conditions other than mitral regurgitation that increase flow or volume in a noncompliant left atrium, such as ventricular septal defect, mitral stenosis, postoperative surgical conditions, or rheumatic alterations of the atrial wall, can produce large V waves without mitral regurgitation. In addition, tachycardia resulting in a shorter diastolic emptying period for the left atrium may also cause large pulmonary capillary wedge V waves.

Contribution of Atrial Systole to Left-Sided V Waves

A 49-year-old woman with combined mitral stenosis and regurgitation underwent right- and left-heart cardiac catheterization prior to consideration of balloon catheter valvuloplasty. Hemodynamic tracings were obtained with fluid-filled catheters in the left ventricular and pulmonary capillary wedge positions (Figure 2.7). Examine the A and V waves of this tracing and explain the "giant" V wave on beat #2. The cardiac rhythm demonstrates a late P wave on beat #2 (seen in the T wave). Late atrial systole markedly increases atrial volume occurring

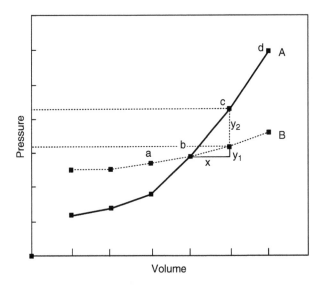

Figure 2.7 Simultaneous pulmonary capillary wedge (PCW) and left ventricular (LV) pressure tracings in a patient with mitral stenosis. Is mitral regurgitation present in this individual?

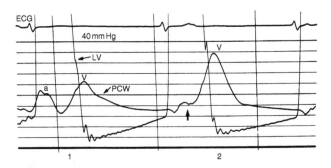

Figure 2.8 Pulmonary capillary wedge (PCW) and left ventricular (LV) pressure tracings in a patient with aortic stenosis; "a" and V wave are denoted on the PCW.

V Wave Morphology

The morphology and, specifically, the downslope of the V wave in Figure 2.7 are also characteristic of mixed mitral stenosis and regurgitation. Compare this V wave downslope to that in Figures 2.1 and 2.6. The downslope of the V wave in the patient with left ventricular failure in Figure 2.6 suggests associated mitral regurgitation. However, quantitation of the severity of regurgitation does not correlate with the V wave downslope. The delayed downslope suggests, but is not directly proportional to the severity (i.e., valve area) of, co-existent mitral stenosis. Use of the pressure half-time method appears to be more predictive of the true valve area in patients with hemodynamic tracings of combined mitral regurgitation and stenosis [14, 15].

A 52-year-old woman had a prosthetic mitral valve implanted four years prior to the recent onset of severe dyspnea and fatigue. A new murmur was appreciated at the clinician's first examination. Because of signs and symptoms of congestive heart failure with a new onset of clinical mitral regurgitation, a complete hemodynamic study was performed. Pulmonary hypertension was present (75/30 mm Hg), but a reliable pulmonary capillary wedge pressure could not be obtained. Because of this difficulty, transseptal catheterization was performed from the right femoral vein. The left atrial pressure was obtained with a Brockenbrough catheter. The left ventricular pressure was obtained with a 7F pigtail catheter (Figure 2.4). Examine the hemodynamic tracing and consider the pressure waves numbered 1, 2, and 3 and assign the A, C, and V designations. As can be seen from the electrocardiogram, the rhythm is atrial fibrillation. There is no atrial activation by P wave on either the electrocardiogram or "a" wave on the left ventricular or left atrial pressure tracings. Therefore, in the absence of any atrial pressure deformity of left ventricular upstroke, waveform #1 is part of waveform #2, the C wave. Waveform #3 is obviously the large, steep V wave characteristic of severe mitral regurgitation. The rapid filling occurs early under the left ventricular pressure wave. Also note that the downslope of the V wave is identical to the left ventricular pressure tracing, indicating no resistance to outflow despite marked regurgitation of blood into the left atrium. As discussed earlier, the timing of the peak of the V wave occurs slightly inside the downslope of the left ventricular pressure tracing, in distinction to the wedge pressure V wave peak occurring with the characteristic delay on or outside the left ventricular pressure (Figures 2.1, 2.7). Compare the downslope of the V wave in this tracing with that of Figure 2.7, in which the downslope of the V wave is markedly delayed due to resistance to outflow from concomitant mitral stenosis. Note also that the left atrial pressure is identical to the diastolic left ventricular

during mid and late ventricular systole. Consider the hemodynamic tracings in Figures 2.2 and 2.8. Both the left atrial (Figure 2.2) and pulmonary capillary wedge pressure (Figure 2.8) A and V waves are large on beat #2 compared to beat #1. As in Figure 2.7, the responsible mechanism for the increase in A and V waves on these tracings is the timing of atrial systole. In Figure 2.2, the astute observer will appreciate the upright P wave on beat #1 compared to beat #2. Beat #2 has an ectopic atrial focus. The late timing of atrial systole increases both the A wave and the V wave. In Figure 2.8, the ectopic and delayed "a" wave on beat #2 did not augment the left ventricular end-diastolic pressure (18 vs. 23 mm Hg). The late atrial systole occurring during the left ventricular systolic period markedly increases the V wave. In this patient without clinical or angiographic mitral regurgitation, the larger V wave does not result from increased regurgitant flow. The augmented atrial volume due to delayed atrial systole produces these large V waves.

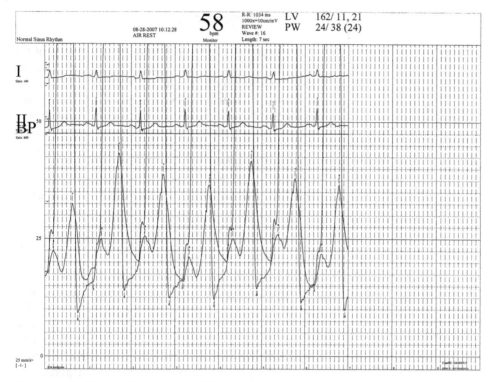

Figure 2.9 Simultaneous left ventricular (LV) and pulmonary capillary wedge (PCW) pressure tracings (0–40 mm Hg scale) in a patient with hypertension.

pressure and is an accurate reflection of left ventricular filling in patients without mitral outflow restriction.

V Wave Alternans

A 69-year-old man was evaluated for advanced congestive heart failure after several prior hospitalizations for atypical chest pain and two remote myocardial infarctions. Right- and left-heart hemodynamics were obtained prior to coronary arteriography (Figure 2.6). The hemodynamic tracings of the left ventricular and pulmonary capillary wedge pressures were obtained with a 7F pigtail catheter and balloon-tipped pulmonary artery catheter through fluid-filled transducers. Consider the following questions: Why are the V waves of different sizes? Where is the pulmonary capillary wedge "a" wave? Does the V wave indicate significant mitral regurgitation or is there some degree of mitral stenosis? Besides an elevated mean pulmonary capillary wedge pressure, what other features of either pressure tracing indicate poor left ventricular function?

On examination of the simultaneous pulmonary capillary wedge and left ventricular pressures, beat #1 shows a left ventricular "a" wave of 28 mm Hg and a pulmonary capillary wedge V wave of 48 mm Hg. On beat #2, the left

ventricular end-diastolic pressure (taken at the end of the A wave) is 34 mm Hg and the corresponding pulmonary capillary wedge V wave exceeds 60 mm Hg. This alternating pattern repeats on beats #3–5. This unusual example of V wave alternans was produced as a function of a failing left ventricle, with pulsus alternans demonstrated in the arterial pressure waveform. As one will see, the function of the left ventricle and its filling pattern (ventricular pressure–volume relationship) have a great influence on V wave generation [3, 16]. Figure 2.9 also shows wave alternans in a patient with left ventricular dysfunction.

Key Points

1) When measured directly, the true left atrial V wave peak should occur within the downslope of the left ventricle tracing.
2) The size of the V wave is determined by the position of the atrial compliance curve during the filling period rather than the degree of the filling that is occurring.
3) A steep V wave downslope (Y descent) suggests the presence of mitral regurgitation, while a delayed V wave downslope suggests the presence of mitral stenosis.

References

1 Kern MJ. Hemodynamic rounds: Interpretation of cardiac pathophysiology from pressure waveform analysis. The left-side V wave. *Cathet Cardiovasc Diagn* 23:211–218, 1991.

2 Connolly DC, Kirklin JW, Wood EH. The relationship between pulmonary artery wedge pressure and left atrial pressure in man. *Circ Res* 2:434–440, 1954.

3 Shaffer AB, Silber EN. Factors influencing the character of the pulmonary arterial wedge pressure. *Am Heart J* 51: 522–532, 1956.

4 Haskell R, French WJ. Accuracy of left atrial and pulmonary artery wedge pressure in pure mitral regurgitation in predicting left ventricular end-diastolic pressure. *Am J Cardiology* 61:136–141, 1988.

5 Lappas D, Lell WA, Gabel JC, Civetta JM, Lowenstein E. Indirect measurement of left atrial pressure in surgical patients: Pulmonary capillary wedge and pulmonary artery diastolic pressures compared with left atrial pressures. *Anesthesiology* 38: 394–397, 1973.

6 Walston A, Kendall ME. Comparison of pulmonary wedge and left atrial pressure in man. *Am Heart J* 86:159–164, 1973.

7 Lange RA, Moore DM Jr, Cigarroa RG, Hillis LD. Use of pulmonary capillary wedge pressure to assess severity of mitral stenosis: Is true left atrial pressure needed in this condition? *J Am Coll Cardiol* 13: 825–829, 1989.

8 Rahimtoola SH, Loeb HS, Ehwani A, Sinno M, Chuquimia R, Lal R, Rosen KM, Gummar RM. Relationship of pulmonary artery to left ventricular diastolic pressures in acute myocardial infarction. *Circulation* 46:283–290, 1972.

9 Pichard AD, Kay R, Smith H, Rentrop P, Holt J, Gorlin R. Large V waves in the pulmonary wedge pressure tracing in the absence of mitral regurgitation. *Am J Cardiol* 50:1044–1050, 1982.

10 Fuchs RM, Henser RR, Yin FCP, Brinker JA. Limitations of pulmonary wedge V waves in diagnosing mitral regurgitation. *Am J Cardiol* 49:849–854, 1982.

11 Braunwald E, Awe WC. The syndrome of severe mitral regurgitation with normal left atrial pressure. *Circulation* 27:29–35, 1963.

12 Schwinger M, Cohen M, Fuster V. Usefulness of onset of the pulmonary wedge V wave in predicting mitral regurgitation. *Am J Cardiol* 62:646–648, 1988.

13 Harshaw CW, Murro AB, McLaurin LP, Grossman W. Reduced systemic vascular resistance as therapy for severe mitral regurgitation of valvular origin. *Ann Intern Med* 83:312, 1975.

14 Libanoff AJ, Rodbard S. Evaluation of the severity of mitral stenosis and regurgitation. *Circulation* 33:281–320, 1966.

15 Fredman C, Pearson AC, Labovitz N, Kern MJ. Comparison of hemodynamic pressure half-time method and Gorlin formula to Doppler and echocardiographic determinations of mitral valve area in patients with combined mitral stenosis and regurgitation. *Am Heart J* 119:121–129, 1990.

16 Yu PN, Murphy OW, Schreiner BF Jr, James DH. Distensibility characteristics of the human pulmonary vascular bed: Study of the pressure/volume response to exercise in patients with and without heart disease. *Circulation* 35:710–723, 1967.

3

Left Ventricular End-Diastolic Pressure (LVEDP)

Morton J. Kern

The end-diastolic filling pressure is often indicative of the hemodynamic health of the ventricle. The left ventricular pressure is available for examination in nearly every catheterization. In some patients undergoing diagnostic angiography, it was thought that right-heart catheterization would add important data, especially regarding the left ventricular filling and pulmonary artery pressures. Right-heart catheterization and measurement of the pulmonary capillary wedge pressure in most patients with coronary artery disease have been replaced by examining the left ventricular end-diastolic pressure (LVEDP) before contrast ventriculography. However, at times even this straightforward-appearing pressure wave can be misinterpreted. Although it is well known and taught that the LVEDP is measured after the A wave at the onset of left ventricular isovolumetric contraction coincident with the R wave, the identification of the true LVEDP may be difficult.

Examine the left ventricular pressure tracing in Figure 3.1 (provided by Dr. G. Alfred Dodds III, Medical College of Ohio, Toledo, Ohio). The LVEDP was recorded in a 43-year-old woman with exertional chest pain and multiple risk factors for coronary artery disease. The tracing demonstrates several different inflection points of the A wave. Note the changing LVEDP of 20 mm Hg (beat #2) with an LVEDP of 42 mm Hg (beats #3–5). On beats #8 and 9, the LVEDP is again at or below 20 mm Hg. What is the true LVEDP and why is this value changing? A multiple-holed catheter (pigtail) may move across the aortic valve and cause the LVEDP to be artifactually higher. With minor differences in positioning over the respiratory cycle, it appears that the pigtail catheter is moving slightly out of the ventricle with one or two of the side holes at the aortic valve (the average pigtail catheter tip is 3 cm in diameter with three side holes). This artifact can be detected by the pressure waveform and identification of the lowest left ventricular pressure at the initiation of diastole. Note in beat #2 that the minimal

diastolic pressure is 10 mm Hg and that in beats #3 and 4 the minimal diastolic pressure is higher, occurring at mid-diastole and not at the initiation of the diastolic period. Also, the initial downstroke of left ventricular pressure is delayed further (beat #3), suggesting aortic pressure contamination, which can sometimes occur when side holes of the catheter have moved out of the left ventricle. Thus, stability of the catheter and acquisition of a reliable pressure wave are required for accurate interpretation of the LVEDP.

LVEDP: Clues to Unsuspected Conditions

In the routine examination of the left ventricular pressure tracing in Figure 3.1, the diastolic waveform, when examined carefully, provided a clue to the error of an abnormally high LVEDP. Myocardial relaxation abnormalities may be suggested by observing the trend of pressure during diastasis. Consider the left ventricular pressure measured in a 42-year-old patient with atypical chest pain syndrome and hypertension (Figure 3.2). Nitroglycerin was given prior to left ventriculography. Note the low LVEDP with a continuing decline of pressure over the mid-diastolic period, with the pressure nadir occurring 50% of the way through the diastolic period. This waveform pattern suggests impaired myocardial relaxation. This patient was found to have severe left ventricular hypertrophy, and an evaluation for an unsuspected obstructive cardiomyopathy was then performed. No inducible intraventricular pressure gradient was demonstrated. In a similar case in another patient (Figure 3.3) without hypertension, the LVEDP waveform was abnormal, with impairment of left ventricular relaxation as described in the previous patient. A Valsalva maneuver with induction of premature ventricular contractions was performed and demonstrated several beats

Hemodynamic Rounds: Interpretation of Cardiac Pathophysiology from Pressure Waveform Analysis, Fourth Edition.
Edited by Morton J. Kern, Michael J. Lim, and James A. Goldstein.

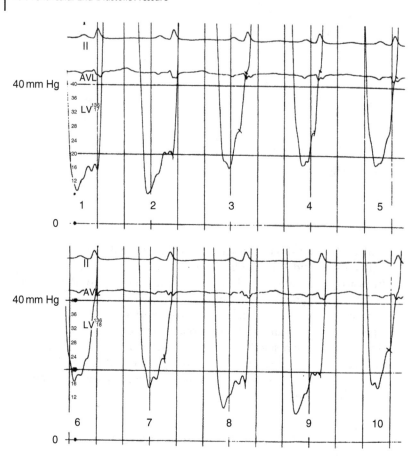

Figure 3.1 Left ventricular pressure (0–40 mm Hg scale). Electrocardiogram (leads II and AVL) are shown at the top of the tracings. *Source:* Kern 1998 [1]. Reproduced with permission of John Wiley & Sons.

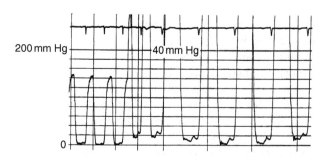

Figure 3.2 Left ventricular pressure (0–200 mm Hg and 0–40 mm Hg scales), demonstrating an abnormal left ventricular diastolic pressure waveform.

in which an intraventricular gradient could be produced (Figure 3.3, bottom). The diagnosis of hypertrophic myopathy with a nonobstructive classification at rest and provocable interventricular gradient during Valsalva and premature ventricular contractions was made, and beta blockers were recommended. Had the abnormal left ventricular pressure waveform not been appreciated, this diagnosis would not have been entertained, identified, or treated.

Insights into the diagnosis of left ventricular dysfunction may be appreciated by examination of simultaneously displayed left and right ventricular pressure waveforms. Abnormalities of ventricular contraction

and relaxation, ventricular conduction abnormalities, and restrictive/constrictive pathophysiologic states are often evident. A collection of simultaneously measured left and right ventricular pressures (Figure 3.4) denotes hemodynamic clues to different common clinical problems. What can one deduce from this collection of waveforms?

In Figure 3.4 (top middle), the LVEDP is 16 mm Hg, and there is a premature atrial contraction (beat #1) which has near-normal filling without apparent influence on right ventricular hemodynamic pressure. Left ventricular relaxation is impaired, which is apparent from the abnormal slope of the LV diastolic pressure. The patient has elevation of right ventricular pressure and pulmonary hypertension. He is being evaluated for congestive heart failure and chronic mitral regurgitation.

In Figure 3.4 (top right), the simultaneous pressure waveforms from the left and right ventricles were obtained in a patient who has exacerbation of known severe congestive heart failure. Note the LVEDP of approximately 35 mm Hg, varying from 30–40 mm Hg over the four beats demonstrated. The extreme elevation of both the minimal diastolic and LVEDP and the high right ventricular systolic and end-diastolic pressures indicates the critical decompensation. In addition, the upslope of contraction is delayed, consistent with severe

Figure 3.3 Left ventricular and aortic pressures obtained before (top) and during (bottom) Valsalva maneuver with stimulation of ventricular premature contractions (PVC). Note the intraventricular gradient during peak Valsalva with PVC (bottom middle).

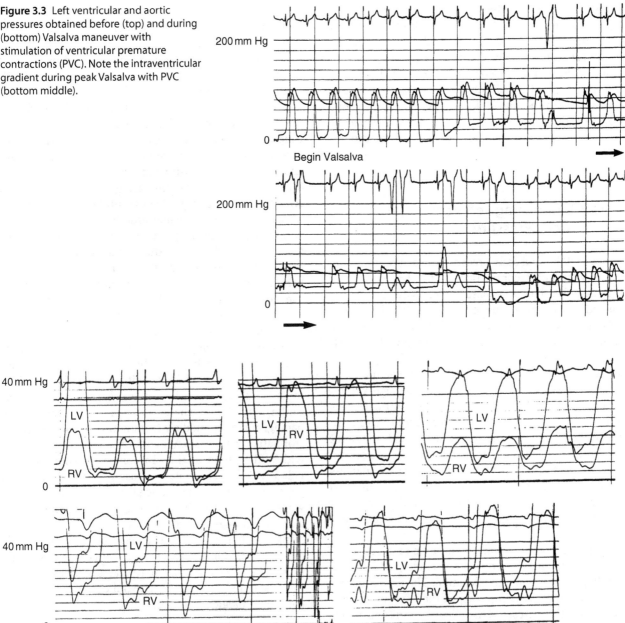

Figure 3.4 Simultaneously recorded left ventricular (LV) and right ventricular (RV) pressures obtained with fluid-filled catheters in a series of patients with cardiovascular abnormalities. (Top left) Patient with low filling pressures. (Top middle and right) Two patients with high end-diastolic pressures. (Bottom left and right) Two patients with conduction abnormalities. Scale is 0–40 mm Hg except at the top right, which is 0–100 mm Hg.

global left ventricular dysfunction (ejection fraction < 20%). Deterioration of this patient's left ventricular function secondary to ischemic cardiomyopathy was confirmed by ventriculography.

Abnormalities of cardiac rhythm can produce marked distortions in the timing relationship between left ventricular and right ventricular pressures. Note the left and right ventricular end-diastolic pressures in a patient with an abnormal rhythm (Figure 3.4, lower left). The LVEDP is 32 mm Hg. Right ventricular end-diastolic pressure is above 22 mm Hg. There is an endocardial pacemaker rhythm that delays and skews the relaxation period of left ventricular pressure, resulting in overlapping of the left ventricular pressure downslope with that of the right ventricular pressure. The unusual alignment of diastolic pressures in this case would provide an additional clue to conduction abnormalities, if these were not evident already from the coincident electrocardiographic tracings. The high filling pressures were due to nonischemic cardiomyopathy.

Similar findings can be observed in a patient with a left-bundle branch block (Figure 3.4, bottom right) in which the LVEDP is 28 mm Hg with a rapid upslope greatly exceeding that of the right ventricular pressure upslope. The compliance of the left ventricle (estimated from the slope of the diastolic filling pressure) can be compared with the rather slow filling rate (higher compliance) of the right ventricle. This patient had hypertensive congestive heart failure with mild pulmonary hypertension.

Factors Influencing Left Ventricular End-Diastolic Pressure

The LVEDP immediately precedes the beginning of isometric ventricular contraction in the left ventricular pressure pulse. This point, also known as the "Z" point, is situated on the downslope of the left ventricular A wave and marks the crossing over of the left atrial and left ventricular pressures. The LVEDP is normally < 12 mm Hg and may be elevated when the left ventricle experiences excessive diastolic volume overload in conditions of mitral or aortic valvular regurgitation or high-volume shunting (left to right) at or distal to the ventricular septum. Impairment of myocardial contractility alters the diastolic pressure–volume relationship and shifts the end-diastolic pressure point upward. Conditions of concentric hypertrophy due to hypertension or valvular stenosis, restrictive or infiltrative cardiomyopathy, or other diseases of the ventricular muscle produce a stiffer chamber and thus alter the pressure–volume curve, elevating the LVEDP.

The interpretation of the LV diastolic pressure waveform has contributed to our understanding of ventricular filling contraction and relaxation. The pressure wave is a reflection of the compliance of the left ventricle and thus indirectly represents the clinical conditions which affect ventricular performance. Clinical studies of hypertrophic cardiomyopathy often emphasize the characteristics of the intraventricular gradient. Echocardiographic information demonstrated that hypertrophic myopathies also have abnormal diastolic function, with prolonged left ventricular isovolumetric relaxation phases and impaired diastolic filling. The patients reviewed in Figure 3.2 and some of the patients in Figure 3.4 have the LV pattern of abnormal ventricular relaxation. The earliest report of improved diastolic function and systolic performance in patients with hypertrophic myopathy after calcium blocker was by Lorell et al. [2] and indicated that nonobstructive hypertrophic cardiomyopathy was responsive to calcium-channel blockers to produce substantial hemodynamic and clinical improvements, with amelioration of the abnormal left ventricular diastolic pressure curve.

Left ventricular function can be assessed by changes in the LVEDP due to the relationship coupling LVEDP to the existing stroke work for that particular pressure. The curvilinear relationship between stroke work and LVEDP has commonly been called the left ventricular function curve and is a measure of the performance of ventricular activity. The ventricular function curves are shifted upward by positive inotropic interventions and downward by those impairing inotropic activity. Afterload also may significantly influence the elevation or decline of the ventricular function curve. Ventricular compliance is the major determinant of the LVEDP. Compliance is defined as the change in volume divided by the change in pressure. Both ventricular volume and pressure must be measured simultaneously to compute the compliance value. The slope of the compliance curve is called stiffness, which is the inverse of compliance. Compliance tends to decrease in chronic conditions involving myocardial hypertrophy, restrictive cardiomyopathy, or other infiltrative processes. The LVEDP can be changed with provocations such as myocardial ischemia. Parker et al. [3] reported their findings on LVEDP changes at rest, during rapid atrial pacing, and on immediate termination of pacing in control patients and patients with coronary artery disease with and without angina. In contrast to normal individuals, left ventricular pressure was elevated in patients with pacing-induced myocardial ischemia, whereas patients without pacing-induced ischemia had a smaller change in LVEDP.

Information about ventricular function, especially diastolic function, can be gleaned from careful examination of the LVEDP waveform. Artifacts of pressure waveforms should be identified to avoid confusion with true pathophysiologic responses.

Key Points

1) The end-diastolic filling pressure (e.g., LVEDP approximately 12 or < 12 mm Hg) is a good tool to assess the hemodynamic health of the ventricle.
2) Myocardial relaxation abnormalities may be suggested by observing the slope of the ventricle pressure during diastole.
3) Elevation of the minimal diastolic pressure and LVEDP along with delay in the upslope of the LV contraction are hemodynamic findings consistent of ventricular diastolic dysfunction.

References

1 Kern MJ. The LVEDP. *Cathet Cardiovasc Diagn* 44:70–74, 1998.

2 Lorell BH, Paulus WJ, Grossman W, Wynne J, Cohn PF, Braunwald E. Improved diastolic function and systolic performance in hypertrophic cardiomyopathy after nifedipine. *N Engl J Med* 303:801–803, 1985.

3 Parker JO, Ledwich JR, West RO, Case RB. Reversible cardiac failure during angina pectoris: Hemodynamic effects of atrial pacing in coronary artery disease. *Circulation* 39:745–757, 1969.

4

Left and Right Ventricular Pressure: Interactions and Influencing Factors

Morton J. Kern

The physiology of ventricular pressure generation is more complicated than simple ventricular contraction and ejection [1–6]. The spiral arrangement of the layers surrounding and forming the thicker muscular left ventricle covered by the thinner right ventricle makes contraction a wiring out movement more than a simple inward movement. The result is that complex vortices are generated as the ventricular chamber shortens and thickens, ejecting their contents into the great vessels.

Ventricular interaction coupled with septal contractile mechanisms plays a major role in the appearance of individual ventricular pressure waveforms. Moreover, differences in compliance between the two ventricles and the timing of activation (conduction) produce interesting hemodynamic records which are reflections of the myocardial diseases affecting one side more than the other. In many cardiac catheterization laboratories, simultaneous measurements of right (RV) and left ventricular (LV) pressures are only performed to evaluate uncommon explanations for cardiac dysfunction, such as constrictive pericardial disease or restrictive cardiomyopathies. Rarely do cardiologists review simultaneous right and left ventricular pressures during routine hemodynamic studies.

As part of many training programs, a comparison of simultaneous right and left ventricular pressures during combined complete hemodynamic studies is routinely performed. The waveforms of constrictive and restrictive physiology are described elsewhere [7]. The characteristic configuration and significance of the diastolic ventricular pressure tracings in such patients will be reviewed here.

Hemodynamic Measurement Technique

Simultaneous right and left ventricular pressures are easily measured during pullback of the balloon-tipped catheter from the pulmonary artery to the right ventricle while a ventriculography (pigtail) catheter remains within the left ventricle. Standard fluid-filled transducers and tubing provide satisfactory pressure waves, which are recorded at a fast (50–100 mm/sec) speed. Although fluid-filled systems provide clinically useful hemodynamic tracing, high-fidelity micromanometer-tipped catheters (or high-fidelity pressure sensor guidewires) are needed to identify small pressure differences or quantitative contraction/relaxation (e.g., dP/dt) data used for research studies.

Right and Left Ventricular Pressures in a Patient with Hypertension

A 65-year-old man with hypertension had routine diagnostic study for dyspnea and atypical chest pain. Cardiac catheterization was performed from the femoral approach as described earlier [8]. Right-heart hemodynamics revealed a mean right atrial pressure of 8 mm Hg, right ventricular pressure of 65/12 mm Hg, mean pulmonary capillary wedge pressure of 20 mm Hg, and pulmonary artery pressure of 65/22 mm Hg. Left ventricular pressure was 162/26 mm Hg. Cardiac output and oxygen saturations were within normal limits. The simultaneous right and left ventricular pressure tracings are shown on Figure 4.1. In assessing the ventricular pressures, examine four features: (i) the A waves; (ii) the rates of systolic pressure rise; (iii) the position of the right ventricular pressure within the left ventricular tracing; and (iv) the rate of diastolic pressure decline and mid-diastolic upslope. Recall that these pressures were obtained immediately prior to left ventriculography, which demonstrated global hypokinesis and moderate mitral regurgitation. Mild, noncritical coronary artery narrowings were also present. The left ventricular compliance is reflected by both the height of the A wave and the diastolic upslope. Note that both findings are lower in the right ventricle compared

Hemodynamic Rounds: Interpretation of Cardiac Pathophysiology from Pressure Waveform Analysis, Fourth Edition.
Edited by Morton J. Kern, Michael J. Lim, and James A. Goldstein.

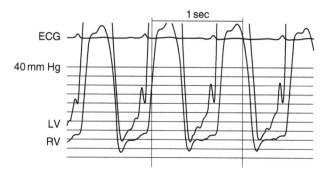

Figure 4.1 Simultaneous right (RV) and left ventricular (LV) pressures in a patient with hypertension.

with the left. The left ventricular diastolic pressure has a steep upsloping diastolic filling period. The A wave is also pronounced. The right ventricular pressure tracing is contained (that is, the upstroke and downstroke occur) equally spaced within the left ventricular pressure waveform. This normal pattern is seen with patients who have normal electrocardiographic conduction and generally normal biventricular function. Despite pulmonary hypertension, the normal diastolic pressure upslope and diminutive A wave suggest that right ventricular compliance is nearly normal.

Effects of Conduction on Right and Left Ventricular Pressures

Examine the tracings in a 77-year-old woman with a prior history of myocardial infarction (Figure 4.2). Normal left-heart hemodynamic values and cardiac output were reported. Right-heart catheterization revealed mild pulmonary stenosis. Note the shift of the right ventricular upstroke to the left earlier under the left ventricular pressure upstroke. The entire right ventricular curve shifted leftward, with an earlier pressure decline shown by the wider-spaced RV–LV downslope tracings during the isovolumetric relaxation period (two arrows). This shift is attributed to a delay in intraventricular

conduction and pressure generation. The QRS complex is consistent with left bundle branch block [9, 10]. The review of the A waves, diastolic upstroke, and rates of pressure rises reveals normal values with low right and left ventricular end-diastolic pressures. Of special interest are the similar observations of Dr. Wiggers over half a century ago using first-generation electromechanical pressure manometers [10]. Wiggers also examined the effects of premature systoles and the subsequent temporary alteration of simultaneous left and right ventricular pressures [10] (Figure 4.3). The precedence of the left over right ventricular contraction force (systole) was noted in a premature beat and that an alteration of systolic pressures of the subsequent beats affected both ventricles (Figure 4.3). Similar findings have been observed more recently with high-fidelity micromanometer-tipped transducers to identify the precise timing, force of contraction, and differences in contractile function between the two ventricles [9].

Compare the positioning of the right ventricular pressure of the middle beat (arrow) of Figure 4.4. Right and left ventricular pressures were obtained during a routine catheterization. The electrocardiogram was normal, but the downstroke of the right ventricular pressure overlies that of the left ventricle on several beats (arrows). Why? This pattern was only intermittently present and was a catheter tip artifact. When the tip of the catheter is occluded by the septal wall, the pressure pattern falls directly with left ventricular pressure. The subsequent beats have a normal spacing of the right ventricle pressure upstroke within the left ventricular pressure tracing and a normal spacing during early diastolic relaxation. These tracings are otherwise remarkable for findings of poor left ventricular compliance (large A wave, high minimum diastolic pressure and diastolic upstroke) and the strikingly low right ventricular filling pattern (negative overshoot in early diastole, small A wave, flat diastolic slope).

Another example of conduction delay on the pressure waveforms was found in a 63-year-old woman with recent chest pain and electrocardiographic findings of

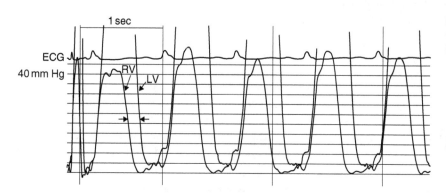

Figure 4.2 Simultaneous right (RV) and left ventricular (LV) pressures in a patient with an intraventricular conduction defect.

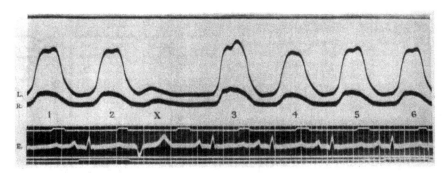

Figure 4.3 Original hemodynamic recordings by Dr. Wiggers of simultaneous right and left ventricular pressures in a dog, showing the effect of a premature systole and subsequent temporary alternation on left and right ventricular pressure curves. Observe the precedence of left over right ventricular contraction in premature beat. The alternation affects both ventricles. L = left ventricle; R = right ventricle; E = electrocardiogram, lead II. 1 and 2, normal beats; X premature ventricular systole of left ventricle; 3–4 and 5–6, alternans couples. *Source:* Wiggers 2005 [10]. Reproduced with permission of John Wiley & Sons.

Figure 4.4 Simultaneous right (RV) and left ventricular (LV) pressures in a patient without an intraventricular conduction defect. Why is pressure overlapping at the arrow?

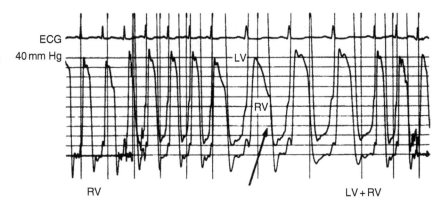

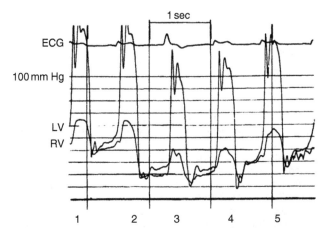

Figure 4.5 Simultaneous right (RV) and left ventricular (LV) pressures in a patient with Intraventricular conduction defect.

acute myocardial infarction. Intermittent hypotension and Wenckebach arrhythmia were noted during the procedure. In the catheterization laboratory, mean right atrial pressure was 25 mm Hg and mean pulmonary capillary wedge pressure was 22 mm Hg. The simultaneous right and left ventricular pressures are shown on Figure 4.5.

An interventricular conduction delay (with ST segment elevation) is associated with a displaced right ventricular pressure downstroke later in the cycle toward the left ventricular pressure diastole on beats #1, 2, 4, and 5.

The interventricular conduction delay of a right bundle branch block pattern has normal early septal excitation contraction of the left ventricle with 40–100 msec delay in right ventricular excitation. From these tracings, why does beat #3 have an early right ventricular upstroke? What is the clinical diagnosis? An acute inferior myocardial infarction with right ventricular involvement is responsible for elevation and near equilibration of diastolic pressures, especially evident on beat #5. The compliance of the ventricles is obscured by the constrictive/restrictive diastolic dip and plateau patterns. Right and left ventricular filling pressures in this patient are elevated due to recent RV infarction. When examining patients with abnormal right ventricular pressures, the concordance (matching) of diastolic waveforms should be placed in the clinical context. Low but matched diastolic pressures may separate after rapid volume administration, indicating normal function, whereas in restrictive myopathy, the diastolic pressure concordance may persist [5]. Beat #3 is a fusion beat with normalized conduction (note the P and T waves). The right ventricular pressure on this beat is different, with the upstroke and downstroke occurring earlier inside the left ventricular pressure.

Pacemaker Pressure Responses

Ventricular pacemaker activation and left bundle branch block may also produce unusual patterns of right and left ventricular pressure waves. Simultaneous right and left ventricular pressures were obtained in an elderly patient with congestive heart failure and a permanent pacemaker undergoing right- and left-heart catheterization (Figure 4.6). The compliance of both ventricles was thought to be similar, with absent "a" waves (due to ventricular pacing) and a normal diastolic upslope. A delayed rate of pressure rise and delayed relaxation of the right ventricular pressure waveform can be seen, with the later part of the right ventricular pressure (arrow) falling outside the left ventricular pressure curve. This abnormal

pattern can be attributed, in part, to the pacemaker rhythm. In addition, the slow upstroke reflects abnormal right ventricular systolic function. Note that the right ventricular pressure is 72/20 mm Hg. A delay of the right ventricular pressure rise could be caused by damping within the right ventricular catheter, but the resonant frequency of the pressure responses seems to be within the normal range (consider the sinusoidal variations during the peak systolic and early diastolic periods). This unusual timing relationship of right and left ventricular pressures is a result of left bundle branch block and a pacemaker in a patient with ventricular dysfunction. In patients with left bundle branch block (Figure 4.7), maximal right ventricular contraction (dP/dt) usually precedes maximal left ventricular contraction, suggesting that the abnormal ventricular activation of the pacemaker has an important action on right and left ventricular function.

First-degree AV block conduction abnormalities can also be reflected in the hemodynamic pressure tracings of both ventricles. The atrial contraction is easily

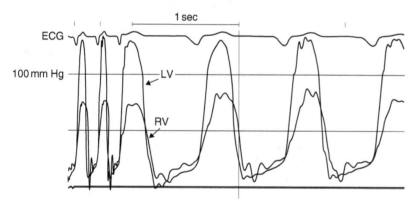

Figure 4.6 Simultaneous right (RV) and left ventricular (LV) pressures in a patient with a permanent pacemaker.

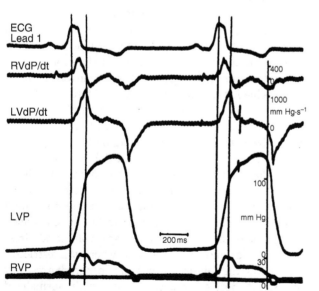

Figure 4.7 Simultaneous right (RV) and left ventricular (LV) pressures and dP/dt recorded from a subject with left bundle branch block. The small right ventricular dP/dt peak precedes the onset of the rise of left ventricular dP/dt, which is delayed. A secondary rapid rise of right ventricular dP/dt occurs after the onset of left ventricular dP/dt and is followed by an unusually slow decline. This pattern reflects the contractile function and interaction between the ventricular chambers. *Source:* Feneley 1985 [9]. Reproduced with permission of Wolters Kluwer Health, Inc.

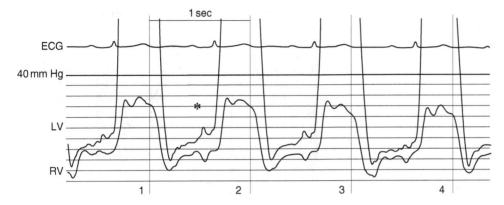

Figure 4.8 Simultaneous right (RV) and left ventricular (LV) pressures in a patient with first-degree atrioventricular block. * = P wave.

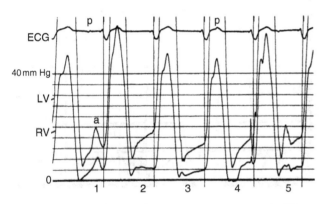

Figure 4.9 Simultaneous right (RV) and left ventricular (LV) pressures in a patient with a pacemaker rhythm.

discernable on simultaneous right and left ventricular pressures in a patient with first-degree block (Figure 4.8). The atrial pressure wave of beat #2 shows up as a positive deflection in the left ventricular pressure, but as a small negative deflection in the right ventricular pressure wave. The right ventricular pressure in this patient is normally located within the left ventricular pressure outline. The explanation for a negative P wave in this tracing is unknown. Compare the A waves in this patient to those in Figure 4.9 with a pacemaker rhythm. The right and left ventricular pressures show striking A waves (beat #1) when P waves occur in normal sequence to ventricular activation. The ventricular pressures also show the contribution of atrial filling by augmented systolic pressure. On beat #2, no "a" waves are seen and differences in diastolic filling slopes are indicative of compliance differences between the two ventricles. As P wave activity occurs again, first on the T wave (beat #4) and then after the T wave (beat #5), the atrial contribution to ventricular pressures can be easily appreciated. The effect of pacing on the timing of right and left ventricular pressure patterns in this patient was minimal.

Ventricular Pressures in a Patient with Mitral Stenosis

Mitral or pulmonary valvular lesions may be associated with markedly different ventricular chamber compliance. Differences in ventricular pressures may become apparent during cardiac arrhythmias with varying RR cycles. Consider the hemodynamic tracings obtained in a 42-year-old woman with mitral stenosis. Simultaneous right- and left-heart pressures (Figure 4.10) demonstrate hemodynamic findings typical of atrial fibrillation. Diastolic filling rates (slopes) differ between ventricles during long pauses (beat #3). The left ventricular diastolic pressure has no "a" wave and a more rapid upstroke compared to the right ventricular pressure tracing, which shows a long plateau before ventricular ejection. On beat #3, filling of the right ventricle appears to be completed by early diastole, whereas filling of the left ventricle continues throughout the cycle because of high left atrial pressure. This pattern also reflects differences in chamber compliance, as well as the influence of a long

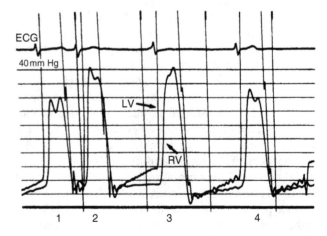

Figure 4.10 Simultaneous right (RV) and left ventricular (LV) pressures in a patient with mitral stenosis.

RR cycle [11]. The flat right ventricular diastolic filling period of beat #3 is affected by respiratory activity on subsequent beats.

Pulsus Alternans

Pulsus alternans [12], first described by Traube in 1872, is the regular alternation of strong and weak cardiac contractions in the absence of respiratory or cycle length variation [13, 14]. It is detected by palpation of a peripheral artery or by sphygmomanometry with a regular alteration of the intensity of the Korotkoff sounds. Total alternans occurs when the left ventricular systolic pressure is less than aortic pressure on alternate beats, so that the aortic valve does not open, with apparent halving of the pulse rate. Pulsus alternans is usually found in patients with severe myocardial disease due to aortic stenosis, systemic arterial hypertension, cardiomyopathy, or coronary heart disease [15]. It has, however, been described in patients with normal hearts for brief periods during or after supraventricular tachycardia.

Pulsus alternans may also be transiently induced by premature ventricular contractions [16], orthostatic factors [17], rapid atrial pacing [18], inferior vena caval occlusion [19], as well as myocardial ischemia [20]. Intracoronary contrast injection during angiography in a patient with hypertensive cardiomyopathy has also been reported to attenuate pulsus alternans [21].

A 52-year-old male was admitted with dyspnea. Shortly after admission, the patient had a respiratory and cardiac arrest and was successfully resuscitated. After two weeks of convalescing, palpation of the peripheral pulses revealed reduced amplitude with every other beat. Jugular veins were 5 cm at 30°. Lungs were clear. In the sixth intercostal space along the anterior axillary line, the apical impulse was enlarged and associated with a soft S3 gallop.

Cardiac catheterization showed significant (>80%) lesions in both the left anterior descending and right coronary arteries. Left ventriculography demonstrated an enlarged chamber with a calculated left ventricular ejection fraction (by area length method) of 16%.

The systolic aortic and left ventricular pressures (Figure 4.11) demonstrated a consistent alternating pattern with a reduced pressure every other beat of approximately 20 mm Hg. Interestingly, the left ventricular waveform on the "weak" beats differs by its reduced peak and time to peak pressure, as well as a subtle alteration of the rapid phase of relaxation. A similar alteration in peak systolic pressure is also noted on every other beat in the right ventricular and pulmonary artery tracings (Figure 4.12). Pulmonary and left ventricular diastolic pressures are significantly elevated, consistent with

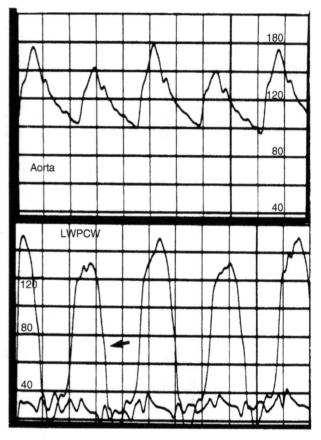

Figure 4.11 Aortic and left ventricular (LV) pressure tracings demonstrate mechanical alternans with peak systolic pressure reduced to 20 mm Hg every other contraction. The left ventricular relaxation pattern of weak beats shows a subtle delay and an altered waveform (arrow). Of note is that the pulmonary capillary wedge (PCW) tracing does not significantly vary during this recording. See text for details.

biventricular dysfunction. The time to peak systolic pressure is also prolonged in the weaker beats of right-sided pressures, consistent with the hypothesized mechanism of alternating diminished contractility. Right ventricular pulsus alternans may occur independently, concordantly or discordantly with left ventricular alternans [22, 23]. Atrial alternans has also been described [24].

This patient demonstrated pulsus alternans by both clinical and hemodynamic criteria. Physical findings associated with pulsus alternans included alternating intensity of heart sounds and an S3 gallop. Pulsus alternans may be augmented by maneuvers which decrease venous return, such as head tilting, standing, or administration of nitroglycerin.

Pulsus alternans must be differentiated from conditions with similar physical examination characteristics. Pulsus bigeminus occurs when the cardiac rhythm is bigeminal, with either atrial or ventricular pairing and with the premature beats having decreased stroke

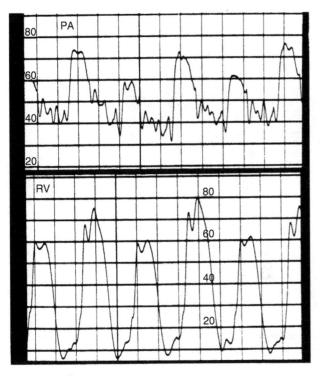

Figure 4.12 Pulmonary artery (PA) and right ventricular (RV) pressure tracings demonstrate mechanical alternans occurring in a similar fashion to the left ventricular hemodynamics of Figure 4.11.

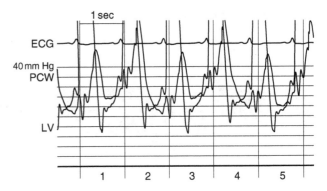

Figure 4.13 Left ventricular (LV) and pulmonary capillary wedge (PCW) pressure tracings in a patient with large A and V waves of alternating magnitude. See text for details.

volume and systolic peak pressure. Pulsus paradoxus is the decrease in pulse amplitude during the inspiratory phase of respiration. In this condition, when a patient has a rapid respiratory rate that is equal to half the pulse rate, the physical findings may resemble pulsus alternans, with an apparent decrease in pulse amplitude every other beat.

Mechanisms of Pulsus Alternans

Weber *et al.* [25] induced pulsus alternans in the canine heart when anaerobic metabolism was reached by increasing the filling volume, heart rate, and contractility and by decreasing coronary perfusion. When the aerobic limit of the myocardium was exceeded, myocardial performance declined, with resultant pulsus alternans [25]. Pulsus alternans is thought to be primarily due to decreased myocardial contractility on alternate beats, with relatively less effect produced by changes in preload, afterload, or diastolic relaxation [16, 18, 26]. Decreased contractility is attributed to deletion of the number of myocardial cells contracting on alternate beats. This reduction in the contractile cell population is thought to be caused by intracellular calcium cycling involving the sarcoplasmic reticulum, leading to localized electrical mechanical dissociation [27]. Another postulated

mechanism for the alternations in pulse pressure evolved from Frank–Starling's mechanism due to alterations in diastolic volume [17, 28]. However, measured diastolic volumes in patient studies [19] suggest that the earlier mechanism may play a more predominant role.

A 62-year-old patient with congestive failure underwent cardiac catheterization for mitral regurgitation and continuing left ventricular dysfunction. Right- and left-heart hemodynamics were obtained in a routine fashion. Examine the hemodynamic tracings of the simultaneous left ventricular and pulmonary capillary wedge pressures (Figure 4.13). Note the differences in the height of the V and A waves during sinus rhythm on the odd-numbered beats. The alternation of V waves was consistent with the pulsus alternans produced in the systemic pressure. The left atrial filling curve (compliance) was appropriately influenced with a greater degree of mitral regurgitation (a larger V wave) for greater systolic ejection (regurgitant pressure).

The theory of pressure generation and alternation of contractility on a beat-to-beat basis with unimpaired diastolic parameters was reported by Bashore *et al.* [19]. Pulsus alternans was induced by preload reduction with balloon occlusion of the inferior vena cava, performed during measurements of left ventricular function. Reduction in preload in 11 patients with nonischemic cardiomyopathy produced sustained pulsus alternans in 5 patients. The strong beats demonstrated systolic characteristics similar to baseline values, despite a decline in both left ventricular end-diastolic diameter and left ventricular end-diastolic pressure (Figure 4.14). The weak beats demonstrated a reduction in peak systolic pressure, fractional shortening, and peak positive dP/dt. Diastolic parameters were not different between baseline beats and strong beats. Left ventricular end-diastolic wall stress differed somewhat between baseline beats and weak beats, but not strong beats. Significant differences in peak systolic pressure, positive dP/dt, and

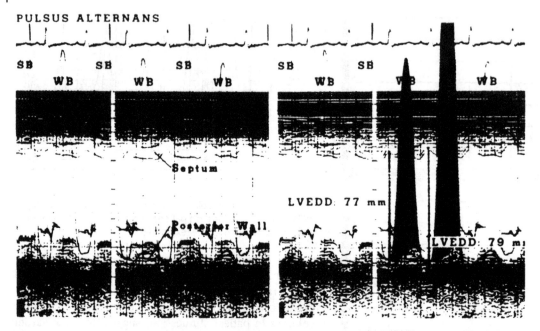

Figure 4.14 Simultaneous echocardiography and pressure measurements during induction of pulsus alternans. Left ventricular pressure and M-mode echocardiography (on left panel) are unretouched, with septal posterior wall and weak beats (WB) and strong beats (SB) shown accentuated in black (on right panel). A small but statistically significant difference in left ventricular end-diastolic dimension (LVEDD) occurs between strong and weak beats. *Source:* Bashore 1988 [19]. Reproduced with permission of John Wiley & Sons.

fractional shortening were present between strong and weak beats (Figure 4.15), but no difference in any measured diastolic parameter was observed. These data were consistent with an augmentation and deletion of intrinsic contractile forces in association with an alternation in preload on a beat-to-beat basis during pulsus alternans.

Of the many associations of pulsus alternans, myocardial ischemia appears to contribute to both the alternation and attenuation of the pressure waveforms. Pulsus alternans observed prior to coronary angiography in a patient with severe cardiomyopathy was significantly attenuated during contrast injection [21]. Pulsus alternans may also disappear after administration of digitalis [29] and during continued deterioration of left ventricular function [30]. Both the new appearance of pulsus alternans and the disappearance of pulsus alternans should alert the clinician to possible deteriorating myocardial function.

Nitroglycerin and Ventricular Unloading

Effects of Nitroglycerin

Nitroglycerin is the most commonly used medication in the cardiac catheterization laboratory [31]. The hemodynamic effects of systemic and coronary vasodilation are often striking and, in general, are therapeutic. Nitroglycerin is routinely administered sublingually, intravenously, or intra-arterially during coronary and left ventricular angiography. Significant increases in the caliber and flow responses of the coronary arteries as well as reduction of left ventricular filling pressures are well documented [32–34]. However, the varied hemodynamic influences of nitroglycerin reported during myocardial ischemia [34, 35] may not be readily apparent from routine responses observed in stable patients. This section will review the hemodynamic effects of nitroglycerin with particular reference to ventricular unloading and acute ischemia. The case examples illustrate the systemic and coronary influence of this potent, short-lived, and important medication.

A 72-year-old woman with severe triple vessel coronary artery disease and hypertension had intermittent chest pain preceding the diagnostic coronary angiogram. At the conclusion of coronary angiography, elevated left ventricular pressure was measured through an 8 F pigtail catheter (Figure 4.16). Before reviewing the hemodynamic tracings, consider the following issues. What is the upper limit of left ventricular end-diastolic pressure (above which the risk of problems increases) for patients undergoing left ventriculography? Based on the pressure tracing and clinical presentation, would this patient likely have a problem during or following left ventriculography? Finally, is volume unloading necessary for this individual?

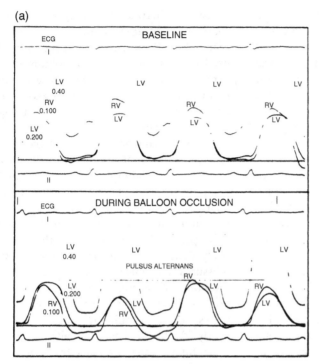

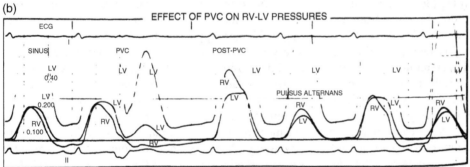

Figure 4.15 (a) Concordant right ventricular (RV) and left ventricular (LV) pulsus alternans. Subtle baseline concordant right and left ventricular alternans is dramatically accentuated during inferior vena caval balloon occlusion. (b) Induction of right ventricular (RV) and left ventricular (LV) pulsus alternans following premature ventricular contractions (PVC) after beat #2. The mild baseline pulsus alternans shown is accentuated following the post-extrasystolic accentuation of the pressure. The concordance of right and left ventricular pulsus alternans is again demonstrated. *Source:* Bashore 1988 [19]. Reproduced with permission of John Wiley & Sons.

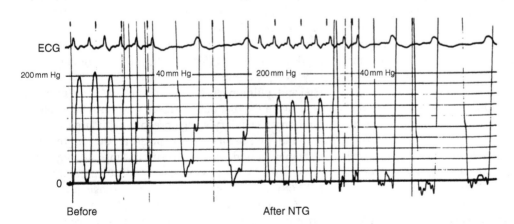

Figure 4.16 Hemodynamic tracings of left ventricular end-diastolic pressure before and after nitroglycerin (NTG). See text for details.

Examine the pressure tracings. Left ventricular systolic pressure is 200 mm Hg and end-diastolic pressure approximately 22 mm Hg (Figure 4.16). Prior to contrast ventriculography, 0.4 mg sublingual nitroglycerin was administered. The effects of nitroglycerin shown on the right side of Figure 4.16 occurred within 2 minutes. Nitroglycerin reduced the systolic pressure from 200 mm Hg to 155 mm Hg and end-diastolic pressure to approximately 2 mm Hg.

It should be obvious from this typical hemodynamic tracing that sublingual nitroglycerin produced a marked reduction in left ventricular preload, dropping the left ventricular filling pressure from 22 mm Hg to 2 mm Hg, with a corresponding reduction in the left ventricular systolic pressure. This is a characteristic response to sublingual nitroglycerin, especially evident in patients with high left ventricular end-diastolic pressure. The decrease in left ventricular filling pressure with vasodilators such as nitroglycerin (and sodium nitroprusside) is characterized by a downward shift in the left ventricular pressure–volume relationship [36, 37]. During rest, nitrates routinely reduce left ventricular systolic pressure by between 10 mm Hg and 15 mm Hg [36], while reducing left ventricular end-diastolic volume by 25–30% and left ventricular end-systolic volume by 30–35%. These effects are also present during ischemia. During the ischemic stress of supine exercise, systemic nitroglycerin also demonstrates a significant reduction in end-diastolic pressures and left ventricular end-systolic volume in comparison to intracoronary nitrates [38]. These findings support the systemic effects of preload reduction more than coronary dilation as predominantly responsible for the anti-ischemic effects of nitroglycerin [33, 35].

Patients with elevated left ventricular end-diastolic pressure may have ongoing ischemia that does not become symptomatic until after left ventriculography. High left ventricular end-diastolic pressures (>30 mm Hg) have been associated in the catheterization laboratory with the development of accelerated angina and congestive heart failure in some patients [39, 40]. Nitroglycerin should be routinely administered (either sublingually or systemically) for left ventricular end-diastolic pressures greater than 20 mm Hg. Depending on the volume status of the individual, preload reduction with small doses of nitroglycerin can result in a significant decrease in filling pressures, as demonstrated in this patient. Patients with hypertension and high left ventricular end-diastolic pressure, especially those with coronary artery disease and hypertrophy, have an increased potential for subclinical ischemia and generally respond favorably to prophylactic nitroglycerin.

To maintain a satisfactory systemic pressure after ventriculography should hypotension occur due to a marked vasodilatory effect of radiographic contrast media, we infuse fluids to increase the left ventricular end-diastolic pressure by between 5 mm Hg and 10 mm Hg. It is not routinely necessary to administer volume after nitroglycerin, but the hemodynamic effect of nitroglycerin can be used as an indicator of the volume status to prevent hypotension, either following contrast-induced vasodilatation or later in the postcatheterization period in which contrast-induced diuresis may further deplete the marginal volume status of such individuals.

A 61-year-old woman with unstable angina was admitted to the hospital for cardiac catheterization. In the catheterization laboratory, routine right- and left-heart hemodynamic measurements were obtained before coronary angiography and ventriculography. During these measurements, the patient complained of her typical chest pain while resting during the mid-portion of the study. Pulmonary capillary wedge and pulmonary artery pressures were measured during and after spontaneous resolution of the angina (Figure 4.17a, left). Examine the pressure tracings during spontaneous ischemia. Giant V waves seen on the pulmonary capillary wedge tracing are nearly 60 mm Hg. The V can also be appreciated on the downslope of the pulmonary artery pressure tracing and be confused with a PA dichrotic notch. The mean pulmonary capillary wedge pressure with chest pain was 35 mm Hg and approximately equal to the pulmonary artery diastolic pressure. While we were preparing to administer nitroglycerin, the chest pain resolved. The ischemia-related pressure changes were dramatically improved. Examine the pressure tracings again (Figure 4.17a, right; pressure scale is 0–40 mm Hg). During myocardial ischemia, the mean pulmonary capillary wedge, V wave, and pulmonary artery pressures were markedly elevated. After spontaneous relief of ischemia, pulmonary artery pressure is 32/16 mm Hg, the pulmonary artery V wave cannot be seen, and the pulmonary capillary wedge pressure is reduced to approximately 10 mm Hg. A few minutes later, ischemia recurred (Figure 4.17b, left). Observe the hemodynamics before administration of nitroglycerin and compare these hemodynamics with those of the spontaneous occurrence and resolution of ischemia. Before nitroglycerin (Figure 4.17b, left; pressure scale 0–200 mm Hg), aortic pressure is 138/64 mm Hg, mean pulmonary capillary wedge pressure 30 mm Hg with V waves to 42 mm Hg, and pulmonary artery pressure is 60/20 mm Hg. Note again the distinct change in waveform between the pulmonary capillary wedge pressure with large V waves and the pulmonary artery pressure during the pre-ischemic period. Nitroglycerin (0.4 mg sublingual) is given and within 3 minutes aortic pressure falls (122/68 mm Hg), mean pulmonary wedge pressure is now 6–8 mm Hg without V waves, and pulmonary artery pressure is 22/10 mm Hg. Nitroglycerin-induced relief of chest pain was dramatic. The most striking difference between spontaneous and nitroglycerin-induced relief of

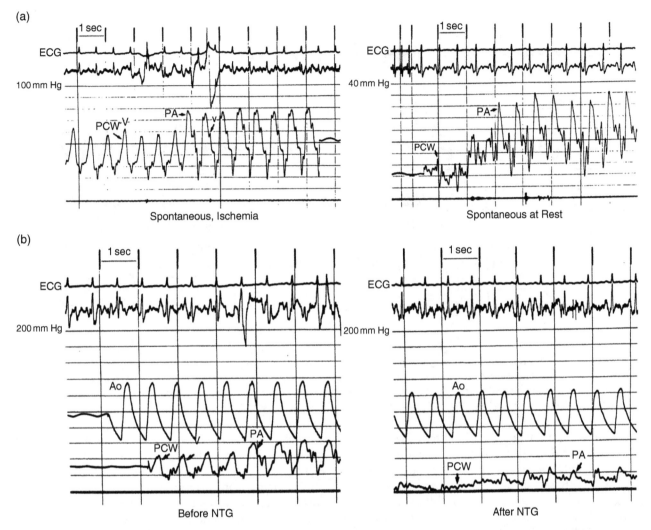

Figure 4.17 (a) Hemodynamic tracing of right-heart pressure during the spontaneous development of ischemia and its spontaneous resolution prior to the administration of nitroglycerin. Note the difference in scale between the left and right panels from 100 mm Hg to 40 mm Hg. (b) Arterial and pulmonary artery pressures prior to nitroglycerin (left) during an episode of ischemia and its relief after nitroglycerin (right). Note that the scale on both tracings is 0–200 mm Hg for both pulmonary artery and aortic pressures. Ao = aortic pressure; NTG = nitroglycerin; PA = pulmonary artery pressure; PCW = pulmonary capillary wedge pressure; V = V wave.

ischemia is the dramatic preload reduction demonstrated by the greater decline in mean pulmonary capillary wedge and pulmonary artery pressures. Spontaneous resolution of ischemia causes less shift in the pressure–volume relationship of the left ventricle than does the nitroglycerin-induced reduction in ischemia.

Nitroglycerin and Coronary Blood Flow

Does sublingual nitroglycerin improve coronary blood flow to relieve myocardial ischemia in patients with coronary artery disease [41]? A 73-year-old man with severe angina refractory to calcium-channel blockers and topical nitroglycerin was admitted for cardiac catheterization. Coronary angiography revealed severe triple-vessel coronary artery disease, with left ventricular ejection fraction of 46% and anterior hypokinesis. After coronary angiography, coronary blood flow response to calcium-channel blockers was measured under an approved research protocol. Coronary sinus thermodilution and high-fidelity dual-micromanometer-tipped left ventricular catheters were positioned for hemodynamic study.

Although unanticipated, hemodynamic measurements were obtained continuously before, during, and after an episode of typical angina. Prior to the onset of chest pain, blood pressure (Figure 4.18, left) was 160/70 mm Hg with a left ventricular end-diastolic pressure of 12 mm Hg. While preparing the study medication, asymptomatic ST depression was observed preceding the onset of chest pain (Figure 4.18, pre-angina). The observed pre-anginal hemodynamic alterations were consistent with a hierarchy of ischemic events later described to occur reproducibly during controlled, transient ischemia produced by angioplasty [42]. Blood pressure was

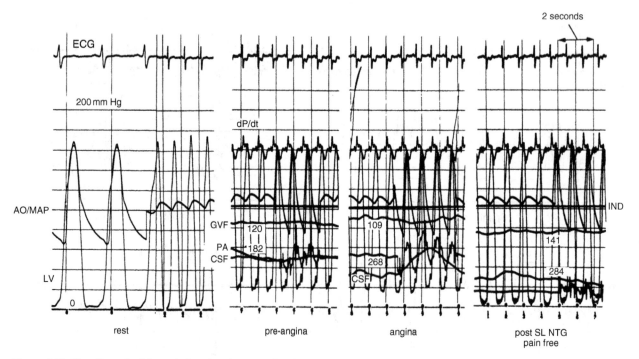

Figure 4.18 The effect of sublingual nitroglycerin on total and regional coronary blood flow during spontaneous ischemia. Increasing coronary flow is directed toward the bottom of the figure. Numbers under the coronary sinus and great vein flow signals are the average flow in milliliters/minute averaged over a 5-second time period. Ao = aortic pressure; CSF = coronary sinus flow; GVF = great vein flow; LV = left ventricular pressure; MAP = mean arterial pressure; PA = pulmonary artery pressure.

unchanged at approximately 160/78 mm Hg, but left ventricular end-diastolic and minimal diastolic pressures were increased to 30 mm Hg and 20 mm Hg, respectively (Figure 4.18, pre-angina). Great cardiac vein flow (an index of anterior left ventricular blood flow) was 120 ml/min with coronary sinus (global left ventricular) flow of 182 ml/min. The mean pulmonary artery pressure was also elevated at 30 mm Hg (0–100 mm Hg scale for pulmonary artery). After 1 minute of ST segment depression, angina occurred, gradually becoming more severe (Figure 4.18, angina). Great cardiac vein flow decreased to 109 ml/min, whereas coronary sinus flow increased to 268 ml/min. Left ventricular end-diastolic, minimal diastolic, and mean pulmonary artery pressures remained elevated as in the pre-anginal period. Nitroglycerin produced the expected result. Within 2 minutes after receiving 0.4 mg sublingual nitroglycerin, the angina abated and ST segment changes returned toward normal, with marked improvement in great cardiac vein flow, which increased to 141 ml/min. Coronary sinus flow increased to 284 ml/min. Coincident with improved blood flow and reduced clinical ischemia, left ventricular end-diastolic pressure declined to normal values. The mean pulmonary artery pressure also fell to 16 mm Hg.

Peripheral venous dilation decreasing myocardial oxygen consumption through preload reduction has been well established [32, 33], but the nitrate-induced increase in coronary blood flow to ischemic myocardium through reversal of coronary vasoconstriction has been a contro-

versial subject [36, 37]. Evident from this case is that the mechanism relieving ischemia is a sum of the two drug actions of both myocardial oxygen demand reduction and augmentation of coronary flow when coronaries can respond to vasodilation. These detailed hemodynamic observations in this third patient demonstrated that coronary blood flow may be significantly, albeit regionally, improved simultaneously with the reduction in the determinants of myocardial oxygen demand in at least some patients with severe coronary artery disease.

Nitroglycerin, Angina, and Aortic Stenosis

Nitroglycerin may reduce angina-like chest pain which is unrelated to coronary artery disease. A 74-year-old man with mild aortic stenosis, increasing fatigue, and angina pectoris underwent diagnostic cardiac catheterization. Simultaneous left ventricular and aortic pressures (Figure 4.19) demonstrated an aortic gradient of approximately 30 mm Hg with a cardiac output of 4.9 L/min, resulting in a calculated aortic valve area of approximately 0.9 cm^2. Coronary arteriography was normal. Left ventriculography showed global hypokinesis with an ejection fraction of 32%. To assess the influence of changing loading conditions and cardiac output on aortic valve gradient, sublingual nitroglycerin and dopamine (5 mcg/kg/min) were administered and the hemodynamics re-examined (Figure 4.19). Nitroglycerin reduced left ventricular end-diastolic and minimal diastolic pressures

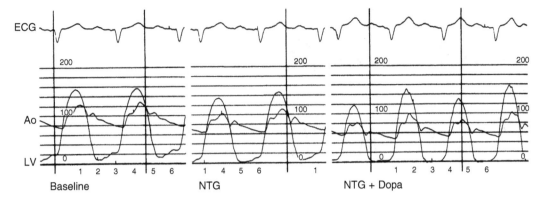

Figure 4.19 Simultaneous aortic and left ventricular pressures in a patient with severe aortic stenosis at baseline, after 0.4 mg sublingual nitroglycerin (NTG) and after sublingual nitroglycerin with low-dose dopamine infusion (5 mcg/kg/min). Note the decline in pressures after nitroglycerin and the pulsus alternans after the administration of dopamine. See text for details.

from approximately 28 mm Hg to 18 mm Hg and from 10 mm Hg to 2 mm Hg, respectively. Left ventricular systolic pressure also fell, without increasing the transvalvular pressure gradient. When low-dose dopamine was infused, augmenting contractility and cardiac output, pulses alternans was observed and was augmented over that seen with nitroglycerin. The aortic stenotic gradient showed alternating pressure gradients with the strong and weak beats. The increase in cardiac output to 6.5 L/min with a mean gradient of 45 mm Hg did not alter the aortic valve area calculation (0.9 cm^2). Note that dopamine and nitroglycerin further decreased left ventricular filling pressures. Nitroglycerin predominantly reduced preload in this patient, but had little effect on the valve area. As a rule, vasodilators should not be employed in patients with significant aortic stenosis. The production of pulsus alternans was unexpected. Pulses alternans occurs in patients with aortic stenosis and has been attributed to alternations in afterload (wall stress) and contractile state, but not to preload [43]. We speculate that the nitroglycerin in this patient produced a reflex increase in sympathetic tone, resulting in pulsus alternans because of the impaired cardiac contractile reserve. However, in the previous studies [43], patients with aortic stenosis and pulsus alternans were given nitroglycerin and did not have this effect based on observable direct or indirect (reflex-mediated) changes in contractile state. Whether this is a finding related to reduced preload reserve or not remains under study.

Nitroglycerin and the Aortic Pressure Waveform

With nitroglycerin, the aortic pressure wave shows a more distinct dichrotic notch and a more prominent secondary reflected wave (Figure 4.20). The changing waveform with nitroglycerin has been reviewed in detail by Nichols and O'Rourke [44]. The ascending aortic pressure wave after nitroglycerin is significantly modified, as shown by a drop in the height of the anachrotic notch and augmentation of the dichrotic notch by wave reflections. This reflected wave physiology is more pronounced as one measures pressure further in the peripheral circulation (Figure 4.21). The mechanism for nitroglycerin's effect on the pressure waveform is not precisely known. Nitroglycerin, an endothelial independent vasodilator, decreases arterial stiffness and improves arterial distensibility, and thus reduces arterial pressure. Nitrates, in low dosages, dilate arteries without effecting arterioles, whereas calcium-channel antagonists and angiotensin-converting enzyme (ACE) inhibitors dilate both arteries and arterioles. Nitrates have little effect on the largest arteries, such as the aorta, or on the smallest arteries, the arterioles, but substantial effects on arteries of medium size. Exactly how dilatation improves distensibility in arteries is currently under investigation [44–48]. A suggested mechanism is that arterial smooth muscle is in series with some stiffer collagen components, but in parallel with the elastic lamini [47]. Contraction of smooth muscle tenses the collagen components, whereas dilation transfers stress to the elastic lamellae, thus improving distensibility. The release of endothelial-derived relaxing factor and the common pathway of nitrate activation of guanylate cyclase have also been proposed [48]. Despite these hypotheses, the exact mechanism of nitroglycerin on the vascular responses remains unresolved. These effects may also be due to the greater dilatation of sub-branches than of the parent branch, with a subsequent reduction in the amplitude of the reflected wave returning from the periphery (Figure 4.22). This explanation is based on nitroglycerin's effect on the caliber of small peripheral arteries minimizing the contribution of arterial distensibility. Probably both caliber and distensibility are altered with nitroglycerin and contribute to the beneficial effect. With regard to cardiac function, a favorable effect is produced as a result of reduced wave reflection in the impedance modulus at various heart rate frequencies, as well as in the peak aortic and left ventricular end-diastolic

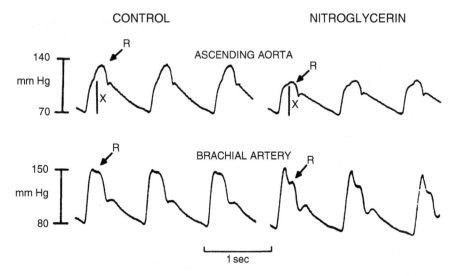

Figure 4.20 Pressure waves recorded in the ascending aorta (top) and brachial artery (bottom) under control conditions and after 0.4 mg sublingual nitroglycerin in a human adult. The right panel demonstrates the effects of nitroglycerin. *Source:* Nichols 1990 [44]. Reproduced with permission of Wolters Kluwer Health, Inc.

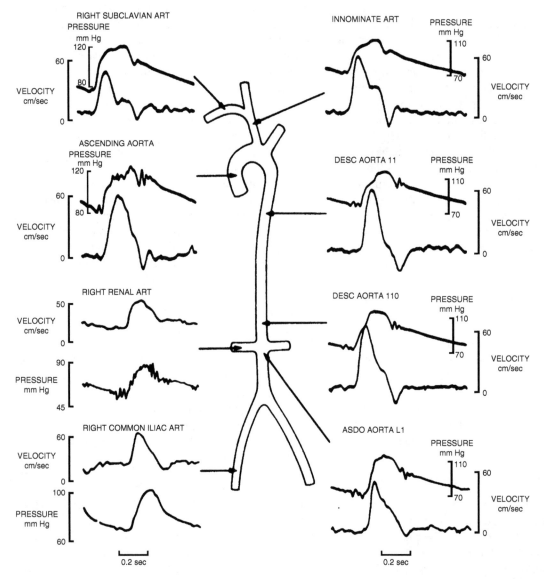

Figure 4.21 Pressure and velocity waveforms in different arteries recorded in a patient undergoing diagnostic cardiac catheterization. Signals were obtained with an electromagnetic catheter transducer. *Source:* Nichols 1990 [44]. Reproduced with permission of Wolters Kluwer Health, Inc.

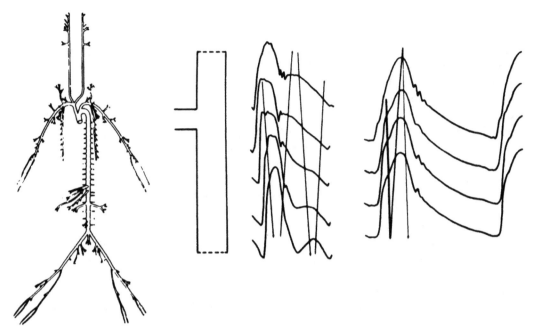

Figure 4.22 Graphic explanation of pressure wave amplitude and contour differences between central aortic and peripheral arteries on the basis of wave travel and reflection. The systemic arterial system (left) is similar to an asymmetric T tube, with the short limb representing all arteries in the upper part of the body and the long limb representing descending aorta and arteries in the lower part of the body. The ends of the T tube represent resultant terminations of individual arteries in both the upper and lower parts of the body. Pressure waves in different arteries of dogs are displayed second to right and in a patient with arteriosclerosis at far right (at half amplitude). The changes in waveform occur based on the reflection and re-reflection of the pulse wave with respect to ventricular ejection. *Source:* Nichols 1990 [44]. Reproduced with permission of Wolters Kluwer Health, Inc.

pressures, independent of the influence on coronary vasodilatation and reduction of myocardial ischemia [38, 44].

To sum up, nitroglycerin has dependable, short-lived venous and arterial vasodilatory effects ameliorating ischemia through both preload reduction and coronary vasodilation. Nitroglycerin should be used prior to left ventriculography in patients with elevated left ventricular end-diastolic pressure. The arterial pressure waveform alteration of nitroglycerin can be explained on the basis of changes in arterial distensibility and reflected wave patterns, and may vary considerably among individuals with different degrees of atherosclerosis.

Key Points

1) In addition to demonstrating constrictive and restrictive cardiac physiology, simultaneous right and left ventricular pressure measurements can be helpful to identify various aspects of myocardial dysfunction.
2) Intracardiac conduction defects will delay the rise of the right ventricular pressure under the left ventricular pressure, shifting both the upstroke and downstroke of the pressure wave rightward due to the differences in the timing of ventricular contraction.

3) Right ventricular dysfunction will also produce abnormal right ventricular pressure waveforms, which may overlap with left ventricular pressure and contribute to abnormalities in right atrial and ventricular pressure waveforms.
4) Pulsus alternans is the regular alteration of strong and weak cardiac contractions in the absence of respiratory or cycle length variation.
5) The physiologic etiology of the reduced muscle contractility of pulsus alternans is thought to be due to a reduction of the number of myocardial cells contracting on alternate beats.
6) There is no difference in the diastolic parameters between baseline beats and strong beats.
7) Administration of sublingual nitroglycerin produces a marked reduction in left ventricular preload, resulting in the reduction of left ventricular end-diastolic pressure and left ventricular end-systolic volume.
8) The systemic effects of nitroglycerin on preload reduction are more significant than with coronary artery dilation, and it is this preload reduction that is the major contributor to the anti-ischemic affects observed with nitroglycerin.
9) Spontaneous resolution of ischemia causes less shift in the left ventricular pressure–volume relationship than nitroglycerin-induced reduction in ischemia.

References

1 Kern MJ, Donohue T, Bach R, Aguirre F. Hemodynamic rounds: Interpretation of cardiac pathophysiology from pressure waveform analysis: Simultaneous left and right ventricular pressure measurements. *Cathet Cardiovasc Diagn* 28:51–55, 1992.

2 Holt JP, Rhode EA, Kines H. Pericardial and ventricular pressure. *Circ Res* 8:1171–1181, 1960.

3 Glantz SA, Parmley WW. Factors which affect the diastolic pressure–volume curve. *Circ Res* 42:171–180, 1978.

4 Goldstein JA, Harada A, Yagi Y, Barzilai B, Cox JL. Hemodynamic importance of systolic ventricular interaction, augmented right atrial contractility and atrioventricular synchrony in acute right ventricular dysfunction. *J Am Coll Cardiol* 16:181–189, 1990.

5 Hoit BD, Dalton N, Bhargava V, Shabetai R. Pericardial influences on right and left ventricular filling dynamics. *Cir Res* 68:197–208, 1991.

6 Janicki JS, Weber KT. The pericardium and ventricular interaction, distensibility, and function. *Am J Physiol* 238(4):H494–H503, 1980.

7 Kern MJ, Aguirre FV. Hemodynamic rounds: Interpretation of cardiac pathophysiology from pressure waveform analysis: Pericardial compressive hemodynamics, Parts I, II and III. *Cathet Cardiovasc Diagn* 25:336–342; 26:34–40; 26:152–158, 1992.

8 Kern MJ, Deligonul D, Gudipati C. Hemodynamic and ECG data. In MJ Kern (ed.), *The Cardiac Catheterization Handbook*. St. Louis: Mosby Year Book, 1991, pp. 98–201.

9 Feneley MP, Gavaghan TP, Baron DW, Branson JA, Roy PR, Morgan JJ. Contribution of left ventricular contraction to the generation of right ventricular systolic pressure in the human heart. *Circulation* 71:473–480, 1985.

10 Wiggers CJ. The pressure pulses under certain abnormal types of ventricular contraction. In *The Pressure Pulses in the Cardiovascular System*. London: Longmans, Green, 1928, pp. 166–181.

11 Thompson CR, Kingma I, MacDonald RPR, Belenkie I, Tyberg JV, Smith ER. Transseptal pressure gradient and diastolic ventricular septal motion in patients with mitral stenosis. *Circulation* 76:974–980, 1987.

12 Schoen WJ, Talley JD, Kern MJ. Hemodynamic rounds: Interpretation of cardiac pathophysiology from pressure waveform analysis: Pulsus alternans. *Cathet Cardiovasc Diagn* 24:315–319, 1991.

13 Traube L. Ein Fall von Pulsus bigeminus nebst Bemerkungen über die Leberschwellungen bei Klappenfehlern und über acute Leberatrophie. *Ber Klin Wochenschr* 9:185–188;221–224, 1872.

14 Laskey WK, St. John Sutton M, Unterecker WJ, Martin JL, Hirschfield JW. Mechanics of pulsus alternans in aortic valve stenosis. *Am J Cardiol* 52:809–812, 1983.

15 Braunwald E (ed.). *Heart Disease: A Textbook of Cardiovascular Medicine*. Philadelphia, PA: McGraw-Hill, 1988, p. 481.

16 Hess OM, Surber EP, Ritter M, Krayenbuehl HP. Pulsus alternans: Its influence on systolic and diastolic function in aortic valve disease. *J Am Coll Cardiol* 4:1–7, 1984.

17 Lewis BS, Lewis N, Gotsman MS. Effect of postural changes on pulsus alternans: An echocardiographic study. *Chest* 75:634–636, 1979.

18 McGaughey MD, Maughan WL, Sunagawa K, Sagawa K. Alternating contractility in pulsus alternans studied in the isolated canine heart. *Circulation* 71:357–362, 1985.

19 Bashore TM, Walker S, Van Fossen D, Schaffer PB, Fontana ME, Unverferth DV. Pulsus alternans induced by inferior vena caval occlusion in man. *Cathet Cardiovasc Diagn* 14:24–32, 1988.

20 Elbaum DM, Banka VS. Pulsus alternans during spontaneous angina pectoris. *Am J Cardiol* 58:1099–1100, 1986.

21 Ring ME, Kern MJ, Genovely H, Serota H, Vandorrmael M. Attenuation of pulsus alternans during coronary angiography. *Cathet Cardiovasc Diagn* 20:193–195, 1990.

22 Hada Y, Wolfe C, Craige E. Pulsus alternans by biventricular systolic time intervals. *Circulation* 65:617–626, 1982.

23 Desser KB, Benchimol A. Phasic left ventricular blood velocity alternans in man. *Am J Cardiol* 36:309–314, 1975.

24 Verheugt FWA, Scheck H, Meltzer RS, Roelandt J. Alternating atrial electro-mechanical dissociation as contributing factor for pulsus alternans. *Br Heart J* 48:459–461, 1982.

25 Weber KT, Janicki JS, Sundram B. Myocardial energetics: Experimental and clinical studies to address its determinants and aerobic limit. *Basic Res Cardiol* 84:237–246, 1989.

26 Miller WP, Liedtke AJ, Nellis SH. End systolic pressure diameter relationships during pulsus alternans in intact pig hearts. *Am J Physiol* 250:H606–H611, 1985.

27 Lab MJ, Lee JA. Changes in intracellular calcium during mechanical alternans in isolated ferret ventricular muscle. *Circ Res* 66:585–595, 1990.

28 Gleason WL, Braunwald E. Studies on Starling's Law of the Heart. VI. Relationship between left ventricular end-diastolic volume and stroke volume in man with observations on the mechanism of pulsus alternans. *Circulation* 25:841–847, 1962.

29 Windle JD. Clinical observations on the effects of digitalis in heart disease with pulsus alternans. *Q J Med* 10:274, 1917.

30 Ryan JM, Schieve JF, Hull HB, Osner BM. The influence of advanced congestive heart failure on pulsus alternans. *Circulation* 12:60–63, 1955.

31 Kern MJ, Aguirre FV, Hilton TC. Hemodynamic rounds: Interpretation of cardiac pathophysiology from pressure waveform analysis: The effects of nitroglycerin. *Cathet Cardiovasc Diagn* 25:241–248, 1992.

32 McGregor M. The nitrates and myocardial ischemia. *Circulation* 66:689–692, 1982.

33 Kaski JC, Plaza LR, Meran DO, Araujo L, Chierchia S, Maseri A. An improved coronary supply: Prevailing mechanisms of action of nitrates in chronic stable angina. *Am Heart J* 110:238–245, 1985.

34 Liu P, Houle S, Burns RS, Kimball B, Warbick-Cecrone A, Johnston L, Gilday D, Weisel RD, McLaughlin PR. Effect of intracoronary nitroglycerin on myocardial blood flow and distribution on pacing-induced angina pectoris. *Am J Cardiol* 55:1270–1276, 1985.

35 Ganz W, Marcus HR. Failure of intracoronary nitroglycerin to alleviate pacing-induced angina. *Circulation* 46:880–889, 1972.

36 Kingma I, Smiseth OA, Belenkie I, Knudtson ML, MacDonald RPR, Tyberg JV, Smith ER. A mechanism for the nitroglycerin-induced downward shift of the left ventricular diastolic pressure diameter relation. *Am J Cardiol* 57:673–677, 1986.

37 Brodie BR, Grossman W, Mann T, McLaurin LP. Effects of sodium nitroprusside on left ventricular diastolic pressure–volume relations. *J Clin Invest* 59:59–68, 1977.

38 DeCoster PMN, Chierchia S, Davies GJ, Hackett D, Fragasso G, Maseri A. Combined effects of nitrates on the coronary and peripheral circulation in exercise-induced ischemia. *Circulation* 81:1881–1886, 1990.

39 Grossman W. Cardiac ventriculography. In *Cardiac Catheterization and Angiography*, 3rd ed. Philadelphia, PA: Lea and Febiger, 1986, p. 204.

40 Deligonul U, Kern MJ, Serota H, Roth R. Angiographic data. In MJ Kern (ed.), *The Cardiac Catheterization Handbook*. St. Louis: Mosby Year Book, 1991, p. 245.

41 Kern MJ, Eilen SD, O'Rourke R. Coronary vasomotion in angina at rest and effect of sublingual nitroglycerin on coronary blood flow. *Am J Cardiol* 56:484–485, 1985.

42 Labovitz AJ, Lewen MJ, Kern MJ, Vandormael M, Deligonul U, Kennedy HL. Evaluation of left ventricular systolic and diastolic dysfunction during transient myocardial ischemia. *J Am Coll Cardiol* 10:748–755, 1987.

43 Laskey WK, Sutton MSJ, Untereker WJ, Martin JL, Hirshfeld JW Jr, Reichek N. Mechanics of pulsus alternans in aortic valve stenosis. *Am J Cardiol* 52:809–812, 1983.

44 Nichols WW, O'Rourke MF. *McDonald's Blood Flow in Arteries: Theoretical, Experimental and Clinical Principles*, 3rd ed. Philadelphia: Lea & Febiger, 1990, pp. 421–432.

45 Cohen MV, Kirk ES. Differential response of large and small coronary arteries to nitroglycerin and angiotensin. *Circ Res* 33:445–453, 1973.

46 Feldman RL, Pepine CJ, Conti CR. Magnitude of dilation of large and small coronary arteries by nitroglycerin. *Circulation* 64:324–333, 1981.

47 O'Rourke MF, Avolio AP, Yaginuma T. Arterial dilation as a mechanism for favorable effects of nitroglycerin in man. In *Proceedings of the 6th International Adalat Symposium*, Geneva, 1985, p. 13.

48 O'Rourke MF, Kelley RP, Avolio AP, Hayward CS. Potential for reversing the ill-effects of angina and of arterial hypertension on central aortic systolic pressure and on left ventricular hydraulic load by arterial dilator agents. *Am J Cardiol* 63:381–441, 1989.

5

Hemodynamics during Arrhythmias

Morton J. Kern, Thomas J. Donohue, and Richard G. Bach

Cardiac pressure waveforms are determined by the underlying cardiac rhythm. Normal sinus rhythm produces the characteristic atrial and ventricular filling patterns, which are further influenced by the cardiac cycle length, chamber compliance, resting circulating volume, and extrinsic factors of pericardial restraint, pulmonary resistance, and ventricular–aorto and ventricular–ventricular interactions [1–3]. Further compounding the interpretation of pressure waves, disturbances of normal impulse conduction will distort or obliterate these waveforms or initiate unique pressure patterns. Some of the most obvious examples of altered hemodynamic pressure patterns occur during cardiac arrhythmias induced during normal pacemaker function, as previously described [4]. Even more unusual rhythms can be observed in cardiac transplant recipients, with the native or donor heart rhythm at times interfering with or, in the case of heterotopic transplantation, potentiating normal pressure waves [5].

Premature Contractions

The most commonly observed cardiac arrhythmia is a premature ventricular contraction (PVC). A naturally occurring or mechanically (catheter) induced PVC causes a systolic beat, which generally ejects a substantially reduced stroke volume, often limiting the arterial pressure pulse and resetting the sinus rhythm with a prolonged, compensatory pause (Figure 5.1). The post-PVC beat generally is stronger than the normal beat due to both enhanced filling (the Frank–Starling mechanism) and an enhanced contractile state. In general, the hemodynamic result of the PVC is of little clinical importance, but may serve a diagnostic purpose in the hemodynamic assessment of hypertrophic cardiomyopathy (recall the

Brockenbrough–Braunwald–Morrow sign; Figure 5.2) [6]. PVCs have also been used to assess contractile reserve and viability of ischemic hypokinetic myocardial segments [7]. In the absence of mechanical stimulation, frequent PVCs may portend serious and life-threatening events, and must be considered a treatable risk factor during diagnostic and therapeutic catheterization laboratory procedures.

Consider the hemodynamics of a 54-year-old woman with a rumbling apical systolic murmur (Figure 5.3). Simultaneous left ventricular and pulmonary capillary wedge pressures were measured with fluid-filled catheters. The pulmonary capillary wedge tracing demonstrated large V waves, consistent with clinically significant mitral regurgitation. Intermittent PVCs produce characteristic changes in the magnitude of both the left ventricular pressure and the V wave. The systolic left ventricular pressure of one sinus beat (#2) is 146 mm Hg with a large V wave (60 mm Hg). The PVC (beat #3) has a left ventricular systolic pressure of 120 mm Hg with a smaller (<40 mm Hg) and delayed V wave. Note also that the V wave peak falls outside the left ventricular downstroke. The post-PVC beat (#4) systole is augmented (152 mm Hg) with a V wave of 44 mm Hg. Of interest is the timing of the PVCs in this example. These beats are late-cycle escape-type PVCs in Figure 5.3. The speed of the recording changes from 10 mm/sec to 25 mm/sec, but the rhythm and associated pressures demonstrate features of grouped beats. The PR interval prolongs with a regular frequency followed by a pause with a PVC. Mobitz type I (Wenckebach) rhythm is present with period 3:2 and 4:3 beats. The P wave without its QRS is likely to be obscured by the late PVC. The influence of a longer ventricular filling period during the sinus arrhythmia (between beats #1 and 2) may account for the larger V wave.

Hemodynamic Rounds: Interpretation of Cardiac Pathophysiology from Pressure Waveform Analysis, Fourth Edition.
Edited by Morton J. Kern, Michael J. Lim, and James A. Goldstein.

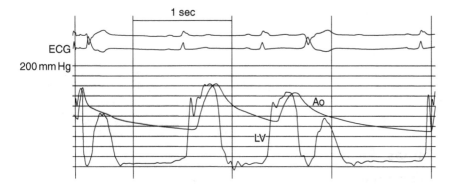

Figure 5.1 Left ventricular (LV) and aortic (Ao) pressures during a premature ventricular contraction. Note the minimal change in aortic pressure and large post-PVC arterial pressure.

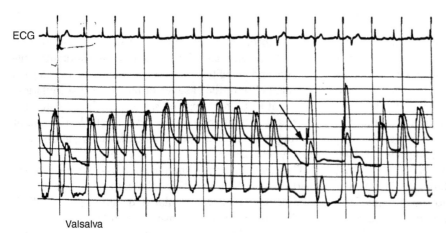

Figure 5.2 Premature ventricular contraction (arrow) in a patient with hypertrophic cardiomyopathy. Note the post-PVC reduction of pulse pressure. *Source:* Brockenbrough 1961 [6]. Reproduced with permission of Wolters Kluwer Health, Inc.

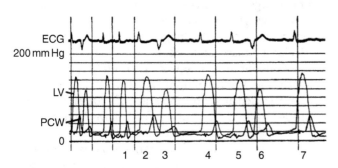

Figure 5.3 Left ventricular (LV) and pulmonary capillary wedge (PCW) pressures in a patient with mitral regurgitation. Left ventricular pressures vary with the cardiac rhythm. Why is the V wave larger on beat #2? See text for details.

Irregular Rhythms

PVCs are often characterized by compensatory pauses and distorted QRS complexes. However, the QRS complex may not be easily distinguishable from a normal beat on physiologic monitors with reduced or poor-quality electrocardiographic waveforms due to loose electrocardiographic leads. Such ECG tracings often require scrutiny of the associated pressure waves, since the electrocardiographic artifacts cause loss of the signal or a signal trigger for an audible beep in the laboratory of the regular rhythm. An audible regular rhythm is helpful, especially at the beginning of a procedure during catheter and sheath placement. The changing, slowing audible beeps may be the only early warning or

evidence of a vagal reaction. Early treatment with atropine (0.6 mg intravenous) can save time and extra procedures (e.g., temporary pacemaker, leg raising) during the catheterization.

Because the electrocardiographic monitor complex is not always detailed enough to see each part of the entire PQRST complex, interpretation of the rhythm can be difficult. Examine the hemodynamic left atrial and left ventricular waveforms obtained in a 39-year-old woman with mixed mitral stenosis and regurgitation (Figure 5.4). Left atrial pressure was obtained by the transseptal technique prior to consideration of mitral balloon valvuloplasty. The rhythm is irregularly irregular without grouped beats. No P waves are evident on the electrocardiographic tracing. No "a" waves are seen on left

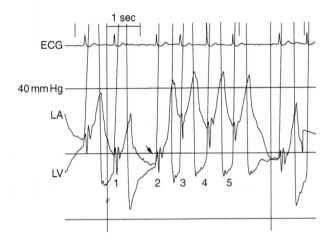

Figure 5.4 Left atrial (LA) and left ventricular (LV) pressures in a patient with an irregular rhythm. Identify A, C, and V waves. See text for details.

ventricular and left atrial pressures. The absence of an A wave is especially evident on beat #2, with a long pause before the next systole. This rhythm is obviously atrial fibrillation and demonstrates that equilibration of left atrial–left ventricular pressure occurs with long cardiac cycles (>900 msec). A run of short RR cycles, shown on beats #3–5, is associated with a substantial left atrial–left ventricular gradient, resulting in the appearance of symptoms during periods of tachycardia (e.g., exercise). With proper heart rate control, valve repair or valvuloplasty may be delayed.

Misleading Atrial Waveforms during Arrhythmias

A 53-year-old woman presented with increasing dyspnea six years after tricuspid and mitral valve replacements. She had a childhood history of rheumatic fever. Consider the right-heart hemodynamics with attention to the cardiac rhythm (Figure 5.5a). Because of suspected tricuspid stenosis, one catheter was positioned in the right atrium and one in the right ventricle to measure the gradient. Before crossing the tricuspid valve, the pressures from both catheters were matched to verify the equivalency of the transducers (Figure 5.5a, left panel). The matched and elevated right atrial pressures show attenuation of the normal A and V waves. The right ventricular–right atrial tracing demonstrates a significant tricuspid valve gradient with an irregular rhythm and grouped beats, with systolic pressures varying with respiration (Figure 5.5a, right panel). The pulmonary capillary wedge and right atrial pressures are displayed at 50 mm/sec paper speed, with the pulmonary capillary wedge pressure showing distinct A and V waves

(Figure 5.5b, beat #1). The electrocardiographic complex has a first-degree AV block with a presumed PR interval of nearly 50% of the RR interval. Consider beat #2. No such A and V waves are present. The QRS is different, with a short PR interval. Note that the right atrial pressure on beat #1 does not show the same striking A or V waves of the pulmonary capillary wedge pressure, but has distinct X and Y descents (X > Y). This pattern repeats itself over the remaining beats.

Further clarification of these findings occurs on examination of the left ventricular–pulmonary capillary wedge pressure tracings (Figure 5.5c). The paired beats are now more clearly displayed, with an abbreviated left ventricular diastolic period (beat #1) and a coupled beat with a longer filling period (beat #2). Beat #1 can now be easily identified as a PVC and beat #2 as a junctional beat (no A wave). The biphasic waveform previously assumed to be A and V waves on the right atrial–pulmonary capillary wedge tracings (Figure 5.5b) can now be seen to be a V wave of an ectopic ventricular beat, with the coupled V wave of the underlying predominant junctional beat. No "a" wave is present either on the left ventricular or pulmonary capillary wedge tracings. This rhythm is then a junctional rhythm with ventricular bigeminy. The patient was receiving digoxin for atrial fibrillation and had developed transient periods of a regular rhythm with coupled beats. Arterial and left ventricular pressures (Figure 5.5d) clearly demonstrate the predominant patterns of this rhythm. This case is an example of how reliance on pressure waves of the pulmonary capillary wedge alone (or any single pressure) may be confusing, resulting in a misinterpretation of the cardiac events.

Rhythm with Wide QRS Patterns

Occasionally an electrocardiographic tracing will look like ventricular fibrillation due to patient movement or a loose lead. Immediately check the patient—"Are you okay, Mr. Jones?"—and the pressure (Figure 5.6). In some patients it may be artifact, in others this may be real (Figure 5.7a, b). Treatment of ventricular fibrillation may be delayed if the operator is not monitoring arterial pressure and assumes the electrocardiographic changes to be an artifact.

Wide complex QRS rhythms also include accelerated junctional rhythms with or without atrial dissociation. Examine the right atrial pressure in a 65-year-old man with dyspnea and coronary artery disease (Figure 5.8a). The rhythm is regular. The peaked waves occur at the ECG T wave downstroke (see arrow). Are these sharp V waves? Review the rhythm again. A P wave may be conducted retrograde to generate a notched ECG T wave and produce a cannon "a" wave. Another clue to this

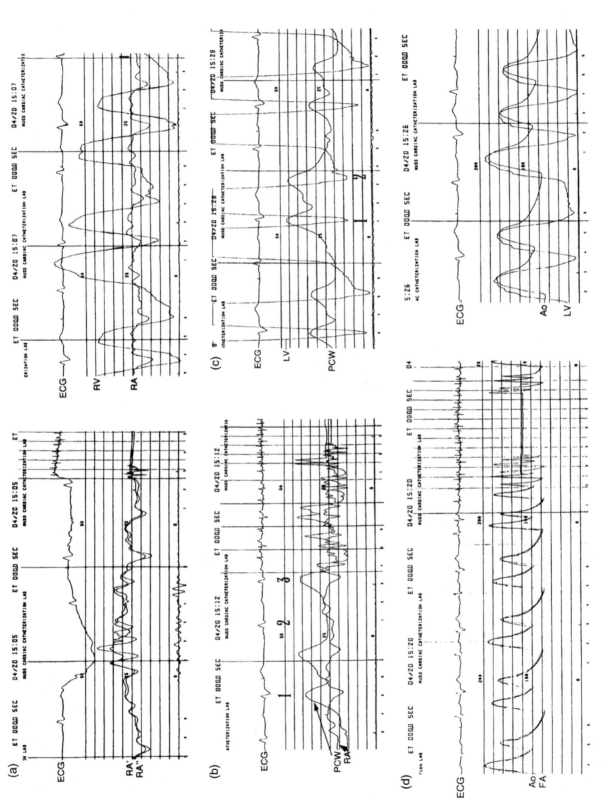

Figure 5.5 (a, left panel) Simultaneous two-catheter measurement of right (RA′, RA″) pressure in preparation to assess tricuspid stenosis. Pressures match during the irregular rhythm. (Right panel) Right ventricular (RV) and right atrial (RA) pressures in the same patient. Note the grouped beating of right ventricular pressure. The magnitude of pressures varies due to respiratory activity. See text for details. (b) Simultaneous pulmonary capillary wedge (PCW) and right atrial (RA) pressures. Note that the right atrial waveform has X and Y descents with smaller A and V waves. Does the PCW pressure waveform have large A and V waves? (c) Left ventricular (LV) and pulmonary capillary wedge (PCW) pressures (0–50 mm Hg scale) demonstrating a coupled rhythm. Note the bigeminal pattern with V waves and no A waves. See text for details. (d, left) Femoral (FA) and central aortic (Ao) pressures (0–200 mm Hg scale) demonstrating coupled beats during the bigeminal rhythm. (Right) The rhythm is atrial fibrillation with periods of coupled beats. See text for details.

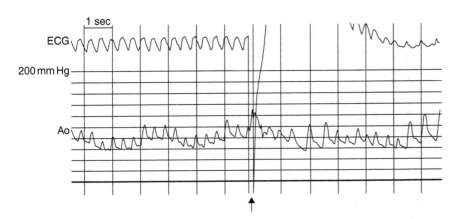

Figure 5.6 Wide complex QRS tachycardia with mild arterial hypotension. Note the pattern changes at the arrow. See text for details.

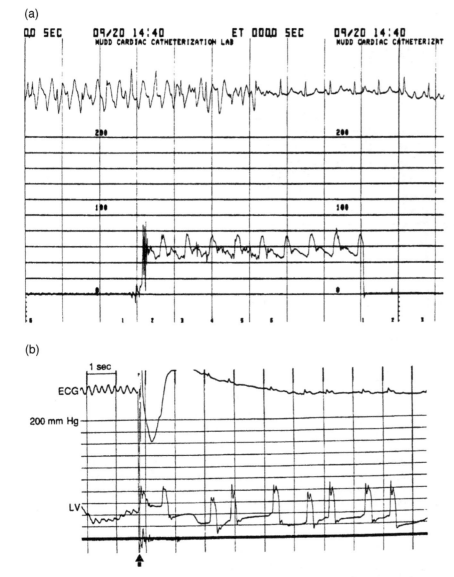

Figure 5.7 (a) Electrocardiogram showing ventricular fibrillation with preserved arterial pressure. (b) Electrocardiogram showing ventricular fibrillation with gradual restoration of a sinus mechanism after electrocardioversion. See text for details.

(a)

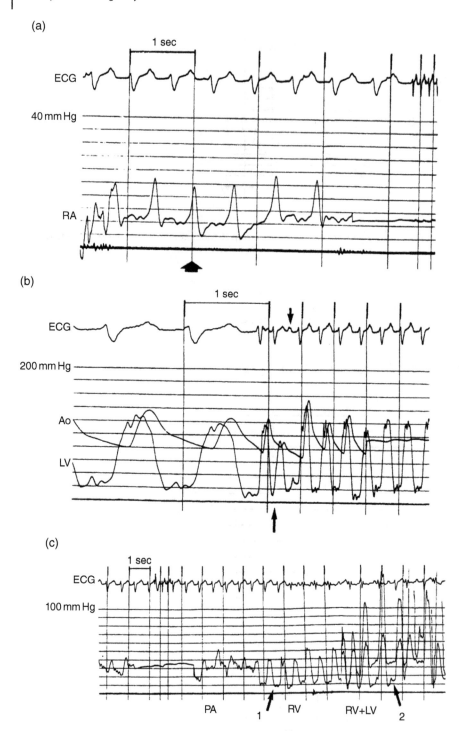

Figure 5.8 (a) Right atrial (RA) pressure with wide complex QRS rhythm. Are the sharp peaks (arrow) V waves? See text for details. (b) Simultaneous left ventricular (LV) and aortic (Ao) pressures. A PVC (bottom arrow) produces a change in the electrocardiogram to reveal a P wave (top arrow). (c) Right-heart catheter pullback from pulmonary artery (PA) to right ventricle (RV) and then simultaneous left ventricle (LV) to right ventricle (0–100 mm Hg scale). Note the rhythm change after right ventricular beat #1.

rhythm is the response to a PVC. Figure 5.8b shows the left ventricular and aortic pressures during a PVC (bottom arrow), which separates the P wave from the QRST complex (top arrow). This rhythm was also exposed as a junctional rhythm during right-heart catheter pullback, which produced a transient right bundle branch block and separated the P waves, demonstrating a brief period of sinus rhythm. Of interest is that the right and left ventricular "a" waves also reflect the changing rhythm, with retrograde P waves contributing notching to right ventricular filling. Compare right ventricular beat #1 to the right ventricular beat three cycles later (Figure 5.8c) and the diastolic portion of the left ventricular beat #2 (Figure 5.8c) with that on Figure 5.8b.

Pacemaker Hemodynamics

Many patients coming into the cardiac catheterization laboratory will have temporary or permanent pacemakers implanted for myocardial diseases related to conduction disturbances. The normal timing of physiologic events is disturbed, with corresponding abnormalities in pressure waveforms. The hemodynamic consequences of sequential atrial ventricular contraction are of interest and often clinical importance relative to the generation of regurgitant waves, arterial pressure, and optimal left ventricular filling. As will be seen, the influence of atrial systole is principally, through the Frank–Starling mechanism [8], on the end-diastolic pressure–volume relationship of both the right and left ventricles. The hemodynamic tracings presented below will illustrate several altered sequences of atrial–ventricular activation and their hemodynamic consequences.

Atrial Waves during Pacemaker Activity

A 63-year-old woman had a pacemaker implanted for syncope and heart failure two years prior to the onset of vague atypical chest pains with increasing dyspnea. Right- and left-heart cardiac catheterization was performed using fluid-filled catheters. Right atrial pressure was recorded during a period of pacemaker activity (Figure 5.9). Examine the ECG rhythm and waveforms of right atrial pressure. Two different waveforms are evident. On the left side of Figure 5.9, atrial pacing is not present. Ventricular activation without associated atrial pacing produces indistinct waveforms which may be confused with artifact and

offer no organized transport of atrial blood to the right ventricle. On the right side of Figure 5.9, AV sequential pacing generates distinct "a" waves (the smaller wave is the V wave) which augment atrial transport and increase right ventricular performance [9–11]. The mean pressure of both atrial wave patterns is equal. In this patient, the right-heart filling pressures were low and tricuspid regurgitation or right ventricular volume overload was not considered important.

In the same patient, the pulmonary capillary wedge pressure was obtained with a balloon flotation pulmonary artery catheter (Figure 5.10). The pacemaker spike artifact on the electrocardiographic signal shows only ventricular activation. Can we explain how the distinct and equivalent A and V waves of pulmonary capillary wedge pressures are produced? The A–V sequential pacemaker with leads placed in the right atrial appendage and right ventricular apex senses P waves to suppress atrial pacing. Although atrial activity is not registering on the electrocardiographic tracing, a P wave is occurring, possibly from only the left atrium, and produces a hemodynamic "a" wave without an electrical P wave or atrial spike being seen on the electrocardiogram. This example serves to illustrate that although the pacemaker activity may *appear* to be functioning in only one mode, nonrecorded (on one lead) atrial contraction can be detected on the hemodynamic tracings.

A more common abnormality of right atrial pressure would be dyssynchronous atrial activity producing atrial contraction against a closed mitral valve. In a patient with mild aortic stenosis, a pacemaker was implanted for lightheadedness and transient sinus arrest. The right atrial pressure of this patient during a paced and sinus rhythm readily demonstrates an alteration in the right atrial pressure waveform (Figure 5.11). Large cannon waves (in the beats preceding the asterisk) show the effect of late or retrograde atrial contraction occurring after ventricular pacing. When the patient moves into sinus rhythm, the pressure waveform changes to a normal A and V wave configuration with the corresponding

Figure 5.9 Right atrial (RA) pressure in a patient with A–V sequential pacing (0–40 mm Hg scale). See text for details.

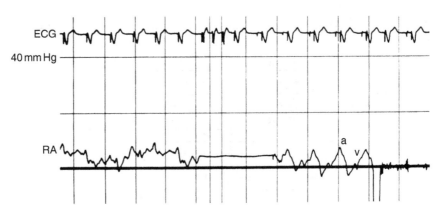

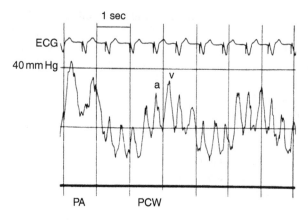

Figure 5.10 Pulmonary capillary wedge (PCW) and pulmonary artery (PA) pressure tracings (0–40 mm Hg scale) in a patient with a pacemaker for heart block. See text for details.

normal X and Y descents. Although the cannon waves are of no significance, the loss of atrial contraction to ventricular filling in this patient was important (see below, Figure 5.15).

Dissociated Atrial Activity and Hemodynamic Function

Pacemakers of a single pacing mode (e.g., VVI) often are associated with dyssynchronous atrial activity which may produce unusual hemodynamic findings. The influence of dissociated atrial contraction on the ventricular filling function is readily apparent when examining the pressure data collected from a 52-year-old woman with a pacemaker inserted for complete heart block. The VVI (ventricular sensed, paced, and inhibited) mode pacemaker was functioning normally. Right and left ventricular and pulmonary capillary wedge pressures were measured with fluid-filled catheters in a routine fashion (Figures 5.12 and 5.13). The hemodynamic results of atrial contraction can be readily seen on beat #1

(Figure 5.12) as a large and early A wave on the left, as well as right ventricular pressure tracings. Note that the right ventricular pressure, normally enclosed evenly within the left ventricular pressure contour, has an earlier and more rapid upstroke than on the following beat #2, occurring without an atrial contribution to ventricular filling. Peak right ventricular (and left ventricular) pressures are higher when atrial systole is appropriately timed. Compare the peak right ventricular systolic pressure on beats #1 and 4 with beats #2 and 3. Also, a difference in the compliance (the pressure–volume relationship) of the two ventricular chambers can be appreciated on beat #2 by comparing the upslope of the diastolic pressures. The left ventricular diastolic pressure slope is steep. The right ventricular diastolic pressure slope is horizontal, with slowed filling in the absence of the atrial contribution. The dissociated atrial activity influences ventricular filling pressures dependent on its timing relative to ventricular ejection. An optimal P–Q interval for ventricular function in experimental animal preparations of complete heart block was 85–125 msec [10]. Very early atrial activity with pressure wave deformity can be seen on beat #3 (Figure 5.12), demonstrated by the notch in the early diastolic period of the right ventricular pressure tracing. Compare the right and left ventricular minimal diastolic pressure waveforms. The P wave is located in the T wave and is not readily appreciated on the electrocardiogram. Beat #4 shows atrial activity superimposed on the T wave, but has less of an effect on right and left ventricular pressures. However, the diastolic filling pattern of both ventricles shows the effect of early atrial contraction, with a continued rise in diastolic pressure and larger peak systolic pressure (beats #1 and 4). The P wave activity in beat #4 occurs much earlier than in beat #5, with the pressure pattern repeating. This example demonstrates two points: (i) the importance of atrial filling to ventricular pressure; and (ii) differences in ventricular filling

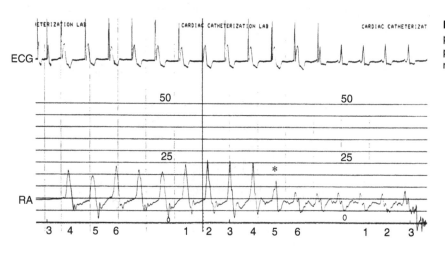

Figure 5.11 Right atrial (RA) pressure in a patient with aortic stenosis and a pacemaker. Asterisk indicates a change in rhythm. See text for details.

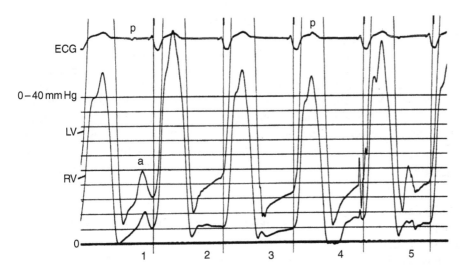

Figure 5.12 Right (RV) and left ventricular (LV) pressures (~O mm Hg scale) demonstrating the influence of atrial activity on left ventricular filling. See text for details.

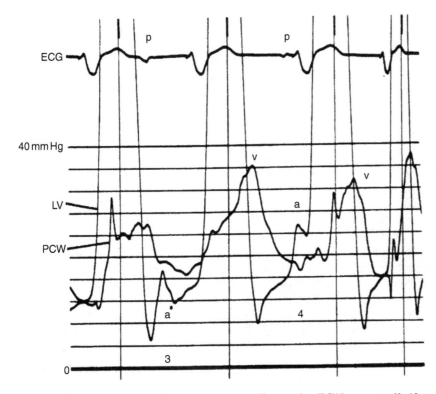

Figure 5.13 Left ventricular (LV) and pulmonary capillary wedge (PCW) pressures (0–40 mm Hg scale) demonstrating the influence of atrial activity on pulmonary capillary wedge waveforms. See text for details.

pattern between the two ventricles. These findings have been extensively studied and were confirmed in both experimental and clinical studies over two decades ago [5, 6].

A similar lesson can be obtained from the simultaneous left ventricular and pulmonary capillary wedge pressures (Figure 5.13) in the patient described above. The atrial and ventricular pacing activity is dyssynchronous.

In beat #3 (Figure 5.13), the P wave produces an atrial contraction occurring earlier in left ventricular diastole. The corresponding A wave on the pulmonary capillary wedge pressure is blunted and the V wave following the paced beat is large. In the next beat #4, the A wave occurs in normal sequential timing, the pulmonary capillary wedge A wave is small, and the V wave is somewhat attenuated. The shape of the V wave downslope is more rapid than the preceding V wave. Does the A wave occurring in beat #3 occur early enough to account for the reduced height of the V wave relative to the following beats in which a more normal A–V synchrony is obtained? This question is difficult to answer from this tracing alone. An A wave superimposed on a V wave should generally increase not decrease the size of the V wave. Why this V wave is altered may be due to artifact.

Normal and Paced Atrial Systoles and Left Ventricular Pressure

A–V sequential pacing usually produces effective atrial contractions. Simultaneous right and left ventricular pressures were measured during A–V sequential pacing in Figure 5.14. However, normal sinus atrial systole remains a more effective mechanism for augmenting left ventricular filling. Examine the rhythm and corresponding left ventricular pressure. Atrial pacing is inhibited in beat #1. The left ventricular "a" wave is normal although elevated. On beats #2 and 3, the A–V sequential pacing spikes can be observed with only minimal alteration in the left ventricular end-diastolic pressure (arrow) upstroke. The atrial contraction in beat #3 produces more of a deformation of the left ventricular end-diastolic pressure which, as the timing of normal atrial systole supervenes (in beats #4 and 5), is even more pronounced. The normal P wave may not be well seen on the electrocardiogram lead displayed during cardiac catheterization and the physiology of active atrial contraction may only be appreciated by noting the alteration of the diastolic left ventricular pressure waveform. Two other features are of interest. First, the atrial contraction does not produce the A wave on this right ventricular pressure tracing; the left ventricular compliance is usually different from the right ventricle. Compare the effect of atrial contraction on a stiffer right ventricle (see Figure 5.12). The second finding of note is the artifact of distorted right ventricular pressure on beat #1 and the last 40 msec of systole on beat #2. Right ventricular pressure is superimposed on the left ventricular pressure downslope and RV systole is distorted. In beat #1, the sharp cutoff of systole indicates a nonphysiologic artifact of the catheter tip touching the ventricular septum, transiently blocking pressure transmission and producing an artificial matching of the left ventricular pressure decline. The normal right ventricular pressure pattern of right bundle branch block conduction includes only a slight delay of right ventricular pressure increase, but the decline should be within the left ventricular pressure decline.

Clinical Significance of Ventricular Pacemaker Hemodynamics

The clinical importance of pacemaker function is related to ventricular compliance and the need for the atrial contribution to filling. Normal sequential atrial–ventricular contraction is particularly important in patients with noncompliant left ventricles. In some patients, loss of atrial contraction has a dramatic influence on systemic pressure and cardiac output [11, 12].

A 78-year-old man had a VVI pacemaker placed for episodic third-degree heart block with near syncope. Noninvasive evaluation suggested mild aortic stenosis. Because of persistent fatigue and vague periods of light-headedness, hemodynamic evaluation was requested. Left ventricular and femoral artery pressures (matched with central aortic pressure) were recorded during a change in the cardiac rhythm (Figure 5.15). The left ventricular–aortic gradient (200 mm Hg – 160 mm Hg = 40 mm Hg) was maintained while both systolic pressures fell after the pacing began (left ventricular–aortic pressures, 140 – 100 mm Hg = 40 mm hg). The decline in pressure during ventricular pacing produced mild symptoms while recumbent. It is interesting to note no change in aortic valve gradient, but a lower cardiac output due to reduced stroke volume (without the atrial contribution to filling) would yield a smaller calculated valve area. The low left ventricular compliance and

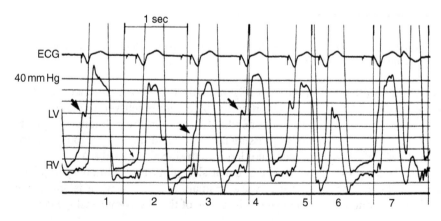

Figure 5.14 Right (RV) and left ventricular (LV) pressures (0–40 mm Hg scale). A–V sequential pacing is occurring at variable times during this hemodynamic tracing. Why is the right ventricular morphology in beat #1 different from beats #3–5? See text for details.

Figure 5.15 Left ventricular (LV) and aortic (Ao) pressures in a patient with aortic stenosis with pacemaker. Asterisk indicates onset of pacemaker activity. See text for details.

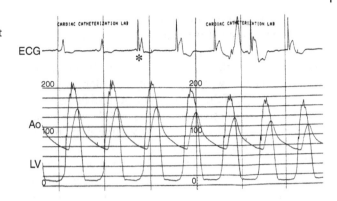

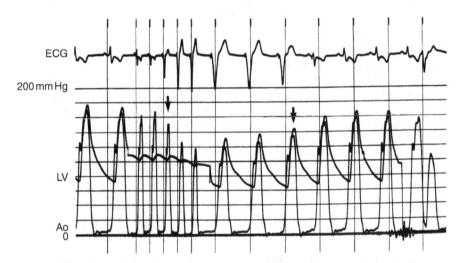

Figure 5.16 Left ventricular (LV) and aortic (Ao) pressures in a patient with hypertension. Pacemaker onset is shown by the first arrow and the return of sinus rhythm shown after the second arrow. Note the decline in systemic pressure. See text for details.

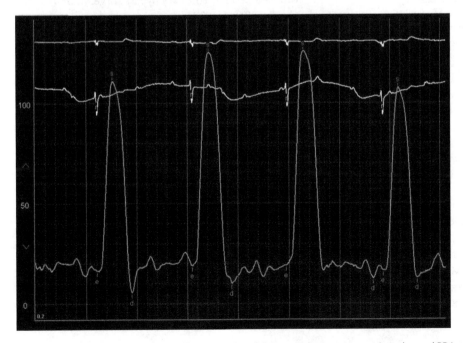

Figure 5.17 Left ventricular pressure with a distinct "a" wave seen in patient with prolonged PR interval of first-degree A–V block.

abnormal relaxation are also suggested by the flat or slightly declining left ventricular diastolic pressure during left ventricular filling. This pattern has been associated with incomplete left ventricular relaxation, as may occur in patients with hypertrophic cardiomyopathy. A similar example of the contribution of atrial filling to systemic pressure is also shown in Figure 5.16 without aortic stenosis. Both of these patients became asymptomatic with A–V sequential pacing.

As noted by Benchimol *et al.* [11], in patients with normal hearts, atrial and ventricular pacing results in nearly identical changes in cardiac output, stroke volume, systemic pressure, ventricular power, and stroke power at any given pacing rate. The contribution of atrial systole to cardiac function in the normal heart is small or relatively unimportant. Furthermore, in impaired ventricles, at any given rate of cardiac pacing, cardiac output, systemic pressure, ventricular power, stroke work, and systolic ejection rate are significantly higher with atrial pacing than with ventricular pacing. These classic observations of over two decades ago are still applicable and evident in hemodynamics obtained in daily practice.

The abnormal sequence of A–V contraction produces alteration of right- and left-heart hemodynamics, reflecting the inappropriate timing of atrial contraction to ventricular filling. Some symptomatic patients may require A–V sequential pacing to improve cardiac output. The clinical effects of the atrial contribution to left ventricular function can be demonstrated by a careful review of hemodynamic tracings in these individuals.

Hemodynamics during First-Degree A–V Block

The left ventricular pressure waveform is altered when the A wave is initiated and completed well before the QRS activates the left contraction. In this circumstance, the LV pressure wave easily identifies a first-degree A–V block (Figure 5.17).

Key Points

1) Various arrhythmias can produce distorted pressure waveforms, which may be confused with benign physiologic events.
2) Delay in the management of serious arrhythmias can be avoided by vigilant monitoring of both ECG and systemic pressures.

References

1 Kern MJ, Donohue T, Bach R, Aguirre F. Hemodynamic rounds: Interpretation of cardiac pathophysiology from pressure waveform analysis: Cardiac arrhythmias. *Cathet Cardiovasc Diagn* 27:223–227, 1992.

2 Meisner JS, McQueen DM, Ishida Y, Vetter HO, Bortolotti U, Strom JA, Peskin CS, Yellin El. Effects of timing of atrial systole on ventricular filling and mitral valve closure: Computer and dog studies. *Am J Physiol* 249(3 Pt 2):H604–H619, 1985.

3 O'Rourke MF. Pressure and flow waves in systemic arteries and the anatomical design of the arterial system. *J Appl Physiol* 23:139–149, 1967.

4 Kern MJ, Deligonul U. Hemodynamic rounds: Interpretation of cardiac pathophysiology from pressure waveform analysis: Pacemaker hemodynamics. *Cathet Cardiovasc Diagn* 24:22–27, 1991.

5 Kern MJ, Deligonul U, Miller L. Hemodynamic rounds: Interpretation of cardiac pathophysiology from pressure waveform analysis. IV. Extra hearts: Part I. *Cathet Cardiovasc Diagn* 22:197–201, 1990.

6 Brockenbrough EC, Braunwald E, Morrow AG. A hemodynamic technique for the detection of hypertrophic subaortic stenosis. *Circulation* 23:189–194, 1961.

7 Popio KA, Gorlin R, Bechtel DJ, Levine JA. Post-extrasystolic potentiation as a predictor of potential myocardial viability: Preoperative analyses compared with studies after coronary bypass surgery. *Am J Cardiol* 39:944, 1977.

8 Linderer T, Chatterjee K, Parmley WW, Sievers RE, Glantz SA, Tyberg JV. Influence of atrial systole on the Frank–Starling relation and the end-diastolic pressure–diameter relation of the left ventricle. *Circulation* 67:1045–1053, 1983.

9 Samet P, Castillo C, Bernstein WH. Studies in P wave synchronization. *Am J Cardiol* 19:207–212, 1967.

10 Brockman SK, Manlove A. Cardiodynamics of complete heart block. *Am J Cardiol* 16:72–83, 1965.

11 Benchimol A, Ellis lG, Dimond EG. Hemodynamic consequences of atrial and ventricular pacing in patients with normal and abnormal hearts. *Am J Med* 39:911–922, 1965.

12 Samet P, Castillo C, Bernstein WH. Hemodynamic consequences of sequential atrioventricular pacing: Subjects with normal hearts. *Am J Cardiol* 21:207–212, 1968.

Part Two

Valvular Hemodynamics

6

Aortic Stenosis

Michael J. Lim and Morton J. Kern

The stenotic aortic valve produces resistance to blood outflow, manifesting as a pressure gradient with highly developed left ventricular pressure and reduced aortic pressure in proportion to certain characteristics of the stenosis and the arterial elastic properties. Measurement of aortic valve pressure gradients and valve areas can be computed by Doppler echocardiography and catheter-based pressure signals. Doppler flow velocity is used to compute the maximal pressure drop across the valve from peak velocity, whereas catheter-based pressures acquire the hemodynamic pressure waves from the left ventricle and the aorta at some distance from the valve orifice. The gradient between the pressures is used to compute the valve area. Figure 6.1 compares the Doppler and catheter-based hemodynamic measurements of the stenotic aortic valve and the pathophysiologic pressure changes over the left ventricular outflow and aorta [1]. Differences between Doppler and catheter hemodynamics are related to a phenomenon called pressure recovery. Pressure recovery occurs when blood flow decelerates after exiting the valve into the wider lumen of the ascending aorta. As the kinetic energy is reconverted to static energy, the pressure rises. This increased pressure relative to the lower pressure exactly in the valve orifice accounts for the fact that the catheter pressure gradient is always less than the maximum Doppler velocity pressure gradient.

Likewise, the valve area or effective orifice area (EOA) derived from the Gorlin formula uses recovered pressures and as such is larger than that obtained using the Doppler EOA derived from the continuity equation. Doppler velocity measures the actual area across which the valvular flow traverses the stenosis. The extent of pressure recovery is determined by the ratio between the valve area and the cross-sectional area of the ascending aorta, a situation important for patients with small aortas.

There are three distinct types of aortic stenosis (AS) encountered in clinical practice and these are distinguished by the anatomic site of obstruction: supravalvular, subvalvular, and (most commonly) valvular AS. Valvular AS can be further subdivided into one of three major etiologies: congenital/bicuspid AS (Figure 6.2), rheumatic AS, and, most commonly, calcific/degenerative AS (formerly known as senile calcific AS). A bicuspid aortic valve is the most common congenital heart condition, occurring in up to 2% of the general population. The bicuspid aortic valve generally does not become stenotic until early adulthood, after years of turbulent flow damage to the valve architecture, leading to leaflet calcification and fibrosis, and ultimately narrowing of the valve orifice.

Calcific/degenerative AS is the most common cause of AS in adults, and its incidence increases with age. It is not surprising, therefore, that aortic stenosis and coronary atherosclerosis share similar risk factors; namely, tobacco use, older age, dyslipidemia, male gender, chronic kidney disease, hypertension, and diabetes mellitus.

A typical patient example can be seen in Figure 6.3. An elderly woman had a "heart murmur," hypertension, and complaint of progressively worsening dyspnea on exertion over the course of one week; aortic stenosis was of primary concern. She had also been having exertional chest pains, primarily substernal and nonradiating. Physical examination revealed a harsh, late-peaking, crescendo–decrescendo III/VI systolic ejection murmur at the right upper sternal border (RUSB), which radiated to both carotid arteries. Her second heart sound was very soft. An S4 gallop was present. Transthoracic echocardiographic images revealed a densely calcified aortic valve with limited mobility of the aortic valve leaflets. Her left ventricular systolic function was at the lower limits of normal. Left

Hemodynamic Rounds: Interpretation of Cardiac Pathophysiology from Pressure Waveform Analysis, Fourth Edition.
Edited by Morton J. Kern, Michael J. Lim, and James A. Goldstein.
© 2018 John Wiley & Sons Ltd. Published 2018 by John Wiley & Sons Ltd.

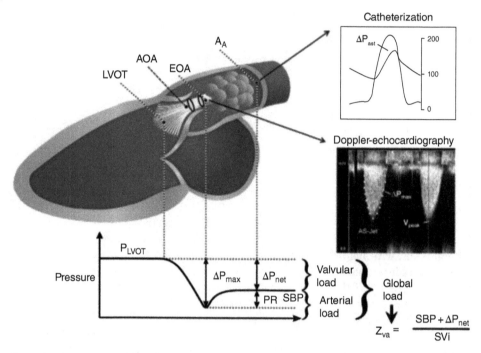

Figure 6.1 Aortic stenosis blood flow and pressure across left ventricular outflow tract, aortic valve, and ascending aorta during systole. When the blood flow contracts to pass through a stenotic orifice (i.e., the anatomic orifice area, AOA), a portion of the potential energy of the blood—namely, pressure—is converted into kinetic energy—namely, velocity—thus resulting in a pressure drop and acceleration of flow. Downstream of the vena contracta (i.e., the effective orifice area, EOA), a large part of the kinetic energy is irreversibly dissipated as heat because of flow turbulences. The remaining portion of the kinetic energy that is reconverted to potential energy is called the "pressure recovery" (PR). The global hemodynamic load imposed on the left ventricle results from the summation of the valvular load and the arterial load. This global load can be estimated by calculating the valvuloarterial impedance. In patients with medium or large ascending aorta, the impedance can be calculated with the standard Doppler mean gradient in place of the net mean gradient. AA = cross-sectional area of the aorta at the level of the sinotubular junction; Pmax = maximum transvalvular pressure gradient recorded at the level of the vena contracta (i.e., mean gradient measured by Doppler); Pnet = net transvalvular pressure gradient recorded after pressure recovery (i.e., mean gradient measured by catheterization); LVOT = left ventricular outflow tract; PLVOT = pressure in the LVOT; SBP = systolic blood pressure; SVi = stroke volume index; Vpeak = peak aortic jet velocity; Zva = valvuloarterial impedance. *Source:* Pibarot 2012 [1]. Reproduced with permission of Elsevier.

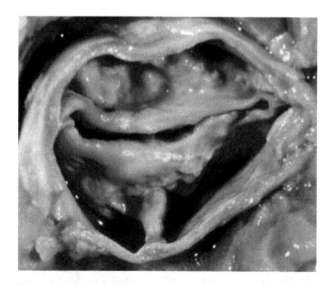

Figure 6.2 This bicuspid aortic valve has only two cusps with atretic raphe and heavily thickened leaflets, with calcification in the leaflets as well as the cusp. Note the irregular orifice responsible for the differences in gradients across this group of valves.

ventricular hypertrophy was present. Right ventricular function was normal and there was no pulmonary hypertension. The peak aortic valve velocity measured by Doppler was 4.7 m/s. The peak instantaneous transvalvular gradient was 90 mm Hg, with a mean transvalvular gradient of 64 mm Hg. The patient was diagnosed with severe aortic stenosis with a calculated aortic valve area of 0.6 cm².

Doppler Hemodynamics of Aortic Stenosis

Doppler echocardiography has supplanted the invasive evaluation of valvular heart disease in modern practice. A more detailed discussion of the echocardiographic assessment of aortic stenosis can be found elsewhere [2], but a brief discussion to illustrate the similarities and differences in the invasively and noninvasively determined aortic valve gradient is provided here.

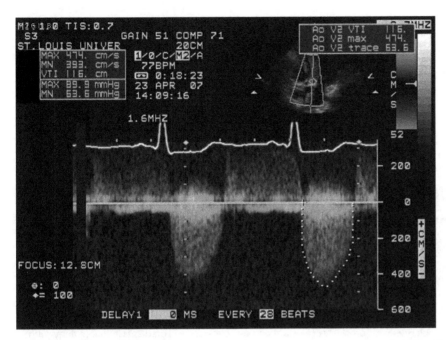

Figure 6.3 Continuous-wave Doppler recording of maximal aortic valve velocity. The dotted line represents the operator tracing of the velocity envelope. From this envelope, the maximal velocity was found to be 4.74 m/sec (474 cm/sec) and the gradients were found to be 89.9 mm Hg (peak) and 63.6 mm Hg (mean). (*See insert for color representation of the figure.*)

The most common hemodynamic parameters obtained by echocardiography include:

- Peak aortic valve velocity (AV_{max})
- Peak instantaneous transvalvular pressure gradient
- Continuity equation for calculation of aortic valve area.

The peak aortic valve velocity is determined using continuous-wave Doppler echocardiography and is thought to represent the most reproducible noninvasive measure of aortic stenosis severity. From this velocity, the modified Bernoulli equation ($4 \times AV_{max}^2$) is used to calculate the peak transvalvular pressure gradient. The mean pressure gradient is derived by integrating the continuous-wave Doppler tracing over the entire systolic ejection period. To calculate the valve area, the continuity equation must be used:

$$AVA = \left(CSA_{LVOT} \times VTI_{LVOT} \right) / V_{AS}$$

where CSA_{LVOT} is the cross-sectional area of the left ventricular outflow tract (LVOT), VTI is the velocity time integral of the left ventricular outflow tract pulsed-wave Doppler tracing, and V_{AS} is the maximal velocity across the valve.

Currie and colleagues [3] simultaneously assessed Doppler-derived aortic pressure gradients and catheter-derived invasive gradients in 100 patients with calcific aortic stenosis. They showed a very strong correlation between the gradients assessed by both techniques, with the strongest correlations when comparing the maximum instantaneous and mean gradients. Figure 6.4 shows several representative patients from their study of the simultaneously obtained catheter- and Doppler-derived gradients.

Accurate echocardiographic hemodynamics depend upon the precise technical performance of the examination and interpretation of the velocity envelopes. Numerous sources of error have been reported that may mislead the clinician and should be appreciated when conflicting information complicates decision-making in the AS patient.

Role of Invasive Hemodynamic Assessment

The most recently published guidelines for patients with valvular heart disease strongly discourage routine invasive hemodynamic measurements to assess the severity of aortic stenosis when there is adequate echocardiographic data that is concordant with the patient's clinical presentation [2]. Assessing the hemodynamics of aortic stenosis at the time of coronary angiography is reserved for those situations when noninvasive testing is inconclusive or there is a discrepancy between noninvasive testing and clinical symptoms.

There are numerous techniques that have been utilized to determine the gradient across the aortic valve (Table 6.1). The best technique currently in routine practice is that of

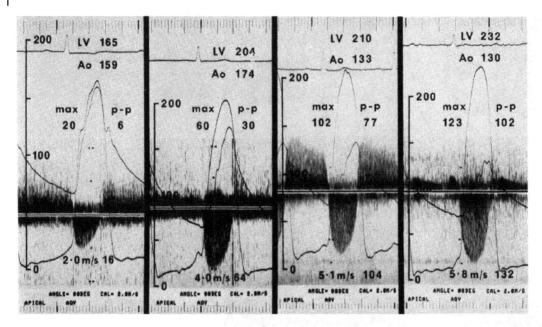

Figure 6.4 Representative comparisons of Doppler-derived aortic valve velocities and catheter-assessed gradients in four patients with varying degrees of aortic stenosis. The left ventricular (LV) and aortic (Ao) pressures are shown at the top of each tracing. Calculated gradients from the invasive data are listed as peak instantaneous (max) and peak to peak (p–p). The continuous-wave Doppler peak velocity is shown on the bottom portion of each tracing, with the associated peak gradient listed immediately to the right of the velocity. As can be seen, the best correlation between measures is the peak instantaneous gradient and the Doppler-derived peak gradient. The Doppler gradient tends to overestimate the peak-to-peak gradient at every degree of stenosis shown. *Source:* Currie 1985 [3]. Reproduced with permission of Wolters Kluwer Health, Inc.

Table 6.1 Methods utilized for invasive assessment of aortic valve gradients.

Left ventricular pressure	Aortic pressure
Single catheter in ventricle	Pullback of catheter to aorta
Catheter in ventricle	Sidearm of arterial sheath
Catheter in ventricle	Sidearm of long arterial sheath in central aorta
Direct apical puncture	Catheter in central aorta
Catheter in ventricle	Catheter in central aorta (second arterial puncture)
Transseptal puncture with catheter in ventricle	Catheter in central aorta
Pressure wire in ventricle	Catheter in central aorta
Dual-lumen pigtail in ventricle	Second lumen of pigtail in ascending aorta
Micromanometer catheter in ventricle	Micromanometer catheter in aorta

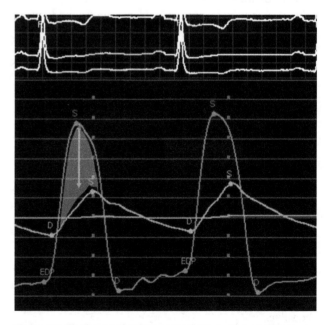

Figure 6.5 The best technique currently in routine practice to measure the aortic valve gradient is with a dual-lumen pigtail fluid-filled catheter. The left ventricular (LV) pressure is shown in yellow and the aortic (Ao) pressure in red. The LV–Ao gradient is shaded, with the arrow showing the peak-to-peak pressure measurement. (*See insert for color representation of the figure.*)

measuring the aortic valve gradient with a dual-lumen pigtail fluid-filled catheter (Figure 6.5). The mean pressure gradient across the aortic valve is determined by planimetry of the area separating the left ventricular and aortic pressure curves. The peak instantaneous gradient is the maximum pressure difference between the left ventricle and the aorta at the same moment in the cardiac cycle, and typically occurs in early systole. The peak-to-peak gradient is the measured difference between the peak aortic pressure and peak left ventricular pressure. The peak-to-peak gradient is often used to assess the severity of aortic stenosis, because it is the easiest to determine based upon initial visual inspection. The peak left ventricular pressure and peak aortic pressures, however, do not occur at the same time, and therefore the peak-to-peak gradient has been stated to have no true physiologic basis.

Historically, operators assessed the aortic valve gradient with two transducers, one connected to the sidearm of the arterial sheath and the other connected to a catheter which crosses the aortic valve and resides in the left ventricular cavity. Modern hemodynamics use a dual-lumen catheter as the most accurate fluid-filled system and this obviates any need to adjust or shift the aortic pressure to match the left ventricular pressure for the best gradient calculations (Figures 6.5 and 6.6). Assey *et al.* [5] evaluated the effect of catheter position on the aortic valve gradients and subsequent calculation of valve area. They showed that utilizing an assessment of aortic pressure from a site distal to the ascending aorta resulted in an underestimate of the valvular gradient. The difference between peripheral arterial pressure and central arterial pressure is largely due to pressure amplification of the peripheral arterial pressure. Amplification usually is found in older patients with calcified, noncompliant vessels, and results from the aortic pressure wave moving in a smaller-diameter conduit (resulting in a greater flow velocity) with decreased arterial compliance.

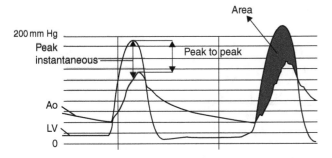

Figure 6.6 Invasive determination of an aortic valve pressure gradient shown with simultaneous aortic (Ao) and left ventricular (LV) waveforms on a 200 mm Hg scale. Three potential gradients can be determined from this tracing: (i) a peak instantaneous gradient occurring at the peak of the left ventricular pressure envelope with the corresponding aortic pressure; (ii) a peak-to-peak gradient which compares the peak left ventricular pressure to the peak aortic pressure; and (iii) a mean pressure gradient determined by the area between the two pressures. *Source:* Kern 1997 [4]. Reproduced with permission of John Wiley & Sons.

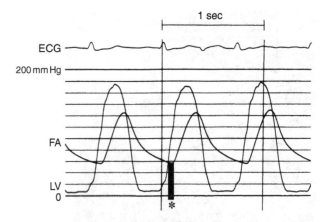

Figure 6.7 Simultaneous recording of the femoral artery (FA) and left ventricular (LV) pressures on a 200 mm Hg scale. As is typical for the comparison of these two pressures, one observes a time delay in the upstroke of the FA tracing compared to the LV tracing of 40–50 msec (depicted by the black column). When comparing this tracing to Figure 6.8, one can infer that the peak instantaneous and mean gradients will be greater in this tracing because of this time delay.

An example of aortic stenosis hemodynamics with arterial sheath pressure and left ventricular pressure is shown in Figure 6.7. There is a time delay (usually 40–50 msec) separating the upstroke of the left ventricular pressure with the upstroke of the peripheral arterial pressure. This antiquated technique has been replaced by the dual-lumen catheter and eliminates the need to "phase shift" the femoral artery pressure tracing to align with the left ventricular tracing prior to the determination of the gradient.

The hemodynamics of a dual-lumen pigtail catheter show the simultaneous rise of the aortic and left ventricular pressure tracings compared to the distal femoral artery pressure (Figure 6.8).

Although single catheter pullback across the aortic valve (Figure 6.9) has been utilized as routine in many laboratories, this method is only useful as "screening" for previously unrecognized left ventricular outflow tract gradients. Accurate estimates of peak pressures may be obscured by catheter whip and the bounce effects of end-hole catheters as they are pulled back across the stenotic valve. Furthermore, ectopic beats invoked during the pullback produce changes in left ventricular filling dynamics which alter the left ventricular and aortic pressures over the first few beats. Finally, there are respiratory effects on ventricular loading conditions that make evaluation of a single beat-to-beat gradient determination by pullback falsely higher or lower than the true gradient [6].

Calculating the Aortic Valve Area

The aortic valve area is calculated using the Gorlin equation. Gorlin and Gorlin first described this equation in 1951 as a means of calculating the mitral valve area in patients

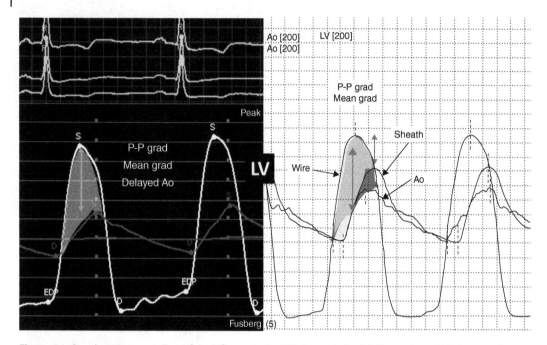

Figure 6.8 Simultaneous recording of the left ventricular (LV), femoral arterial (FA), and aortic (Ao) pressures in a patient with aortic stenosis on a 200 mm Hg scale. One can observe that the peak instantaneous pressure gradient occurs early in systole, as is typical with more severe valvular narrowing. Furthermore, when comparing the FA and Ao tracings, there is a similar systolic pressure but a larger difference in the diastolic pressure. This difference will overestimate the peak instantaneous and mean pressure gradients in this patient. (*See insert for color representation of the figure.*)

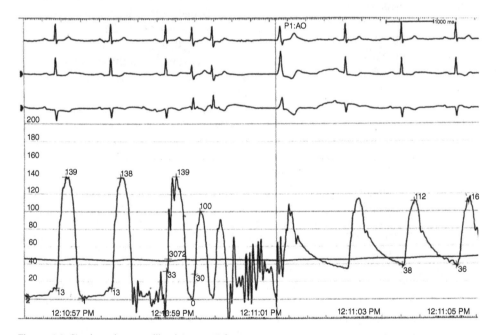

Figure 6.9 Single catheter pullback is unsatisfactory to measure precise aortic valve gradients, 0–200 mm Hg scale.

with mitral stenosis [7]. The Gorlin equation is based on Torricelli's law ($F = AVC_C$), where flow, F, across a round orifice is equal to the area (A) of the orifice times the velocity of flow (V) times the coefficient of orifice contraction (C_C). After rearranging and substituting terms, the Gorlin equation for determining the aortic valve area (AVA) is:

$$AVA = \left[CO / \left(SEP \times HR \right) \right] / \left(44.3 \times \sqrt{G} \right)$$

where CO is cardiac output in L/min, SEP is systolic ejection period in seconds, HR is heart rate in beats per minute, and G is the mean pressure gradient across the

(a)

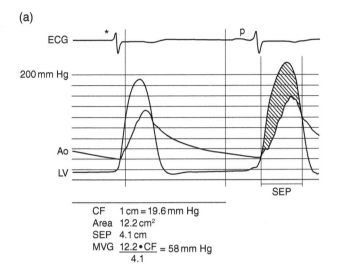

CF   1 cm = 19.6 mm Hg
Area   12.2 cm²
SEP   4.1 cm
MVG $\dfrac{12.2 \cdot CF}{4.1}$ = 58 mm Hg

(b)

Calculating Aortic Valve Area

• AVA: Gorlin equation

$$\text{Valve Area (cm}^2) = \frac{\boxed{\text{Cardiac Output }\left(\frac{ml}{min}\right)}}{\text{Heart rate}\left(\frac{beats}{min}\right).\text{ Systolic ejection period (s) .44.3. }\sqrt{\text{mean Gradient (mm Hg)}}}$$

• AVA: Hakke formula ("poor man's Gorlin")
  • Assumes HR*SEP*44.3 = 1000 in most patients
  • Valid for HR ~65–100

  AVA= cardic output (L/min)/√Peak-Peak Pressures

Figure 6.10 (a) Factors needed for use of the Gorlin formula to compute an aortic valve area. Ao = aortic pressure; Area = derived from the cross-hatched portion of the tracing; CF = correct factor from cm of tracing height to mm Hg; LV = left ventricular pressure; MVG = mean valve gradient; SEP = systolic ejection period. *Source:* Kern 2003 [8]. Reproduced with permission of Elsevier. (b) Formulas used for calculation of valve area.

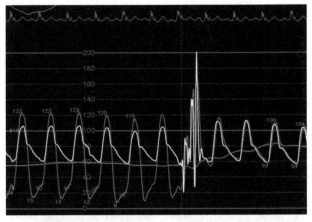

Figure 6.11 Left ventricular and aortic pressures during pullback. Peak-to-peak gradient is 45 mm Hg. Systolic pressures correspond on pullback, but disparity of diastolic pressure suggests sheath damping. (*See insert for color representation of the figure.*)

obstruction in mm Hg (Figure 6.10). It should be noted, however, that although the Gorlin equation is reasonably accurate in calculating the aortic valve area, it has only been validated in patients with mitral stenosis.

A simplified estimation of the aortic valve area has been validated by Hakki *et al.* [9]. This formula is based on the fact that the systolic ejection period, heart rate, and constant portion of the Gorlin equation approximate 1 under resting conditions. Therefore, the estimated aortic valve area can be calculated as:

$$\text{AVA} = \text{Cardiac Output}\left(\text{liters / min}\right) /$$
$$\sqrt{\text{peak} - \text{to} - \text{peak LV} - \text{Aortic pressure}}$$

Figure 6.11 shows left ventricular–aortic pressure pullback. The peak-to-peak gradient is only 20 mm Hg. A cardiac output of 4.0 L/min would yield an aortic valve area of 0.9 cm² = (4 L/min)/ √20 mm Hg.

The Gorlin equation for calculating AVA is flow dependent, and varies directly with flow across the aortic valve; that is, the calculated AVA depends upon the patient's cardiac output. In most patients with severe AS and a large transvalvular gradient, the Gorlin equation accurately calculates a critically stenotic aortic valve. The Gorlin equation is less accurate in patients with a low cardiac output and low transvalvular gradient. In this scenario, the AVA is calculated to be severely stenotic, when in reality no significant aortic stenosis exists, setting the stage for the paradoxical situation of low-flow, low-gradient, severe AS.

Low-Flow, Low-Gradient, Paradoxically Severe Aortic Stenosis

Aortic stenosis patients with low ejection fraction and a low LVOT–AS gradient can have a very small valve area calculation. This conundrum highlights whether the patient's low flow due to weak LV ejection cannot generate enough force to open the valve, or whether the low flow due to the valve severity is the limiting factor. To resolve this dilemma, transvalvular hemodynamics can be examined during dobutamine infusion to increase transaortic flow. If the flow increases and the valve area remains the same, then one can conclude the valve stenosis is fixed. If, on the other hand, the flow increases and the valve area increases as well, then the valve stenosis is variable, the problem is the myocardial function, and valve surgery would be of little help. Figures 6.12, 6.13, and 6.14 illustrate a case of low-flow, low-gradient, paradoxically severe AS.

Aortic stenosis is graded as mild, moderate, or severe (Table 6.2), with the normal aortic valve area being between 3.0 and 4.0 cm². In general, patients do not develop symptoms until the valve area is less than or equal to 0.7 cm². Exceptions obviously exist, and a

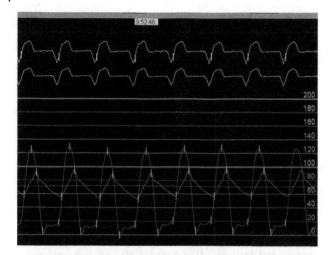

Figure 6.12 A 68-year-old man with low ejection fraction of 25% and cardiac output of 3.2 L/min. Peak-to-peak left ventricular–aortic pressure gradient was 25 mm Hg with an aortic valve area calculation of 0.7 cm². (*See insert for color representation of the figure.*)

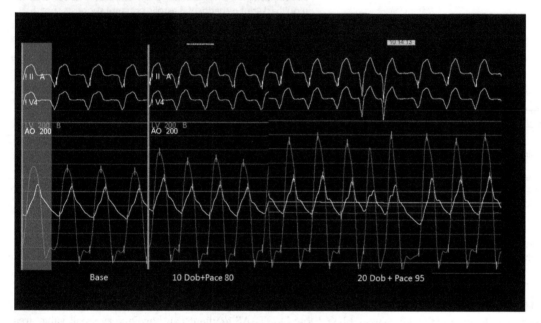

Figure 6.13 Hemodynamics during dobutamine infusion. Left panel is baseline, middle panel 10 mcg/min dobutamine infusion and paced rhythm 80 bpm. Right panel is 20 mcg/min infusion of dobutamine with pacing at 95 bpm. Hemodynamics at peak dobutamine show increased cardiac output of 4.2 L/min, peak-to-peak left ventricular (LV)–aortic (AO) pressure of 50 mm Hg, with a calculated aortic valve area of 0.6 cm². The valve area is fixed and the patient will likely benefit from aortic valve replacement or transcatheter aortic valve replacement. (*See insert for color representation of the figure.*)

correlation must be made between a patient's aortic valve area, gradient, and the clinical symptoms.

Disappearing Gradients during Data Collection

A 49-year-old man with mild early fatigue, vague atypical chest pain syndrome, and systolic murmur underwent hemodynamic study (Figure 6.15) [4]. The femoral (sheath) and left ventricular pressures (pigtail catheter) were matched at the central aortic position prior to crossing into the left ventricle. In panel a, significant aortic stenosis is demonstrated. Within a few minutes after inserting the

pigtail catheter into the left ventricle, the hemodynamic pressures on panel b were obtained. On fluoroscopy, the pigtail catheter appeared to be in nearly the identical position within the ventricle on both tracings. How can one explain the loss of gradient? If panel b was your initial tracing, is there significant aortic stenosis?

Observe the left ventricular–end-diastolic pressure on panel b. The left ventricular pressure continues to decline throughout diastole and increases just at the A wave. Compare this pressure tracing to panel a. The left ventricular diastolic waveform is flat or slightly increasing before the prominent A wave. The aortic (FA) pressure is unchanged in both panels, so this cannot account for the change in the stenotic gradient. The explanation for the

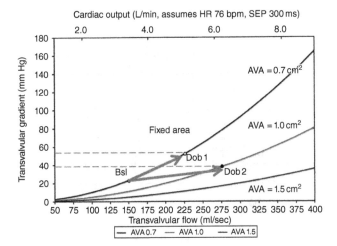

Figure 6.14 Plot of the relationship between mean gradient (y axis) and transvalvular flow (x axis, bottom) according to the Gorlin formula for three different values of aortic valve area (AVA): 0.7, 1.0, and 1.5 cm². Cardiac output (x axis, top) is also shown, assuming a heart rate of 75 bpm and systolic ejection period of 300 ms. At low transvalvular flows, mean gradient is low at all three valve areas. Two different responses to dobutamine challenge are illustrated for a hypothetical patient (Bsl) with a baseline flow of 150 mL/s, mean gradient of 25 mm Hg, and calculated AVA of 0.7 cm². In one scenario (Dob 1), flow increases to 225 mL/s, mean gradient increases to 52 mm Hg, and AVA remains at 0.7 cm², consistent with fixed aortic stenosis (AS). In the second scenario (Dob 2), flow increases to 275 mL/s, mean gradient increases to 50 mm Hg, and AVA increases to 1.0 cm². This patient has changed to a different curve, consistent with relative or pseudo-AS. HR = heart rate; SEP = systolic ejection period. *Source:* Grayburn 2006 [10]. Reproduced with permission of Wolters Kluwer Health, Inc. (*See insert for color representation of the figure.*)

Table 6.2 Classification of aortic valve disease.

Indicator	Mild	Moderate	Severe
Vmax (m/sec)	<3.0	3.0–4.0	>4.0
Mean gradient (mm Hg)	<25	25–40	>40
Valve Area (cm²)	>1.5	1–1.5	<1.0

Source: Excerpted from Nishimura 2017 [11].

loss of gradient is that one of the side holes of the pigtail catheter is now residing in the aorta, evidenced by the continual decline of diastolic left ventricular pressure. This highly abnormal diastolic pressure configuration may be rarely seen in patients who have hypertrophic cardiomyopathy [12]. Had panel b been the first tracing recorded, one might have concluded that aortic stenosis was not significant. For this reason, repositioning the pigtail catheter within the ventricle in all cases, especially those with questionable pressure tracings relative to clinical findings, is mandatory. This catheter artifact is easily recognized if more side holes have their opening in the aorta with the left ventricular diastolic pressure even more elevated, approaching that of aortic diastolic pressure.

Cardiac Rhythms and Aortic Pressure Gradients

Review Figure 6.6. What role does the cardiac rhythm play with respect to aortic–left ventricular gradients? Atrial contraction increases left ventricular–end-diastolic volume and results in increased peak left ventricular pressure, as well as the aortic pressure. Beat #2 is a junctional beat (no P wave) without atrial contraction. Beat #3 is a normal sinus beat (P wave on the electrocardiographic tracing) and an A wave is visible on the left ventricular pressure. The atrial contribution to left ventricular filling increases the aortic pressure by approximately 25% (for aortic pressure from 134 mm Hg to 160 mm Hg and for left ventricular pressure from 190 mm Hg to 220 mm Hg). In the full cycle beat (#3), the valve area calculation, however, does not change appreciably, since both the left ventricular pressure and the aortic pressure increase together. A post-extrasystolic beat with an augmented filling period also has a marked increase in the left ventricular systolic pressure with no change or a slight increase in the aortic pressure. In view of the junctional beat and its hemodynamics, it would

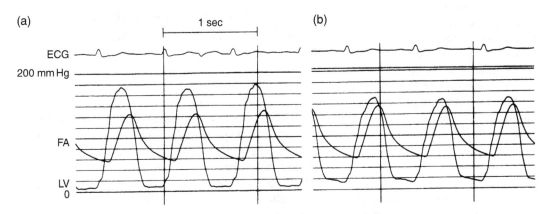

Figure 6.15 Simultaneous femoral artery (FA) and left ventricular (LV) pressure tracings (0–200 mm Hg scale) in a patient with systolic murmur. (a) before catheter movement, (b) after catheter movement. (see text for description)

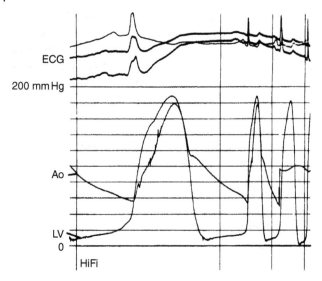

Figure 6.16 Simultaneous measurements of aortic (Ao) and left ventricular (LV) pressures (0–200 mm Hg scale) in a patient with hypertension.

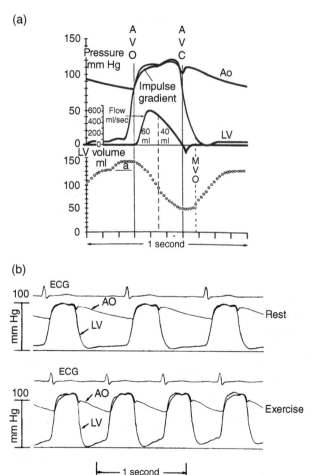

Figure 6.17 (a) Impulse-type gradient in a normal left ventricle. Left ventricular (LV) and aortic (Ao) pressures, aortic outflow, and ventricular volumes are displayed. Solid vertical lines indicate aortic valve opening (AVO) and aortic valve closure (AVC). Dashed lines indicate midpoint of systole and mitral valve opening (MVO). a = atrial contribution to ventricular filling. (b) Representative aortic (AO) and left ventricular (LV) micromanometer pressures at rest and during exercise in normal human left ventricle. An impulse gradient can be seen during exercise. *Source:* Pasipoularides 1990 [15]. Reproduced with permission of Elsevier.

be unlikely if this patient decompensated in atrial fibrillation if the ventricular response could be controlled.

One of the most precise hemodynamic methods of measuring aortic valvular gradients was used in a 55-year-old woman with a systolic murmur and longstanding hypertension (Figure 6.16). An 8 F dual-micromanometer-tipped catheter with two miniaturized pressure transducers separated by approximately 5–7 cm was inserted across the aortic valve. The precisely defined upstroke of both the aortic and left ventricular pressures accurately demonstrates an early pressure gradient of minimal aortic stenosis. The upstroke of aortic pressure with a high frequency vibration coincides precisely with the left ventricular pressure upstroke during ejection of blood from the left ventricle. Simultaneous high-fidelity pressures may detect the early systolic gradients of an "impulse type" [13] (Figure 6.17a), which may be normal in many younger patients with vigorous hearts, especially during high flow states such as exercise [14, 15] (Figure 6.17b). The peak-to-peak gradient on Figure 6.16 is obviously much smaller than the mean or peak instantaneous gradient.

The peak instantaneous gradient is more difficult to obtain from the hemodynamic data alone, but occurs early in ejection (Figure 6.16, just after the J point of the electrocardiogram, well before the peak pressure) and is the maximal distance (pressure) between left ventricular and aortic pressures [16]. This value is most easily obtained by Doppler techniques and correlates with aortic valve planimetered areas [17]. Peak instantaneous gradients can be estimated as planimetered mean gradient/0.70 [17]. Similarly, the mean planimetered gradient can be estimated as 0.71 × peak-to-peak gradient + 17 mm Hg [17].

Aortic Stenosis with Low Aortic–Left Ventricular Gradients and Low Aortic Flow

A continuing dilemma exists in patients with low cardiac output and small aortic–left ventricular gradients (e.g., the patient with dyspnea, poor left ventricular function, and a 20 mm Hg aortic–left ventricular gradient, with cardiac output of 3 L/min; aortic valve area = 0.7 cm^2). Should this valve be replaced with a prosthetic valve which has an intrinsic gradient of 10–20 mm Hg? As Carabello [18] discusses, the Gorlin formula for aortic valve area calculations uses an empiric constant (K) which now must be considered a variable under low-flow

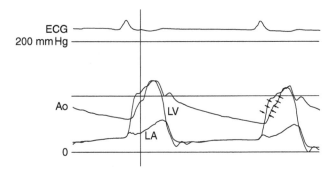

Figure 6.18 Aortic (Ao) and left ventricular (LV) pressure tracings in a patient with an intrinsic "impulse-type" aortic valve gradient (arrow). Left atrial (LA) pressure was obtained through a sheath.

conditions. Although some laboratories attempt to increase cardiac output and reassess gradients (and valve areas) under low- and high-flow states, there are no data indicating that augmented cardiac output calculations are better than those at rest.

A 62-year-old man underwent cardiac catheterization five years after implantation of a prosthetic mechanical aortic valve. On examination of the hemodynamic tracings (Figure 6.18), a small (and predominantly early) systolic left ventricular–aortic gradient is apparent. Cardiac output is 4.0 L/min. One can appreciate the intrinsic "impulse-type" left ventricular–aortic gradient and clinical limitations of a tilting disc prosthesis in patients with small gradients of the aortic valve. This gradient occurs in a well-functioning valve and has no significant pathologic implications. Dyspnea was due to development of new mitral regurgitation (V wave on left atrial pressure).

Aortic Regurgitation Complicating Aortic Stenosis

Hemodynamic characteristics consistent with chronic aortic regurgitation may only include wide pulse pressure. A wide pulse pressure can commonly be seen during a long cardiac cycle (Figure 6.19). The aortic diastolic pressure declines toward left ventricular pressure so that at the end of diastole (45 mm Hg), the pulse pressure is 70 mm Hg. This wide pulse pressure is consistent with aortic insufficiency, but can also be due to bradycardia alone in patients with noncompliant vascular beds (e.g., systolic hypertension) without aortic regurgitation. The slow heart rate (60 bpm) is indicated by the long RR interval.

Hemodynamic Artifacts of Aortic and Left Ventricular Pressures

Whenever fluid-filled systems are used, artifacts from the transducer chambers, catheters, pressure tubing, or manifolds may confound waveform analysis. The tracing on

Figure 6.20 demonstrates a prominent high-frequency "overshoot" of the left ventricular tracing in early systole and a marked overshoot on the early diastolic portion. The overshoot is characteristically called "ringing," representing the resonating frequency of the pressure system. The tracing on the right is obtained after manipulation of the fluid-filled system. What artifact produced the overshoot? The left-hand tracing is characteristic of an underdamped (i.e., too much ringing) fluid-filled system with a bubble in the fluid line to the transducer. On flushing the bubble, the system now shows the normal, correctly damped, resonant pattern of left ventricular pressure.

Examine the left ventricular pressure tracing on Figure 6.21. The pressure waveform on the left was obtained through the pigtail catheter immediately after contrast ventriculography. There is no evidence of ringing as shown earlier. The waveform is slightly rounded. After flushing the catheter, the continuous tracing to the right shows the ringing artifact. What conditions explain this transition in pressure waveform? The contrast media in the catheter remaining after ventriculography has a higher viscosity than saline, thus damps the system. On flushing the catheter through with saline, the underdamped ringing pattern of the left ventricular pressure appears. When using fluid-filled systems and these pressure tracings, assess the degree of ringing that is acceptable. Flush the catheter to purge bubbles or, if needed, instill contrast media to provide a higher-quality pressure signal for more accurate interpretation of the waveforms.

Peripheral Arterial Wave Summation and Zero Drift

Whenever using the femoral artery pressure to assess aortic valve gradients, always match pressures in both transducers prior to obtaining aortic–left ventricular gradients. Zero alignment of both systems and simultaneous pressure recording (both phasic and mean) with a zero-position check against transducer drift from baseline after recording will insure accuracy. A discrepancy should be reconciled or the transducers changed.

Femoral and central aortic pressures were measured in a 30-year-old woman (Figure 6.22). A pressure difference was evident, with significantly lower femoral artery pressure (left panel). (Remember that the later upstroke of the pressure wave marks the more distal location.) To reconcile these differences, carefully flush both systems (catheters, manifolds, transducers, zero lines) with special attention to the arterial sheath. After flushing (right panel), the tracings were more closely matched and were used for hemodynamics. Note that the femoral artery (A′) is now higher than central aortic (A) pressure, despite underdamped waveforms.

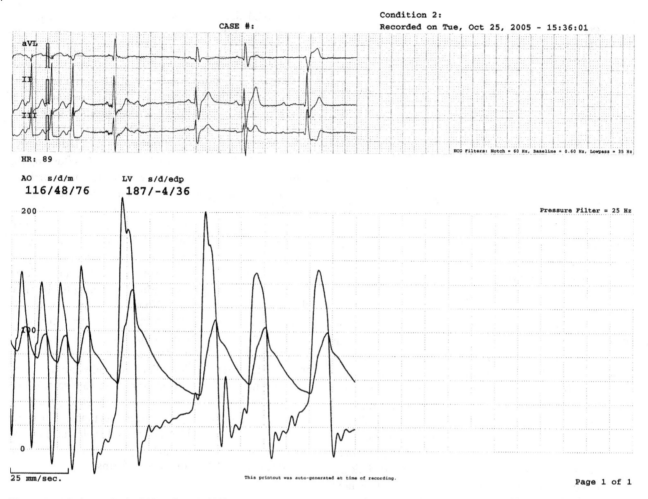

Figure 6.19 Left ventricular (LV) and aortic (AO) pressure tracing in patient with aortic stenosis and aortic insufficiency. After a period of supraventricular tachycardia, beat #5 demonstrates an increased pressure gradient with a peak-to-peak difference of 65 mm HG with a long diastolic phase. There is an equilibration of left ventricular end diastolic pressure with aortic pressure. This wide pulse pressure is consistent with aortic insufficiency.

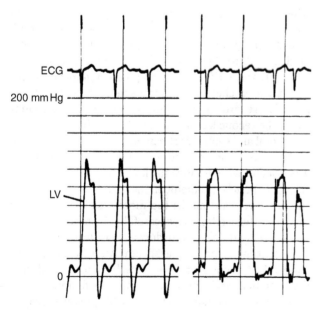

Figure 6.20 Left ventricular (LV) pressure tracings before (left) and after (right) pressure system manipulation.

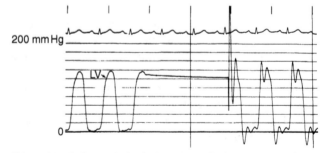

Figure 6.21 Left ventricular (LV) pressure after ventriculography.

Although matching of pressures at the beginning of the study is precise, some transducers may drift from zero. Figure 6.23 (top) shows matched femoral artery–aortic pressures. Femoral artery pressure did not match left ventricular pressure during simultaneous measurements (first and second lower panels). Reflushing after initial pressures produced satisfactory measurements, with both pressures returning to zero (right edge, bottom middle panel). However, on pullback a drift of femoral

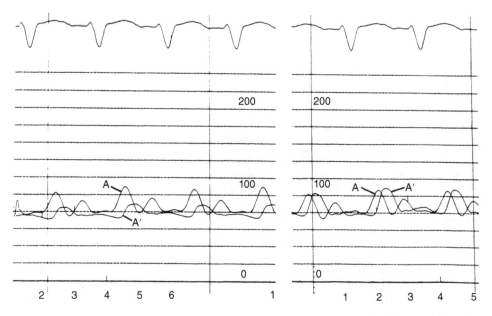

Figure 6.22 Simultaneous central aortic pressure measurement (A) with pigtail catheter and femoral artery sheath (A′). Zero pressures ("checks") are the same. Note differences in delay and overshoot of femoral artery tracing.

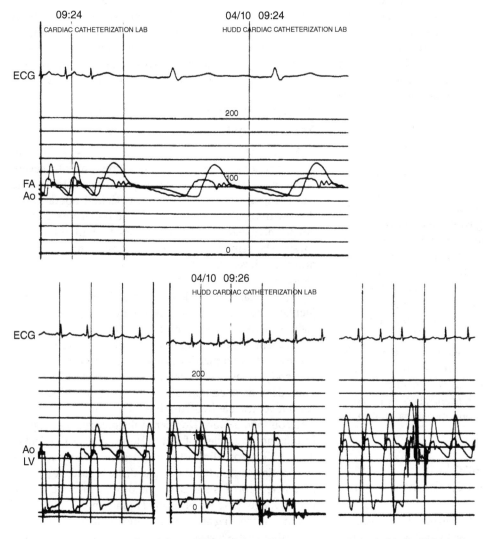

Figure 6.23 Simultaneous femoral artery (FA) and aortic (Ao) pressures measured with the 5F femoral artery sheath and 7F pigtail catheter before crossing the aortic valve (top panel). Note the delay in femoral artery pressure and marked overshoot of the peripheral pressure. Both zero and mean pressures were matched. (Lower panel, left) Aortic pressure markedly higher than left ventricular pressure. Re-zero indicated zero drift of the transducer. (Middle panel) Matching of left ventricular and aortic pressures, both zeros are now again correct (last beat, right-hand side of middle panel). Prior to pullback from left ventricle to aorta, there is again drift of the aortic pressure, and on pullback the disparity between peripheral arterial pressure and aortic pressure can be seen. This is an example of a drifting and faulty transducer.

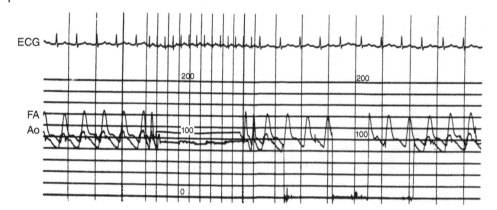

Figure 6.24 Simultaneous SF femoral artery (FA) sheath pressure and central aortic (Ao) pressure measured through a 7F pigtail catheter. The disparity between pressures is evident on both phasic and mean differences of pressure, despite an accurate "zero" of both transducers. The disparity remained after recalibration. This tracing demonstrates the differences in sensitivity of pressures due to a faulty transducer, which was replaced.

artery pressure (last panel, bottom) was again evident due to a faulty transducer and zero baseline drift.

Femoral or peripheral arterial pressure is not, and usually should not be, equal to central aortic pressure. The overshoot of femoral artery pressure is due to summation of the pressure wave reflections generated by the expansion and recoil characteristics of the central aortic and large artery elasticity. The peripheral or femoral artery pressure is almost always higher than the central aortic pressure.

Unequal sensitivity of transducers may cause differences in femoral artery–aortic pressures (Figure 6.24). Despite precise zeros, the femoral artery–aortic pressures could not be matched. Recalibrate both transducers with a mercury manometer as a standard to identify a faulty transducer.

A damped arterial sheath pressure can be due to (i) pressure artifact with damping within the sheath; (ii) significant arterial disease with aortic coarctation or iliac or femoral arterial disease; or (iii) inadequate pressure transmission outside the sheath. In this patient with peripheral vascular disease and no clinical or echocardiographic signs of aortic stenosis other than an ejection murmur, a second arterial catheter insertion was not performed. Reflushing the sheath rectified the problem.

However, if there is a major discrepancy between the femoral artery and central aortic pressure tracings after all steps to insure good pressures are taken, introduction of a second arterial catheter to the central aortic position for precise transvalvular gradient measures should be performed.

Prosthetic Aortic Valve and Left Ventricular Outflow Tract Gradients

Determining the significance of a higher than expected pressure gradient measured across an aortic valve prosthesis is challenging. Certain diagnoses, such as prosthetic valve dysfunction, severe aortic regurgitation, and severe prosthesis–patient mismatch, may necessitate a high-risk intervention or surgery. In contrast, some situations resulting in a high, noninvasively measured gradient do not require valve surgery. These include the presence of high-flow states or intrinsic artifacts of noninvasive testing leading to overestimation of the gradient [19–23].

Case Examples of Hemodynamics across a Prosthetic Aortic Valve

A 68-year-old woman with coronary bypass surgery in 1991 developed heart failure symptoms due to severe aortic valve stenosis with aneurysmal dilatation of the ascending aorta. She underwent a second operation in 2004 with repair of the aneurysm and replacement of the aortic valve using a 23 mm Hancock II stented bioprosthesis. She remained mildly symptomatic for two years and then developed progressive and severe dyspnea on exertion with atypical chest pain.

On physical examination, she was obese, with elevated jugular venous pressure and clear lung fields, a prominent right ventricular heave, a normal S1, and a loud pulmonic component of the second heart sound, with a crescendo–decrescendo, mid-peaking systolic murmur over the aortic area and no diastolic murmur. A transthoracic echocardiogram demonstrated normal systolic function with concentric left ventricular hypertrophy and a normal mitral valve. The continuous-wave Doppler evaluation revealed a peak instantaneous gradient of 55 mm Hg and a mean gradient of 32 mm Hg across the aortic prosthesis. These values were substantially higher than anticipated; the reported expected parameters for this size and type of valve include a peak instantaneous gradient of 25 mm Hg and a mean gradient of 17 mm Hg, yielding an effective orifice area of 1.4 cm^2 [24].

Cardiac catheterization was performed to exclude prosthetic valve dysfunction as a cause of the patient's symptoms and abnormally elevated transvalvular gradient. Hemodynamic findings are summarized in Table 6.3, with right heart pressures documenting severe pulmonary hypertension and elevated pulmonary vascular resistance (6.6 Woods units). The aortic prosthesis was crossed using a 0.035" straight wire followed by a dual-lumen 6 F catheter. Simultaneous left ventricular and aortic pressures were recorded (Figure 6.25). A 25 mm Hg peak-to-peak and 28 mm Hg mean gradient were observed. The effective orifice area using Gorlin's equation was calculated as 1.08 cm^2; indexed to body surface area, the effective orifice area index was 0.53 cm^2/m^2.

Aortography showed no regurgitation and left ventriculography confirmed normal left ventricular function. Coronary angiography showed no luminal obstruction except for severe proximal disease of the left anterior descending artery, which was bypassed with a widely patent left internal mammary artery graft. In light of these findings, the prosthetic valve appeared to be functioning normally and the patient's symptoms were attributed to a combination of severe pulmonary hypertension

Table 6.3 Hemodynamic findings, Case #1.

Chamber	Pressure (in mm Hg)
Right atrium	a = 17, v = 16, mean = 13
Right ventricle	83/17
Pulmonary artery	83/28, mean = 50
Pulmonary capillary wedge	a = 22, v = 20, mean = 18
Aorta	138/64, mean = 93
Left ventricle	163/18
Thermodilution cardiac output = 4.87 L/min	

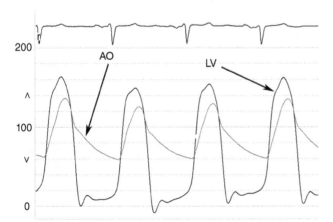

Figure 6.25 Simultaneous left ventricular (LV) and aortic (AO) pressures obtained from the patient in Case #1 using a dual-lumen pigtail catheter. demonstrating a 25 mm Hg peak-to-peak systolic gradient across a bioprosthetic aortic valve.

and prosthesis–patient mismatch. The patient declined consideration for a third surgical procedure. An exhaustive search for the cause of her pulmonary hypertension was unrevealing and she was prescribed medical therapy with sildenafil, with some symptomatic improvement.

Another example of LVOT gradients across a prosthetic aortic valve is demonstrated by a 60-year-old man with a type I aortic dissection repaired at an outside hospital in 2002 with valve-sparing surgery and a Dacron prosthetic graft. He developed congestive heart failure four years later and was found to have severe aortic regurgitation and depressed left ventricular function. He underwent aortic valve replacement with a 21 mm St. Jude bileaflet aortic valve early in 2006. Several months postoperatively, he again developed congestive heart failure. A transthoracic echocardiogram demonstrated moderate, global left ventricular systolic dysfunction, with an ejection fraction of 35–40%. The aortic prosthesis appeared to function normally, but continuous-wave Doppler interrogation recorded a peak instantaneous gradient of 80 mm Hg and a mean gradient of 50 mm Hg. He was treated with diuretics and an angiotensin receptor blocker, with improvement in symptoms. Transthoracic echocardiograms obtained during the follow-up period showed improvement in left ventricular function with an estimated ejection fraction of 50–55%, but persistently elevated peak instantaneous gradients by continuous-wave Doppler measuring 80–90 mm Hg and mean gradients of 50–60 mm Hg with no evidence of aortic regurgitation.

The patient again presented with increasing shortness of breath. On physical examination, he was an obese man with normal jugular venous pressure and clear lungs, normal prosthetic closing clicks, a harsh, mid-to-late-peaking crescendo–decrescendo systolic murmur over the aortic area, and no diastolic murmur. It was believed that the marked transvalvular gradient noted on echocardiography was due to severe patient–prosthesis mismatch and he was referred for cardiac catheterization prior to consideration for repeat aortic valve surgery.

Fluoroscopic examination of the St. Jude aortic prosthesis confirmed normal opening and closing and aortography showed no regurgitation. A radiolucent ridge appeared at the distal end of the aortic prosthesis (Figure 6.26). Right-heart pressures are presented in Table 6.4. A right-heart and transseptal catheterization was performed, both to assess the transvalvular hemodynamics and to perform left ventriculography. Simultaneous left ventricular pressure (via a transseptal approach) and aortic pressure was obtained and confirmed a peak-to-peak systolic gradient of 60 mm Hg and a mean pressure of 49 mm Hg (Figure 6.27). The aortic pressure waveform exhibited a delayed upstroke consistent with severe obstruction. The operator noted that this recording of aortic pressure was

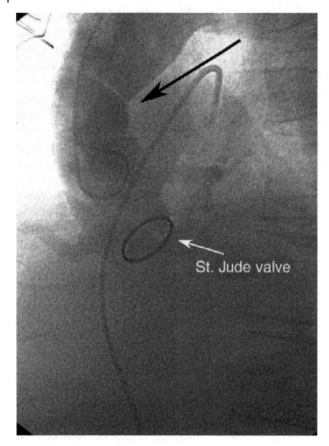

Figure 6.26 Left anterior oblique aortogram from case #2. A radiolucent ridge can be seen at the distal end of the aortic conduit (arrow).

Table 6.4 Hemodynamic findings, Case #2.

Chamber	Pressure (in mm Hg)
Right atrium	a = 13, v = 13, mean = 8
Right ventricle	36/11
Pulmonary artery	36/19, mean = 26
Pulmonary capillary wedge	a = 14, v = 12, mean = 11
Aorta	118/67, mean = 87
Left ventricle	187/15
Thermodilution cardiac output = 9.48 L/min	

obtained with the pigtail catheter high in the arch of the aorta and distal to the radiolucent ridge. The aortic pigtail catheter was repositioned 2 cm above the aortic prosthetic valve. At this location, the upstroke of the aortic waveform appeared to be less delayed and the left ventricular–aortic pressure gradient was smaller (peak-to-peak systolic gradient of 38 mm Hg and mean of 36 mm Hg; Figure 6.28). The effective orifice area using Gorlin's equation on this set of pressures was calculated as 1.52 cm^2; indexed to

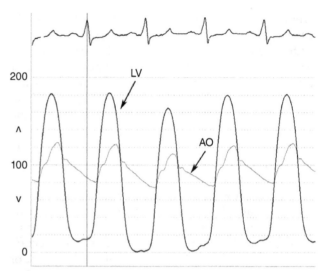

Figure 6.27 Simultaneous left ventricular (LV) and aortic (AO) pressure obtained from the patient in Case #2. The left ventricular pressure was obtained via a transseptal approach; the aortic pressure was obtained from a pigtail catheter placed at about the aortic arch. Note the delayed upstroke of the aortic pressure wave and the large (60 mmHg peak to peak) transvalvular gradient.

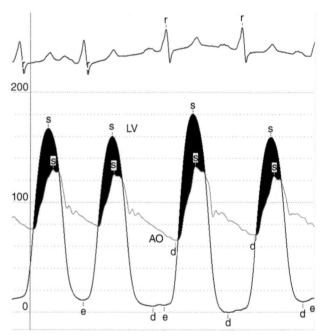

Figure 6.28 Simultaneous left ventricular (LV) and aortic (AO) pressures obtained as described in Figure 6.27. The pigtail catheter was positioned 2 cm above the aortic prosthesis in the ascending aorta. Note that the aortic pressure wave is not as delayed as the one shown in Figure 6.27 and the transvalvular gradient is lower (average of 38 mm Hg peak to peak).

body surface area, the effective orifice area index was 0.59 cm^2/m^2. A dual-lumen multipurpose catheter was then positioned in the ascending aorta, with the distal tip placed above the valve and the proximal port just distal to the radiolucent ridge seen on the aortogram. Simultaneous

(a)

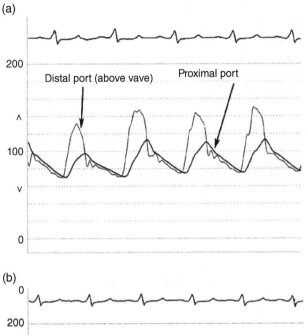

(b)

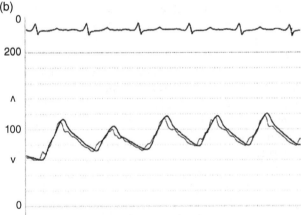

Figure 6.29 (a) Pressure obtained in the ascending aorta with a dual-lumen multipurpose catheter. The distal port of the catheter recorded pressure in the aorta directly above the aortic valve prosthesis (arrow); the proximal port recorded pressure at the arch of the aorta just distal to the translucent ridge. A 30 mm Hg gradient was noted across this ridge. (b) The catheter tip was pulled back distally, confirming equal pressures from both lumens of the catheter.

aortic pressure recording from these two locations confirmed supravalvular aortic stenosis with a 30 mm Hg peak systolic gradient within the ascending aorta (Figure 6.29). Based on these findings, optimal relief of outflow tract obstruction would necessitate not only a repeat aortic valve replacement using a larger prosthesis, but also surgical repair of the acquired supravalvular aortic stenosis, a procedure with a much greater surgical risk.

Prosthetic Valve Hemodynamics: Invasive versus Noninvasive Methods

Following valve surgery, the function of a prosthetic valve is usually assessed noninvasively by Doppler echocardiography. Normally functioning prosthetic valves obstruct blood flow to some degree, usually

resulting in a transvalvular gradient. In addition, there may be high-velocity jets around the complex orifices associated with some prostheses, resulting in turbulence and localized gradients. The challenge facing a clinician lies in determining whether the observed Doppler gradient is entirely normal and represents a well-functioning prosthesis, or is due to prosthetic valve malfunction.

In general, Doppler gradients across aortic prosthetic valves exceed catheter gradients, particularly in St. Jude valves [19–23]. This was clearly observed in both cases presented above. In addition to the fact that catheter techniques report gradients differently than Doppler techniques (i.e., peak-to-peak versus peak instantaneous gradients), Doppler measurements are higher than catheter gradients primarily because of the phenomenon of pressure recovery, not because Doppler techniques are erroneous [20]. It is important to note that for both Doppler and a catheter-based technique, the magnitude of the gradient depends not only on the type and size of the prosthetic valve, but also on the flow across the valve. Therefore, although there are published "normal values" for Doppler indices of prosthetic valve function based on the type and size of the prosthesis [24], these data may not reconcile with an individual patient existing at either extreme of blood flow across the valve. The flow across the valve is not known when Doppler methods are employed, but is readily available during invasive techniques.

Invasive interrogation of a prosthetic valve offers greater accuracy, but requires several considerations. As exemplified by patient #1, a bioprosthetic aortic valve (but not mechanical) can be crossed with a catheter and the transvalvular pressure gradient assessed similar to a native aortic valve. A mechanical prosthesis should not be crossed with a catheter, since entrapment or severe regurgitation may result, with catastrophic consequences [25]. Alternative catheterization techniques involve the placement of a catheter in the aorta above the valve and another catheter in the left ventricle via a transseptal catheterization. Direct apical puncture is another method of accessing the left ventricle, used exclusively when there is also a mechanical valve in the mitral position [26]. A recently described, easy, and safe method to measure left ventricular pressure in the presence of a mechanical aortic valve involves the use of a pressure wire [27, 28]. This method has been used with great success in the cardiac catheterization laboratory to assess many different mechanical aortic valves, including the Starr–Edwards valve, and both single and bileaflet tilting disc valves. The main limitation of this technique is that it does not allow for ventriculography; for this reason, a transseptal catheterization was chosen for patient #2 instead of the pressure-wire technique.

Prosthesis–Patient Mismatch

A prosthetic valve too small for an individual patient may function entirely normally yet cause substantial obstruction. The term "prosthesis–patient mismatch" was coined to describe this phenomenon and is generally defined as present when "the effective prosthetic valve area, after insertion into the patient, is less than that of a normal human valve" [29]. More precise definitions of prosthesis–patient mismatch have been recently offered [30, 31]. These are based on indexed orifice areas which take into account the patient's body surface area. Since at least moderate aortic stenosis is present in a native valve if the indexed orifice area is $\leq 0.90 \, cm^2/m^2$, the indexed orifice area of a prosthetic valve should be no less than $0.85–0.90 \, cm^2/m^2$ [30]. Accordingly, severe prosthesis–patient mismatch is present when the indexed effective orifice area of a prosthesis is $\leq 0.60 \, cm^2/m^2$, moderate mismatch is present when the indexed effective orifice area is between 0.60 and $0.85 \, cm^2/m^2$, and no significant mismatch is present if the index effective orifice area is $> 0.85 \, cm^2/m^2$. When these criteria are used, the presence of severe prosthesis–patient mismatch has been shown to be an independent predictor of adverse outcome [32].

In both cases presented, catheterization was performed to exclude prosthetic valve dysfunction. In patient #1, the bioprosthesis was without regurgitation and it is unlikely that a 2-year-old tissue valve would develop significant stenosis. By catheterization data, the indexed effective orifice area of $0.53 \, cm^2/m^2$ is consistent with severe prosthesis–patient mismatch. Similarly, in patient #2, the mechanical prosthesis had normal opening and closing characteristics on fluoroscopy and no regurgitation. Using the gradient obtained with the aortic catheter directly above the prosthetic valve, the indexed effective orifice area was $0.59 \, cm^2/m^2$, which is also consistent with severe prosthesis–patient mismatch. Both patients presented were significantly obese and thus received valves too small for their body habitus. Re-operation was deemed to be of excessive risk in both cases, which emphasizes the importance of choosing the largest valve possible at the time of valve replacement surgery to avoid prosthesis–patient mismatch and the dreaded prospect of another operation.

Other Sources of a Transvalvular Gradient

In addition to prosthetic valve dysfunction or prosthesis–patient mismatch, there are other sources of a transvalvular gradient that need to be explored. High-flow states associated with anemia, thyrotoxicosis, or fever may result in high gradients. Similarly, it is important to exclude the presence of severe aortic regurgitation. An unusual finding in patient #2 was the presence of a gradient within the ascending aorta due to a ridge of tissue or kink in the conduit. This "acquired supravalvular aortic stenosis" is probably very rare, although the actual incidence of this finding is difficult to glean from the literature. It has been reported at least one other time in a patient after aortic surgery [33], and has been observed as a consequence of an aortic dissection and after surgery for congenital heart disease and heart transplantation [34–36]. In the case presented, the degree of obstruction by itself was not severe; however, it contributed to the gradient due to prosthesis–patient mismatch, so that, in summation, a substantial degree of outflow tract obstruction existed. Importantly, an aortic valve replacement alone with a larger prosthesis in this case would not have rectified all the outflow tract obstruction and would have provided little patient benefit.

Another important lesson from this case lies in the fact that the diagnosis of acquired supravalvular stenosis might have been missed if the operator had not been attentive to the careful collection of hemodynamic data. One of the important tenets of catheterization states that the most accurate method of measuring a transvalvular gradient requires simultaneous pressure measurement with a catheter positioned directly above and below the valve. In patient #2, the aortic catheter was inadvertently positioned in the arch of the aorta. Had this improper catheter position been overlooked, the large observed pressure gradient would have been attributed solely to the prosthetic valve; the supravalvular stenosis would have gone undetected and the patient may have had an inappropriate surgery.

Key Points

1) The approach to the patient with the stenotic aortic valve should remain highly individualized, dependent upon the specific clinical symptoms and comorbidities of the patient as well as the expertise of the catheterization operator.
2) Regardless of the method used to interrogate the aortic valve gradient (invasive or noninvasive), similar principles are involved in understanding the pathophysiology represented by the gradient.
3) Care must be taken to insure that the sources of error that are common in assessing this gradient do not lead to improper patient decision-making.

References

1 Pibarot P, Dumesnil JG. Improving assessment of aortic stenosis. *J Am Coll Cardiol* 60:169–180, 2012.

2 Otto CM. Valvular aortic stenosis: Disease severity and timing of intervention. *J Am Coll Cardiol* 47: 2141–2151, 2006.

3 Currie PJ, Seward JB, Reeder GS, Vlietstra RE, Bresnahan DR, Bresnahan JF, Smith HC, Hagler DJ, Tajik AJ. Continuous-wave Doppler echocardiographic assessment of severity of calcific aortic stenosis: A simultaneous Doppler-catheter correlative study in 100 adult patients. *Circulation* 71:1162–1169, 1985.

4 Kern M, Deligonul U. The stenotic aortic valve. In MJ Kern (eds), *Hemodynamic Rounds*, 2nd ed. New York: Wiley-Liss, 1997, Chapter 3.

5 Assey ME, Zile MR, Usher BW, Karavan MP, Carabello BA. Effect of catheter position on the variability of measured gradient in aortic stenosis. *Cathet Cardiovasc Diagn* 30:287–292, 1993.

6 Brogan WC, Lange RA, Hillis LD. Accuracy of various methods of measuring the transvalvular pressure gradient in aortic stenosis. *Am Heart J* 123:948–953, 1992.

7 Gorlin R, Gorlin SG. Hydraulic formula for calculation of the area of the stenotic mitral valve, other cardiac valves, and central circulatory shunts. *Am Heart J* 41:1–29, 1951.

8 Kern MJ, Serajja P, Lim, MJ. *The Cardiac Catheterization Handbook*, 4th ed. St. Louis: Mosby-Year Book, 2003.

9 Hakki AH, Iskandrian AS, Bemis CE, Kimbiris D, Mintz GS, Segal BL, Brice C. A simplified valve formula for the calculation of stenotic cardiac valve areas. *Circulation* 63:1050, 1981.

10 Grayburn PA. Assessment of low-gradient aortic stenosis with dobutamine. *Circulation* 113:604–606, 2006.

11 Nishimura RA, Otto CM, Bonow RO, Carabello BA, Erwin JP III, Fleisher LA, *et al.* 2017 AHA/ACC/AHA 2006 focused update of the 2014 AHA/ACC Guideline for the Management of Patients with Valvular Heart Disease: A report of the American College of Cardiology/American Heart Association Task Force on Clinical Practice Guidelines for the management of patients with valvular heart disease. *Circulation* 135:e1159–e1195, 2017.

12 Lorell BH, Paulus WJ, Grossman W, Wynne J, Cohn PF, Braunwald E. Improved diastolic function and systolic performance in hypertrophic cardiomyopathy after nifedipine. *N Engl J Med* 303:801803, 1980.

13 Criley JM, Siegel RI. Has "obstruction" hindered our understanding of hypertrophic cardiomyopathy? *Circulation* 72:1148–1154, 1985.

14 Murgo JP, Altobelli SA, Dorethy JF, Logdson JR, McGranahan GM. Left ventricular ejection dynamics in man during rest and exercise. *Am Heart Assoc Monogr* 46:92, 1975.

15 Pasipoularides A. Clinical assessment of ventricular ejection dynamics with and without outflow obstruction. *J Am Coll Cardiol* 15:859–882, 1990.

16 Oh JK, Taliercio CP, Holmes DR Jr, Reeder GS, Bailey KR, Seward JB, Tajik AJ. Prediction of the severity of aortic stenosis by Doppler aortic valve area determination: Prospective Doppler catheterization correlation in 100 patients. *J Am Coll Cardiol* 11:1227–1234, 1988.

17 Gordon IB, Folland ED. Analysis of aortic valve gradients by transseptal technique: Implications for noninvasive evaluation. *Cathet Cardiovasc Diagn* 17:144–151, 1989.

18 Carabello BA, Barry WH, Grossman WG. Changes in arterial pressure during left heart pullback in patients with aortic stenosis: A sign of severe aortic stenosis. *Am J Cardiol* 44:424–427, 1979.

19 Rothbart RM, Smucker ML, Gibson RS. Overestimation by Doppler echocardiography of pressure gradients across Starr–Edwards prosthetic valves in the aortic position. *Am J Cardiol* 61: 475–476, 1988.

20 Baumgartner H, Khan S, DeRobertis M, Czer L, Maurer G. Discrepancies between Doppler and catheter gradients in aortic prosthetic valves in vitro: A manifestation of localized gradients and pressure recovery. *Circulation* 82:1467–1475, 1990.

21 Laske A, Jenni R, Maloigne M, Vassalli G, Bertel O, Turina MI. Pressure gradients across bileaflet aortic valves by direct measurement and echocardiography. *Ann Thorac Surg* 61:48–57, 1996.

22 Bech-Hanssen O, Gjertsson P, Houltz E, Wranne B, Ask P, Loyd D, Caidahl K. Net pressure gradients in aortic prosthetic valves can be estimated by Doppler. *J Am Soc Echocardiogr* 16:858–866, 2003.

23 Bech-Hanssen O, Caidahl K, Wallentin I, Ask P, Wranne B. Assessment of effective orifice area of prosthetic aortic valves with Doppler echocardiography: An in vivo and in vitro study. *J Thorac Cardiovasc Surg* 122:287–295, 2001.

24 Rosenhek R, Binder T, Maurer G, Baumgartner H. Normal values for Doppler echocardiographic assessment of heart valve prostheses. *J Am Soc Echocardiogr* 16:1116–1127, 2003.

25 Kober G, Hilgermann R. Catheter entrapment in a Bjork–Shiley prosthesis in aortic position. *Cathet Cardiovasc Diagn* 13:262–265, 1987.

26 Walters DL, Sanchez PL, Rodriguez-Alemparte M, Colon-Hernandez PJ, Hourigan LA, Palacios IF. Transthoracic left ventricular puncture for the assessment of patients with aortic and mitral valve prostheses: The Massachusetts General Hospital Experience, 1989–2000. *Cathet Cardiovasc Intervent* 58:539–544, 2003.

27 Parham W, Shafei AE, Rajjoub H, Ziaee A, Kern MJ. Retrograde left ventricular hemodynamic assessment across bileaflet prosthetic aortic valves: The use of a high-fidelity pressure sensor angioplasty guidewire. *Cathet Cardiovasc Intervent* 59:509–513, 2003.

28 Doorey AJ, Gakhal M, Pasquale MJ. Utilization of a pressure sensor guidewire to measure bileaflet mechanical valve gradients: Hemodynamic and echocardiographic sequelae. *Cathet Cardiovasc Intervent* 67:535–540, 2006.

29 Rahimtoola SH. The problem of valve prosthesis–patient mismatch. *Circulation* 58:20–24, 1978.

30 Pibarot P, Dumesnil JG. Hemodynamic and clinical impact of prosthesis–patient mismatch in the aortic valve position and its prevention. *J Am Coll Cardiol* 36:1131–1141, 2000.

31 Pibarot P, Dumesnil JG. Prosthesis–patient mismatch: Definition, clinical impact and prevention. *Heart* 92:1022–1029, 2006.

32 Mohty-Echahidi D, Malouf JF, Girard SE, Schaff HV, Grill DE, Enriquez-Sarno ME, Miller FA. Impact of prosthesis–patient mismatch on long-term survival in patients with small St. Jude: Medical mechanical prostheses in the aortic position. *Circulation* 113:420–426, 2006.

33 Kern MJ, Aguirre FV, Guerrero M. Hemodynamic rounds series II: Abnormal hemodynamics after prosthetic aortic root reconstruction: Aortic stenosis or insufficiency? *Cathet Cardiovasc Diagn* 44:336–340, 1998.

34 Rose AG, Park SJ, Shumway SJ, Norton D, Miller LW. Acquired supravalvar aortic stenosis following heart transplantation: Report of 2 cases. *J Heart Lung Transplant* 21:499–502, 2002.

35 Vilacosta I, San Roman JA, Aragoncillo P, Ferreiros J, Mendez R, Graupner C, Stoermann, W, Batlle E, Baquero M. Supravalvular aortic stenosis in aortic dissection. *Am J Cardiol* 81:1271–1273, 1998.

36 Williams WG, Mathieu J, Culham GA, Trusler GA, Olley PM. Acquired supravalvular aortic stenosis. *Ann Thorac Surg* 27:335–339, 1979.

7

Aortic Regurgitation

Morton J. Kern and Michael J. Lim

Aortic regurgitation (AR) occurs when there is inadequate closure or malcoaptation of the aortic valve leaflets, allowing blood to enter the left ventricular cavity from the aorta during diastole. It is one of the most common valvular lesions encountered in the cardiac catheterization laboratory, with an estimated prevalence of approximately 10%. Patients with aortic regurgitation may present under dramatically different circumstances with, at times, confusing clinical findings and symptoms. Table 7.1 categorizes the general mechanisms and corresponding etiologies of aortic regurgitation. Depending on the primary cause and extent of disease of the aortic valve leaflets and/or aortic root, some patients may require only valve replacement, while others undergo a combined procedure replacing both the aortic root and the valve.

Angiographic and invasive hemodynamic evaluation of aortic regurgitation was the historical gold standard and is now supplanted by Doppler echocardiography, because the determination of the severity of aortic regurgitation is equal to and, at times, even more sensitive than angiographic and hemodynamic characteristics used for daily decision-making [1]. The hemodynamic alterations of aortic regurgitation form the basis for understanding the clinical, invasive, and echocardiographic manifestations of the disease and have practical applications to appreciating complications during transcatheter aortic valve replacement (TAVR).

Chronic Aortic Insufficiency

Etiology

The most common causes of chronic aortic insufficiency (AI) include the degeneration of congenital bicuspid valves and atherosclerotic aortic valve disease. Infective endocarditis is certainly a common cause of acute regurgitation, but also can be associated with the chronic form of the condition. With the advent of the prevention and treatment of rheumatic fever (and subsequent decline in rheumatic valve disease), connective tissue disorders such as Marfan's syndrome or Ehlers–Danlos syndrome, aortic valve prolapse, sinus of Valsalva aneurysm, and aortic annular fistula have become relatively more common. Other etiologies include inflammatory and vasculitic diseases (Takayasu's arteritis, ankylosing spondylitis, Reiter syndrome, rheumatoid arthritis, lupus, Bechet's disease), primary aortic root and ascending aorta abnormalities or infection, trauma associated with jet lesion such as sub-aortic stenosis, and those cases considered idiopathic.

Pathophysiology

The pathophysiology of aortic regurgitation hinges on complete systolic left ventricular (LV) emptying, with an increase in left ventricular end-diastolic volume providing the major hemodynamic compensatory mechanism [2]. To better appreciate the flow dynamics of aortic valvular disease, combined Doppler echocardiographic and hemodynamic data were obtained in a 72-year-old woman with mixed aortic stenosis and regurgitation (Figure 7.1). Simultaneous femoral artery and left ventricular pressures were patched into the Doppler echocardiographic recorder. Flow-velocity signals were recorded at the left ventricular outflow tract from the suprasternal notch. Aortic pressure is 130/50 mm Hg and left ventricular pressure 190/40 mm Hg. A significant 50 mm Hg aortic gradient remains when a 10 mm Hg femoral pressure overshoot (not shown) is considered. High systolic aortic flow (area marked by **), with peak velocities of 3.5 m/sec yielding a pressure gradient from Doppler calculations of 49 mm Hg [1], corresponds to the systolic aortic–left ventricular gradient. Equally striking are the continuous diastolic flow velocities (area marked by *) corresponding to the left ventricular–aortic diastolic gradient. The velocity slope (from the initial elevated peak diastolic velocity of 4 m/sec, which rapidly

Hemodynamic Rounds: Interpretation of Cardiac Pathophysiology from Pressure Waveform Analysis, Fourth Edition.
Edited by Morton J. Kern, Michael J. Lim, and James A. Goldstein.
© 2018 John Wiley & Sons Ltd. Published 2018 by John Wiley & Sons Ltd.

Table 7.1 Mechanisms and etiologies of aortic regurgitation.

Mechanism	Etiology
Cusp abnormality or perforation	Endocarditis
	Rheumatic or rheumatoid disease
	Ankylosing spondylitis
Aortic root dilatation with malcoaptation or aortic cusps	Ankylosing spondylitis
	Rheumatoid disease
	Syphilis
	Ehlers–Danlos
	Pseudoxanthomas elasticum
Lack of commissural support with malcoaptation of aortic cusps	Tetralogy of Fallot
	Ventricular septal defect
	Aortic dissection
	Aortitis
	Trauma

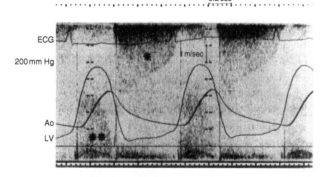

Figure 7.1 Combined echo-Doppler and hemodynamic study in a patient with mixed aortic valve disease. Aortic (Ao) and left ventricular (LV) pressures. Flow velocities were obtained with continuous mode Doppler from the left ventricular outflow tract. Scale marks for Doppler are 1 m/sec. Scale marks for pressure are 40 mm Hg per division. * = diastolic velocity integral; ** = systolic velocity integral. See text for details.

tapers to 1.5 m/sec at end-diastole) parallels the severity of the left ventricular–aortic gradient. The more rapid (>2 m/sec) the downslope of the diastolic flow velocity, the more severe the aortic regurgitation [3].

Severe aortic regurgitation can occur with normal effective forward flow and a normal ejection fraction coupled with elevated end-diastolic pressure and volume. With time, left ventricular dilation increases. The left ventricular systolic tension required to maintain the same pressure (or stress) also increases, as determined by

Laplace's law. The clinical course is then dependent on compensated left ventricular wall stress with replication of sarcomeres in series, stretching of myocardial fibers, and wall thickening sufficient to maintain systolic wall stress at a normal level [2, 4]. The ventricular thickness to cavity ratio remains normal (e.g., eccentric hypertrophy). This process occurs in distinction to that developing in aortic stenosis, in which replication of myocardial sarcomeres occurs in parallel with an increased ratio of wall thickness to cavity radius (e.g., concentric hypertrophy). Left ventricular mass in patients with aortic regurgitation is usually greatly elevated, exceeding values reported in isolated aortic stenosis [2].

The clinical course of aortic regurgitation involves left ventricular deterioration when the left ventricular end-diastolic volume (LVEDV) increases without further elevation of left ventricular ejection volume. The left ventricular end-diastolic radius to wall thickness ratio increases with increasing systolic tension and often with afterload mismatch, producing a decline in ejection fraction for any additional level of ventricular stress. Ultimately, left ventricular ejection fraction and forward stroke volume diminish, producing congestive symptomatology. The advance stages of decompensation of aortic regurgitation involve elevation of left atrial, pulmonary artery wedge, pulmonary arterial, right ventricular, and right atrial pressures with reduction of cardiac output. A proposed physiologic scheme for chronic aortic regurgitation as conceptualized by Borrow and Marcus [2] is depicted in Figure 7.2.

Regurgitation of blood from the aorta into the left ventricle results in an increase in left ventricular end-diastolic volume (preload). This is manifest by a rapid fall in measured central aortic diastolic pressure. LVEDV increases and, initially, there is an augmented stroke volume. Often, this creates an elevated systolic pressure and, when coupled with the reduced diastolic pressure, results in a substantial pulse pressure. Close examination of the left ventricular diastolic pressure will reveal a relatively flat slope and a prominent early A wave, which characterize mild regurgitation (Figure 7.3). Left ventricular end-diastolic pressure (LVEDP), left atrial pressure, and pulmonary capillary wedge pressure (PCWP) usually remain in the normal range during the early stages of chronic aortic insufficiency because of preserved LV wall diastolic compliance. As chronic LV overload leads to myocardial fibrosis, impaired compliance, and compromised contractility, the left ventricle begins to progressively decompensate [4, 5]. The clinical course is then dependent on compensated left ventricular wall stress with replication of sarcomeres in series, stretching of myocardial fibers, and wall thickening sufficient to maintain systolic wall stress at a normal level [1–4, 6, 7]. The ventricular thickness to cavity ratio remains normal

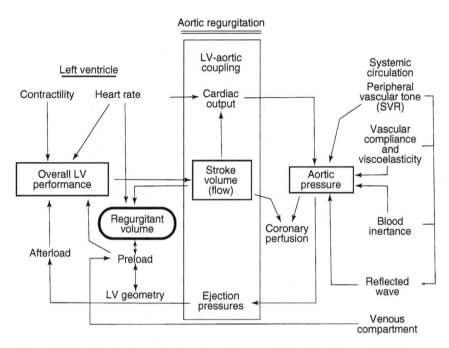

Figure 7.2 Physiologic scheme for chronic aortic regurgitation. LV = left ventricle; SVR = systemic vascular resistance.

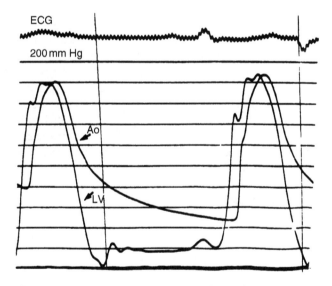

Figure 7.3 Hemodynamics in a patient with hypertension. LV = left ventricular pressure; Ao, aortic pressure. See text for details.

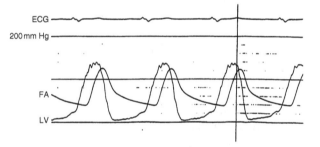

Figure 7.4 Femoral artery (FA) and left ventricular (LV) pressures in a patient with systolic and diastolic murmurs. See text for details.

(e.g., eccentric hypertrophy). This process occurs in distinction to that developing in aortic stenosis, in which replication of myocardial sarcomeres occurs in parallel with an increased ratio of wall thickness to cavity radius (e.g., concentric hypertrophy). Left ventricular mass in patients with aortic regurgitation is usually greatly elevated, exceeding values reported in isolated aortic stenosis [2].

The decompensated LV is marked by an elevated LV end-systolic volume, LV end-diastolic pressure, and ele-

vated pulmonary pressures as the progression of valvular incompetence exceeds the ability of the LV to remodel. The severity of aortic regurgitation can be estimated by evaluating the diastolic pressure difference between the aorta and left ventricle, with special attention to the slope of the ventricular diastolic waveform. As the LV diastolic pressure waveform increases its rate of rise, the regurgitation through the aortic valve is more severe, leading to earlier equalization of the aortic and ventricular pressures in diastole (Figure 7.4). The natural progression leads to progressive LV cavity dilatation, with a subsequent reduction in stroke volume and eventual signs and symptoms of heart failure and pulmonary edema. The natural history of this valvular lesion has also been well studied and is shown in Table 7.2.

Table 7.2 Natural history of aortic regurgitation.

Asymptomatic patient with normal LV systolic function	
Progression to symptomatic +/or LV dysfunction	<6%/yr
Progression to asymptomatic LV dysfunction	<3.5%/yr
Sudden death	<0.2%/yr
Asymptomatic patient with LV dysfunction	
Progression to symptoms	>25%/yr
Symptomatic patient	
Mortality rate	>10%/yr

LV = left ventricular.

Physical Findings

A decrescendo diastolic murmur can often be heard over the second through fourth left intercostal spaces (this may not be present in acute AR). This usually is heard best with the patient sitting or standing and leaning forward. A high-frequency early diastolic murmur primarily occurs in mild AR, whereas a harsh holo-diastolic or decrescendo diastolic murmur occurs more frequently in severe regurgitation. With careful auscultation in moderate or severe AR, a concomitant systolic ejection murmur caused by increased stroke volume and outflow can be heard. Less often, an apical diastolic rumble (Austin–Flint murmur) or an S3 (if there is LV dysfunction) is identified. Moreover, the apical impulse is found to be diffuse, hyperdynamic, and displaced inferolaterally. With advanced aortic valve disease and limited movement of the leaflets, S2 softens or disappears. Other signs and findings of severe chronic AR exist (Table 7.3).

Peripheral Pulse Amplification

The physical examination signs are a result of the hyperdynamic state of the arterial pressure wave, which is manifested more in the peripheral circulation rather than the proximal larger vessels, producing findings of peripheral arterial pressure amplification hemodynamically observed as the overshoot in femoral artery sheath pressure [7].

Peripheral arterial systolic pressure amplification may occur in any patient with high left ventricular ejection velocities. In aortic regurgitation, peak femoral artery systolic pressure may exceed central aortic pressure by 20–50 mm Hg. The mechanism of the arterial pressure amplification has been previously described as the result of the summation of pressure wave reflections returning from smaller peripheral arteries [7]. The use of central aortic pressure measurement for accurate computation of the hemodynamic findings,

Table 7.3 Physical findings in severe chronic aortic regurgitation.

Sign	Description
Quincke's sign	Fingernail capillary pulsations
Traub's sign	Pistol-shot sounds heard over compressed femoral artery
Muller's sign	Pulsating uvula
Corrigan's pulse	Bounding carotid pulse
deMusset's sign	Head bobbing
Hill's sign	Popliteal cuff systolic pressure exceeds brachial cuff pressure by > 60 mm Hg
Duroziez's sign	Systolic murmur heard over the femoral artery when compressed proximally and diastolic murmur heard when compressed distally
Water-hammer pulse	Bounding radial pulse with elevation of the patient's arm
Bisferiens pulse	Two systolic peaks of equal or unequal magnitudes separated by a mid-systolic trough detected in the carotid, brachial, or femoral pulses

especially in combined aortic regurgitation and stenosis, is optimal. The femoral arterial pressure may be used if previously matched to central aortic pressure, as shown in Figure 7.5a. The peripheral (femoral) pressure shows the normal delay in pressure upstroke, with a 15 mm Hg pressure overshoot compared to central aortic pressure (note the well-defined dichrotic notch and anachrotic shoulder of the central pressure). These pressures are considered matched and the overshoot can be excluded from calculations after the central catheter is positioned in the left ventricle (Figure 7.5b and 7.5c).

Acute Aortic Insufficiency

Acute aortic insufficiency is often associated with rapid cardiovascular deterioration, necessitating early identification, evaluation, and treatment. Most commonly, infective endocarditis causes destruction or perforation of valve leaflets or malcoaptation because of associated vegetation. Similarly structurally damaging is a proximal aortic dissection (type A), which undermines the commissural suspensions of the aortic valve leaflets, resulting in altered coaptation, prolapse, and acute regurgitation. Direct traumatic damage or rupture to the valve structure, post-balloon valvuloplasty complications, and malfunction of a mechanical valve all likewise generate situations of acute aortic insufficiency.

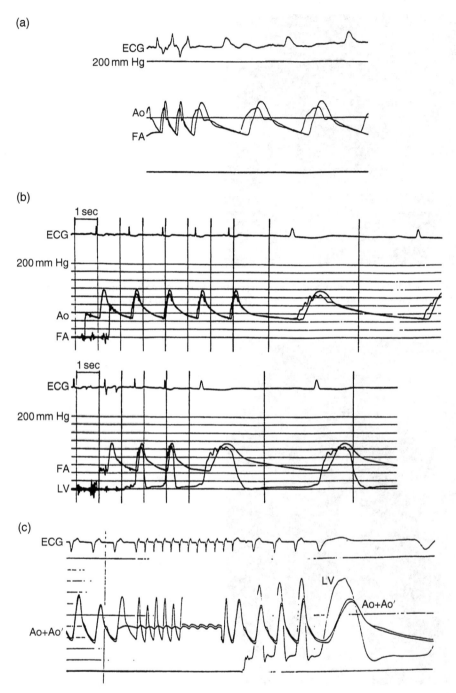

Figure 7.5 (a) Central aortic (Ao) and femoral artery (FA) pressures in a normal subject. A 15 mm Hg femoral pressure overshoot is acceptable. See text for details. (b) Central aortic and peripheral pressures are matched before recording left ventricular (LV)–aortic pressures. See text for details. (c) Systemic hemodynamics obtained with two catheters, one in the central aortic position (Ao) and a second through the arterial sheath (Ao′). These pressures match, with no signs of peripheral pressure amplification. The left ventricular pressure was obtained via a transseptal catheter. See text for details.

Pathophysiology

The hemodynamic environment of acute aortic regurgitation is comparable to chronic regurgitation, except the LV does not have the time for adaptation to the large increase in diastolic blood volume. Compliance is relatively low, so the increased volume in acute regurgitation therefore results in a swift and marked increase in LVEDP (Figures 7.6 and 7.7). Acute aortic regurgitation exposes the unconditioned left ventricle to large diastolic volumes. The immediate and rapid increase in diastolic pressure in the left ventricle with or without a wide aortic pulse

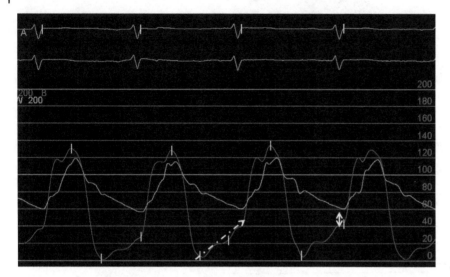

Figure 7.6 Hemodynamic tracing of acute aortic insufficiency. Relatively normal pulse pressure, but a marked increase and rapid rise of diastolic pressure and narrow end diastolic left ventricular–aortic pressures. (*See insert for color representation of the figure.*)

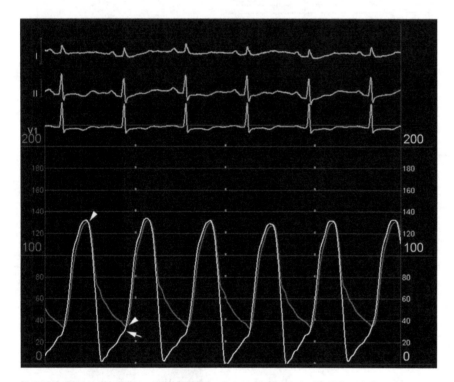

Figure 7.7 Hemodynamic tracing showing elevated left ventricular (LV) end-diastolic pressure (arrow), widened aortic pulse pressure (arrowheads), and near equalization of LV and aortic end-diastolic pressures. *Source:* Ren 2012 [8]. Reproduced with permission of Wolters Kluwer Health, Inc. (*See insert for color representation of the figure.*)

pressure is one of several findings which distinguishes acute from chronic aortic regurgitation (see Table 7.4). Early closure of the mitral valve with rapid left ventricular filling limits the increase in pulmonary capillary wedge pressure substantially below LVEDP (Figure 7.8) [9].

Ultimately in this acute scenario of aortic insufficiency, progressive ventricular decompensation and the rising LV volume and pressure will generate concomitantly high left atrial and pulmonary pressures. These abnormally prominent pressures may even be potentiated by associated diastolic mitral regurgitation. All of these components of decompensation contribute to the significant signs and symptoms of pulmonary edema, cardiogenic shock, or death.

Table 7.4 Grading for aortic regurgitation.

Indicator	Mild	Moderate	Severe
Qualitative			
Angiographic grade	1+	2+	3–4+
Color Doppler: % of central jet width to LVOT size	<25%	>25% and <65%	>65%
Doppler vein contracta width (cm)	>0.3	0.3–0.6	>0.6
Quantitative			
Regurgitant volume (ml/beat)	<30	30–59	≥60
Regurgitant fraction (%)	<30	30–49	≥50
Regurgitant orifice area (cm^2)	<0.10	0.10–0.29	≥0.3
Left ventricular size	–	–	Increased

LVOT = left ventricular outflow tract.

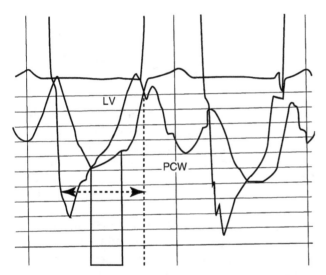

Figure 7.8 Simultaneous left ventricular (LV) and pulmonary capillary wedge (PCW) pressure recording on a 40 mm Hg scale. The PCW pressure falls beneath the LV pressure at the first third of the diastolic period. This suggests premature closure of the mitral valve.

Angiographic Determination of Aortic Regurgitation

Despite good quantitation by echocardiography of the amount of regurgitant flow, angiographic regurgitation differs at times and is dependent on a variety of factors [10–13]. In general, the severity of the angiographic aortic regurgitation correlates with the regurgitant volume index [13]. However, the regurgitant volume index could only differentiate the combined minimal and mild (1+ and 2+) grades from the combined moderate and severe (3+ and 4+) grades [14]. In grading a particular degree of regurgitation, the qualitative angiographic system is influenced by the volume of the chamber into which the contrast is injected, the volume of the chamber that receives regurgitant flow (aorta), pressure gradients across regurgitant values, heart rate, cardiac output, angiographic injector rates, as well as factors related to subjective angiographic image interpretation.

Because no practical way exists to measure regurgitant volume directly, indirect measurements are used in the cardiac catheterization laboratory. Specialized studies involving flow velocity transducers and aortic cross-sectional area are not practical for routine clinical purposes. Use of quantitative angiography to measure the total strike volume and net forward stroke volume computed by cardiac output (either by the Fick or indicator dilution methods) yields the regurgitant volume calculated as the difference between stroke volume by angiography and stroke volume by cardiac output. Dividing the regurgitant volume by the body surface area produces the regurgitant volume index (in ml/min/m^2). Regurgitant volume indexes of < 700 mL/min/m^2 are mild, 700–1700 ml/min/m^2 moderate, and 1700–3000 ml/min/m^2 severe; > 3000 mL/min/m^2 represents very severe valvular insufficiency. The regurgitant fraction is the regurgitant volume divided by the stroke volume obtained by angiography as a percentage (0–20% mild, 20–40% moderate, 40–60% moderately severe, and > 60% severe insufficiency). Regurgitant fraction calculations are not widely used in routine clinical studies because of the complexity of making accurate measurements. Sources of error include independent and accurate determination of cardiac output and stroke volume simultaneously. Left ventricular volume is dependent on optimal radiographic image, chamber opacification, chamber border identification, normal geometry, and stable cardiac cycle, with an accurate correction for image magnification and validation within the laboratory obtaining the ventriculogram.

Many of these conditions are not satisfactory in clinical laboratories, and thus the computation of regurgitant volume and regurgitation fraction remains elusive [15].

Calculation of Aortic Valve Area in Patients with Aortic Regurgitation

The Gorlin formula for the aortic valve area [16], systolic flow / √gradient, uses the systolic ejection period (SEP) to obtain the mean valve gradient without a correction factor for aortic or mitral regurgitation. How should we account for the regurgitant lesion in aortic stenosis? Aortic regurgitation increases left-sided forward flow, which is underestimated by both Fick and thermodilution cardiac output methods. In our laboratory, aortic valve area is computed in the traditional manner and reported as the worst case, with liberalization of the valve area by 20% for each degree of angiographic regurgitation.

Regardless of the nature of the regurgitant lesion, several key indications have been described which allow the clinician to grade the severity of the leak. These primarily focus on echocardiographic criteria, but include quantitative catheterization data as well. In particular, left ventricular size and function play an extremely important role in determining proper surgical replacement timing in these patients (Table 7.5).

Different Presentations of Aortic Regurgitation

Several hemodynamic waveform patterns provide clues to the various clinical presentations and help gauge the severity of the regurgitant aortic valve.

Patient #1 is a 63-year-old man with symptoms of left ventricular failure and a loud decrescendo aortic diastolic

Table 7.5 Major hemodynamic features of severe aortic regurgitation.

	Acute	Chronic
Left ventricular compliance	↔	↑
Regurgitant volume	↑	↑
Left ventricular end-diastolic pressure	↑↑↑	May be normal
Left ventricular dp/dt	↔	↑↑↑
Aortic systolic pressure	↔	↑
Aortic diastolic pressure	↔ to ↓	↓↓↓
Systemic arterial pressure	↑ to ↑↑	↑↑↑
Ejection fraction	↔	↑
Effective stroke volume	↓	↔
Effective cardiac output	↓	↔
Heart rate	↑	↔
Peripheral vascular resistance	↑	↔

↑increased or augmented value, ↓decreased or diminished value, ↔, no change or unaffected.
Source: Morganroth 1977 [5]. Reproduced with permission of The American College of Physicians.

murmur. Patient #2 is a 78-year-old woman with a brief diastolic murmur at the left sternal border and mild fatigue. Patient #3 is a 48-year-old man with fever, a diastolic murmur, and dyspnea at rest. Femoral artery and left ventricular pressures were obtained in all three patients (Figures 7.3, 7.4, and 7.9, not in order of patients described).

Which pressure tracing is associated with the most and least decompensated patient? Which has the longest, loudest, and softest murmurs? Which tracing has the highest and lowest degree of angiographic aortic insufficiency? Finally, in which tracing would the patient most likely have peripheral vascular disease?

Examine Figure 7.9. The femoral arterial pressure is 140/45 mm Hg with the left ventricular pressure

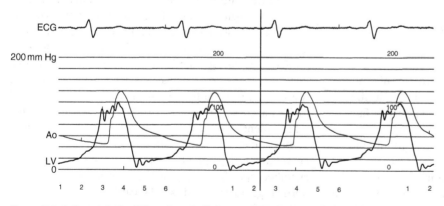

Figure 7.9 Left ventricular (LV) and aortic (Ao) pressures using an 8F femoral sheath and 7F pigtail catheter with fluid-filled transducers in a patient with a diastolic murmur.

118/39 mm Hg. The pulse pressure is nearly 100 mm Hg (normally 40 mm Hg) and the end-diastolic difference between aortic diastolic and left ventricular pressure is about 5–6 mm Hg, the normal difference between end-diastolic aortic (80 mm Hg) and left ventricular end-diastolic pressure (10 mm Hg). The wide pulse pressure, rapidly rising slope and elevation of left ventricular diastolic pressure, and near end-diastolic equilibration between aortic and left ventricular pressures with the left sternal border diastolic murmur are classic findings for aortic insufficiency. The marked elevation of end-diastolic pressure (40 mm Hg) suggests a poorly compensated left ventricle and probably recent acute onset of aortic regurgitation associated with severe symptoms.

Now examine Figure 7.4. The femoral artery pressure tracing also demonstrates a widened pulse pressure (122 – 40 mm Hg = 82 mm Hg), but less (40 – 24 = 16 mm Hg) than in Figure 7.9; the left ventricular diastolic pressure slope also exhibits a more gradual increase over the course of diastole with a less prominent A wave before an end-diastolic pressure of only 24 mm Hg. The hemodynamics demonstrated in this patient are also compatible with severe aortic regurgitation, but are more compensated than in Figure 7.9, with a lower left ventricular end-diastolic pressure and slower left ventricular diastolic pressure rise. One other major difference is the systolic gradient. Note the higher left ventricular systolic pressure (138 mm Hg) compared to aortic pressure (122 mm Hg). This tracing suggests combined mild aortic stenosis and moderate to severe regurgitation.

Consider Figure 7.3. Aortic pressure is 180/48 mm Hg, with left ventricular pressure 180/20 mm Hg. The pulse pressure is 132 mm Hg, with a 28 mm Hg difference between aortic and left ventricular end-diastolic pressures. Note the exact matching of femoral artery and left ventricular systolic pressures, flat left ventricular diastolic pressure slope, and prominent early A wave. From this tracing one might conclude that if aortic regurgitation were present at all, it would be hemodynamically compensated, probably chronic, and not associated with significant left ventricular dysfunction. A brief diastolic murmur and symptoms of fatigue due to hypertension might be a logical association. The prominent A wave, which is completed before left ventricular ejection, is a clue to first degree AV block, which is generally of no clinical significance.

Signs of Peripheral Pressure Amplification in Aortic Regurgitation

Before matching the pressure tracings to the three patients, recall that the common clinical manifestations of severe isolated aortic regurgitation, which one or more of our patients may have demonstrated, include the striking increase in pulse pressure, with an accelerated velocity of ventricular ejection which may cause head bobbing with each heart beat (DeMusset's sign), a collapsing-type pulse with abrupt distension and quick collapse (Corigan's pulse), booming systolic and diastolic sounds over the femoral artery (Tralp's sign), or systolic pulsations of the uvula (Muller's sign). A systolic murmur heard over the femoral artery with proximal compression and diastolic murmur when the compression is released (Duroziez's sign), as well as capillary pulsations (Quincke's pulse), can be detected in some patients. These signs are a result of the hyperdynamic state of the arterial pressure wave, which is manifested more in the peripheral circulation than in the proximal larger vessels, producing findings of peripheral arterial pressure amplification hemodynamically observed as the overshoot in femoral artery sheath pressure [7].

Returning to the descriptions of the pressure waveforms in Figures 7.3, 7.4, and 7.9, let us match the tracings with patients #1, 2, and 3. Figure 7.9 was obtained in patient #3, with recent acute bacterial endocarditis and decompensated congestive heart failure from severe aortic insufficiency. This patient had the longest and loudest murmur and the most severe degree of angiographic aortic regurgitation. Figure 7.4 was obtained in patient #1, with moderately severe aortic insufficiency, mild aortic stenosis, and compensated congestive heart failure. The matching of central aortic and femoral pressures would permit discrimination between the stenotic gradient and reduced femoral arterial pressure due to peripheral vascular disease. Figure 7.3 was obtained in patient #2 with hypertension, minimal aortic insufficiency (the least by angiography), and no signs of congestive heart failure. This tracing is also consistent with bradycardia alone, which can produce an exaggerated pulse pressure as well as a diastolic pressure plateau.

Acute Aortic Insufficiency with Large A Wave: A Rare Finding

A 59-year-old morbidly obese man presented with nine hours of abdominal and chest pain. The pain was severe, nonradiating, and associated with shortness of breath. He had systemic arterial hypertension, type II diabetes mellitus, alcoholism, hepatitis, and a history of medical noncompliance. He was diaphoretic and awake with waning consciousness. The blood pressure was 76/26 mm Hg and bounding pulses were felt in all extremities. There were diffuse crackles in both lungs and heart sounds were not audible. There was no edema or cyanosis.

A central venous catheter with a side port extension was placed in the right internal jugular vein and intravenous lactated Ringer's, dobutamine, and dopamine were begun. The central venous pressure was 30 mm Hg.

(a)

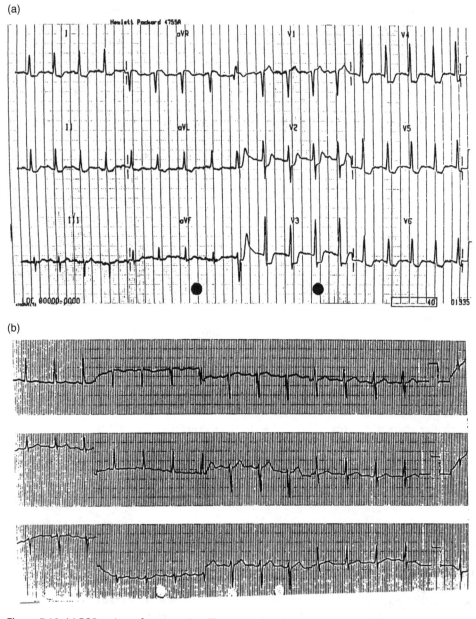

(b)

Figure 7.10 (a) ECG at time of presentation. There is sinus tachycardia and deep ST segment depressions in anterolateral leads. The patient had no evidence of coronary artery disease on postmortem examination, and the changes were related only to the presence of acute aortic insufficiency. (b) ECG one year prior to presentation, with no evidence of myocardial ischemia.

The patient was intubated. Chest X-ray revealed mediastinal dilatation, cardiomegaly, and pulmonary edema. An echocardiogram was technically difficult, with only nondiagnostic, limited views obtained. The ECG showed sinus tachycardia at 104 beats/min and diffuse ST segment depression of 2–4 mm (Figure 7.10a). An ECG from one year earlier was normal (Figure 7.10b).

With the differential diagnosis of acute myocardial infarction or acute AI, cardiac catheterization was performed using the standard Judkins technique. A 6 F

sheath was inserted in the right femoral artery and a 6 F angled pigtail placed in the ascending aorta. The aortic pressure was 200/60 mm Hg. This rapid rise in blood pressure was primarily attributed to volume repletion or to pre-existent "pseudohypotension" [17, 18] and represented the pharmacological response to the intravenous fluids and inotropes begun in the emergency department. Treatment with intravenous nitroglycerin at an initial rate of 10 mcg/min was started to achieve pre- and afterload reduction while sodium nitroprusside was being prepared. An ascending aortogram demonstrated aortic root dilatation (5 cm) and 4+ AI (Figure 7.11). The left ventricular–aorta "pullback" pressure tracing showed "a" waves preceding the anachrotic limb of the pressure curve (Figure 7.12). Coronary angiography was attempted, but the ostia could not be engaged due to catheter "whip."

While awaiting transfer to the surgical suite, the patient suddenly became hypotensive and expired despite resuscitative efforts. Postmortem examination revealed dissection involving the entire length of the aorta (DeBakey class I), with an intimal flap 3 cm distally from the aortic

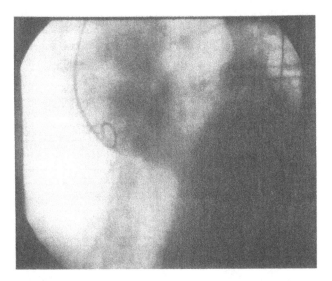

Figure 7.11 Ascending aortogram in the left anterior oblique position revealing 4+ aortic insufficiency.

valve. Dissection extended retrogradely and caused a 3 cm hematoma surrounding the left anterior descending artery (LAD) with 200 ml of pericardial hemorrhage. There was no evidence of LAD, circumflex, or right coronary artery compression. The aortic valve was structurally normal and did not appear to prolapse or to be weakened. Coronary vessels were free of atherosclerosis. The left ventricle was hypertrophied, with no evidence of recent or remote myocardial infarction. The cause of death was cardiac tamponade.

This patient's presentation illustrates three important but seldom appreciated features of acute AI: (i) the physical findings of acute AI may mimic chronic AI; (ii) the endocardial injury pattern on the ECG may have several potential etiologies; and (iii) the A wave in the aortic tracing is highly specific for acute AI.

Chronic AI is characterized by bounding pulses and a wide arterial pulse pressure. These findings are seldom seen with acute AI, especially when it co-exists with left ventricular hypertrophy, due to poor left ventricular compliance and the rapid rise of the left ventricular end-diastolic pressure [19, 20]. Our patient demonstrates that there are exceptions to this rule. The bounding pulses of chronic AI were clearly present and pressure recording from the left ventricular–aorta pullback demonstrated pulse pressure of 140 mm Hg (Figure 7.3). The ascending aorta was dilated and the left ventricle hypertrophied, probably related to longstanding systemic arterial hypertension. There was no evidence, either by history or physical examination, to suggest pre-existing chronic AI. Therefore, signs of chronic AI may be present in the

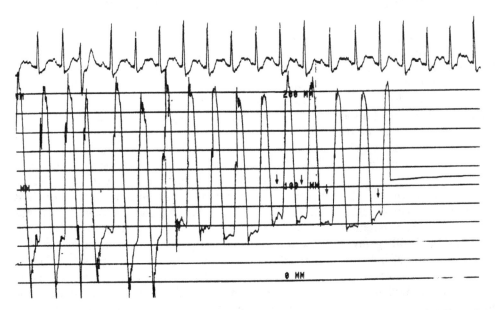

Figure 7.12 Pressure recording from the left ventricular (LV) pullback to ascending aorta (Ao). The pulse pressure is 140 mm Hg and the Ao diastolic pressure is approximately equal to LV end-diastolic pressure. Preceding the anachrotic limb of the Ao pressure tracing, there are positive deflections correlating with the P waves on the ECG (arrow). These A waves are due to premature opening of the Ao valve in acute aortic insufficiency. (Recording speed is 25 mm/sec.)

most severe cases of acute AI, which is precisely where they may be of the greatest diagnostic value [17].

The electrocardiogram in acute AI is frequently described as showing nonspecific changes [19]. The ST segment depressions in this case were profound and were noted to have occurred within the last year when compared to the previous tracing. The mechanism responsible for these changes in our patient was the sudden increase in left ventricular end diastolic pressure, producing subendocardial ischemia. Other mechanisms postulated to produce ischemia which were not present in our patient include (i) an epicardial hematoma surrounding the coronary arteries compressing the vessels, leading to the impaired coronary flow; (ii) the coincidental presence of coronary atherosclerotic lesions, leading to decreased perfusion; (iii) impaired systolic performance, leading to a decreased coronary perfusion gradient; and (iv) experimental data suggesting that acute AI caused by an incompetent left coronary cusp is associated with more severe hemodynamic consequences and worse LV dysfunction than when other cusps are involved [21]. It can be postulated that the regurgitant flow caused by the failure of the left coronary cusp causes a Venturi effect at the left coronary artery ostium and decreases or reverses the normal antegrade coronary flow. Therefore, while acute ST segment abnormalities may represent a subendocardial injury pattern due to epicardial coronary artery lesions, they may have many other potential mechanisms.

The presence of an "a" wave in the aortic pressure tracing has been reported in a patient with acute AI complicating balloon aortic valvuloplasty [22]. Figure 7.12 shows presystolic waves which coincide with P waves of the ECG. Echocardiographic studies have shown that in the setting of acute but not chronic AI, the rapid rise in left ventricular end-diastolic pressure causes diastolic mitral regurgitation, premature closure of the mitral valve, and premature opening of the aortic valve [23, 24]. The premature opening of the aortic valve allows for the atrial impulse to be transmitted to the aorta. Therefore, this finding has high specificity for acute AI, although its sensitivity is unclear. The finding can be expected only when sinus rhythm is present.

The demonstration of an "a" wave on the arterial pulse transmitted from the left ventricular end-diastolic pressure into the aorta is specific for an acute decompensation with markedly increased left ventricular filling pressures. The normal valvular chamber separation between the left ventricle and aorta is virtually eliminated. Although only a single pressure tracing is available, the matching of aortic and left ventricular end-diastolic pressures is easily appreciated. Features which usually differentiate acute from chronic aortic insufficiency are somewhat mixed, confounding interpretation of the pressure waveform. Acute aortic insufficiency is characterized by tachycardia, lower end-diastolic, end-systolic, and total stroke volume, as well as markedly reduced systolic, diastolic, and mean arterial pressures. This patient had tachycardia, but high pressure on vasopressors. The pulse pressure in acute aortic insufficiency is usually significantly less than that with chronic aortic insufficiency. This patient's pulse pressure was 140 mm Hg. Systemic vascular resistance may be the same in both presentations. One of the findings not shown in the current hemodynamic rounds is that of left ventricular and pulmonary capillary wedge pressures, indicating premature mitral valve closure. The massive reflux of blood from the aorta enters the left ventricle in diastole and rapidly increases end-diastolic volume and pressure, closing the mitral valve prematurely. An unusually steep increase on the left ventricular diastolic pressure with the loss of a clear A wave and a markedly elevated left ventricular end-diastolic pressure is suggestive. The wedge pressure is consistently lower than left ventricular end-diastolic pressure for nearly half of the diastolic interval in this setting.

Combined Aortic Stenosis/Aortic Insufficiency after Prosthetic Aortic Root Reconstruction

The hemodynamics associated with aortic root disease mostly involve induction of severe valvular incompetence. Replacement of the aortic root often cures the abnormality at hand. The restored hemodynamics after treating aortic insufficiency with prosthetic aortic root replacement may deteriorate over time and present with unusual findings. The unique hemodynamics of a new onset of aortic stenosis and insufficiency demonstrate one complication of aortic root replacement.

A 38-year-old man had proximal aortic dissection and underwent aortic repair in January 1997. There was no prior history of aortic valvular disease, connective tissue disease, or trauma before the surgery. In postoperative recovery he had been symptom free, with rare episodes of palpitations, but denied dyspnea on exertion or chest discomfort. The aortic root was replaced with a #32 replacement Dacron graft. As part of routine follow-up six months after surgery, echocardiography demonstrated marked aortic dilatation with a question of aortic pseudoaneurysm and severe aortic insufficiency. A chest computed tomography (CT) scan demonstrated possible aortic root aneurysm. The patient was asymptomatic.

The blood pressure was 120/60 mm Hg in both arms, pulse 60 beats/min, respirations 14 breaths/min. There was 6–7 cm of jugular venous distension. There were no

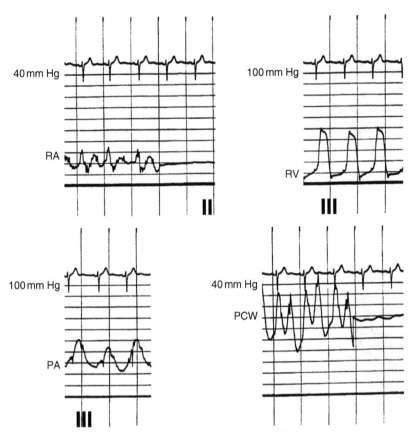

Figure 7.13 Right-heart hemodynamics showing the right atrial (RA), right ventricular (RV), pulmonary artery (PA), and pulmonary capillary wedge (PCW) pressures. The RA and PCW pressures are on a 0–40 mm Hg scale. The RV and PA pressures are on a 0–100 mm Hg scale. Note the well-defined A and V waves in the RA and PCW pressure tracings.

carotid bruits. The heart sounds (both S_1 and S_2) were normal. There was a thrill along the left sternal border, with a III/VI mid-peaking holosystolic murmur and a III/VI early to mid-diastolic murmur along the left sternal border. The peripheral pulses were bounding and bilaterally symmetric. There was no peripheral edema or peripheral arterial bruits. The electrocardiogram showed a normal sinus rhythm with nonspecific intraventricular conduction defect. Cardiac catheterization was performed. The right-heart hemodynamics showed mildly elevated right atrial pressure with a mean of 8 mm Hg, a right ventricular pressure of 50/25 mm Hg, pulmonary artery pressure of 50/25 mm Hg, and a mean pulmonary capillary wedge pressure of 28 mm Hg (Figure 7.13). The A and V waves are well demarcated on both the right atrial and pulmonary capillary wedge pressures. Of interest is that this tracing illustrates the classically described relationship that the A wave is greater in the right (atrial) compared to the pulmonary capillary wedge pressure, where the V wave is usually predominant.

The left ventricular and aortic pressures initially demonstrated aortic stenosis, with an aortic pressure of 130/60 mm Hg and a left ventricular pressure of

150/40 mm Hg (Figure 7.14). The pulse pressure is 70 mm Hg. The high LVEDP and the rate of pressure rise across diastole suggested only moderately decompensated aortic insufficiency.

However, during pullback of the left ventricular catheter to the aorta, the presumed aortic valve stenosis was shown to be, in reality, a supravalvular narrowing. The pressure gradient between the left ventricular and femoral artery persisted when the catheter was positioned in the central aorta (Figure 7.14, middle panel). On further retraction of the pigtail catheter from the central aortic position to the lower abdominal aorta, the gradient disappeared and was appreciated only in the grafted region of the prosthetic conduit (Figure 7.14, right panel). There was no mitral valve gradient and no significant mitral regurgitation. When comparing pulmonary capillary wedge pressure to left ventricular pressure (Figure 7.15), it can be appreciated that the pressure crossover between the pulmonary capillary wedge and the left ventricular diastolic pressure occurs in the first one-third of diastole, consistent with premature closure of the mitral valve associated with severe aortic insufficiency.

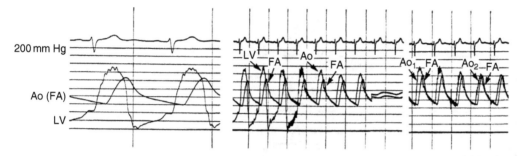

Figure 7.14 (Left panel) Simultaneous femoral artery (FA) and left ventricular (LV) pressures (0–200 mm Hg scale). (Middle panel) Pseudoaortic stenosis on pullback of the LV pressure to the central aortic (Ao) position. The transprosthetic gradient can be detected, and on further pullback (far right panel) the prosthetic graft gradient (Ao_1–FA) disappears as the pigtail catheter is positioned in the lower abdominal aorta (Ao_2–FA).

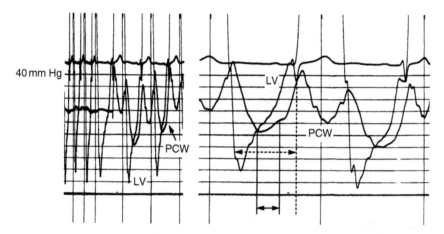

Figure 7.15 Simultaneous left ventricular (LV) and pulmonary capillary wedge (PCW) pressures (0–40 mm Hg scale). The PCW pressure falls beneath the LV pressure at the first third of the diastolic period. It is more common to have the LV/PCW crossover occur after the mid-point of the diastolic period. This configuration suggests premature closure of the mitral valve, which was confirmed by two-dimensional echocardiography.

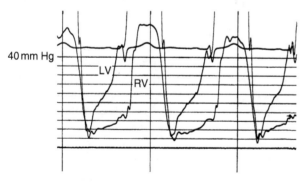

Figure 7.16 Simultaneous left (LV) and right ventricular (RV) pressure tracings (0–40 mm Hg scale) demonstrating rapid filling of the left ventricle compared to the right ventricle and reduced compliance of the left ventricular pressure, with the large A wave having an end-diastolic pressure of approximately 40 mm Hg.

To assess the compliance differences between the left and right ventricles, a simultaneous measurement of left and right ventricular pressures was made (Figure 7.16), demonstrating a marked increase in the end-diastolic pressure slope of the left ventricle relative to that of the right ventricle. The conduction delay in the excitation and relaxation timing of ventricular contraction can also be appreciated by the position of the right ventricular pressure beneath the left ventricular pressure curve.

On completion of the hemodynamics, left ventriculography and aortography were performed in the right and left anterior oblique projections, respectively. The left ventricle had mild anterior hypokinesis with an ejection fraction of 59%. There was no mitral regurgitation. The unusual configuration and dilated aortic root can be appreciated from the ventriculogram (Figure 7.17). Aortography also demonstrated the marked enlargement of the aortic root and an aneurysmal formation near the origin of the coronary ostia. A kink and linear lucency at the insertion of the prosthetic conduit into the native aorta are likely the site of the intragraft stenosis and pressure gradient. There was 4+ aortic insufficiency by contrast angiography.

LAO   RAO

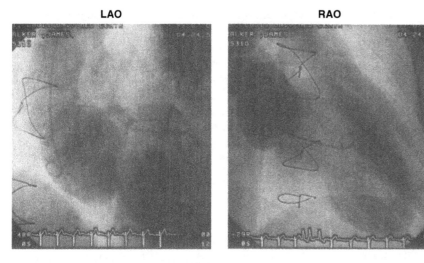

Figure 7.17 Cineangiographic frames of aortography performed in the left anterior oblique (LAO, left panel) and left ventriculography performed in the right anterior oblique (RAO, right panel) projection. There is marked dilatation of the aortic root, with an indentation noted above the globular configuration of the aneurysm.

Acquired Mixed Aortic Stenosis/Aortic Insufficiency

This case demonstrates unusual hemodynamics associated with prosthetic aortic root replacement. The dilatation of the basal part of the native aortic root resulted in aortic insufficiency and, in conjunction with a kink and bend in the elongated graft portion, produced an intragraft gradient that was initially mistakenly identified as aortic stenosis. Graft deformation was likely associated with the continuous alterations of the native ungrafted aorta. The abnormal connective tissue of the great vessels requiring the initial repair suggests a Forme Fruste of Marfan's syndrome [25].

The chronic nature of this insidious change in aortic geometry can be contrasted with the presentation of acute aortic insufficiency. Acute aortic regurgitation often precludes necessary myocardial adaptation and, thus, pressure in the left ventricle rises rapidly, producing a steep diastolic pressure–volume relationship, a marked elevation of left ventricular end-diastolic pressure, and often premature closure of the mitral valve [26, 27]. There is minimal increase in left ventricular end-diastolic volume. The left ventricular stroke volume cannot increase sufficiently to compensate for the regurgitant volume and, thus, stroke volume and cardiac output may be diminished. The high left ventricular end-diastolic pressure minimizes left ventricular runoff, and diastolic pressure in the aorta may remain near normal despite having severe aortic insufficiency. This physiologic response contrasts with that of chronic aortic regurgitation, wherein the left ventricle adapts to the extensive volume experienced by the left ventricle [28]. Left ventricular end-diastolic pressure does not rise rapidly

as the left ventricle can expand to accommodate the volume and, thus, the slope of the left ventricular end-diastolic pressure has a gradual incline. The aortic pulse pressure continues to be wide, however, since compensation and runoff permit the fall of the aortic pressure to decrease both in the peripheral circulation and back into the left ventricle.

The right-heart pressures were also elevated in this individual despite minimal congestive symptoms. Although left ventricular hemodynamics suggested only moderately or minimally compensated aortic insufficiency, the elevated pulmonary artery pressure (50 mm Hg) and pulmonary capillary wedge pressure (28 mm Hg) suggested the effects of adverse compensatory left ventricular hemodynamics on right ventricular function. It is interesting to note that Friedberg, in his classic text entitled *Diseases of the Heart* in 1958, reported that "The symptoms of left-sided heart failure and aortic insufficiency are eventually combined with or overshadowed by those of failure of the right ventricle" [29]. As the right ventricle dilates, tricuspid regurgitation, right atrial enlargement with reflux, and an increase of vena caval pressure are evident. The degree of decompensation of the ventricle precedes that of the clinical complaints, as is evident in the right-heart hemodynamics measured in this individual [30].

Premature closure of the mitral valve may affect the extreme of left ventricular end-diastolic pressure increases and may be associated with the presence of an Austin–Flint murmur [31]. Recall that a low, rumbling late diastolic or pre-systolic apical murmur in patients with aortic insufficiency may be indistinguishable from the characteristic murmur of mitral stenosis. In those patients without organic mitral stenosis, such a murmur has been termed an Austin–Flint murmur [31]. This murmur may be associated with a diastolic thrill, which was identifiable in this case. The murmur is generally associated with left ventricular failure, evident by hemodynamics but not a symptom in our patient. The frequency of the murmur has been variously estimated, although in routine clinical practice it appears to be rare. Although the etiology of the Austin–Flint murmur is disputed, the mechanism is that of the mitral leaflet nearest the aortic valve being forced toward the closing position, producing a functional mitral stenosis, impeding inflow to the left ventricle. The disappearance of the Austin–Flint murmur after relief of cardiac failure suggests that the mechanism of ventricular volume and chamber size relates to the degree of insufficiency. In this individual, no Austin–Flint murmur was reported even though a diastolic thrill was palpable.

Despite the angiographic and hemodynamic degree of aortic regurgitation, the peripheral signs of aortic insufficiency, including low diastolic and high pulse pressure, the Corrigan or radial pulse (water hammer sign), capillary pulsations disproportionate to femoral systolic hypertension (Hill's sign), and a sharp femoral murmur (pistol shot), were lacking, which is possibly attributable to the stenotic component of the prosthetic graft blunting the rate of left ventricular ejection or to the relative lack of chronicity of the disease process.

The determination of premature mitral valve closure from hemodynamics in patients with aortic insufficiency may be difficult. However, as suggested in Figure 7.15, the "crossover point" of the pulmonary capillary wedge pressure and left ventricular end-diastolic pressure occurs within the first one-third to one-half of diastole. It can be noted that the crossover of the pulmonary capillary wedge pressure occurs at the first third of diastole,

and a continued rapid rise of left ventricular end-diastolic pressure occurs to the point of left ventricular ejection. There is evidence of a lower pulmonary capillary wedge A wave pressure than the left ventricular A wave. The expected crossover point of these two pressures is normally in the last one-third of diastole. The association of the early crossover of pulmonary capillary wedge pressure and left ventricular pressure likely reflects the premature closure of the mitral valve, which was easily demonstrated by two-dimensional echocardiography.

Key Points

1) The hemodynamics of aortic regurgitation are related to the chronicity and severity of the regurgitant volume. Characteristic waveforms of aortic regurgitation can be used to differentiate acute from chronic aortic regurgitation in the appropriate clinical settings.
2) Currently, there is no consensus on how best to report aortic valve area in patients with mixed valvular lesions.
3) The classical physical findings of chronic aortic insufficiency, wide pulse pressure, and bounding pulses may help in identification of acute aortic insufficiency, especially in severe cases.
4) The ECG may be misleading, suggesting anatomically significant coronary artery lesions when other mechanisms are operative, such as dramatic elevation of the left ventricular end-diastolic pressure, vessel compression by an epicardial hematoma, and decreased or reversed flow in the coronary artery due to Venturi effect caused by regurgitant flow at the left coronary ostium.
5) The presence of "a" waves in the aortic pressure tracing is virtually diagnostic of acute aortic insufficiency.

References

1 Hatle L, Angelsen B. *Doppler Ultrasound in Cardiology: Physical Principles and Clinical Applications.* Philadelphia, PA: Lea and Febiger, 1985, pp. 188–205.
2 Borow KM, Marcus RH. Aortic regurgitation: The need for an integrated physiologic approach. *J Am Coll Cardiol* 17:898–900, 1991.
3 Labovitz AJ, Ferrara RP, Kern MJ, Bryg RJ, Mrosek DG, Williams DA. Quantitative evaluation of aortic insufficiency by continuous wave Doppler echocardiography. *J Am Coll Cardiol* 8:1341–1347, 1986.
4 Gaasch WH, Andrias CW, Levine HJ. Chronic aortic regurgitation: The effect of aortic valve replacement on left ventricular volume, mass and function. *Circulation* 58:825–836, 1978.
5 Morganroth J, Perloff JK, Zeldis SM, Dunkman WB. Acute severe aortic regurgitation: Pathophysiology, clinical recognition, and management. *Ann Intern Med* 87:223–232, 1977.
6 Abdulla AM, Frank MJ, Endin RA Jr, Canedo MI. Clinical significance and hemodynamic correlates of the third heart sound gallop in aortic regurgitation: A guide to optimal timing of cardiac catheterization. *Circulation* 64:464–471, 1981.
7 Nichols WW, O'Rourke MF. *McDonald's Blood Flow in Arteries: Theoretical, Experimental and Clinical*

Principles, 3rd ed. Philadelphia, PA: Lea and Febiger, 1990, pp. 421–432.

8 Ren X, Banki NM. Classic hemodynamic findings of severe aortic regurgitation. *Circulation* 126:e28–e29, 2012.

9 Mann T, McLaurin LP, Grossman W, Craige E. Assessing the hemodynamic severity of acute aortic regurgitation due to infective endocarditis. *N Engl J Med* 293:108, 1975.

10 Deligonul U, Kern MJ. Hemodynamic rounds: Interpretation of cardiac pathophysiology from pressure waveform analysis: Percutaneous balloon valvuloplasty. *Cathet Cardiovasc Diagn* 24(2):111–120, 1991.

11 Rigaud M, Dubourg O, Luwaert R, Rocha P, Hamoir V, Bardet J, Bourdarias JP. Retrograde catheterization of left ventricle through mechanical aortic prostheses. *Eur Heart J* 8:689, 1987.

12 Kober G, Hilgermann R. Catheter entrapment in a Bjork–Shiley prosthesis in aortic position. *Cathet Cardiovasc Diagn* 13:262, 1987.

13 Croft CH, Lipscomb K, Mathis K, Firth BG, Nicod P, Tilton G, Winniford MD, Hillis LD. Limitations of qualitative angiographic grading in aortic or mitral regurgitation. *Am J Cardiol* 53:1593–1598, 1984.

14 Sandler H, Dodge HT, Hay RE, Rackley CE. Quantitation of valvular insufficiency in man by angiocardiography. *Am Heart J* 65:501–513, 1963.

15 Bolger AF, Eigler NL, Maurer G. Quantifying valvular regurgitation: Limitations and inherent assumptions of Doppler techniques. *Circulation* 78:1316–1318, 1988.

16 Gorlin R, Gorlin SG. Hydraulic formula for calculation of stenotic mitral valve, other cardiac valves, and central circulatory shunts. *Am Heart J* 41:1–29, 1951.

17 Eagle KA, DeSanctis RW. Diseases of aorta. In E. Braunwald (ed.), *Heart Disease: A Textbook of Cardiovascular Medicine*. Philadelphia, PA: WB Saunders, 1988, pp. 1554–1562.

18 Wheat MW. Acute dissecting aneurysms of aorta. In E. Goldberger, MW Wheat (eds), *Treatment of Cardiac Emergencies*. St. Louis: Mosby, 1990, pp. 221–236.

19 Kereiakes DJ, Ports TA. Emergencies in valvular heart disease. In BH Greenberg (ed.), *Valvular Heart Disease*. Littleton, MA: PSG, 1987, pp. 215–233.

20 Dalen JE, Pape LA, Conn LH, Koster JK Jr, Collins JJ Jr. Dissection of the aorta: Pathogenesis and treatment. *Prog Cardiovasc Dis* 23:237–245, 1980.

21 Nakao S, Nagatomo T, Kiyonaga K, Kashima T, Tanaka H. Influence of localized aortic valve damage on coronary artery blood flow in acute aortic regurgitation: An experimental study. *Circulation* 76:201–207, 1987.

22 Alexopulos D, Sherman W. Unusual hemodynamic presentation of acute aortic regurgitation following percutaneous balloon valvuloplasty. *Am Heart J* 116:1622–1623, 1988.

23 Meyer T, Sareli P, Pocock WA, Dean H, Epstein M, Barlow J. Echocardiographic and hemodynamic correlates of diastolic closure of mitral valve and diastolic opening of aortic valve in severe aortic regurgitation. *Am J Cardiol* 559:1144–1148, 1987.

24 Downes TR, Nomeir AM, Hackshaw BT, Kellam LJ, Watts LE, Little WC. Diastolic mitral regurgitation in acute but not chronic aortic regurgitation: Implications regarding the mechanism of mitral closure. *Am Heart J* 117:1106–1112, 1989.

25 Gott VL, Pyeritz RE, Magovern GJ Jr, Cameron DE, McKusick VA. Surgical treatment of aneurysm of the ascending aorta in the Marfan syndrome: Results of composite-graft repair in 50 patients. *N Engl J Med* 314:1070–1074, 1986.

26 Goldschlager N, Pfeifer J, Cohn K, Popper R, Selzer A. The natural history of aortic regurgitation: A clinical and hemodynamic study. *Am J Med* 54:577–588, 1973.

27 Osbakken M, Bove AA, Spann JR. Left ventricular function in chronic aortic regurgitation with reference to end-systolic pressure, volume and stress relations. *Am J Cardiol* 47:193–198, 1981.

28 Borow KM, Marcus RH. Aortic regurgitation: The need for an integrated physiologic approach. *J Am Coll Cardiol* 17:898–900, 1991.

29 Friedberg CK. *Diseases of the Heart*. Philadelphia, PA: WE Saunders, 1958, pp. 684–692.

30 Mann T, McLaurin LP, Grossman W, Craige E. Assessing the hemodynamic severity of acute aortic regurgitation due to infective endocarditis. *N Engl J Med* 293:108, 1975.

31 Flint A. On cardiac murmurs. *Am J Med Sci* 44:29–54, 1862.

8

Mitral Valve Stenosis

Morton J. Kern and Michael J. Lim

Patients with the classic findings of severe rheumatic mitral stenosis have typical pathology with thickened and rolled-back leaflets, shortened and thickened cordae tendinea, and a fish mouth orifice (Figure 8.1). While such patients are relatively uncommonly encountered in either urban and rural medical centers in North America, they are usually older (>45 years), with calcified annular and subvalvular structures. In distinction to younger patients, the poorly mobile valve leaflets and heavy calcification make these older individuals at higher risk for complications of mitral valve balloon catheter commissurotomy [1–4]. Regardless of the clinical presentation, the determination of the mitral valve gradient with its characteristic atrial and left ventricular (LV) pressure waveforms is often critical to both diagnostic and therapeutic considerations.

The use of echo-Doppler and flow velocity in determination of the mitral valve area is the hemodynamic standard, developed by validation from invasive hemodynamic methods used in calculating valve area [5, 6]. A typical hemodynamic tracing of mitral stenosis is shown in Figure 8.2. Because of changes in the pressure–volume relationship, computation of the valve area after mitral balloon valvuloplasty based on hemodynamics, as well as echocardiographic techniques, has been questioned [7]. Figure 8.3 shows hemodynamics before and after mitral balloon valvuloplasty. Discrepancies in these results are likely due to differences in atrial and ventricular chamber volume and flow characteristics (compliance) in a setting of a changing valve orifice area. This chapter will examine examples of mitral valve gradients and discuss features of the pressure waveforms and factors which influence the determination of the mitral valve area for clinical decision-making.

Mitral Stenosis and V Waves

A 47-year-old woman with progressive exertional dyspnea and fatigue has a diastolic murmur of a low rumbling quality, with a narrow opening snap and a brief systolic murmur. The patient reported a history of rheumatic fever as a child, but physicians did not diagnose the heart murmur until four years prior to this examination. Echocardiography confirmed that severe mitral stenosis was present. The patient underwent cardiac catheterization using fluid-filled catheters prior to consideration for definitive valve repair. The right atrial pressure, measured with a balloon flotation catheter, was 6 mm Hg, right ventricular pressure 45/6 mm Hg, and pulmonary artery pressure 45/25 mm Hg. The pulmonary capillary wedge pressure was elevated and equal to the left atrial pressure obtained with a transseptal puncture. The mitral valve gradient was obtained from the simultaneously recorded left ventricular and left atrial pressures obtained through 7 F pigtail and Brockenbrough catheters, respectively (Figure 8.4). The cardiac output, measured by both Fick and thermodilution techniques, was 3.5 L/min. From the brief clinical data and pressure waveforms, address the following: Does the patient have longstanding mitral stenosis? Is there co-existent mitral regurgitation? Identify the A, C, and V waves on the left atrial pressure tracing. What is the valve area from the available data?

In the examination of every pressure tracing, review the cardiac rhythm. Atrial fibrillation is the underlying rhythm, often associated with longstanding and severe mitral stenosis. This rhythm is also associated with loss of the A wave on both left atrial and left ventricular pressure tracings. The V waves are large. However, the presence of large V waves in mitral stenosis is common,

Hemodynamic Rounds: Interpretation of Cardiac Pathophysiology from Pressure Waveform Analysis, Fourth Edition.
Edited by Morton J. Kern, Michael J. Lim, and James A. Goldstein.
© 2018 John Wiley & Sons Ltd. Published 2018 by John Wiley & Sons Ltd.

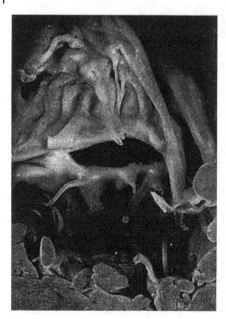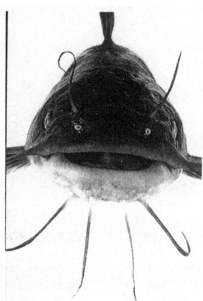

Figure 8.1 Rheumatic mitral stenosis has been described as producing a fish mouth orifice due to the rolled-back, thickened, and shortened leaflets (left). An actual fish mouth is shown on the right.

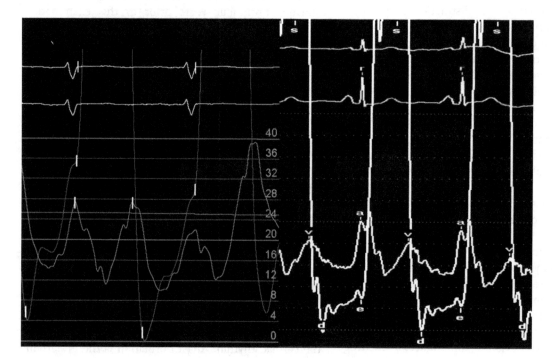

Figure 8.2 Hemodynamic tracings of (left) normal left atrial (LA, blue) and left ventricular (LV, red) pressures compared to those of mitral stenosis hemodynamics with LA in orange and LV in yellow (right). Note diastolic gradient and large "a" wave in mitral stenosis. Scale 0–50 mm Hg. (*See insert for color representation of the figure.*)

often reflecting a low compliance (stiff) chamber, and does not necessarily indicate clinically significant mitral regurgitation. Recall that large V waves result from factors altering chamber compliance, with pressure changes occurring due to flow volume and chamber dimensions acting together, as discussed in earlier rounds [9]. Mitral regurgitation is determined by clinical examination, angiography, and echo-Doppler studies. This patient's systolic murmur was due to aortic ejection and not mitral regurgitation.

(a)

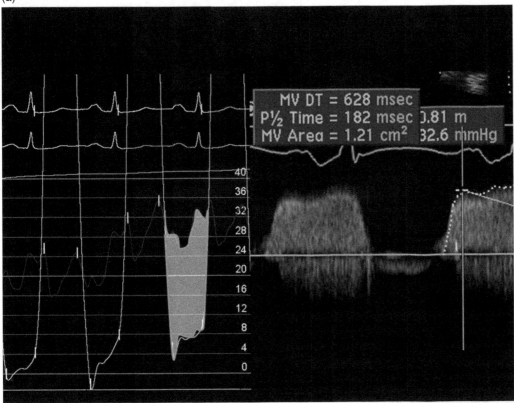

(b)

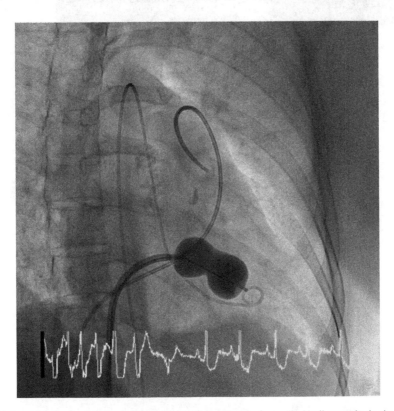

Figure 8.3 (a) Combined echo and hemodynamic data for patient before mitral balloon valvuloplasty with mitral stenosis (left), hemodynamic tracings with simultaneous left atrial (LA, red) and left ventricular (LV, blue) pressures, with diastolic gradient shaded in yellow. (Right) Doppler flow across mitral valve showing pattern of flat E–A slope and delayed chamber emptying. There is a significant mitral gradient. (b) Cine frame showing Inoue mitral balloon valvuloplasty catheter partially inflated in the mitral valve to perform commissurotomy. (c) Combined echo and hemodynamic data for the patient after mitral balloon valvuloplasty with mitral stenosis. (Left) Hemodynamic tracings with simultaneous LA (red) and LV (blue) pressures, with markedly reduced diastolic gradient shaded in yellow. (Right) Doppler flow across mitral valve showing normalized pattern of LA flow consistant with marked reduction in LA–LV. These comparisons indicated mitral gradient. (*See insert for color representation of the figure.*)

(c)

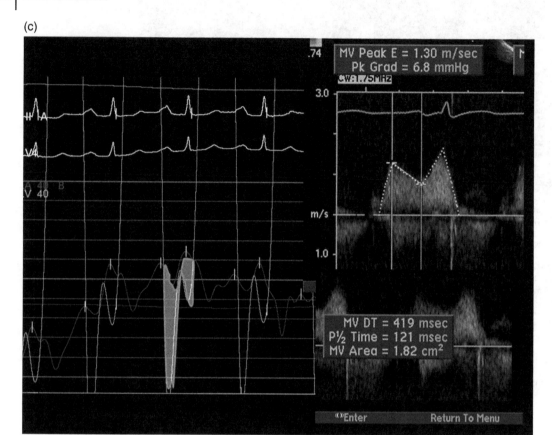

Figure 8.3 (Cont'd)

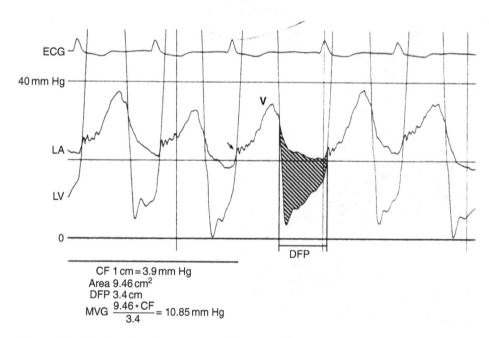

Figure 8.4 Left atrial (LA) and left ventricular (LV) pressures (0–40 mm Hg scale) in a patient with dyspnea on minimal exertion. Shaded area is mitral valve gradient (MVG). CF = correction factor to convert paper distance to pressure value; DFP = diastolic filling period. "Notch" at arrow. *Source:* Kern 2015 [8]. Reproduced with permission of Elsevier.

Technical Notes for Mitral Valve Area Calculation

For the most accurate results, use the waveforms of directly measured chamber pressures. Although technically more difficult to obtain, the left atrial pressure by transseptal puncture resolves any doubt about small but significant mitral gradients. The left atrial and pulmonary capillary wedge pressures are matched in the majority of cases [10]. In patient #1 (Figure 8.4), the left atrial pressure is differentiated from the pulmonary capillary wedge pressure by the abrupt pressure notch at the C wave, with left ventricular ejection and continued pressure rise (left atrial filling) across systole and the peak V wave occurring within the left ventricular pressure downstroke. The pulmonary capillary wedge tracing, although equal to the left atrial pressure in many patients, will always be delayed by 40–120 msec (Figure 8.5), with the peak V wave being inscribed after the left ventricular pressure downslope (Figure 8.6).

In patients in whom the pulmonary capillary wedge pressure is used to measure mitral valve gradients, phase shift the peak of the V wave to the downslope of the left ventricular pressure before planimetering the gradient area. Note that when phase shifting the pulmonary capillary wedge tracing to the left ventricular pressure on Figure 8.6, the gradient becomes even smaller. The pulmonary capillary wedge pressure should not be used when there is an unreliable tracing, when there are known causes of abnormally high pulmonary capillary wedge pressure, or when there is a mitral valve prosthesis. However, in most cases the pulmonary capillary wedge pressure can be used to measure mitral valve gradients [10]. The correspondence of typical left atrial and pulmonary capillary wedge pressures in a patient without mitral stenosis (Figure 8.5) also shows the slightly higher left atrial (2–4 mm Hg) pressure difference which can normally be expected.

To calculate mitral valve gradient, average 10 consecutive mitral valve gradient areas (Figure 8.4, shaded area)

Figure 8.5 Simultaneous pulmonary capillary wedge (PCW) and left atrial (LA) pressures in a patient in sinus rhythm. Pressure transmission from the left atrial to pulmonary capillary wedge is delayed by 40–120 msec and reduced by 2–4 mm Hg. a′, v′ = pulmonary capillary wedge pressure waves. *Source:* Kern 2015 [8]. Reproduced with permission of Elsevier.

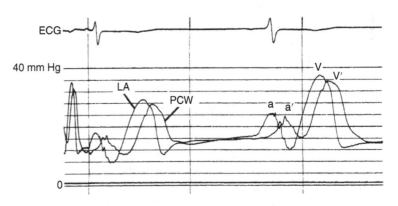

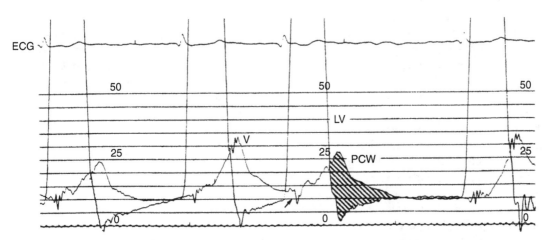

Figure 8.6 Pulmonary capillary wedge (PCW) and left ventricular (LV) pressures in a patient with mild mitral stenosis/regurgitation in atrial fibrillation. Note the position of the C and V waves relative to left ventricular pressure and the equilibration of pulmonary capillary wedge–left ventricular pressures by the first one-half of diastole on long RR intervals. Cardiac output = 4.5 L/min; mitral valve gradient = 8.4 mm Hg; mitral valve area = 1.1 cm^2.

when data is obtained from patients in atrial fibrillation or 5 gradient areas from sinus rhythm. The fastest paper recording speed (usually 100 mm/sec) with the pressure gradient displayed on the largest scale possible (usually a 0–40 mm Hg scale) is optimal.

In the patient in Figure 8.4, assuming the cardiac output is 3.5 L/min and heart rate 80 beats/min, the valve area by available data could be estimated as transvalvular flow/√gradient = (CO/√p-p gradient, or Hakki "quick" formula for valvular stenosis[11] as $3.5/\sqrt{11} = 3.5/3.3 = 1.1\,cm^2$). The computation of valve area by the Gorlin formula is:

$$MVG = \frac{CO/DFP * HR}{K\sqrt{MVG}}$$

where CO = cardiac output (mL/minute); DFP = diastolic filling period (sec); MVA = mitral valve area; MVG = mean valve gradient (mm Hg); and K = constant from Gorlin's empiric data [12] for mitral values (44.3*0.8 = 38).

$$MVA = \frac{\dfrac{3.500}{0.34} * 80}{38\sqrt{10.85}} = \frac{129}{38*3.3} = \frac{129}{125} = 1.0\ cm^2$$

In mitral stenosis, the "quick" valve area estimate should be used with caution, if at all, especially in patients with tachycardia [13].

Pathophysiology of Mitral Stenosis

The fundamental hemodynamic lesion of mitral stenosis is the increased left atrial pressure due to restriction of normal outflow. Normal mitral valve flow patterns can be precisely described by Doppler-echocardiography (Figure 8.7a). In sinus rhythm, mitral flow velocity has an initial peak filling wave occurring in early diastole (PE = peak early filling wave). This flow pattern is the result of passive filling from left ventricular relaxation and a "negative" left atrial–left ventricular gradient in early diastole [14]. Passive left atrial filling slows until atrial contraction produces the active flow velocity (peak A, PA). The PA wave corresponds to the left atrial and left ventricular A wave pressure.

In patients with mitral stenosis, the normal flow velocity pattern is dramatically altered (Figure 8.7b, 8.7c). The mitral flow velocity pattern parallels the left atrial–left ventricular gradient, with a sustained increase in flow velocity occurring across all of diastole. The peak early velocity occurs earlier than the normal PE at the highest gradient point. The decline of flow velocity (and pressure) creates a characteristic velocity envelope with a flattened slope. The slope of diastolic flow is proportional to the severity of the stenosis [5].

In some patients with mitral stenosis in sinus rhythm, mitral flow velocity may increase with contractions, producing acceleration of blood at the wave (Figure 8.7c). In other patients, the atrial flow wave is often abolished due to high pressure or atrial fibrillation. The mitral valve gradient (15 mm Hg, Figure 8.7b, asterisk) shows the characteristic diastolic velocity envelope with a maximal flow velocity of 1.8 m/sec. The diastolic slope of flow velocity is used to compute mitral valve area by the left atrial pressure half-time method, as described elsewhere [5, 6]. The shape of the mitral velocity envelope and the absolute flow velocity values are influenced by both the pressures in the left atrium and in the receiving left ventricular chamber and the net compliance of the individual chambers [7].

Mitral Stenosis and Regurgitation

In patients with concomitant mitral regurgitation, reversed high-velocity flow can be identified occurring under the systolic ejection period (Figure 8.7c). The highest left atrial–left ventricular pressure gradient and flow velocity occurred at end-diastole after atrial systole (Figure 8.7c), with a regurgitant mitral flow velocity jet in a reversed direction seen immediately at the initiation of systole. Although the Gorlin method of calculating mitral valve area in patients with pure mitral stenosis is universally accepted, in patients with co-existing valvular regurgitation, the formula underestimates the true valve area. Forward cardiac output is used in the numerator of the formula and does not account for the regurgitant fraction contributing to the total transmitral diastolic flow. Qualitative correction for angiographic degree of valvular regurgitation has significant limitations and, therefore, is not generally used. Quantitative cineangiographic left ventricular stroke volume provides a more precise value in the numerator of flow in the Gorlin formula and has improved the accuracy of valve area calculation [15], but requires meticulous technique. Left ventricular volume calculations may be distorted in patients with atrial fibrillation or extra systoles during ventriculography.

Alternative Methods for Valve Area Calculations

Three alternative methods, the pressure half-time method of Libanoff and Rodbard [16], the Doppler mitral velocity half-time method, and two-dimensional echo planimetry, are currently available for computing mitral valve area (Figure 8.8a).

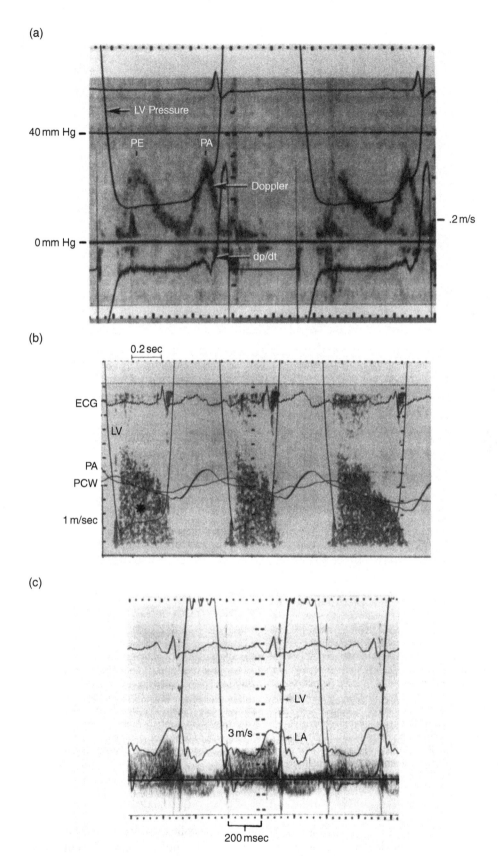

Figure 8.7 (a) Combined hemodynamic and Doppler flow velocity signals demonstrating normal mitral flow physiology. PA = peak atrial filling wave; PE = peak early filling wave velocity. (Velocity scale is 0.2m/sec per division.) (b) Combined hemodynamic and Doppler echocardiographic data demonstrating severe mitral stenosis. LV = left ventricular pressure; PA = pulmonary artery pressure; PCW = pulmonary capillary wedge (pressure scale 0–40 mm Hg). * denotes mitral flow velocity envelope with classical appearance of mitral stenosis. The highest flow velocity (approximately 1.8 m/sec) corresponds to the largest left ventricular–pulmonary capillary wedge gradient in early diastole. (c) Left atrial (LA) and left ventricular (LV) pressures in a patient with mitral stenosis and regurgitation. Note reversal of flow velocity during systole (arrow) due to mitral regurgitation. *Source:* Kern 2015 [8]. Reproduced with permission of Elsevier.

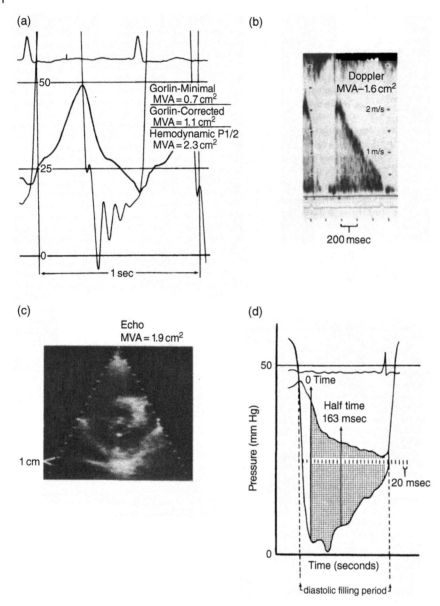

Figure 8.8 Hemodynamic, Doppler, and two-dimensional echocardiographic data from a single patient with mitral stenosis and 4+ mitral regurgitation. (a) Simultaneous left atrial and left ventricular pressures showing diastolic transmitral pressure gradient. The mitral valve areas (MVA) calculated by the Gorlin formula, Gorlin formula corrected for mitral regurgitation, and the hemodynamic pressure half-time ($P_{1/2}$) method are shown. (b) Doppler velocity tracings of transmitral flow. The mitral valve area calculated by the Doppler half-time method is shown. (c) Parasternal short-axis view of the mitral valve orifice frozen during diastole. The mitral valve determined by planimetry is shown. (d) Simultaneous left atrial and left ventricular diastolic pressures in a patient with combined mitral stenosis and regurgitation. The maximal transmitral gradient occurring during the initial 120 msec of the diastolic filling period is measured. From this point, marked "0 time," the diastolic pressure gradient is measured at 20 msec intervals until the onset of ventricular systole. The shaded area shows the diastolic transmitral pressure gradient diminishing with time from the initial peak level. The pressure half-time for this diastolic period is shown. *Source:* Fredman 1990 [17]. Reproduced with permission of Elsevier.

Pressure Half-Time Methods

Using the simultaneous left atrial and left ventricular diastolic pressures in patients with combined mitral stenosis and regurgitation, the maximal transmitral valve gradient occurring during the 120 msec of diastolic filling period is measured (Figure 8.8b). From this point (marked 0 time), the diastolic pressure gradient is measured in 20 msec intervals until the onset of ventricular systole. The log rhythm of each transmitral diastolic pressure difference measured at 20 msec intervals is plotted against time. Using a linear extrapolation to the y axis, the time required for pressure difference to decrease from the extrapolated maximal gradient to one-half that value is the hemodynamic pressure half-time. Pressure half-time in mild mitral stenosis is 100–200 msec, moderate 200–300 msec, and severe > 300 msec. Normal valves have a pressure half-time of < 25 msec [16]. In patients with combined mitral stenosis and regurgitation, the mitral valve area by the hemodynamic pressure half-time method correlated closely with valve areas determined by Doppler echocardiography (r = 0.90) [17].

Doppler Method

The Doppler methodology employs a slightly different technique where the flow velocity is substituted for pressure [18]. The pressure half-time from Doppler is computed as $220/T_{1/2}$, where $T_{1/2}$ is the time from peak to one-half of peak (peak $_{1/2}$) velocity. Peak$_{1/2}$ velocity is the peak mitral velocity divided by 1.4, representing the velocity at which the diastolic transvalvular pressure gradient has fallen by one-half. The Doppler pressure half-time value has been shown to correlate well with the severity of mitral stenosis at catheterization [17, 18]. A modification of this technique has been proposed by Halbe *et al.* [6] with an equally reliable determination of Doppler-derived mitral valve area. The Gorlin formula with and without correction for mitral regurgitation did not correlate as well with the Doppler estimated valve areas (r = 0.47 and r = 0.56, respectively) [17].

Two-Dimensional Echocardiographic Planimetry

The correlation between Doppler-derived mitral valve area and planimetered valve area from two-dimensional echocardiography was satisfactory (r = 0.84) compared to the hemodynamic pressure half-time method with planimetry (r = 0.78) [17]. The Gorlin formula, even with correction for mitral regurgitation, did not correlate well with two-dimensional echocardiographic planimetered valve areas (r = 0.30 and r = 0.35, respectively). These comparisons indicated that in patients with combined mitral valve disease, the hemodynamic pressure half-time method was more accurate than the Gorlin formula, and pressure half-time should be considered for hemodynamic assessment of mitral valve area orifice in patients with mixed mitral valve disease given the limitations of the method [16–18].

Influence of Heart Rate on Determination of Valve Area

The Gorlin formula works best in patients in sinus rhythm with no mitral regurgitation, normal left ventricular function, and no other valve lesions. Mitral valve

area calculation using hemodynamic parameters may be especially difficult in patients with atrial fibrillation, tachycardia, mitral regurgitation, or low cardiac output states. In these patients, numerous studies [18, 19] indicate that clinical correlation with Doppler echocardiography will provide additional information enhancing clinical decision-making.

The effect of heart rate on the mitral valve gradient is evident from the hemodynamic data obtained in a 39-year-old woman with systolic and diastolic murmurs (Figure 8.9). Echocardiography confirmed moderate to severe mitral stenosis with mild regurgitation. Note the dramatic difference in gradient areas between the short and long RR intervals. In Figure 8.9, end-diastolic equilibration of left atrial and left ventricular pressure occurs only during the longest RR interval. Compare this gradient to that in Figure 8.6, which achieves equilibration by mid-diastole in a patient with only mild mitral stenosis and moderate regurgitation. The gradient at mid-point in the longest diastolic cycle of Figure 8.9 is 12 mm Hg, compared to 0 mm Hg in the longest cycle in Figure 8.6. The pressure gradient areas between beats may differ by more than 30% depending on the RR interval. Since the square root of the mean valve gradient is used in the calculation, these differences have less effect on valve area, but for increased accuracy, the average of more than five consecutive beats is used.

Mitral Stenosis with Pulsus Alternans

A 73-year-old woman with dyspnea on exertion presented with complaints of progressive fatigue, breathlessness, weakness, and pedal edema over the last several months [20]. She had known heart murmurs since childhood and had avoided medical attention for many years. She had had cardiac valve replacements for aortic stenosis 12 years ago and mitral stenosis 9 years ago, both with porcine valves. Physical examination demonstrated neck vein distension with prominent A waves and sinus tachycardia. Blood pressure was 123/77 mm Hg. There was a diastolic murmur of mitral stenosis and II/VI murmur at the upper left sternal border. There was a short S_1–OS interval. There was no S_4 gallop. The abdomen was benign and the peripheral pulses were normal, without evidence of edema in the extremities.

Doppler echocardiography identified moderate prosthetic mitral stenosis without significant aortic stenosis or insufficiency. Hemodynamic evaluation was performed for continued dyspnea prior to consideration of a second mitral valve replacement. Left ventriculography showed mild (1+) mitral regurgitation with a normal ejection fraction (75%) and calcification of one mitral valve leaflet. Coronary angiography was normal. The

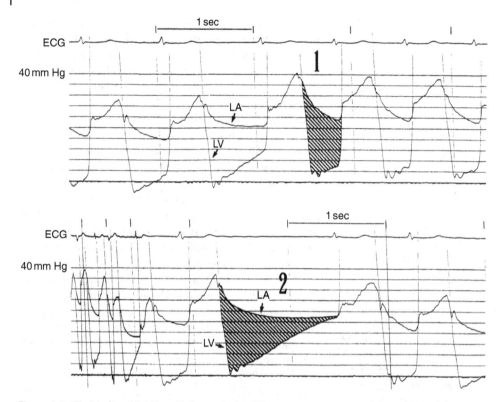

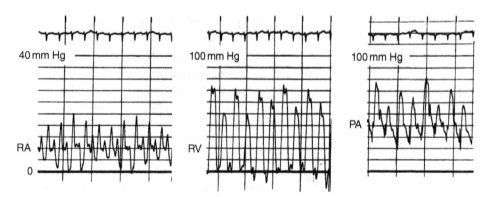

Figure 8.9 (Top) Left atrial (LA) and left ventricular (LV) pressures in a patient with atrial fibrillation. Beat #1 with short RR interval produces large gradient (mitral valve gradient = 22 mm Hg) with reduced mitral valve area. (Bottom) Beat #2 with long RR interval (mitral valve gradient = 29 mm Hg) demonstrates left atrial–left ventricular pressure equilibration at end-diastole.

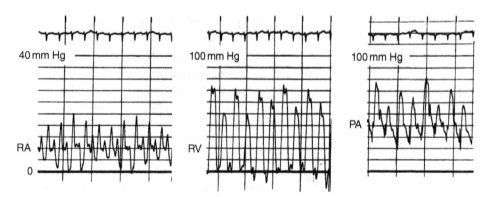

Figure 8.10 Right atrial (RA) pressure on a 0–40 mm Hg scale and right ventricular (RV), and pulmonary artery (PA) pressures on 0–100 mm Hg scale. RV pressure mean is approximately 8 mm Hg, with large V waves. PA and RV pressures demonstrate alternating systolic pressures.

mean right atrial pressure was 8 mm Hg, with large V waves and prominent Y descents (Figure 8.10, left). The right ventricular and pulmonary artery pressures were elevated, with a peak systolic pulmonary pressure of 70 mm Hg. Interestingly, there was pulmonary systolic pressure wave alternans (Figure 8.10, middle and right). Pulsus alternans was also observed in the initial aortic (Figure 8.11, left) and pulmonary capillary wedge pressure tracings (Figure 8.12, top). The systolic right ventricular

pressure (70 mm Hg) alternated with 50 mm Hg, despite evident respiratory variation (Figure 8.10, middle). Similarly, the pulmonary artery pressure alternans (Figure 8.10, right) could be seen within the normal cycle of respiration. Arterial and left ventricular pressures also demonstrated pulsus alternans, with a systolic pressure of 180 mm Hg and a left ventricular end-diastolic pressure of 12 mm Hg, alternating with systolic pressures lower than 140 mm Hg (Figure 8.11, left). In reviewing the left

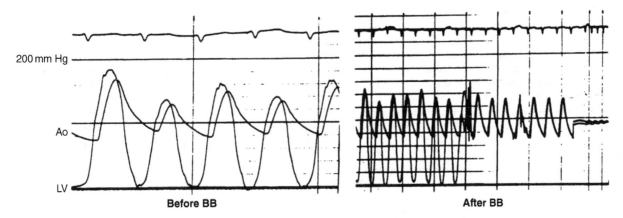

Figure 8.11 Aortic (Ao) pressure before and after beta blockade (BB) on a 0–200 mm Hg scale. Before beta blockade, hemodynamic tracings were recorded at a paper speed of 100 mm. After beta blockade, hemodynamic tracings are shown at a 25 mm paper speed. Note the attenuation of alternans after beta blockade.

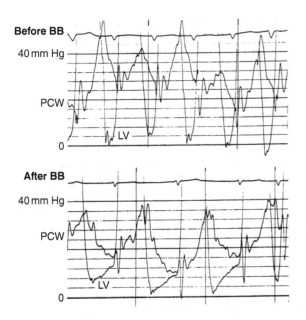

Figure 8.12 Pulmonary capillary wedge (PCW) and left ventricular (LV) pressures on a 0–40 mm Hg scale before and after beta blockade (BB).

ventricular hemodynamics, there was a 20 mm Hg peak-to-peak aortic valve gradient, which is consistent with a 12-year-old calcified valve prosthesis.

In assessing the mitral valve hemodynamics, the pulmonary capillary wedge pressure was measured simultaneously with left ventricular end-diastolic pressure (Figure 8.12, top). The mean pulmonary capillary wedge pressure was 34 mm Hg, with V waves to 50 mm Hg. The pulmonary capillary wedge pressure, in addition to demonstrating alternans of the large V wave, produced a mean transmitral gradient of 22 mm Hg. To assess the effect of heart rate reduction, hemodynamics, including the mitral valve gradient, were measured before and again

after intravenous esmolol, a short-acting IV beta blocker (Figure 8.12, bottom). Beta blockade slowed the heart rate from 120 to approximately 70 beats/min and reduced the mean pulmonary capillary wedge pressure from 32 mm Hg to 24 mm Hg and the transmitral gradient from 22 mm Hg to 9 mm Hg. It is also noteworthy that in addition to reducing heart rate and mitral gradient, beta blockade abolished the pulsus alternans in the left ventricular and pulmonary capillary wedge pressures. The hemodynamic data are summarized in Table 8.1.

To confirm the accuracy of the initial gradient using the pulmonary capillary wedge pressure, direct left atrial pressure measurements were made using the standard transseptal technique (Figure 8.13). Compare the left atrial and pulmonary capillary wedge pressures (Figure 8.13, right). After the administration of beta blockade, the mean mitral gradient was calculated (using the left ventricular and direct left atrial pressure measurement) as 8 mm Hg. With a cardiac output of 4 L/min, the mitral valve area was calculated at 1.3–1.5 cm². The normalization of the arterial pulse (without alternans) and reduction of the pulmonary capillary wedge pressure, an unusual response, suggested improved cardiac function. The patient was treated medically.

This case demonstrates several interesting hemodynamic phenomena, including (i) in the setting of mitral stenosis, the presence of pressure alternans and its elimination with beta blockade; (ii) the improvement in mitral valve gradient after beta blockade; and (iii) the confirmatory gradient measurement with the transseptal approach.

When compared to the typical case described by Dr. Wood [21], the early clinical similarities remain striking, with a history of rheumatic fever in childhood, symptoms of dyspnea, a history of pulmonary edema, and paroxysmal nocturnal dyspnea. Most mitral stenosis cases [21] have elevations of the left atrial pressure

Table 8.1 Hemodynamic data.

	Heart rate (beats/min)	Right atrial pressure (mm Hg)	Right ventricular pressure (mm Hg)	Pulmonary artery pressure (mm Hg)	Pulmonary capillary wedge pressure (mm Hg)	Left atrial pressure (mm Hg)	Left ventricular pressure (mm Hg)	Aortic pressure (mm Hg)	Cardiac output (L/min)	Mean gradient (mmHg)	Mitral Valve area (cm²)
Baseline	120	8	70/8	70/35	32	—	150/14	144.80	3.3	22	0.93
After beta blockade	70	—	—	—	24	22	140/10	132/78	4.0	9	1.50

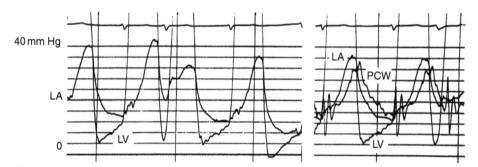

Figure 8.13 (Left) Left atrial (LA) and left ventricular (LV) pressures on a 0–40 mm Hg scale after beta blockade. (Right) LA, pulmonary capillary wedge (PCW), and LV pressures on a 0–40 mm Hg scale simultaneously recorded.

(22–23 mm Hg), with cardiac outputs ranging from 3.5–4.6 L/min. The most common level of pulmonary resistance units is usually under 4 Wood units, with an average of 2.9 for patients with a history of pulmonary edema, 4.7 with paroxysmal nocturnal dyspnea, and 9.2 in patients without such symptoms.

Pulsus alternans is an unusual phenomenon in mitral valve disease and especially in mitral stenosis [22–25]. Pulsus alternans is most commonly associated with decreased left ventricular function, a condition not present by ventriculography or echocardiography. More interesting is the abolition of pulsus alternans after beta blockade, which suggests a heart rate–related phenomenon and/or an improvement in ventricular function, perhaps related to right ventricular contractility. We can only speculate on the mechanisms resulting in this unusual hemodynamic response. The reduced heart rate without pulsus alternans also permitted a more accurate calculation of mitral valve gradients [26–28].

The atrial waveforms are also interesting when compared to indirect left atrial tracings reported by Dr. Wood, who noted A waves higher than V waves in one-third of patients, A and V waves of equal amplitude in 39%, and V waves greater than A waves in 29%. Giant A waves, considered more than 5 mm Hg above the V wave, were a rare occurrence. The difference between A and V is one of Wood's initial observations that we continue to discuss when presenting hemodynamics. He remarked

that the difference between left and right atrial hemodynamics pertained principally to the height of the A and V waves [26]. The A wave was greater in the right than in the left atrium. Wood [26] also noted considerable overlap between the size of V waves and stated, "It is fair to say that a V wave over 15 mm Hg in amplitude nearly always meant mitral incompetence and a V wave under 5 mm Hg nearly always excluded it." The V wave in the case example was 40 mm Hg, with only mild mitral regurgitation. Certainly, postoperative chamber compliance can account for large V waves in the absence of significant valvular regurgitation [26], and such is the case in the patient example.

Left Atrial versus Pulmonary Capillary Wedge Pressure

No one will dispute that the most precise way to assess the mitral gradient is by the left atrial versus left ventricular pressures via the transseptal approach. However, when pulmonary capillary wedge pressure is low and normal, the clinical difference obtained using left atrial pressure to diagnose significant mitral stenosis is negligible. For several practical reasons, the pulmonary capillary wedge pressure remains a first-line tool for hemodynamic evaluation of mitral valve gradients. However, for patients with elevated pulmonary capillary

Figure 8.14 Pulmonary capillary wedge (PCW, red) and left ventricular (LV, yellow) tracings (left) compared to left atrial (LA, orange) and LV (yellow) tracings (right) in patient with mitral stenosis. Note the underdamped PCW tracing and large PCW–LV gradient compared to LA–LV gradient. The LA waveform is correctly damped without an "a" wave but a clear "c" notch and "v" wave. There is a much smaller mitral gradient, with end-diastolic pressure matching. Heart control is indicated over valvuloplasty from these data. (*See insert for color representation of the figure.*)

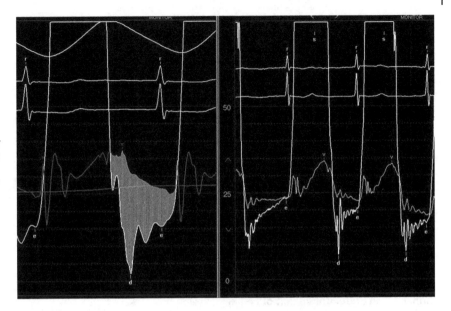

wedge pressures or those with marginal pulmonary capillary wedge pressure waveforms, transseptal left atrial pressure will increase clinical confidence in the accuracy of measurements [29, 30]. Figure 8.14 shows mitral gradients measured by pulmonary capillary wedge compared to left atrial pressures from a transseptal approach.

It is interesting to note that the pulmonary capillary wedge and left atrial pressures, although different in magnitude by 4 mm Hg, yielded nearly identical gradient measurements because the left atrial V wave peak, although higher than that of the pulmonary capillary wedge pressure, had a more rapid V wave decline. Thus, the area under the two pressure curves is similar [27, 28].

A Simplified Mitral Valve Gradient

Cui *et al.* [31] reported a method of simplifying the calculation of mitral valve area from the hemodynamic tracings. Since the mean mitral valve gradient (MVG) is the pressure difference between the mean left atrial (MLAP) and mean left ventricular pressure (MLVP) during diastole (i.e., MLVG = MLAP − MLVP), the computation of the mean mitral valve gradient is simple when the MLVP is known. The MLAP is easily obtained from the electronically meaned signal on the hemodynamic recorder. Cui *et al.* [31] noted that the area under the left ventricular pressure during diastole is roughly a triangle, with the three corners formed from the intersections of the diastolic filling period (DFP) starting and ending points (mitral valve closure and opening) marking the vertical lines intersecting with the LV pressure line (rising diagonally across diastole, see Figure 8.15). This triangular area can be estimated from the rectangular area LVEDP × DFP

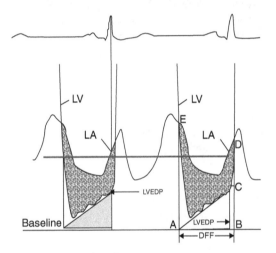

Figure 8.15 The area of triangle ABC approximates the area under the LV pressure tracing during diastole (area LVD). The LVEDP approximates the height of the triangle ABC. So the mean diastolic LV pressure (MDLVP) can be calculated as (area of triangle ABC)/DFP = (DFP×LVEDP/2)/DFP = LVEDP/2, where DFP is diastolic filling period; LA is left atrial pressure tracing; LV is left ventricular pressure tracing; LVEDP is left ventricular end-diastolic pressure. The horizontal line is my estimate of mean left atrial pressure (MLAP), since no MLAP is shown and the dotted arrow is the late LA A wave. *Source:* Cui 2007 [31]. Reproduced with permission of John Wiley & Sons.

divided by 2. Thus, the MLVP is equal to the LVEDP/2. From this key calculation, the mean valve gradient is therefore simplified as MVG = MLAP − LVEDP/2.

There was a strong correspondence among the mitral valve areas calculated by the Gorlin [12] and Hakki [11] formulae and that by Cui, with r values greater than 0.9 and SEE of 1.6 mm Hg. It was also notable that the greatest difference between the Cui and Gorlin methods was only 4 mm Hg in 3/210 calculations. When comparing

Table 8.2 Comparisons of mitral valve area formulas.

MVA	Gorlin	Hakki
Standard method	1.27 +/− 0.61	1.24 +/− 0.33
Cui method	1.26 +/− 0.36	1.23 +/− 0.35

MVA = mitral valve area before valvuloplasty, cm².

Cui MVG to the standard methods of Gorlin and Hakki, mitral valve areas were nearly identical (Table 8.2).

The Cui mitral valve gradient slightly overestimated the standard calculation of mitral valve gradient before but not after mitral valvuloplasty. Hakki significantly underestimated mitral valve gradients after mitral balloon valvuloplasty. The Cui MVG was not affected by mitral regurgitation, aortic insufficiency, atrial fibrillation, or heart rate, unlike that of Hakki.

Although simple, the Cui MVG calculation still has potential problems. Heart rate changes will change the shape of the triangular area under the LV pressure curve, and thus tachycardia may cause a potential overestimation of valve severity. There is one very interesting advantage of this simplified method. The MVG can be estimated easily from a pressure pullback from LV to the left atrium without necessarily making simultaneous two-chamber tracings. Thus mitral valve area could be calculated without entering the LV.

Hemodynamic Evaluation of a Stenotic Bioprosthetic Mitral Valve

The evaluation of the severity of prosthetic valve stenosis may be complicated by differences between hemodynamic and Doppler estimates of the degree of obstruction to flow [32, 33]. Since postoperative and recuperative changes alter myocardial function and compliance, left atrial pressure–volume curves, and responses to exercise status, a precise determination of both resting and exercise-induced hemodynamic function requires careful examination. To illustrate the difficulty of assessing valve function based on hemodynamic and Doppler data, the hemodynamic data from a patient with prosthetic mitral valve stenosis evaluated several years after valve implantation will be reviewed below.

A 74-year-old woman reported progressive symptoms of dyspnea on exertion and decreasing exercise tolerance for the past year. She had a history of rheumatic mitral stenosis and two porcine mitral valve replacements, the first 20 years earlier and the second valve replacement 12 years earlier. She had chronic atrial fibrillation, but denied orthopnea or paroxysmal nocturnal dyspnea.

A two-dimensional echocardiogram revealed thickened bioprosthetic mitral valve leaflets and moderate to severe mitral stenosis, with an estimated valve area of 1.3 cm² without valvular regurgitation. Doppler flow velocity data suggested mild mitral stenosis with a peak velocity of 2 m/sec. Estimated pulmonary artery pressure of 30 mm Hg was also reported.

To evaluate the coronary artery disease and progression of hemodynamic valvular dysfunction, a right- and left-heart cardiac catheterization (including a transseptal approach) using fluid-fined catheters was performed. Right-heart hemodynamics demonstrated a mean right atrial pressure of 12 mm Hg with prominent Y descent (Figure 8.16, top left), with an absent A wave or X descent due to the atrial fibrillation. The right ventricular pressure was 48/12 mm Hg (Figure 8.16, middle top), pulmonary artery pressure was 48/16 mm Hg, and mean pulmonary capillary wedge pressure was 16 mm Hg, with prominent V waves (Figure 8.16, bottom middle). A transseptal puncture using the Brockenbrough technique provided left atrial pressure averaging 16 mm Hg, with prominent V waves to 22 mm Hg (Figure 8.16, top right and bottom left). Simultaneously recorded pulmonary artery and left atrial pressures (Figure 8.16, top right) and left atrial and left ventricular pressures (Figure 8.16, bottom left) are shown. Simultaneous aortic and left ventricular pressures (Figure 8.16, bottom right) showed an aortic pressure of 125/70 mm Hg and left ventricular pressure of 125/18 mm Hg. There was no aortic valve gradient.

The mitral valve pressure gradient was obtained from simultaneous recordings of left ventricular pressure using a 7 F pigtail catheter and left atrial pressure using an 8 F Brockenbrough catheter. For comparison, pulmonary capillary wedge pressure was also recorded (Figure 8.16, bottom left).

After recording hemodynamics and thermodilution cardiac output at rest, data were then obtained during symptom-limited dynamic arm exercise. During exercise, heart rate increased from 55 to 65 beats/min, with a moderate increase in pulmonary artery pressure (48/18 mm Hg to 60/30 mm Hg) and left ventricular end-diastolic pressure (16 mm Hg to 24 mm Hg) (Figure 8.17).

There was no significant change in the mean mitral valve gradient (6 mm Hg to 8 mm Hg) (Figure 8.18) or in the calculated prosthetic mitral valve area (1.30 cm²). The left ventricular, left atrial, and pulmonary artery pressures at rest and at peak dynamic arm exercise are compared in Figures 8.17 and 8.18. The hemodynamic data are summarized in Table 8.3.

Based on the above findings, it was suspected that left ventricular dysfunction (evidenced by exercise-induced increased left ventricular end-diastolic pressure without

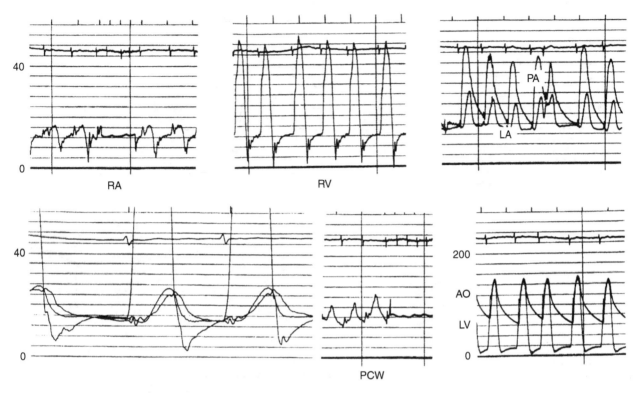

Figure 8.16 Right- and left-heart hemodynamics at rest, demonstrating right atrial (RA, top left), right ventricular (RV, top right), and pulmonary artery (PA, top middle) pressures on a 0–40 mm Hg scale. Also shown are left atrial (LA), pulmonary capillary wedge (PCW), and left ventricular (LV) pressures on a 0–40 mm Hg scale (bottom left), and pulmonary capillary wedge (bottom middle, PCW) and aortic (Ao) and left ventricular (LV) pressures on a 0–200 mm Hg scale (bottom right).

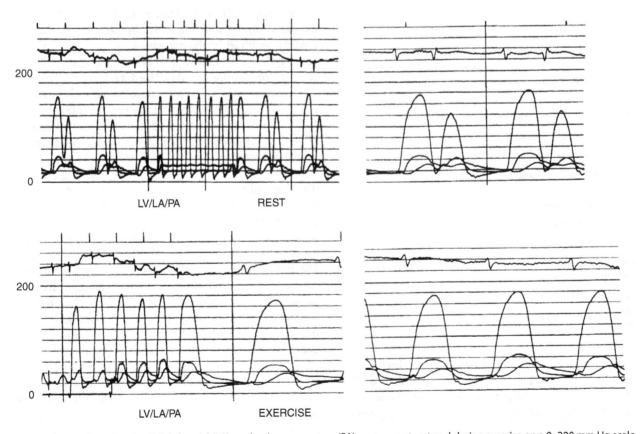

Figure 8.17 Left ventricular (LV), left atrial (LA), and pulmonary artery (PA) pressures at rest and during exercise on a 0–200 mm Hg scale.

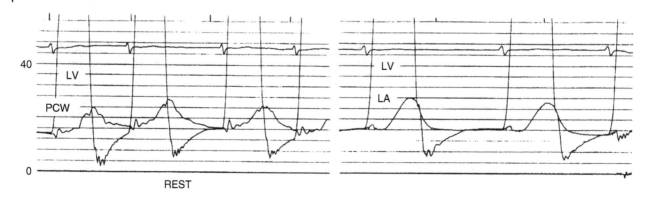

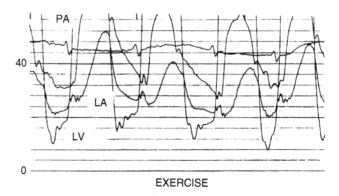

Figure 8.18 Left ventricular (LV), pulmonary capillary wedge (PCW), left atrial (LA), and pulmonary artery (PA) pressures on a 0–40 mm Hg scale at rest and during exercise.

Table 8.3 Hemodynamic data.

	Rest	Exercise
Heart rate (beats/min)	55	64
Right atrial mean pressure (mm Hg)	12	
Right ventricular pressure (mm Hg)	48/12	
Pulmonary artery pressure (mm Hg)	48/18	60/30
Pulmonary artery mean pressure (mm Hg)	26	40
Pulmonary capillary wedge mean pressure (mm Hg)	18	30
Left ventricular pressure (mm Hg)	150/16	190/24
Aortic pressure (mm Hg)	150/70	
Cardiac output (L/min)	3.2	3.6
Pulmonary vascular resistance (dynes · sec · cm^{-5})	200	222
Mitral valve gradient (mm Hg)	6	8
Mitral valve area (cm^2)	1.30	1.27

significant decrease in mitral valve area or increase in mitral valve gradient) was, in part, responsible for the patient's symptoms. The patient was started on oral afterload reduction therapy. Repeat two-dimensional echocardiography was planned in 3–6 months. This patient example illustrates typical hemodynamics frequently required in the assessment of prosthetic mitral valve dysfunction, and highlights several potential limitations of conclusions based on the data.

Prosthetic valves have different natural histories due to characteristics of durability, thrombogenicity, and hemodynamics. Prosthetic valves are classified as either bioprosthetic or mechanical. Mechanical valves are composed of metal or carbon alloys and have mechanisms described as caged-ball, single-tilting disks, or bileaflet-tilting disks. Bioprosthetic valves may be manufactured from heterografts, composed of porcine or bovine tissue (either pericardial or valvular) which is supported by metal struts. Homograft bioprostheses are preserved human aortic valves. Mechanical valves have been documented to last 20–30 years. In contrast, 10–20% of homograft bioprostheses fail within 10–15 years. For heterograft bioprosthesis, 30% may fail within the same time period [33–35]. It is well known that patients under age 40 years have a high incidence of premature heterograft bioprosthetic valve failure. Bioprosthetic valves are preferred in patients who are elderly, who have a life expectancy of less than 10–15 years, or who cannot take anticoagulants.

Valve Areas

For any given valve size, the heterograft bioprosthesis and caged-ball mechanical valves have the smallest effective orifice areas, whereas homograft bioprostheses have valve areas similar to those of native valves [36, 37]. The data in the current case suggest a moderately narrowed mitral valve (1.3 cm^2). This valve area may be compared to caged-ball valve areas for mitral prostheses ranging from 1.4 cm^2 to 3.1 cm^2, for single-tilting discs ranging from 1.9 cm^2 to 3.2 cm^2, and for heterograft bioprostheses ranging from 1.3 cm^2 to 2.7 cm^2 [36, 37].

Mechanisms of Prosthetic Valve Failure

The symptom complex associated with bioprosthetic valve failure usually involves the gradual onset of dyspnea and symptoms of heart failure, as noted in the case example. The structural failure of bioprosthetic valve material may occur in 30% of heterografts within 10–15 years of replacement [38, 39]. The incidence of bioprosthetic valve failure is particularly high in younger patients, as previously noted. The most common mechanism of bioprosthetic valve failure appears to be a tear or rupture of one or more valve cusps, resulting in severe regurgitation. Calcification and increased rigidity promote the destruction of the valve. Few patients develop severe valvular stenosis [40]. Bioprosthetic valve stenosis is initially detected by auscultation. The magnitude of valve dysfunction is principally assessed by echocardiography and cardiac catheterization before consideration of valve replacement.

Methods to Assess Valve Dysfunction

Several nonhemodynamic methods complement the assessment of prosthetic valve dysfunction. Cinefluoroscopy is a rapid, inexpensive, and often overlooked technique. Although the leaflets of a bioprosthetic valve cannot be visualized, the structural integrity of a mechanical valve, especially the motion of the disk ring or poppet, can indicate dysfunction due to tissue ingrowth or thrombus. Excessive rocking of the base ring may suggest partial dehiscence [41, 42]. Cinefluoroscopy has been used to detect the separation of the outlet strut of a Bjork–Shiley tilting disk valve before complete strut fracture occurs [43].

Two-dimensional and Doppler transthoracic echocardiograms are the most popular modalities to assess sewing-ring stability, leaflet motion, and valve orifice area. In contrast to the transthoracic approach, transesophageal echocardiography (TEE) provides an improved viewing window for atrial and mitral valve planes and higher image resolution. The TEE technique is highly recommended for the assessment of prosthetic mitral valve dysfunction. However, because of flow masking, transesophageal echocardiography is somewhat limited in detecting aortic prosthetic valve obstruction or regurgitation, especially when a concomitant mitral prosthesis is present [44, 45]. Doppler echocardiography easily identifies prosthetic valve obstruction and valvular or perivalvular regurgitation, and provides vital comparative data for serial evaluations.

Hemodynamics of Prosthetic Valve Dysfunction

Transvalvular hemodynamic data from catheterization are used as a gold standard in calculating the effective valve orifice area. Although a catheter can be safely passed through a bioprosthetic valve without adverse hemodynamic effects, the most accurate method of obtaining hemodynamic data is that which does not interfere with valvular motion. For tilting disc valves, catheter entrapment in the minor orifice has been associated with complications and, rarely, the requirement of surgical catheter removal. Hemodynamic evaluation of valvular dysfunction is indicated when noninvasive methods remain inconclusive or contradictory, and is confirmatory when performed in the routine course of preoperative coronary angiography.

Despite initial noninvasive evaluation, diagnostic hemodynamics, performed at the time of coronary angiography, add to the considerations for valve replacement. In the case example, the symptoms during initial evaluation were not attributed to the severity of mitral stenosis. However, the Doppler evaluation prompted further investigation. Hemodynamics of mild mitral stenosis of either native or prosthetic valves may not be representative of the conditions during daily activity which produce symptoms. Exercise-induced hemodynamic alterations during cardiac catheterization may be required to associate symptoms with the corresponding hemodynamics. In some cases, exercise hemodynamics may separate valvular from left ventricular dysfunction. In the present case, during exercise, the left ventricular, pulmonary capillary wedge, and pulmonary artery pressures increased substantially with no change in mitral valve gradient or calculated area. The exercise cardiac output failed to increase normally and may explain why the patient reported dyspnea on exertion without alteration in the calculated mitral valve area. It remains unclear whether such a patient may also show improvement after mitral valve replacement.

Pulmonary Capillary Wedge versus Left Atrial Pressure

When pulmonary capillary wedge pressure is low and normal, transseptal left atrial pressure is generally unnecessary. When it is abnormal, pulmonary capillary wedge pressure may be erroneously high and elevate the calculation of the mitral gradient [46]. Misinterpretation of the pressure gradient based on an improperly (usually overly damped) wedged or misleading pulmonary artery pressure results in an overestimation of left atrial pressure and higher transmitral gradient. The use of the transseptal technique to measure left atrial pressure directly has significant importance and probably should be considered the technique of choice for prosthetic mitral valve pressure measurements.

Exercise Hemodynamics

The absence of a significant increase in mean mitral valve gradient during dynamic arm exercise argues against the presumption that the patient's progressive dyspnea on exertion is solely attributable to severe mitral stenosis. Constant pulmonary vascular resistance with exercise (Table 8.3) also suggests that the development of a "second stenosis"—that is, organic obliterative changes in the pulmonary vascular bed, which are a complication of longstanding severe mitral stenosis—was not advanced.

Hemodynamics of Mitral Regurgitation

The filling or "v" wave of the LA is a reflection of the compliance of the LA. A noncompliant LA after a cardiac operation, infection, or from an infiltrative myopathic process can produce a large "v" wave even for normal filling (Figure 8.19). In cases where the mitral

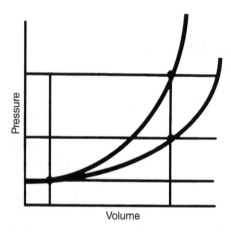

Figure 8.19 Compliance curves of pressure and volume. The chamber compliance or stiffness is represented by the change in pressure for any given change in volume. The upper curve has low compliance (i.e., is stiff), so that a small change in volume produces a large pressure response. The converse is true of the lower curve of high compliance. Thus a "v" wave may not necessarily represent a high volume of regurgitation, but rather a stiff or low-compliant chamber.

Figure 8.20 Left atrial (LA, blue) and left ventricular (LV, red) tracings show large "v" waves of mitral regurgitation. 0–40 mm Hg scale. (*See insert for color representation of the figure.*)

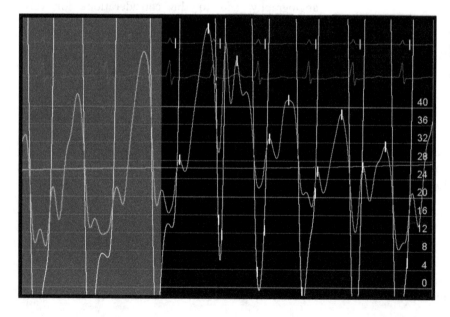

valve leaflets, chordae, or papillary muscle fail, the high pressure in the left is transmitted into the LA, resulting in a large "v" wave such as may occur during mitral balloon valvuloplasty in a patient with severe mitral stenosis (Figures 8.20, 8.21). Since the "v" is a function of the LA compliance, the finding of a large "v" wave from a pulmonary capillary wedge pressure waveform is of limited value in the prediction of mitral regurgitation.

Freihage *et al.* [47] reviewed the invasive assessment of mitral regurgitation. Transseptal left atrial pressure in patients with various degrees of mitral regurgitation was assessed using the simultaneous LA and LV pressure curves. Correlation was performed between these parameters and mitral regurgitation grade by ventriculography. The ratio under the V wave to the LV systolic area—that is, V_a/LV_a—best correlates with the degree of mitral regurgitation (Figures 8.22, 8.23, and 8.24).

The ratio was significantly lower in patients with 0–1+ mitral regurgitation compared to those with greater than or equal to 2+ mitral regurgitation; 0.14 versus 0.23, $P = .002$. The authors concluded that the ratio V_a to LV_a accounts for the LV work that is lost to the atrial regurgitation, with a proportional decrease in forward flow, and is useful in determining the severity of mitral regurgitation over that of ventriculography.

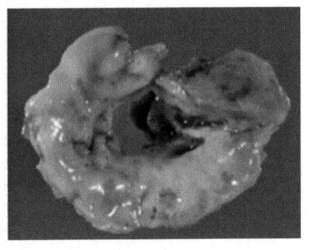

Figure 8.21 Pathologic specimen of torn mitral valve after balloon valvuloplasty. Courtesy of Dr. Zoltan Turi.

Figure 8.22 Simultaneous left atrial (LA) and left ventricular (LV) pressure recordings. Dotted area represents the area under the curve of LV systole. Dark gray shading represents the area under the curve of the "c" wave. Light gray shading represents the area under the curve of the V wave. Dark gray and light gray shaded areas represent total left atrial area during LV systole. Periods labeled 1, 2, 3 are the duration of LV systole, the time to onset of the V wave from the beginning of LV systole, and the duration of the V wave during LV systole, respectively. c = height of "c" wave; V = height of V wave. *Source:* Freihage 2007 [47]. Reproduced with permission of John Wiley & Sons.

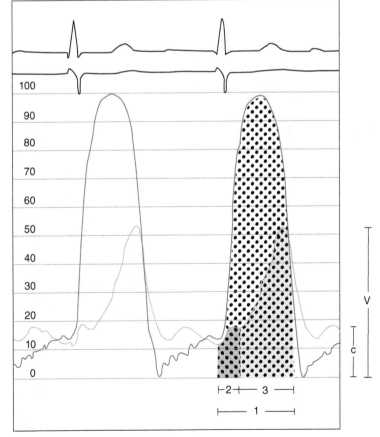

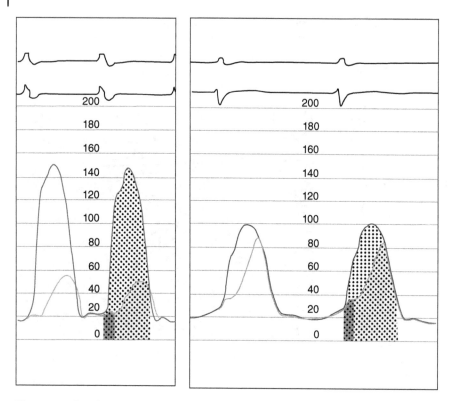

Figure 8.23 Simultaneous left atrial and left ventricular pressure recording in the same patient from 2002 (left) and 2006 (right). In 2002 the patient had 2+ mitral regurgitation by Sellers Classification, whereas the patient has 4+ mitral regurgitation in 2006. See text for details.

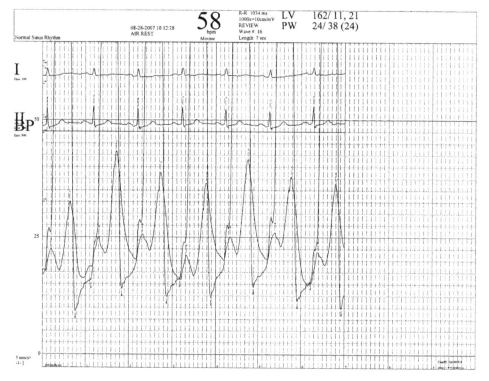

Figure 8.24 Example of respiratory variation with large V waves in a patient with dyspnea. Shows left ventricular pressure tracing with superimposed left atrial pressure on a 0–50 mm Hg scale. Note that the changing left ventricular end-diastolic pressure corresponds to the height of the waves over the respiratory cycle, beginning on beat #2 and extending to beat #5. The V wave falls and then rises again in parallel with the "a" wave. The patient has moderate regurgitation with elevated left ventricular end-diastolic pressure. Note that this is indeed a left atrial pressure rather than wedge pressure due to the timing of the peak of both the A wave and the V wave.

Key Points

1) The evaluation of prosthetic valves requires accurate and, at times, dynamic hemodynamic measurements.
2) The operator's confidence in the data can be increased by using the transseptal technique for prosthetic valves in both the mitral and aortic positions.
3) The hemodynamics of mitral stenosis continue to provide interesting material on the subject of valvular heart disease.
4) Careful inspection of the pressure waves will confirm previous observations and lead to insights into the pathophysiologic aspects of each individual patient.
5) The mitral valve gradient is dependent on the precise measurement of left atrial (or pulmonary capillary wedge) and left ventricular pressures.
6) Artifacts involving either pressure measurement will produce inaccuracies which may have clinical significance.
7) Several methods and formulas using both invasive and noninvasive techniques should verify clinical findings and confirm the severity of mitral valve disease prior to definite therapy.

References

1 Kern MJ, Aguirre F. Hemodynamic rounds: Interpretation of cardiac pathophysiology from pressure waveform analysis: Mitral valve gradients, Part I. *Cathet Cardiovasc Diagn* 26:308–315, 1992.

2 McKay CR, Kawanishi DT, Kotlewski A, Parise K, Odom-Maryon T, Gonzales A, Reid CL, Rahimtoola SH. Improvement in exercise capacity and exercise hemodynamics 3 months after double-balloon catheter balloon valvuloplasty treatment of patients with symptomatic mitral stenosis. *Circulation* 77:1013–1021, 1988.

3 Palacios IF, Block PC, Wilkins GT, Weyman AE. Follow-up of patients undergoing percutaneous mitral balloon valvotomy. *Circulation* 79:573–579, 1989.

4 Turi ZG, Reyes VP, Raju S, Raju AR, Kumar DN, Rajagopal P, Sathyanarayana PV, Rao DP, Srinath K, Peters P, Connors B, Fromm B, Farkas P, Wynne J. Percutaneous balloon versus surgical closed commissurotomy for mitral stenosis: A prospective, randomized trial. *Circulation* 83:1179–1185, 1991.

5 Hatle L, Angelsen B, Tromsdal A. Noninvasive assessment of atrioventricular pressure half-time by Doppler ultrasound. *Circulation* 60:1096–1104, 1979.

6 Halbe D, Bryg RJ, Labovitz AJ. A simplified method for calculating mitral valve area using Doppler echocardiography. *Am Heart J* 116:877–879, 1988.

7 Thomas JD, Wilkins GT, Choong CYP, Abascal VM, Palacios IF, Block PC, Weyman AE. Inaccuracy of mitral pressure halftime immediately after percutaneous mitral valvotomy: Dependence on transmitral gradient and left atrial and ventricular compliance. *Circulation* 78:980–993, 1988.

8 Kern MJ. *The Cardiac Catheterization Handbook*, 6th ed. St. Louis, MO: Mosby-Year Book, 2015.

9 Kern MJ. Hemodynamic rounds: Interpretation of cardiac pathophysiology from pressure waveform analysis: The left-sided V wave. *Cathet Cardiovasc Diagn* 23:211–218, 1991.

10 Lange RA, Moore DM, Cigarroa RG, Hillis LD. Use of pulmonary capillary wedge pressure to assess severity of mitral stenosis: Is true left atrial pressure needed in this condition? *J Am Coll Cardiol* 13:825–829, 1989.

11 Hakki AH, Iskandrian AS, Bemis CE, Kimbiris D, Mintz GS, Segal BL, Brice C. A simplified valve formula for the calculation of stenotic cardiac valve areas. *Circulation* 63:1050–1055, 1981.

12 Gorlin R, Gorlin G. Hydraulic formula for calculation of the area of the stenotic mitral valve, other cardiac valves, and central circulatory shunts. *Am Heart J* 41:1–29, 1951.

13 Brogan WC III, Lange RA, Hillis LD. Simplified formula for the calculation of mitral valve area: Potential inaccuracies in patients with tachycardia. *Cathet Cardiovasc Diagn* 23:81–83, 1991.

14 Courtois M, Kovacs SJ Jr, Ludbrook PA. The transmitral pressure–flow velocity relationship: The importance of regional pressure gradients in the left ventricle. *Circulation* 78:661–671, 1988.

15 Grossman W. Profiles in valvular heart disease. In W Grossman (ed.), *Cardiac Catheterization and Angiography*, 4th ed. Philadelphia, PA: Lea and Febiger, 1991, pp. 565–566.

16 Libanoff AJ, Rodbard S. Atrioventricular pressure half-time: Measure of mitral valve orifice area. *Circulation* 38:144–150, 1968.

17 Fredman CS, Pearson AC, Labovitz AJ, Kern MJ. Comparison of hemodynamic pressure half-time method and Gorlin formula with Doppler and echocardiographic determinations of mitral valve area in patients with combined mitral stenosis and regurgitation. *Am Heart J* 119:121–129, 1990.

18 Smith MD, Wisenbaugh T, Grayburn PA, Gurley JC, Spain MG, DeMaria AN. Value and limitations of Doppler pressure half-time in quantifying mitral stenosis: A comparison with micromanometer catheter recordings. *Am Heart J* 121:480–488, 1991.

19 Bryg RJ, Williams GA, Labovitz AJ, Aker U, Kennedy HL. Effect of atrial fibrillation and mitral regurgitation on calculated mitral valve area in mitral stenosis. *Am J Cardiol* 57:634–638, 1986.

20 Kern MJ. Mitral stenosis and pulsus alternans. *Cathet Cardiovasc Diagn* 43:313–317, 1998.

21 Wood P. An appreciation of mitral stenosis: Part I. Clinical features. *Brit Med J* 1:1051–1064, 1954.

22 Laskey WK, St John Sutton M, Unterecker WJ, Martin JL, Hirschfield JW. Mechanics of pulsus alternans in aortic valve stenosis. *Am J Cardiol* 2:809–812, 1983.

23 Hess OM, Surber EP, Ritter M, Krayenbuehl HP. Pulsus alternans: Its influence on systolic and diastolic function in aortic valve disease. *J Am Coll Cardiol* 4:1–7, 1984.

24 Gleason WL, Braunwald E. Studies on Starling's law of the heart. VI. Relationship between left ventricular end-diastolic volume and stroke volume in man with observations on the mechanism of pulsus alternans. *Circulation* 25:841–847, 1962.

25 Ryan JM, Schieve FJ, Hull HB, Osner BM. The influence of advanced congestive heart failure on pulsus alternans. *Circulation* 12:60–63, 1955.

26 Thomas JD, Wilkins GT, Choong CYP, Abascal VM, Palacios IF, Block PC, Weyman AE. Inaccuracy of mitral pressure half-time immediately after percutaneous mitral valvotomy: Dependence on transmitral gradient and left atrial and ventricular compliance. *Circulation* 78:980–988, 1988.

27 Bryg RJ, Williams GA, Labovitz AJ, Aker U, Kennedy HL. Effect of atrial fibrillation and mitral regurgitation on calculated mitral valve area in mitral stenosis. *Am J Cardiol* 57:634–638, 1986.

28 Brogan WC III, Lange RA, Hillis LD. Simplified formula for the calculation of mitral valve area: Potential inaccuracies in patients with tachycardia. *Cathet Cardiovasc Diagn* 23:81–83, 1991.

29 Lange RA, Moore DM, Cigarroa RG, Hillis LD. Use of pulmonary capillary wedge pressure to assess severity of mitral stenosis: Is true left atrial pressure needed in this condition? *J Am Coll Cardiol* 13:825–829, 1989.

30 Kern MJ, Aguirre FV. Mitral valve gradients: Part II. In Kern MJ (ed.), *Hemodynamic Rounds: The Interpretation of Cardiac Pathophysiology from Pressure Waveform Analysis*. New York: Wiley-Liss, 1993, pp. 43–47.

31 Cui W, Dai R, Zhang G. A new simplified method for calculating mean mitral pressure gradient. *Catheter Cardiovasc Interv* 70:754–757, 2007.

32 Vongpatanasin W, Hillis LD, Lange RA. Prosthetic heart valves. *N Engl J Med* 335:407–416, 1996.

33 Yacoub M, Rasmi NRH, Sundt TM, Lund O, Boyland E, Radley-Smith R, Khaghani A, Mitchell A. Fourteen-year experience with homovital homografts for aortic valve replacement. *J Thorac Cardiovasc Surg* 110:186–194, 1995.

34 O'Brien MF, Stafford EG, Gardner MA, Pohlner PG, Tesar PJ, Cochrane AD, Mau TK, Gall KL, Smith SE. Allograft aortic valve replacement: Long-term follow-up. *Ann Thorac Surg* [Suppl I] 60:65–70, 1995.

35 Bloomfield P, Wheatley DJ, Prescott RJ, Miller HC. Twelve-year comparison of a Bjork–Shiley mechanical heart valve with porcine bioprostheses. *N Engl J Med* 324:573–579, 1991.

36 Gray RJ, Chaux A, Matloff JM, DeRobertis M, Raymond M, Stewart M, Yoganathan A. Bi-leaflet, tilting disc and porcine aortic valve substitutes: In vivo hydrodynamic characteristics. *J Am Coll Cardiol* 3:321–327, 1984.

37 McAnulty JH, Morton M, Rahimtoola SH, Kloster FE, Ahuja N, Starr AE. Hemodynamic characteristics of the composite strut ball valve prostheses (Starr–Edwards track valves) in patients on anticoagulation. *Circulation* [Suppl 1] 58:159–161, 1978.

38 Grunkemeier GL, Jamieson WRE, Miller DC, Starr A. Actuarial versus actual risk of porcine structural valve deterioration. *J Thorac Cardiovasc Surg* 108:709–718, 1994.

39 Gallo I, Ruiz B, Nistral F, Duran CMG. Degeneration in porcine bioprosthetic cardiac valves: Incidence of primary tissue failures among 938 bioprostheses at risk. *Am J Cardiol* 53:1061–1065, 1984.

40 Scohen EJ, Hobson CE. Anatomic analysis of removed prosthetic heart valves: Causes of failure of 33 mechanical valve and 58 bioprostheses, 1980 to 1983. *Hum Pathol* 16:549–559, 1985.

41 Czer LSC, Matloff J, Chaux A, DeRobertis M, Yoganathan A, Gray RJ. A 6 year experience with the St. Jude medical valve: Hemodynamic performance, surgical results, biocompatibility and follow-up. *J Am Coll Cardiol* 6:904–912, 1985.

42 Vogel W, Stoll HP, Bay W, Frohlig G, Schieffer H. Cineradiography for determination of normal and abnormal function in mechanical heart valves. *Am J Cardiol* 71:225–232, 1993.

43 O'Neill WW, Chandler JG, Gordon RE, Bakalyar DM, Abolfathi AH, Castellani MD, Hirsch JL, Wieting DW, Bassett JS, Beatty KC. Radiographic detection of strut separation in Bjork–Shiley convexo-concave mitral valves. *N Engl J Med* 333:414–419, 1995.

44 Mohr-Kahaly S, Kupferwasser I, Eerbel R, Wittlich N, Iversen S, Oelert H, Meyer J. Valve and limitations of transesophageal echocardiography in the evaluation of aortic prostheses. *J Am Soc Echocardiog* 6:12–20, 1993.

45 Karalis DG, Chandrasekaran K, Ross JJ Jr, Micklin A, Brown BM, Ren JF, Mintz GS. Single-plane transesophageal echocardiography for assessing function of mechanical or bioprosthetic valves in the aortic valve position. *Am J Cardiol* 79:1310–1315, 1992.

46 Lange RA, Moore DM Jr, Cigarroa RG, Hillis LD. Use of pulmonary capillary wedge pressure to assess severity of mitral stenosis: Is true left atrial pressure needed in this condition? *J Am Call Cardiol* 13:825–831, 1989.

47 Freihage JH, Joyal D, Arab D, Dieter RS, Loeb HS, Steen L, Lewis B, Liu JC, Leya F. Invasive assessment of mitral regurgitation: Comparison of hemodynamic parameters. *Catheter Cardiovasc Interv* 69:303–312, 2007.

9

Multivalvular Regurgitant Lesions

Morton J. Kern

The majority of classic hemodynamic descriptions of valvular lesions have characteristics which are unique for that lesion as a single or isolated entity. Although significant multivalvular disease is infrequent, many patients may have mild to moderate impairment of one valve, while an associated severe valve lesion appears to be responsible for the major clinical symptomatology. The clinical severity of the presentation depends on the severity of each individual lesion [1, 2]. However, the characteristic and "classical" findings may thus be modified when accompanied by lesions in other valves, producing changes in blood flow which may act synergistically with or nullify the usual perturbations of hemodynamic waveforms. In general, the clinical manifestations are produced by the more upstream or proximal lesion [3]. Characteristic hemodynamic waveforms of isolated lesions of the aortic, mitral, tricuspid, and pulmonary valves have been discussed elsewhere [4–9]. The hemodynamic findings in several patients who have multivalvular regurgitant lesions will be presented in this chapter.

Multiple Heart Murmurs after Mitral Valve Replacement

A 63-year-old woman had a porcine mitral valve replacement 15 years ago for mitral stenosis. In the last 3 years, the patient reported increasing exertional dyspnea. In the last 6 months, progressive orthopnea and paroxysmal nocturnal dyspnea were noted. There has been no history of chest pain or myocardial infarction. Medications at the time of the current evaluation included Lasix and digoxin. Physical examination revealed a blood pressure of 130/80 mm Hg and a pulse of 75 beat/min. There were no carotid bruits. The examination of the lungs was clear. S_1 and S_2 were diminished, with an associated S_3 gallop. There was a grade III/VI holosystolic murmur at the left sternal border radiating to the axilla, with a grade IIVI left-sided diastolic murmur and a variable diastolic murmur over the right sternal border. Echocardiographic (transesophageal) examination revealed mild to moderate mitral regurgitation (among other regurgitant valve lesions to be discussed) and an enlarged left atrium.

Because of the suspected progression of prosthetic mitral valve dysfunction, cardiac catheterization was performed using routine fluid-filled catheters from the femoral approach. An 8 F arterial sheath, a 7 F pigtail catheter, and an 8 F balloon-tipped flotation catheter were initially used for the right- and left-heart catheterizations.

Hemodynamic data were obtained prior to angiography and are summarized in Table 9.1. These data were obtained before changes due to contrast ventriculographic alterations of myocardial function and peripheral vasodilation; however, the angiogram in this patient offers insight into the abnormal hemodynamic findings. A frame from the cineangiogram of the left ventriculogram (Figure 9.1) has been selected to show the characteristic bioprosthetic struts, which can be clearly seen in the mitral position. Multiple metal roentgenographic shadows of wires and pacemakers further demonstrate the extensive prior surgical procedures. On the single-frame angiogram the motion of this strut cannot be appreciated, but a rocking motion suggested a perivalvular leak, often co-existent with prosthetic leaflet degeneration. The left atrium is larger than the ventricle and is well opacified due to severe angiographic mitral regurgitation. Although not seen on this angiogram, left atrial appendage filling during left ventriculography is an additional indicator of severe mitral regurgitation. The left ventricular function appeared normal despite the severe angiographic regurgitation.

Hemodynamic Rounds: Interpretation of Cardiac Pathophysiology from Pressure Waveform Analysis, Fourth Edition.
Edited by Morton J. Kern, Michael J. Lim, and James A. Goldstein.
© 2018 John Wiley & Sons Ltd. Published 2018 by John Wiley & Sons Ltd.

Table 9.1 Hemodynamic data.

	Pressure (mm Hg)	Oxygen Saturation %
Right atrial pressure (mean)	14	46
Superior vena cava	—	48
Inferior vena cava	—	48
Right ventricular pressure	85/8	—
Pulmonary artery pressure (mean)	85/25 (45)	48
Arterial pressure (mean)	145/76 (92)	87
Left ventricular pressure	140/20	—
Left atrial pressure (mean)	40/20 (26)	—
Body surface area	1.54 m^2	
Heart rate (beats/min)	70	
Oxygen consumption (mL/min)	256	
Cardiac output—thermodilution (L/min)	3.2	
Cardiac output—Fick (L/min/m^2)	4.0	
Cardiac index—thermodilution (L/min/m^2)	2.0	
Cardiac index—Fick (L/min/m^2)	2.6	
Systemic vascular resistance (dynes.sec.cm^{-5})	1560	
Pulmonary vascular resistance (dynes.sec.cm^{-5})	380	
Mitral valve gradient (mm Hg)	16	
Mitral valve area (cm^2)	0.9	

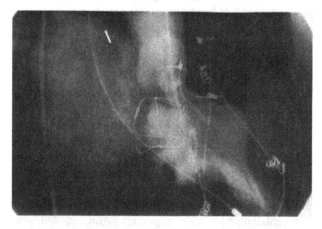

Figure 9.1 A still frame from a cine left ventriculogram showing end-systolic contraction of the left ventricle and the large left atrium well opacified. The left atrial appendage is not seen. Multiple metal roentgenographic shadows can be identified, showing the bioprosthetic struts and pacemaker wires of the epicardial and endocardial leads.

The Regurgitant Tricuspid Valve

Consider the abnormal right atrial pressure waveforms (Figure 9.2). The elevated pressure, large systolic fused V wave, and absent A wave occur during the VVI pacemaker rhythm and complete heart block. (Note the P wave after the T wave on beat #3.) The abnormally large V wave without a clear A wave with a mean pressure exceeding 20 mm Hg varies with inspiration. The waveform abruptly and consistently increases during systolic contraction (immediately after or at the R wave) in this paced rhythm. Occasional P waves appear to deform the right atrial pressure waveform. There are no consistent A waves because of the dissociated rhythm. The V wave is combined with the S wave, producing the characteristic pattern of severe tricuspid regurgitation. To confirm the severity of tricuspid regurgitation, simultaneous right ventricular and atrial pressures were recorded (0–100 mm Hg scale) using a double-catheter technique (Figure 9.3). The degree of tricuspid regurgitation is demonstrated by the height of right atrial pressure rise under the enclosure of the right ventricular systolic waveform [8]. There is no tricuspid stenosis, as is evident by matching of the diastolic pressure waveforms of both tracings. Systolic pulmonary artery pressure was equal to right ventricular systolic pressure (Table 9.1).

Tricuspid regurgitation in the setting of clinical mitral regurgitation with severe pulmonary hypertension is not an uncommon combination of valvular lesions. Longstanding mitral regurgitation produces left ventricular dysfunction with elevated left atrial and ultimately pulmonary artery pressures. Mitral regurgitation begets functional tricuspid regurgitation with right ventricular pressure overload. The interaction of high right ventricular pressures on left ventricular septal wall motion is probably the only significant interaction between the two hemodynamic presentations. The tricuspid valve generally has no influence on left-sided valvular function.

The Stenotic Prosthetic Aortic Valve

The aortic pressure tracings, obtained from a 7 F pigtail catheter in the left ventricle and the side arm of the 8 F femoral artery sheath with fluid-filled transducers, were matched. Prior to crossing the aortic valve, there was a 10 mm Hg overshoot of the femoral artery pressure. With consideration of the normal phase delay of the femoral artery pressure, peak systolic left ventricular pressure exceeds femoral artery pressure by approximately 20–25 mm Hg (Figure 9.4). Although Doppler echocardiography suggested moderate mixed aortic valve disease hemodynamically, the left ventricular aortic gradient demonstrated only minimal aortic obstructive narrowing, a finding further supported when consideration of

Figure 9.2 Right atrial (RA) pressure (G–40 mm Hg scale) demonstrating altering waveforms during paced rhythm. Arrow is large V. See text for details.

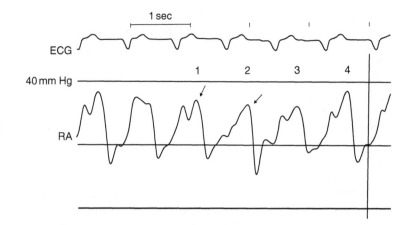

Figure 9.3 Simultaneous right ventricular (RV) and atrial (RA) pressures (0–100 mm Hg scale). Note systolic upstroke of right atrial pressure and matching of pressures in diastole. See text for details.

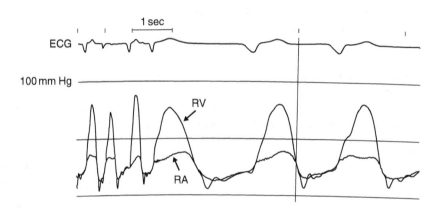

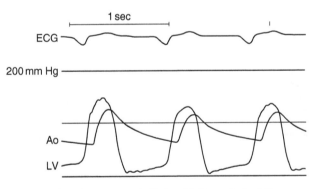

Figure 9.4 Simultaneous aortic (Ao) and left ventricular (LV) pressures (0–200 mm Hg scale) in a patient with a diastolic murmur.

femoral overshoot has been made. From this tracing, is significant aortic regurgitation present?

Based on our previous demonstrations of the spectrum of insufficient aortic valve hemodynamics [5], the aortic pressure decline and left ventricular diastolic pressure rise do not suggest aortic insufficiency. The features suggesting severe aortic insufficiency of wide pulse pressure, rapidly rising left ventricular end-diastolic pressure, and significant overshoot of the femoral artery are missing. However, mild aortic regurgitation would not be unexpected in a patient such as this with a sclerotic aortic valve and prior mitral valve replacement.

As indicated by Doppler echocardiography and later angiography, mild aortic insufficiency was present. Does the mild degree of aortic insufficiency in this patient contribute to the severity of mitral regurgitation? Reflux of blood into the left ventricle from the insufficient aortic valve produces extra left ventricular end-diastolic volume, enlarging the left ventricle. One could postulate that over time, mild mitral regurgitation would more rapidly become severe with the extra load produced by chronic aortic insufficiency. The increased left ventricular end-diastolic volume would increase the regurgitant volume prior to left ventricular decompensation. After left ventricular decompensation, the aortic insufficiency might appear to reduce mitral regurgitation backflow velocity compared to a prior echocardiographic study. Unfortunately, these considerations remain unproven observations, since serial studies in such patients are generally unavailable.

The Prosthetic Mitral Valve

In this patient, regurgitant lesions of the tricuspid and aortic valves, identified by clinical, echocardiographic, and hemodynamic examination, appear with the findings of the predominant mitral valve lesion. To identify the abnormal hemodynamics of the prosthetic mitral valve, and because a pulmonary capillary wedge would not be reliably obtained (due to severe pulmonary hypertension), direct measurement of left atrial pressure was obtained with a transseptal puncture. Crossing the prosthetic mitral valve into the left ventricle was not necessary with the pigtail catheter in the left ventricle. Figure 9.5 shows simultaneous left atrial and left ventricular pressures during the paced cardiac rhythm. Note the variable but consistent pattern of atrial contraction. There is a large V wave to 40 mm Hg and a rapid Y descent characteristic of mitral regurgitation. The left atrial pressure, however, does not decline to match the left ventricular diastolic pressure. Also, the changing position of the A wave reflects the dissociated sinus mechanism more clearly than the electrocardiogram as previously described [10]. On beat #1 (Figure 9.5), the left atrial pressure shows no A wave, but a fused A wave and systolic regurgitant V waveform differentiated from separated waves on the following beats. On beat #2, the A wave appears to fall just inside the left ventricular upstroke. On beat #3, the A wave precedes left ventricular upstroke. A small P wave can be appreciated on the electrocardiogram and appears in mid-diastolic cycle. Beat #5 has a minimal A wave and the largest V wave. This cycle repeats itself every fifth beat and demonstrates the dissociated atrial and ventricular rhythms (Figure 9.6). The mitral valve gradient is approximately 16 mm Hg with a cardiac output of 3.2 L/min, yielding a valve area of $0.9 \, cm^2$. In the setting of 4+ angiographic mitral regurgitation, this calculation is an estimate of only the minimal valve area.

Of special interest is the comparison of the simultaneous left and right atrial pressures measured after pullback of the pulmonary artery catheter. The matching left and right atrial pressures (Figure 9.7) demonstrate slight differences in A and V wave activity, with the large, broad tricuspid regurgitant waves maintained on the right atrial pressure and less striking mitral regurgitant V waves on the left atrial pressure. Left atrial pressure more clearly demonstrates the intermittent activity of A waves than do the right atrial pressure waveforms (Figure 9.8). Equivalency of the left and right atrial pressure transducers is appreciated on transseptal catheter pullback from the left to right atrium, as shown on the far right of Figure 9.8.

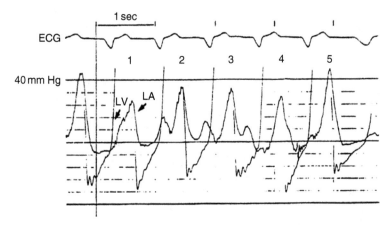

Figure 9.5 Simultaneous left atrial (LA) and left ventricular (LV) pressures (0–40 mm Hg scale) with transseptal technique. Note the changing A waves during paced rhythm. See text for details.

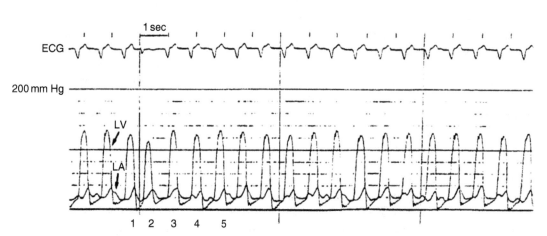

Figure 9.6 Left atrial (LA) and left ventricular (LV) pressures (0–200 mm Hg scale) as in Figure 9.5. Note repetitive pattern of atrial waveform in a patient with paced rhythm.

Figure 9.7 Simultaneous left atrial (LA) and right atrial (RA) pressures (G–100 mm Hg scale) prior to transseptal catheter pullback.

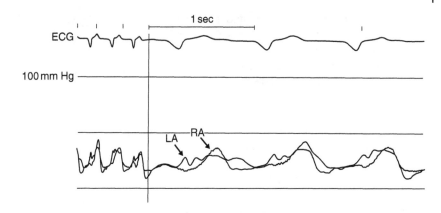

Figure 9.8 Simultaneous left atrial (LA) and right atrial (RA) pressures (G–100 mm Hg scale) showing matching of pressure waveforms on pullback to the right atrium.

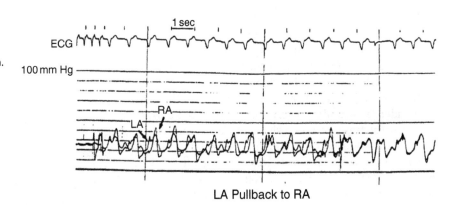

LA Pullback to RA

Figure 9.9 Simultaneous left ventricular (LV) and right ventricular (RV) pressure tracings (G–100 mm Hg scale). Note the delay in upstroke and downstroke of right ventricular pressure under left ventricular pressure envelope in paced rhythm with bundle branch block pattern. See text for details.

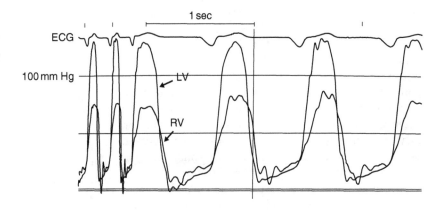

Postsurgical Hemodynamics

Although it is several years after open heart surgery in this patient, evidence of constrictive or restrictive physiology should be checked by comparing the simultaneously recorded right and left ventricular diastolic pressures (Figure 9.9). The ventricular waveforms clearly show normal filling patterns with separation in diastole. Of note is the delay in right ventricular upstroke and fall in right ventricular pressure, consistent with pulmonary hypertension and bundle branch block activity discussed previously [9].

Pulmonary hypertension, as well as the abnormal conduction delay, produces this unusual waveform where the right ventricular downstroke is delayed by 40–120 msec and falls outside the left ventricular pressure downstroke. Normally the right ventricular waveform is completely contained inside the left ventricular tracing.

Recognition of multivalvular lesions preoperatively is important, since failure to correct these lesions at the time of surgery increases surgical mortality. In such patients the relative severity of each lesion may be difficult to estimate by clinical and noninvasive techniques alone, as one lesion may mask the manifestations of another. Complete clinical and hemodynamic evaluation with right- and left-heart catheterization and angiography is often mandatory. At times, questions concerning the presence of significant aortic stenosis in patients with mitral valve disease require direct valve inspection. Palpation of the tricuspid valve at the time of mitral valve replacement may also identify significant, previously unappreciated valvular disease [3]. The frequency of concomitant paired valve lesions is hard to estimate. Two-thirds of patients with severe mitral stenosis may have mitral regurgitation. This degree of regurgitation is usually clinically insignificant. However, in 10% of patients with rheumatic mitral stenosis, rheumatic aortic regurgitation has been recognized [11]. Mitral stenosis masks the hemodynamic detection of left ventricular volume overload, which is characteristic of aortic insufficiency [12]. The combination of mitral stenosis and aortic insufficiency is slightly greater than the 8% incidence of combined aortic and mitral valve disease with pure stenosis of both valves [2]. Aortic and mitral regurgitation are more frequently combined [13] than other lesions, since rheumatic disease may often affect both valves. In some patients, connective tissue disorders may be an apparent cause of multivalvular regurgitation. In combined mitral and aortic regurgitation, the clinical features of aortic regurgitation may predominate and it is difficult to determine whether mitral regurgitation is secondary to ventricular dilatation or a primary organic lesion. With combined regurgitant lesions, regardless of the etiology, reflux of blood from the aorta into both left ventricle and left atrium produces high pulmonary venous pressures. When mitral regurgitation occurs secondary to the left ventricular dilatation of deteriorating aortic regurgitation, mitral regurgitation may be diminished following aortic valve replacement. Severe mitral regurgitation may require annuloplasty at the time of aortic valve replacement [3].

The surgical outcome for treatment of multivalvular disease has been reviewed by Kirklin *et al.* [14], who report a five-year survival rate of 70% after double valve replacement compared to 80% for single valve replacement. Long-term survival is dependent on ventricular functional status prior to surgery. Patients who had combined aortic and mitral insufficiency had poorer outcomes than those receiving valves for other multilesion combinations. Triple valve replacement is a complex procedure associated with a mortality of at least 18% for patients in functional class III and 40% in patients in functional class IV [15]. Substantial clinical improvement has been demonstrated to occur in these patients in the early postoperative period, with arrhythmias and congestive heart failure complicating the late postoperative course.

Combined Native Mitral and Aortic Stenosis

Accurate assessment of valvular hemodynamics is essential in the decision-making process when referring a patient for cardiac surgery who has suspected co-existent aortic and mitral valve disease. Often, one valvular lesion dominates the clinical picture and is worse than the other. The question of "prophylactically" replacing the less severe valve at the time of surgery is controversial. In these situations, and because of uncertainty regarding noninvasive assessment, hemodynamic evaluation in the cardiac catheterization laboratory provides critical information in guiding therapy.

The case of a 56-year-old woman with acute onset of palpitations and shortness of breath will illustrate this dilemma. A 12-lead electrocardiogram revealed atrial fibrillation with rapid ventricular response. Cardiac examination was notable for normal first and second heart sounds and a grade III/VI, mid-peaking systolic ejection murmur best heard over the right upper sternal border. A diastolic murmur was not appreciated because of tachycardia. With intravenous diltiazem, she converted to normal sinus rhythm and her dyspnea resolved.

A transthoracic echocardiogram was performed and showed normal left ventricular (LV) size, moderate concentric LV hypertrophy, hyperdynamic LV systolic function with an ejection fraction of 73%, calcified and thickened aortic valve leaflets, mild aortic regurgitation, calcified and thickened mitral valve leaflets, and moderate mitral stenosis and regurgitation. Doppler echocardiography estimated the mitral valve mean gradient to be 11 mm Hg. The pressure half-time was 116 ms, which estimated the mitral valve area (MVA) at 1.9 cm^2. The aortic valve peak velocity was measured at 3.9 m/s, giving an estimated peak gradient of 62 mm Hg and a mean gradient of 34 mm Hg. The aortic valve area (AVA) was calculated to be 1.1 cm^2 by the continuity equation; this is considered moderate aortic stenosis (AS). An MVA of 1.9 cm^2 is considered mild mitral stenosis (MS), but a mean gradient of 11 mm Hg would qualify as severe stenosis.

To clarify the significance of the valvular lesions, the patient was referred to exercise stress echocardiography. The patient exercised for 3 minutes and 47 seconds, and the test was terminated because of profound dyspnea. The mitral valve gradient rose significantly to 21 mm Hg. The estimated pulmonary pressure also rose from a baseline of 47 mm Hg to 77 mm Hg. Hemodynamically severe MS was diagnosed by these results. From the transthoracic imaging, a Wilkins score [16] in anticipation of potential mitral balloon commissurotomy, with heavy calcification and subvalvular distortion, was calculated to be 10, and therefore valvuloplasty was not offered to the patient.

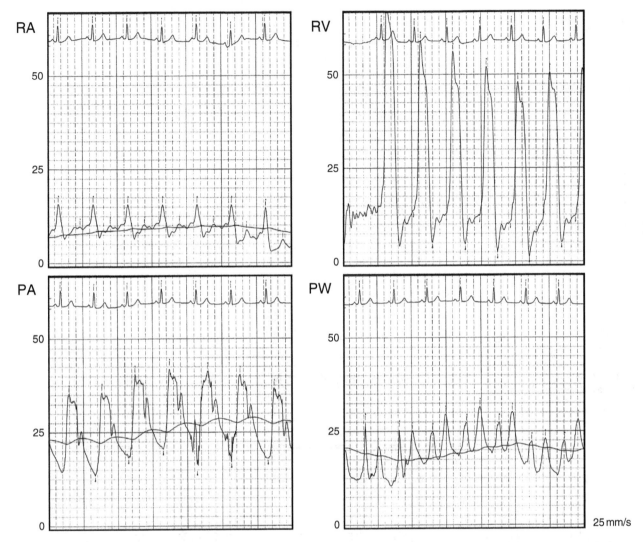

Figure 9.10 Pressure tracings from right-heart catheterization (0–50 mm Hg scale). Right atrial (RA) mean pressure is 9 mm Hg. Right ventricular (RV) pressure is 50/10 mm Hg. Pulmonary artery (PA) pressure is 40/18 mm Hg. Mean pulmonary wedge (PW) pressure is 20 mm Hg. Note V < A on PW compared to RA.

The patient was referred to cardiac surgery for mitral valve replacement. Prior to surgery she underwent cardiac catheterization, both to confirm the stenosis severity of the mitral and aortic valves and to evaluate epicardial coronary artery disease, which may require bypass surgery at the time of valve replacement.

A complete hemodynamic evaluation was performed with simultaneous right- and left-heart hemodynamic measurements. A 6 F sheath was inserted into the right femoral artery, and a 7 F sheath was inserted in the right femoral vein. A 7 F thermodilution pulmonary artery (PA) catheter was used for right-heart catheterization. Pressures were measured in the right atrium, the right ventricle, the main pulmonary artery, and the wedge position (Figure 9.10). Oxygen saturations were obtained in the inferior vena cava, the main pulmonary artery, and

the femoral artery. Cardiac outputs were determined by cold saline thermodilution and the Fick equation (with assumed O_2 consumption at 3 mL/kg, 4.4 L/min, and 15 L/min, respectively). The phasic pulmonary wedge pressure (PW) waveforms appeared adequate, indicating that the mean wedge pressure could be used as a surrogate for left atrial pressure. A 5 F angled pigtail catheter was placed into the left ventricle. The pigtail catheter was flushed and connected to a power contrast injection system. Simultaneous pressures were measured from the LV and PW (Figure 9.11). The transmitral mean gradient was estimated to be 10 mm Hg. Using the Hakki method [17], the MVA was estimated to be 1.5 cm^2.

Next, femoral artery (FA) sheath pressure was connected and measured. Simultaneous LV and FA pressures were then recorded (Figure 9.12). Note that the upstrokes in LV

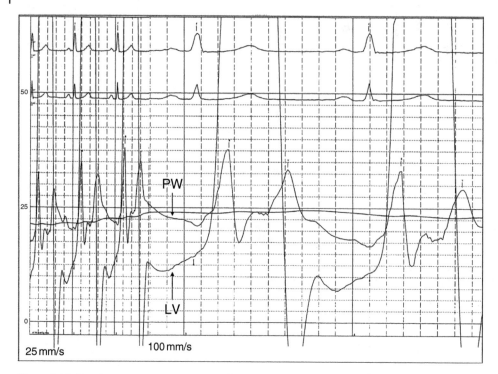

Figure 9.11 Simultaneous pressure tracings of the pulmonary wedge (PW) and left ventricle (LV; 0–50 mm Hg scale). There is a 10 mm Hg PW–LV diastolic gradient.

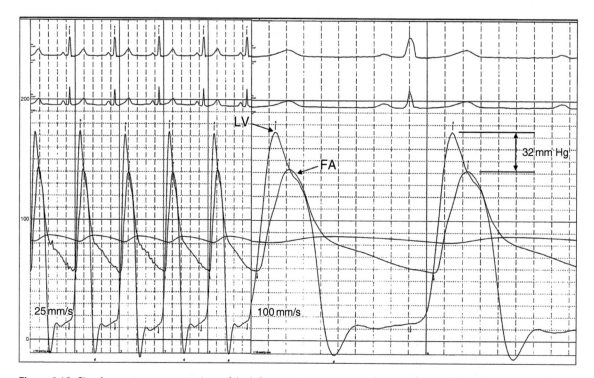

Figure 9.12 Simultaneous pressure tracings of the left ventricle (LV) and femoral artery (FA; 0–200 mm Hg scale). The peak-to-peak gradient is 32 mm Hg. Note crossover point of FA pressure with LV systolic ejection.

Figure 9.13 Simultaneous left ventricle (LV) and femoral artery (FA) pressures before and after pullback (0–200 mm Hg scale). The solid black line demonstrates the course of pressure recovery after a premature systole (*).

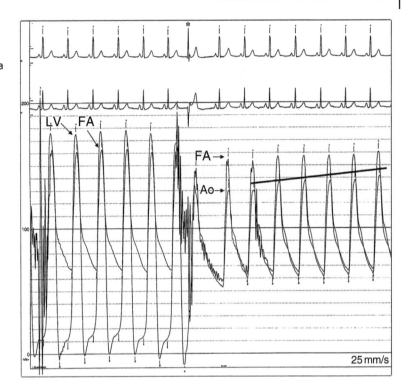

Figure 9.14 Simultaneous pressure tracings of the ascending aorta (Ao) and femoral artery (FA; 0–200 mm Hg scale). Note that there is nearly no delay on the FA tracing. The femoral artery pressure is higher due to distal pulse amplification.

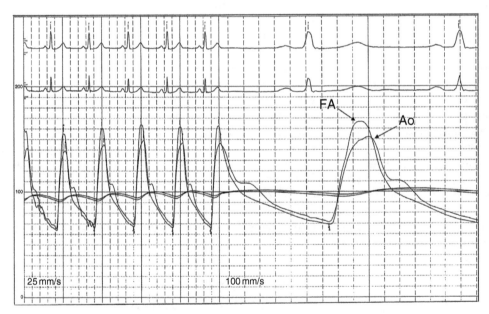

and FA pressures are essentially occurring at the same time, which is physiologically impossible. Normally, FA tracing would be delayed in time after the LV upstroke, since the impulse must travel down the aorta to reach the femoral artery. It was discovered that the power injection transducer of the ACIST system has a built-in 30–40 ms delay, shifting the LV pressure tracing to the right. The peak-to-peak gradient in this tracing is approximately 32 mm Hg, which would suggest moderate aortic stenosis.

The LV pullback provided more information (Figure 9.13). A premature beat occurs with pullback and both pressures after this premature beat are lower. Pressure recovers after seven cardiac cycles. LV pressure was higher than FA pressure prior to pullback, but afterward Ao pressure is lower than FA pressure. The peak-to-peak difference is approximately 15 mm Hg (Figure 9.14). FA pressure is normally higher than Ao pressure secondary to distal pulse amplification. This 15 mm Hg difference needs to be added to the 32 mm Hg gradient seen in Figure 9.12, making the transvalvular peak-to-peak gradient 47 mm Hg. Using the Hakki method [17], AVA was estimated to be 0.64 cm^2, which is much smaller than the AVA of 1.1 cm^2 obtained by echocardiography.

Coronary angiography revealed a 95% stenosis of the mid-left anterior descending artery (LAD). The remainder of the coronary arteries were without significant disease. Based on the data obtained at cardiac catheterization, the patient was referred for simultaneous aortic and mitral valve replacements, as well as an internal mammary graft bypassing the LAD stenosis.

Replacement of Two Valves?

Replacing both aortic and mitral valves in the same surgical procedure increases the morbidity and mortality to the patient when compared to single valve replacement [18]. Therefore, an accurate assessment of valvular lesions is of the utmost importance, and the clinician must carefully interpret every piece of data obtained. Two-dimensional, Doppler, and transesophageal echocardiography are very useful noninvasive techniques in assessing valvular disease. Hemodynamic data obtained from Doppler echocardiography have been shown to correlate well with direct pressure measurements. However, discrepancies may occur among the echocardiogram, clinical presentation, and physical examination. When this happens, cardiac catheterization rises as an old "gold standard" test to directly evaluate the hemodynamics of valvular disease.

It is impossible to attribute symptoms to either valve alone in this patient. The natural history of asymptomatic AS can be widely variable. In some patients, the valve area can decrease by as much as 0.3 cm^2 per year and the transvalvular gradient can increase by as much as 10–19 mm Hg per year. However, in the majority of patients, there will be no significant change. Otto *et al.* [19] performed a prospective study examining aortic jet velocities in 123 patients with asymptomatic AS. They found that patients with an aortic jet velocity of less than 3.0 m/s were unlikely to progress to symptomatic AS in the next five years, and patients with velocities between 3.0 m/s and 4.0 m/s were at intermediate risk of developing symptoms. It is reasonable then for patients with aortic jet velocities between 3.0 m/s and 4.0 m/s to undergo aortic valve replacement (AVR) at the time of other cardiac surgery, and this is a class IIa recommendation by ACC/AHA guidelines [20]. Those patients with velocities greater than 4.0 m/s were at the highest risk, and more than 50% would develop symptoms or die within two years. AVR at the time of other cardiac surgery is an ACC/AHA class I recommendation in patients with severe AS who meet the criteria for valve replacement [20].

Table 9.2 Methods of measuring left ventricular–aortic pressure gradients (in order of least to most accurate).

- Single-catheter LV–Ao pullback
- LV and femoral sheath
- LV and long aortic sheath
- Bilateral femoral access
- Double-lumen pigtail catheter
- Transseptal LV access with ascending Ao
- Pressure guidewire with ascending Ao
- Multitransducer micromanometer catheters

LV = left ventricle; Ao = aortic pressure.

In our patient, the aortic jet velocity was 3.9 m/s, and therefore it is a class IIa recommendation to replace her aortic valve at the time of mitral valve surgery.

The guidelines for replacing isolated stenotic aortic valves may not entirely apply in the setting of concomitant MS, since the reduced cardiac output through the stenotic mitral valve alters the hemodynamics on the aortic valve. The reduced cardiac output lowers the left ventricular systolic pressure and transaortic valvular pressure gradient. Recognizing hemodynamically significant AS is critical prior to mitral valve surgery, because the once protected LV may suddenly be subjected to significantly higher preload conditions after correction of the MS, leading to acute LV failure and flash pulmonary edema. For this reason, right- and left-heart catheterization is recommended in all patients with multivalve disease, especially combined aortic and mitral valve disease, if there is a question of the severity of either valve by two-dimensional and Doppler echocardiography. For most accurate simultaneous pressure measurements, high-fidelity micromanometer catheters or pressure sensor guidewires can be used, but this method is expensive and often impractical (see Table 9.2 for list of methods for LV–Ao pressure gradients).

Double Prosthetic Valve Stenosis Assessment by Left Ventricular Puncture

Catheter access to the left ventricle is limited by the presence of prosthetic valves in the mitral and aortic positions [21]. Retrograde catheterization of the left ventricle with certain mechanical prosthetic valves may be hazardous [22, 23] and has been unsuccessful in some individuals with homograft, xenograft, or severely calcified native aortic valves. Transseptal left atrial access to the left ventricle is similarly inhibited by prosthetic or mechanical mitral valves and, thus, only one approach, direct percutaneous left ventricular puncture, remains to assess cardiac hemodynamics in individuals with both aortic and mitral mechanical prostheses. Although infrequent, critical hemodynamic assessment for the severity of valvular compromise in patients with double-valve prostheses is especially important before interventions. Although the technique and methodology have been well described [24–26], their infrequent application makes periodic review worthwhile.

We review the hemodynamics of a patient who presented with congestive heart failure attributed to a possible stenotic prosthetic mitral valve after replacement of a stenotic prosthetic aortic valve. The approach by direct left ventricular puncture was instrumental in the chemical decision for a second operation.

To illustrate the complex assessment of a patient with two prosthetic valves, the hemodynamics obtained with direct LV puncture will be examined. The patient was a 61-year-old woman with rheumatic heart disease who had had aortic and mitral valve replacements in 1977. A pacemaker was inserted for tachy-brady syndrome in 1996. In May 1997, transesophageal echocardiography demonstrated a normal mitral valve prosthesis with severe prosthetic aortic stenosis. A second valve replacement (22 mm St. Jude Medical, Minneapolis, MN) for aortic stenosis was performed, leaving the mitral valve (29 mm Bjork–Shiley, Baxter Co., Los Angeles, CA) in place based on near-normal echocardiographic data. In the postoperative period the patient had congestive heart failure and was unable to be weaned from mechanical ventilation. She required both vasopressor and vasodilatory support without decreasing the elevated (>60 mm Hg systolic) pulmonary artery pressures. Repeat echocardiographic examination did not identify the etiology of pulmonary hypertension and showed only minimal mitral regurgitation with a small transmitral gradient, normal left ventricular function, no pericardial effusion, and a normally functioning aortic valve. There was no left atrial thrombus. Hemodynamic evaluation was requested to assess whether the mitral prosthetic valve function was

associated with continued pulmonary hypertension and the failure to resolve the congestive symptoms.

Right- and left-heart catheterization was performed using the right femoral artery and vein access by the standard Seldinger technique. A balloon-tipped pulmonary artery catheter was advanced to the pulmonary artery. A 6 F pigtail catheter was positioned in the central aorta above the prosthetic valve. Transseptal catheterization by the standard Brockenbrough technique was performed, placing the catheter in the left atrium.

On completion of the initial catheter placements, the transapical approach to the left ventricle was then undertaken. Two-dimensional echocardiography in the cardiac catheterization laboratory identified the true position of the left ventricular apex between the fourth and fifth intercostal space, lateral to the mid-clavicular line. This position was marked with a pen. The area was prepared in a sterile fashion. An 18-gauge pericardial needle was connected to a pressure monitoring line. The needle was advanced in the plane of the echocardiogram and on the line of the left ventricular apex to the aortic outflow. The needle was introduced slowly, with intermittent administration of additional lidocaine. The pulsations of the left ventricle could be felt, transmitted through the needle during puncture. Under pressure monitoring, the apex of the ventricle was punctured. After confirmation of left ventricular pressure, a 0.035" standard I-wire was advanced into the left ventricular cavity and exchanged for a 4 F pigtail catheter (Figure 9.15). Left- and right-heart hemodynamic data were then acquired in a standard fashion. Following hemodynamic data collection, left ventriculography was performed in the right anterior oblique projection, using 42 cc of contrast at 12 cc/sec. The left ventriculogram showed only trace mitral regurgitation and an ejection fraction of 50% with normal wall motion (left ventricular score = 5).

The hemodynamic data showed that the right atrial pressure was 22 mm Hg with an "M" configuration (Figure 9.16, left). Note the A wave on the pressure tracing, without a visible P wave in the paced QRS ECG

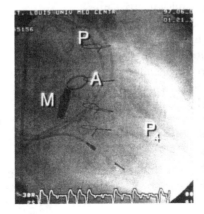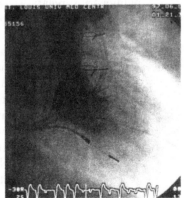

Figure 9.15 Cineangiographic frames before (left) and during (right) left ventriculography through the pigtail catheter (P4) positioned from the left ventricular apex. The supervalvular pigtail catheter (P) is positioned above the aortic ring (A), which is adjacent to the mitral ring (M). There are multiple pacing leads and two pulmonary artery catheters positioned near the superaortic pigtail catheter. Contrast injection during ventriculography shows no mitral regurgitation.

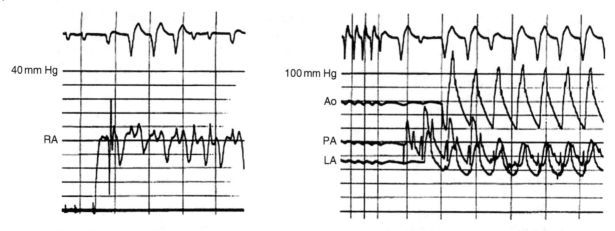

Figure 9.16 (Left) Right atrial (RA) pressure wave (0–40 mm Hg) showing a distinct "M" configuration, with an elevated mean pressure of approximately 20 mm Hg. (Right) Aortic (Ao), pulmonary artery (PA), and left atrial (LA) pressures (0–100 mm Hg scale). There is fair concordance of the pulmonary capillary wedge (after three beats of pulmonary artery pressure) and left atrial pressures.

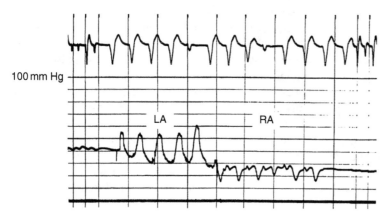

Figure 9.17 Pressure recorded during catheter pullback from the left atrium (LA) to the right atrium (RA; 0–100 mm Hg scale). The left atrial mean pressure is approximately 42 mm Hg, with a mean right atrial pressure of 25 mm Hg. The left atrial V waves exceed 50 mm Hg. Is this consistent with constrictive physiology?

complex. Right ventricular pressure was 75/24 mm Hg, and pulmonary artery pressure was 75/40 mm Hg (Figure 9.16, right). Mean pulmonary capillary wedge pressure was 40 mm Hg, with V waves to 50 mm Hg. Mean left atrial pressure was 38–42 mm Hg, with V waves to 50 mm Hg (Figures 9.16 and 9.17). On matching of the pulmonary capillary wedge and left atrial pressures (Figure 9.16), there was good correspondence of the V wave peak, but a slight delay of the pulmonary capillary wedge V wave decline, resulting in a higher mean value (and left ventricular–pulmonary capillary wedge gradient). Figure 9.17 compares the left and right atrial pressures during catheter pullback. Note the large left atrial V waves, despite only minimal mitral regurgitation by left ventriculography. As an aside, the initial ventricular systolic pressure was lower than the aortic pressure (Figure 9.18). This pressure matched the right ventricular pressure recorded during right-heart catheterization. The needle was then withdrawn and reintroduced at a

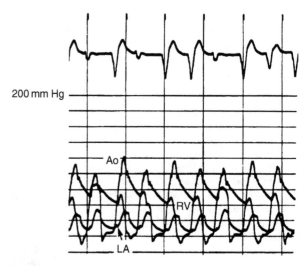

Figure 9.18 Simultaneous aortic (Ao), right ventricular (RV), and left atrial (LA) pressures (0–200 mm Hg scale). The long needle was withdrawn and repositioned.

Figure 9.19 Left ventricular (LV), left atrial (LA), and aortic (Ao) pressures (0–200 mm Hg scale), demonstrating the aortic and mitral prosthetic valve gradients. Note the influence of the paced beats on the valve gradients.

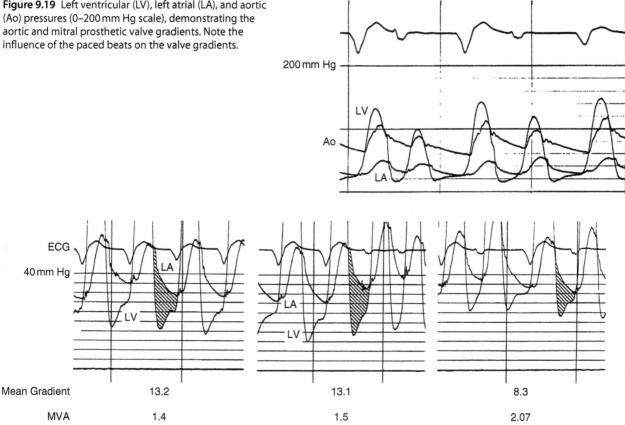

| Mean Gradient | 13.2 | 13.1 | 8.3 |
| MVA | 1.4 | 1.5 | 2.07 |

Figure 9.20 Left ventricular (LV) and left atrial (LA) pressure tracings during changing ventricular rhythms. The variation of the mitral valve area (MVA, cm²) is shown. Shaded area represents the diastolic pressure gradient. Elevation of the left ventricular end-diastolic pressure (far right) during the procedure decreases the gradient, despite lack of significant change in the left atrial pressure. Variation of the MVA occurred without change in cardiac output.

more posterior angle, with immediate achievement of the left ventricular pressure waveform (Figure 9.19). The left ventricular pressure was 140/28 mm Hg, and aortic pressure was 120/76 mm Hg. There was a peak-to-peak left ventricular–aortic gradient which varied from 15 mm Hg to 30 mm Hg. In addition, there was a left ventricular–mitral gradient which varied from 8 mm Hg to 13 mm Hg (Figure 9.20). Cardiac output was 4.4 L/min. Note the influence of RR cycle length on the left atrial–left ventricular gradient, with equilibration before end-diastole. The reduction of the mitral gradient was followed by an increased aortic–left ventricular gradient following the sinus beat (Figure 9.19, third beat). The aortic valve area thus varied from 0.8 (4.4 L/min √30) to 1.1 cm² (4.4 L/min √15).

The mitral valve area also demonstrated variation from 1.4 cm² to 2.07 cm² (Figure 9.20). It is interesting to note the higher left ventricular end-diastolic pressure in Figure 9.20 (far right), which resulted in the lowest mitral gradient. The left atrial pressure was lower during the paced rhythm as compared to sinus beats (Figure 9.20, middle).

The right and left ventricular end-diastolic pressures were elevated and identical, suggesting some degree of restrictive physiology (Figure 9.21). There was no oximetric or angiographic evidence of intracardiac shunts.

After left ventriculography, the pigtail catheter was withdrawn over a guidewire. The patient was monitored in the laboratory for 20 minutes. A repeat echocardiogram was performed which showed no pericardial effusion. The patient underwent reoperation for mitral valve replacement. Recovery was complicated by prolonged ventilatory support, but hemodynamics were improved.

Discussion

The precise calculation of valve areas remains critically dependent on pressure gradients and cardiac output, both of which are subject to variation in patients with arrhythmias or fluctuating hemodynamic baseline conditions [27]. Both factors were present in this patient and resulted in variability in the valve area results.

The aortic valve stenosis was thought to be the principal cause of pulmonary hypertension and congestive

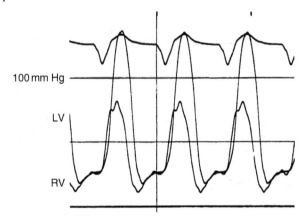

Figure 9.21 Simultaneous left ventricular (LV) and right ventricular (RV) pressure tracings during paced rhythm. The matching and elevation of the diastolic periods suggest some degree of restrictive or constrictive physiology, concomitant with the valvular dysfunction. Note the early rise of right, relative to left, ventricular pressure due to the paced ventricular activation.

heart failure. However, after valve replacement, the mitral valve was suspected of being dysfunctional. The aortic outflow obstruction was also considered partly contributory, since the intrinsic gradient of a newly positioned 22 mm St. Jude was at least 15–20 mm Hg. The valve size was limited by the aortic root in this small woman.

The changing left atrial and left ventricular pressures (Figure 9.20) suggested moderate mitral stenosis and, given the limited options and poor response to aggressive pharmacotherapy, also suggested that mitral valve replacement would be the best therapeutic approach. After the mitral valve was replaced, a slow and gradual reduction of pulmonary artery pressures to 45–50 mm Hg systolic and cessation of intermittent hemoptysis were noted.

The simultaneous use of transseptal left atrial and transapical left ventricular hemodynamics was required to identify a hemodynamically compromised mitral valve. This approach has obvious clinical value, although the computation of valve area is still the parameter with the greatest variance. The interesting question of restrictive physiology (Figure 9.21) remains unanswered. Cardiac constriction appeared to be excluded by the separation of the left atrial/right atrial pressures (Figure 9.17).

Complications of Left Ventricular Puncture

Evaluation of the left ventricular cavity by the direct percutaneous method was first described in 1933 by Reboul and Racine [28] in experimental canines and in 1949 by Buchbinder and Katz [29] in humans.

Other investigators [24–26] have provided the cardiology community with clinical examples in larger series involving over 300 patients, and have demonstrated the major complication rates, estimated to be at 3–4%.

The use of a long 18-gauge pericardiocentesis needle to place a guidewire followed by the 4 F catheter has been described [25, 26, 30] and is associated with minimal complications. The reported complications of direct left ventricular puncture have included transient hypotension, vasovagal symptoms, pneumothorax, ventricular arrhythmias, coronary laceration, and postpericardiotomy syndrome. In children, a death was reported with this technique when assessing complex congenital heart disease, including transposition of the great vessels [26]. Death was related to intramural contrast injection. A relatively low incidence of pericardial bleeding is thought to be reduced in patients with myocardial hypertrophy and by the systolic contraction, which is thought to seal the puncture site on removal of catheters. Previous thoracic surgery limits the active pericardial space and often is associated with lung-tissue adhesion to the anterior heart. This technique, described by Semple *et al.* [30], Wong *et al.* [31], and others [18–20], has used even larger catheters with similarly low complication rates.

Placement of catheters across the Bjork–Shiley or Starr–Edwards valves has been performed safely in some individuals [22, 23]. However, retrograde cannulation of tilting mechanical discs may result in potential catheter entrapment. The possible creation of false valvular regurgitation by propping open the prosthetic occluder limits the confidence in some observations. The risk of valve emboli is also increased for the tilting disc valves.

The largest experience of direct left ventricular access was summarized by Morgan *et al.* [26], who examined the results of the technique in 112 patients from 20,000 catheterizations performed between 1973 and 1987. Of these, 39 patients had mechanical prosthetic aortic valves, 25 with additional mechanical mitral valves. The remainder of the patients studied had severe native aortic valve stenosis (70 patients), xenograft aortic prosthetic stenosis (1 patient), and homograft aortic valve stenosis (2 patients). Direct left ventricular puncture was used to study mitral valve disease or prosthetic mitral valve dysfunction in 17 patients (16%). In contrast to more recent studies [25], their most common technique involved fluoroscopic identification of apical marker placed on the chest at the point of maximal impulse, with subsequent fluoroscopically guided insertion of a 19-gauge needle connected to pressure tubing [26]. The Seldinger technique for catheter insertion was then performed, using a guidewire and short 6 F catheters. In this series [26], there was one death four days after direct left ventricular puncture in a patient with severe aortic stenosis. No death was attributed to the direct left ventricular puncture itself. Two patients subsequently died during hospitalization. Two patients had pericardial tamponade, one whose international normalized ratio (INR) was greater than 2.1. One patient had pneumothorax, and two patients had pericardial effusion, which did not cause hemodynamic compromise. Pericardial and pleuritic pain was present in seven patients, and five patients had vagal episodes. Six patients had left ventricular cavities which could not be entered, and the study was terminated uneventfully. Major complications occurred in 3% of patients with a successful direct percutaneous left ventricular puncture (95% of patients). These data are similar to those on transseptal punctures reported by Lew *et al.* [32] in 207 patients, with morbidity in only 5% and major complications in 1%, with failure to enter the left ventricle in 15%.

Key Points

1) Multivalvular regurgitant lesions may have a common etiology, such as an underlying connective tissue disorder, Marfan's disease, or cardiomyopathy.

2) Careful collection of routine simultaneous left- and right-heart hemodynamics will document the individual valvular lesions.

3) Combined echocardiography and angiographic data will further support the interpretation of the hemodynamic waveforms.

4) Clinical decisions for valve repair or replacement will be based on the severity of associated lesions, myocardial function, and other patient-specific characteristics indicating the acceptable limits of surgical risk.

5) Combined aortic and mitral valve disease is a diagnostic and therapeutic dilemma which can be clarified by hemodynamics.

6) Careful interpretation of hemodynamics with multiple simultaneous pressure recordings is critical in clinical decision-making.

7) Direct left ventricular puncture is generally a safe and simple method with minimal mortality and morbidity, comparing favorably to the transseptal approach, and it offers unique angiographic and hemodynamic data, especially in the setting of abnormal prosthetic mitral or aortic valve involvement.

References

1 Kern MJ, Aguirre FV, Donohue TJ, Bach RG. Hemodynamic rounds: Interpretation of cardiac pathophysiology from pressure waveform analysis: Multivalvular regurgitant lesions. *Cathet Cardiovasc Diagn* 28:167–172, 1993.

2 Paraskos JA. Combined valvular disease. In JE Dalen, JS Alpert (eds), *Valvular Heart Disease*, 2nd ed. Boston, MA: Little, Brown, 1987, pp. 439–508.

3 Braunwald E. Valvular heart disease. In E Braunwald (ed.), *Heart Disease: A Textbook of Cardiovascular Medicine*. Philadelphia, PA: WB Saunders, 1988, pp. 1023–1992.

4 Kern MJ, Deligonul U. Hemodynamic rounds: Interpretation of cardiac pathophysiology from pressure waveform analysis: 1. The stenotic aortic valve. *Cathet Cardiovasc Diagn* 21:112–120, 1990.

5 Kern MJ, Aguirre FV. Hemodynamic rounds: Interpretation of cardiac pathophysiology from pressure waveform analysis: Aortic regurgitation. *Cathet Cardiovasc Diagn* 26:232–240, 1992.

6 Kern MJ, Aguirre F. Hemodynamic rounds: Interpretation of cardiac pathophysiology from pressure waveform analysis: Mitral valve gradients, Part 1. *Cathet Cardiovasc Diagn* 26:308–315, 1992.

7 Kern MI, Aguirre F. Hemodynamic rounds: Interpretation of cardiac pathophysiology from pressure waveform analysis: Mitral valve gradients, Part II. *Cathet Cardiovasc Diagn* 27:52–56, 1992.

8 Kern MJ, Deligonul U. Hemodynamic rounds: Interpretation of cardiac pathophysiology from pressure waveform analysis: II. The tricuspid valve. *Cathet Cardiovasc Diagn* 21:278–286, 1990.

9 Kern MJ. Hemodynamic rounds: Interpretation of cardiac pathophysiology from pressure waveform analysis: The pulmonary valve. *Cathet Cardiovasc Diagn* 24:190–213, 1991.

10 Kern MJ, Deligonul U. Hemodynamic rounds: Interpretation of cardiac pathophysiology from pressure waveform analysis: Pacemaker hemodynamics. *Cathet Cardiovasc Diagn* 24:22–27, 1991.

11 Segal J, Harvey WP, Hufnagel CA. Clinical study of one hundred cases of severe aortic insufficiency. *Am J Med* 21:200, 1956.

12 Gash AK, Carabello BA, Kent RL, Frazier JA, Spann JF. Left ventricular performance in patients with coexistent mitral stenosis and aortic insufficiency. *J Am Coll Cardiol* 3:703, 1984.

13 Melvin DB, Tecklenberg PL, Hollingsworth JF, Levine FR, Glancy DL, Epstein SE, Morrow AG. Computer-based analysis of preoperative and postoperative factors in 100 patients with combined aortic and mitral valve replacement. *Circulation* [suppl III] 48:58, 1973.

14 Kirklin JW, Barratt-Boyes BG. Combined aortic and mitral valve disease with or without tricuspid valve

disease. In *Cardiac Surgery*. New York: John Wiley & Sons, 1986, pp. 431–446.

15 Stephenson LW, Kouchoukos NT, Kirklin JW. Triple valve replacement: An analysis of eight years' experience. *Ann Thorac Surg* 23:327, 1977.

16 Wilkins GT, Weyman AE, Abascal VM, Block PC, Palacios IF. Percutaneous balloon dilatation of the mitral valve: An analysis of echocardiographic variables related to outcome and the mechanism of dilatation. *Br Heart J* 60:299–308, 1988.

17 Hakki AH, Iskandrian AS, Bemis CE, Kimbiris D, Mintz GS, Segal BL, Brice C. A simplified valve formula for the calculation of stenotic cardiac valve areas. *Circulation* 63:1050–1055, 1981.

18 Remadi JP, Baron O, Tribouilloy C, Roussel JC, Al-Habasch O, Despins P, Michaud JL, Duveau D. Bivalvular mechanical mitral-aortic valve replacement in 254 patients: Long-term results—a 22-year follow-up. *Ann Thorac Surg* 76:487–492, 2003.

19 Otto CM, Burwash IG, Legget ME, Munt BI, Fujioka M, Healy NL, Kraft CD, Miyake-Hull CY, Schwaegler RG. Prospective study of asymptomatic valvular aortic stenosis: Clinical, echocardiographic, and exercise predictors of outcome. *Circulation* 95:2262–2270, 1997.

20 Bonow RO, Carabello BA, Chatterjee K, de Leon AC Jr, Faxon DP, Freed MD, *et al.* ACC/AHA 2006 guidelines for the management of patients with valvular heart disease: A report of the American College of Cardiology/American Heart Association Task Force on Practice Guidelines (Writing Committee to Revise the 1998 guidelines for the management of patients with valvular heart disease) developed in collaboration with the Society of Cardiovascular Anesthesiologists endorsed by the Society for Cardiovascular Angiography and Interventions and the Society of Thoracic Surgeons. *J Am Coll Cardiol* 48:e1–e148, 2006.

21 Kern MJ. Left ventricular puncture for hemodynamic evaluation of double prosthetic valve stenosis. *Cathet Cardiovasc Diagn* 43:466–471, 1998.

22 Rigand M, Dubourg O, Luwaert R, Rocha P, Hamoir Y, Bardet J, Bourdarias JP. Retrograde catheterization of the left ventricle through mechanical aortic prosthesis. *Eur Heart J* 8:689–696, 1987.

23 Karsh DL, Michaelson SP, Langou RA, Cohen LS, Wolfson S. Retrograde left ventricular catheterization in patients with an aortic valve prosthesis. *Am J Cardiol* 41:893–896, 1978.

24 Levy LJ, Lillehei WC. Percutaneous direct cardiac catheterization. *N Engl J Med* 271:273–280, 1964.

25 Cata CJ, Grassman ED, Johnson SA. Technique of apical left ventricular puncture revisited: A case report of double-valve prothesis evaluation. *J Invas Cardiol* 6:251–255, 1994.

26 Morgan JM, Gray HH, Geeder C, Miller GA. Left heart catheterization by direct ventricular puncture: Withstanding the test of time. *Cathet Cardiovasc Diagn* 16:87–90, 1989.

27 Cannon SR, Richard KL, Crawford M. Hydraulic estimation of stenotic orifice area: A correction of the Gorlin formula. *Circulation* 71:1170–1178, 1985.

28 Reboul H, Racine M. Ventriculographic cardiaque experimentale. *Presse Med* 37:763, 1933.

29 Buchbinder WC, Katz LN. Intraventricular pressure curves of the human heart obtained by direct transthoracic puncture. *Proc Soc Exp Biol Med* 71:673, 1949.

30 Semple T, McGuiness JB, Gardner H. Left heart catheterization by direct ventricular puncture. *Br Heart J* 30:402–406, 1968.

31 Wong CM, Wong PH, Miller GA. Percutaneous left ventricular angiography. *Cathet Cardiovasc Diagn* 7:425–432, 1981.

32 Lew AS, Harper RW, Federman J, Anderson ST, Pitt A. Recent experience with transseptal catheterisation. *Cathet Cardiovasc Diagn* 9:601–609, 1983.

10

The Pulmonary Valve

Morton J. Kern

Abnormalities of the pulmonary valve occur most frequently in children, with rare individuals having clinically significant pulmonary valve disease in adulthood [1]. The hemodynamics of pulmonary valve disease most often reflect that of a congenitally narrowed, domed valve of pulmonic stenosis. A minority of individuals may have a thickened or dysplastic valve. Infundibular hypertrophy may present as pulmonic stenosis with normal valve structures. Occasionally, ventricular septal defects will also accompany the deformed valve. The diagnosis of pulmonary valvular (and sub- and supra-) lesions is made from echocardiography, right-heart pressure recordings, and right ventricular angiography [2–5]. Although uncommon, it is important to recognize the different waveforms associated with pulmonary stenosis and regurgitation, and conditions which may mimic or be confused with pulmonary stenosis in the absence of true valvular abnormalities. This hemodynamic round will deal with right-heart pressure tracings reflecting abnormalities of the pulmonary valve.

Pulmonary Stenosis: Valvular or Nonvalvular?

A 23-year-old woman with a history of congenital disease developed progressive exertional shortness of breath with atypical chest pain. At 8 months of age, the patient had repair of an atrial septal defect with pulmonary artery banding. The ventricular septal defect was not repaired. At age 14 years, the patient had debanding of the pulmonary artery and ventricular septal patch repair. Despite a small residual ventricular septal defect, right ventricular volume overload and increased right ventricular pressures were identified by echocardiography.

Because of increasing dyspnea on exertion with normal exercise tolerance, repeat echocardiography on the current examination revealed normal left ventricular systolic function, right ventricular enlargement with right ventricular overload, biatrial enlargement, and a small muscular persistent ventricular septal defect. Echocardiography suggested an increased pulmonary flow velocity and a pressure gradient across the pulmonary artery. Systemic blood pressure was 120/80 mm Hg. Pulse was 60 beats/min. There was no jugular vein distension. Heart examination revealed normal S_1 and S_2 without gallops. A III/VI systolic murmur was heard across the precordium with radiation to the back. Lungs were clear. Electrocardiogram showed normal sinus rhythm and pseudoinferior infarction pattern.

Right- and left-heart catheterization was performed. The mean pulmonary capillary wedge pressure was 14 mm Hg. There was no systolic gradient across the aortic valve. There was no clinically detectable shunt by oxygen saturation measurements through the right heart. Left ventriculography revealed a left ventricular ejection fraction of 53% without mitral regurgitation. Right ventriculography revealed a trace of right-to-left ventricular contrast flow.

To assess the right-heart pressures, two catheters were placed in the pulmonary artery and pressures zeroed, matched, and recorded. Examine the pressure waveforms in Figure 10.1. The pressure tracings are superimposed from two fluid-filled catheters. On pullback of the first catheter into the right ventricular cavity, a pressure gradient is easily identified, with right ventricular pressure equal to 95/10 mm Hg and pulmonary artery pressure equal to 30/12 mm Hg. This finding is consistent with pulmonary stenosis. Does this patient have pulmonary stenosis? Examine the pressure tracings in Figure 10.2 from the same patient. A large gradient is obvious between the higher pressure (PP) and the pulmonary artery pressure. From examining this tracing, localize where the gradient is produced. This patient does not have valvular but supravalvular stenosis. On Figure 10.2, the tracing labelled PP is a proximal pulmonary (PP) artery pressure obtained above the pulmonary valve, but

Hemodynamic Rounds: Interpretation of Cardiac Pathophysiology from Pressure Waveform Analysis, Fourth Edition.
Edited by Morton J. Kern, Michael J. Lim, and James A. Goldstein.

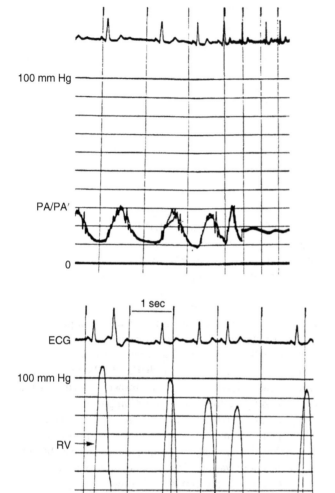

100 mm Hg

PA/PA'

0

1 sec

ECG

100 mm Hg

RV →

PA

0

Figure 10.1 (Top) Two simultaneously matched pressures measuring pulmonary artery pressure beyond the pulmonary valve (0–100 mm Hg scale). The mean pressures also matched. Peak pulmonary artery pressure was 30 mm Hg. (Bottom) Right ventricular (RV) pressure and simultaneous pulmonary artery (PA) pressure. Note the prominent systolic gradient. See text for details.

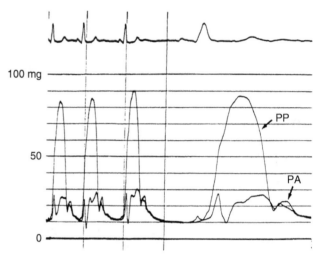

100 mg

50

0

Figure 10.2 Simultaneous pressures from patient example in Figure 10.1 measured as in Figure 10.1. Note the decline in peak systolic pressure. Is this pulmonic valve stenosis? PA = pulmonary artery; PP = proximal pulmonary. See text for details.

below the area of narrowing (the site of the prior pulmonary banding) just proximal to the bifurcation of the left and right pulmonary arteries. The pressures in the distal pulmonary artery were 34/12 mm Hg at the proximal site of narrowing, which was the previous location of the pulmonary artery band (85/12 mm Hg) and right ventricular pressure (95/10 mm Hg). Clues to the fact that this proximal pulmonary artery pressure was not the right ventricular pressure were evident by the reduction in peak systolic pressure and the matching of the diastolic to the pulmonary artery diastolic pressure. The diastolic

pressures of both tracings are superimposable. The finding of valvular pulmonary artery disease is excluded by this tracing. In all patients with suspected pulmonary valvular stenosis, a careful pullback of pressures measured from the distal pulmonary artery to the left main and to the pulmonary valve, and then careful matching of the pressure to the right ventricle, is essential. Compare this tracing to that of the next patient.

Pulmonary Stenosis and ECG Abnormalities

Examine the right-heart hemodynamics (Figure 10.3) of a 77-year-old woman who had a myocardial infarction in April 1984. Because of new-onset chest pain in July 1990, the patient returned to the cardiac catheterization laboratory. This pain was similar to that of the previous myocardial infarction. Because of signs of dyspnea and a systolic murmur heard in the left parasternal area, simultaneous right- and left heart catheterization was performed prior to coronary arteriography. On passage of the balloon-tipped pulmonary artery catheter, a right ventricular systolic pressure of 40 mm Hg was recognized, and on passage into the pulmonary artery beyond the pulmonic valve, the pulmonary artery pressure was 20/10 mm Hg. Simultaneous pressures were then obtained using a second right-heart catheter to identify the pulmonary artery–right ventricular gradient. Cardiac output was 4.9 L/min and the planimetered mean pulmonary artery gradient was 20 mm Hg. Compare the right ventricular and pulmonary artery pressures

Figure 10.3 (Top) Hemodynamics in a patient with a systolic pulmonic murmur. Right ventricular (RV) pressure is 42 mm Hg, pulmonary artery (PA) systolic pressure is 20 mm Hg. On continuous pullback from the pulmonary artery into the right ventricle, the two pressures match. There is no subpulmonic gradient identified. (Bottom) Right ventricular and pulmonary artery pressures (100 mm Hg paper speed). Note that the end-diastolic pressures for both pulmonary artery and right ventricular tracings are separated by 4 mm Hg. Also evident is the "a" wave on right ventricular tracing due to first degree A–V block (arrow). See text for details.

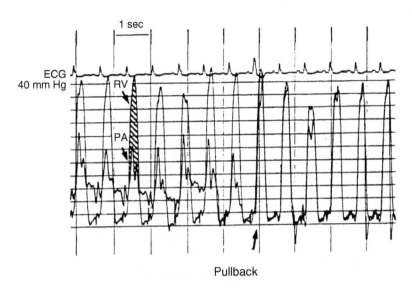

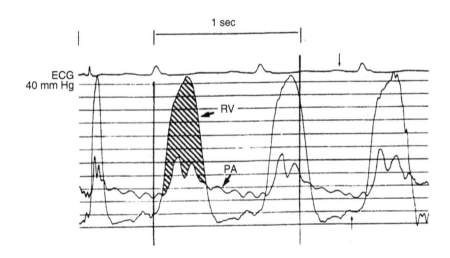

obtained in Figure 10.3 with the tracings in Figures 10.1 and 10.2. Note that the pulmonary artery pressure upstroke is slightly delayed and that the right ventricular pressure on pullback across the right ventricular infundibular area into the right ventricle (Figure 10.3, top) shows no supra- or subpulmonic gradient. The demonstration of the matching right ventricular pressures on pullback across the pulmonary artery valve is needed to identify unsuspected infundibular narrowing as a cause of the murmur.

An aside of special interest is the effect of pulmonary stenosis with right ventricular hypertrophy and bundle branch block on the right ventricular and left ventricular pressure patterns. The normal timing of the right ventricular pressure rise relative to left ventricular pressure (shown in Figure 10.4) can be delayed by abnormal impulse conduction to the right (or left) ventricle. Simultaneous right and left ventricular pressure measurements were made in patient #2 with pulmonary ste-

nosis and myocardial ischemia (Figure 10.5). Note the early onset of the right ventricular pressure relative to the left ventricular pressure, and the leftward shift of right ventricular pressure beneath the left ventricular pressure curve. This timing shift may reflect the intraventricular conduction abnormality. However, with bundle branch block, a delay in right ventricular pressure would be expected. The earlier right ventricular pressure seems to indicate an earlier excitation pathway. Alternatively, one might also attribute this earlier pressure rise to a different mechanism. The widened QRS is a nonspecific conduction defect.

The possible left ventricular hypertrophy with QRS widening may cause a delay in the onset of the left ventricular upstroke, delaying the timing of left ventricular relative to right ventricular pressure. Compared to the normal simultaneous right and left ventricular pressures in Figure 10.4, the left ventricular pressure upstroke in Figure 10.5 occurs later, after the R wave, suggesting

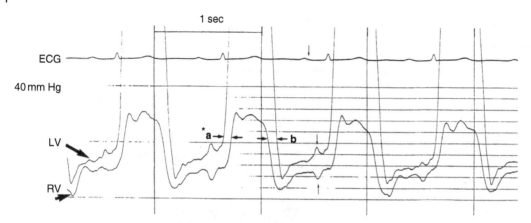

Figure 10.4 Simultaneous left ventricular (LV) and right ventricular (RV) pressures in a patient with ischemic heart disease without intraventricular conduction delay on electrocardiogram. The time intervals between left and right ventricular pressures (a and b) are normal and nearly identical. Because of first-degree heart block, note the prominent A wave on both left ventricular and right ventricular diastolic pressures (arrows) and the unusual configuration of the right ventricular A wave.

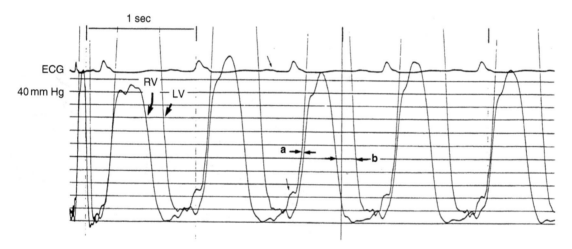

Figure 10.5 Simultaneous right ventricular (RV) and left ventricular (LV) pressures in the patient in Figure 10.3. Note the early onset of right ventricular pressure upstroke as indicated by the distance between arrows (a) on beat #3. During ventricular relaxation, the right ventricular pressure declines earlier and more rapidly than the left ventricular pressure. The time interval between decline in right and left ventricular pressures is indicated by the distance between arrows (b) and is markedly prolonged. See text for discussion.

delay of left ventricular pressure rather than earlier activation of right ventricular pressure. The clinical significance of these findings is unknown.

Combined Pulmonary Stenosis and Insufficiency

A 36-year-old woman had progressive shortness of breath, systolic heart murmur, and combined diastolic murmur. Echocardiography revealed high-velocity jets across the pulmonary valve in systole and diastole. Simultaneous hemodynamics measuring the pulmonary artery, right ventricular, and right atrial pressures (0–50 mm Hg scale) are shown in Figure 10.6. These

pressure waves show a modest gradient between right ventricular and pulmonary artery systolic pressures, with matching of low pulmonary artery and right ventricular end-diastolic pressures. There is a normal decline in pulmonary artery pressure across the diastolic period. Compare this tracing to Figure 10.3 (bottom), in which the pulmonary artery pressure declines across the diastolic period, but is maintained and elevated above right ventricular end-diastolic pressure, analogous to the hemodynamics of aortic stenosis without insufficiency, in which aortic diastolic pressure is maintained at levels well above left ventricular end-diastolic pressure, in distinction to the reduced aortic diastolic pressure seen in chronic aortic insufficiency. The wide pulmonary pulse pressure of Figure 10.6

Figure 10.6 Simultaneous right ventricular (RV), pulmonary artery (PA), and right atrial (RA) pressures (0–50 mm Hg scale) in a patient with systolic and diastolic murmurs. See text for details.

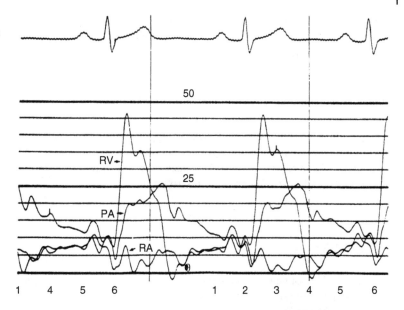

was associated with echocardiographically demonstrated pulmonic insufficiency. From these tracings (Figure 10.6), we can also deduce that there is no tricuspid stenosis or regurgitation. The pulmonary stenosis (and less so insufficiency) can be well characterized by the combined techniques. These findings correlated angiographically with an insufficient pulmonic valve, as well as a mild doming and deformation of the pulmonary valve leaflets.

Diastolic Murmur and Elevated Right Ventricular End-Diastolic Pressure

In a 45-year-old woman, elevated and matching pulmonary artery systolic pressures (Figure 10.7) were observed with continuous diastolic murmur across the right upper

sternal border. There was no right ventricular–pulmonary artery systolic gradient. The end-diastolic right ventricular pressure is elevated (25 mm Hg) and matches the pulmonary artery diastolic pressure at the onset of right ventricular contraction. Compare the waveforms of Figure 10.7 to Figures 10.3 and 10.6. The elevated pulmonary artery diastolic pressure does not normally indicate pulmonary insufficiency, but the marked distortion of the diastolic right ventricular pressure, especially at end-diastole, suggests continued filling of the right ventricle or a very noncompliant chamber. Coupled with clinical and echocardiographic findings, the diagnosis is clear. Less obvious would be the hemodynamic pulmonic insufficiency of Figure 10.6 without the striking right ventricular pressure increase during diastole. These tracings (Figure 10.7) might well correspond to those

Figure 10.7 Simultaneous right ventricular (RV) and pulmonary artery (PA) pressures in a patient with continuous diastolic murmur (0–100 mm Hg scale). See text for details.

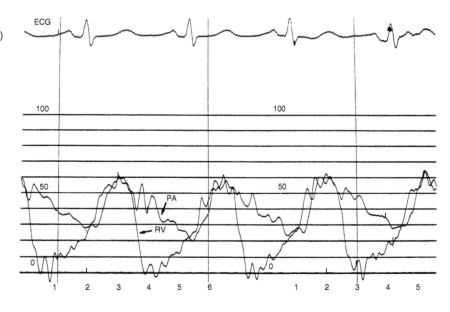

seen for acute aortic insufficiency, where end-diastolic left ventricular pressure increases to nearly equal that of aortic diastolic pressure.

Key Points

1) Although an uncommon lesion, when pulmonary stenosis is considered, pulmonary artery and right ventricular pressures should be assessed simultaneously on two-catheter pullback to appreciate the precise location of pulmonary–right ventricular pressure gradients.

2) Peripheral pulmonic stenosis can mimic pulmonary valve stenosis and pulmonary artery insufficiency may be difficult to delineate on pressure alone (as is often the case with the hemodynamics of aortic insufficiency).

3) Conduction defects or ventricular hypertrophy can affect the right ventricular pressure tracing and either delay or increase the timing of pressure rise and decline, depending on the conduction disturbance and abnormality of myocardial contraction.

References

1 Kern MJ. Hemodynamic rounds: Interpretation of cardiac pathophysiology from pressure waveform analysis: The pulmonary valve. *Cathet Cardiovasc Diagn* 24:209–213, 1991.

2 Grossman W. Profiles in valvular heart disease. In W Grossman (ed.), *Cardiac Catheterization and Angiography*. Boston, MA: Lea and Febiger, 1986, pp.359–381.

3 Freed MD, Keane JR. Profiles in congenital heart disease. In W Grossman (ed.), *Cardiac Catheterization and Angiography*. Boston, MA: Lea and Febiger, 1986, pp. 446–469.

4 Hirshfeld JW. Valve function: Stenosis and insufficiency. In CJ Pepine (ed.), *Diagnostic and Therapeutic Cardiac Catheterization*. Baltimore, MD: Williams & Wilkins, 1989, pp. 390–410.

5 Conti CR. Cardiac catheterization and the patient with congenital heart disease. In CJ Pepine (ed.), *Diagnostic and Therapeutic Cardiac Catheterization*. Baltimore, MD: Williams & Wilkins, 1989, pp. 508–522.

11

Hypertrophic Obstructive Cardiomyopathy (HOCM)

Morton J. Kern

The hemodynamic evaluation of hypertrophic obstructive cardiomyopathy (HOCM) centers on the degree of left ventricular outflow tract (LVOT) obstruction, which is dynamic and exquisitely sensitive to ventricular loading conditions and changes in contractility [1–3]. Figure 11.1 shows the pathologic hypertrophy of both the septum and posterior wall, and the relationship of the anterior leaflet of the mitral valve in proximity to the aortic outflow tract. The dynamic nature of LVOT pressures often produces disparate findings between echocardiographic and invasive measurements occurring at different times and under different conditions [4–8]. The LVOT pressure should be assessed at rest and during provocable maneuvers (e.g., variation with respiration, post-premature ventricular contraction [PVC] accentuation). Since patients may have symptoms during activity, this demonstration is especially important in the low LVOT gradient finding before committing to alcohol septal ablation.

A typical HOCM pressure waveform at rest is shown in Figure 11.2. The demonstration of LVOT obstruction as compared to intrinsic aortic valve obstruction is made by pullback of the left ventricular (LV) catheter from apex to base. The large LV–aortic gradient disappears when the catheter is positioned just above the mid-cavity obstruction (Figure 11.2).

Because of the dynamic nature of HOCM obstruction and its sensitivity to loading conditions, the hemodynamic recordings during a PVC can unmask the pathophysiology. The post-PVC hemodynamic tracings in a patient with HOCM (Figure 11.3) are associated with three distinct features: (i) the rapid upstroke of aortic pressure; (ii) a narrow aortic pulse pressure; and (iii) a "spike and dome" configuration of early vigorous LV ejection followed by delay in ejection of the remaining LV volume, with the resulting outflow gradient. Another method to demonstrate the severity of LVOT obstruction in HOCM patients is to perform a Valsalva maneuver.

At the beginning of the Valsalva strain phase, there is an increase in left ventricular end-diastolic pressure (LVEDP) and reduced arterial pulse pressure. The LVOT gradient begins to appear and is most pronounced during the plateau phase, and may be dramatic during a PVC in this setting.

Both aortic stenosis (AS) and HOCM are associated with systolic outflow obstruction with systolic murmurs. AS can be easily differentiated from HOCM by examining the response to a PVC. A comparison of the post-PVC hemodynamic responses between HOCM and AS is shown in Figure 11.4a. In aortic stenosis, the post-PVC hemodynamic tracings show a larger pulse pressure, a consistently slow aortic upstroke of fixed valve obstruction, and no change in the aortic waveform, all in contrast to the HOCM hemodynamics, which show a reduced pulse pressure, brisk aortic pressure upstroke (parallel to LV pressure), and deformation of the aortic waveform, with a spike and dome of rapid early ejection and secondary outflow obstruction.

Mechanical treatment to relieve the LVOT obstruction includes alcohol septal ablation or surgical myomectomy. Both techniques are effective in this regard, but surgery is favored in the younger (<75 years) patients compared to the elderly [5]. With either technique, the classic hemodynamic abnormalities of the LVOT are abolished when the septum is infarcted, thus reducing or eliminating its contribution to outflow obstruction. Figure 11.4b shows the hemodynamic results of a successful alcohol septal ablation procedure. Note the elimination of the LVOT gradient, along with the spike and dome configuration of the arterial pulse tracing. Further reduction in the LVOT gradient occurs over 3–6 months following the procedure due to ventricular remodeling and basal septal thinning.

The discussion of HOCM hemodynamics begins with an analysis of cases presenting with LVOT pressure gradients.

Hemodynamic Rounds: Interpretation of Cardiac Pathophysiology from Pressure Waveform Analysis, Fourth Edition.
Edited by Morton J. Kern, Michael J. Lim, and James A. Goldstein.
© 2018 John Wiley & Sons Ltd. Published 2018 by John Wiley & Sons Ltd.

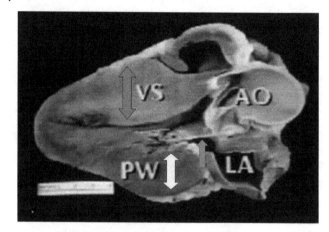

Figure 11.1 The pathologic hypertrophy of both the septum (VS) and posterior wall (PW) and the relationship of the left atrium (LA) and the anterior leaflet of the mitral valve in proximity to the aortic outflow tract (AO).

Disappearing Aortic Stenosis?

A 44-year-old woman is admitted with episodic shortness of breath, occasional episodes of palpitations, and a loud harsh systolic murmur, thought to be aortic stenosis. The electrocardiogram revealed left ventricular hypertrophy. Chest X-ray was normal. Physical examination demonstrated a loud crescendo/decrescendo systolic murmur at rest. The echocardiogram demonstrated left ventricular hypertrophy and normal aortic valve excursion. Cardiac catheterization was performed to clarify the conflicting noninvasive findings. Immediately after crossing the aortic valve, a large pressure gradient between the left ventricle and aorta was seen (Figure 11.5). As the pigtail catheter was repositioned, the aortic–left ventricular gradient disappeared. On pullback of the pigtail catheter from the left ventricular apex, the

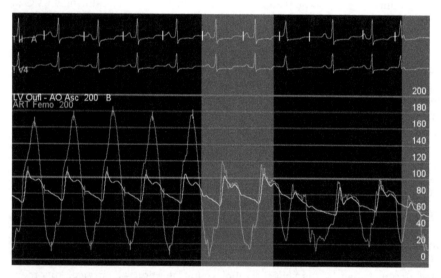

Figure 11.2 Hemodynamic left ventricular (LV, blue) and aortic (Ao, red) pressure tracings in a patient with hypertrophic cardiomyopathy. The LV catheter is pulled back from the distal LV (left side) to subaortic position (right side). Note the reduction in LV–Ao pressure gradient while still recording LV pressure. In addition, one can appreciate the configuration of the aortic pressure with a typical "spike and dome" appearance. (*See insert for color representation of the figure.*)

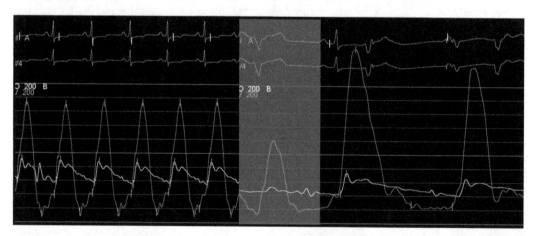

Figure 11.3 Hemodynamics in a patient with hypertrophic obstructive cardiomyopathy (HOCM). Left ventricular (blue) and aortic (red) pressure tracings demonstrate the vertical upstroke of aortic pressure, with a rapid early ejection and mid-systolic delay (spike and dome pattern). Following a PVC (shaded bar), the post-PVC reduction of the aortic pulse pressure is evident (called the Brockenbrough–Braunwald–Morrow sign), with a marked increase in the LVOT pressure gradient. (*See insert for color representation of the figure.*)

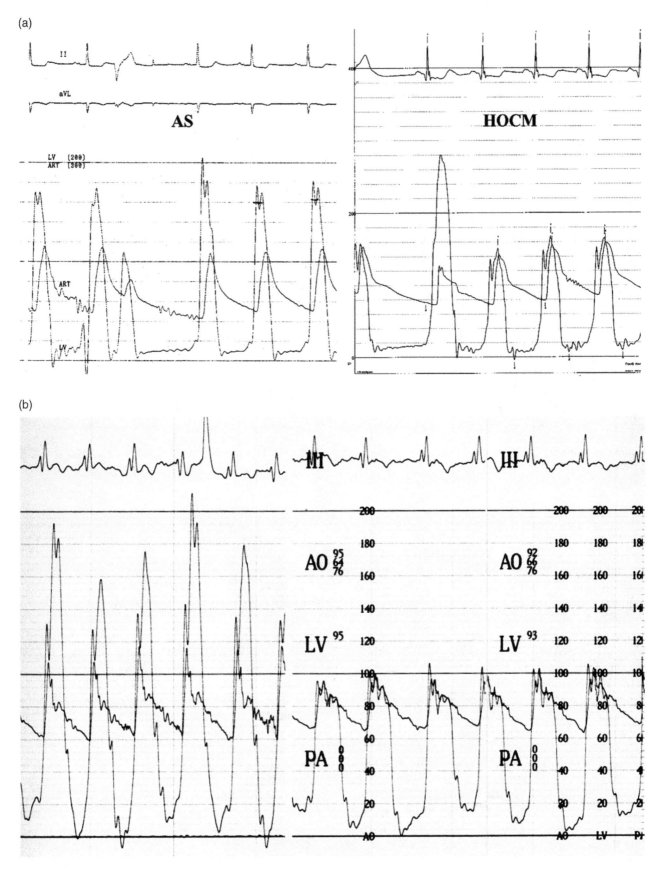

Figure 11.4 (a) Hemodynamic tracings in a patient with aortic stenosis (AS, left) compared to one with hypertrophic obstructive cardiomyopathy (HOCM, right). In AS, the post-PVC beat of the aortic pressure wave has a slow upstroke, wide pulse pressure, and the same waveform as normal beats. In HOCM, the post-PVC aortic pressure wave has a vertical upstroke, narrow pulse pressure, and the typical alteration of the aortic pressure of obstruction with the spike and dome contour. (b) Hemodynamics of HOCM before (left) and after (right) alcohol septal ablation. Note that the arterial waveform before transluminal ablation of septal hypertrophy (TASH) has a spike and dome configuration, which is eliminated after TASH. The left ventricular outflow tract (LVOT) gradient as rest is abolished as well.

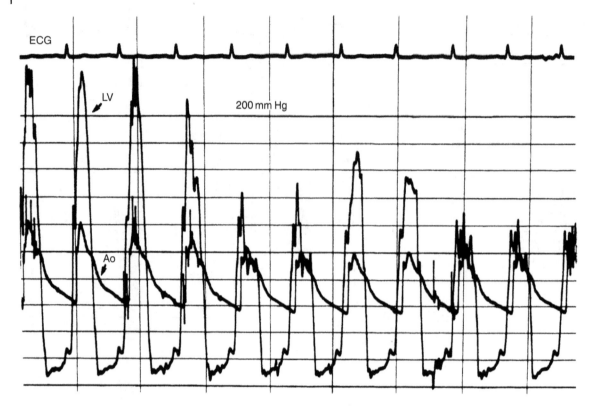

Figure 11.5 Simultaneous left ventricular (LV) and aortic (Ao) pressures (0–200 mm Hg scale) in a patient with "disappearing aortic stenosis." See text for details.

intraventricular gradient is abolished (beats #5 and 6), can be seen to reappear on slight advancement of the catheter (beats #7 and 8), and is again fully absent when the catheter is moved to a more proximal left ventricular position (beats #9 and 10). The left ventricular–aortic gradient is due entirely to an area of obstruction below the normal aortic valve within the mid-proximal portion of the ventricle. Several features clearly distinguish this tracing from that of aortic stenosis. The most diagnostic finding is the loss of aortic–left ventricular gradient on catheter repositioning within the ventricle while still beneath the aortic valve, locating the gradient as truly subvalvular (i.e., intraventricular but not valvular). Secondly, the upstroke of aortic pressure is nearly vertical and parallel with LV pressure, with a very early peak. Compare this waveform and that of Figure 11.6 to the late and slow upstroke in aortic stenosis. In HOCM, the largest left ventricular–aortic pressure gradient occurs in mid-systole, whereas in aortic stenosis, the largest gradient usually occurs in early systole. The third finding is that the distorted aortic pressure wave has a spike and dome configuration of early obstruction and delayed LV ejection (see below). Other more subtle differences between valvular and subvalvular gradients, such as timing changes of left ventricular volume, velocity of

left ventricular flow, and characteristic aortic pressure waves, are illustrated in Figures 11.7 and 11.8.

Methods to Provoke Intracavitary Pressure Differences in HOCM

Three mechanisms augment intraventricular gradients: (i) decreasing ventricular end-diastolic volume (i.e., lowering left atrial filling or reducing length of diastole [10]); (ii) increasing force or duration of ventricular contraction; and (iii) decreasing aortic outflow resistance. Whether the intraventricular gradients of HOCM represent true flow obstruction has been the source of considerable controversy [9, 11]. In human studies when no resting gradients are evident, use of isoproterenol infusions to produce a hypercontractile state has been proposed and applied by White *et al.* [10]

Four common maneuvers to elicit HOCM gradients have been employed in the catheterization laboratory: the Valsalva maneuver, nitroglycerin, post-extra-systolic potentiation [11, 12], and the now obsolete isoproterenol infusion [10].

The hemodynamic technique for assessment of the LVOT gradient is identical to that used for the

Figure 11.6 Simultaneous aortic (Ao) and left ventricular (LV) pressures (0–200 mm Hg scale). Note the influence of premature ventricular contractions. See text for details.

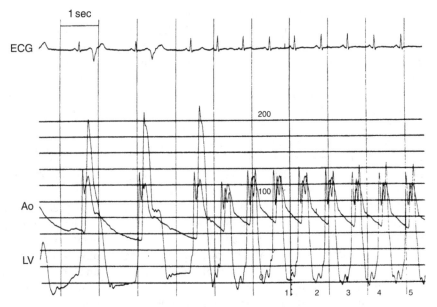

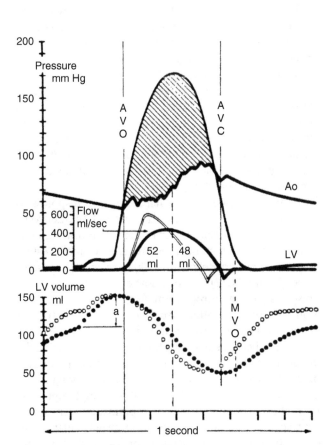

Figure 11.7 Hemodynamic examples of a patient with discrete obstructive gradient with aortic stenosis. Ao = aorta; LV = left ventricle; MVO = mitral valve opening; AVC = aortic valve closure; AVO = aortic valve opening; a = atrial contribution to ventricular filling. See text for details. *Source:* Criley 1985 [9]. Reproduced with permission of Wolters Kluwer Health, Inc.

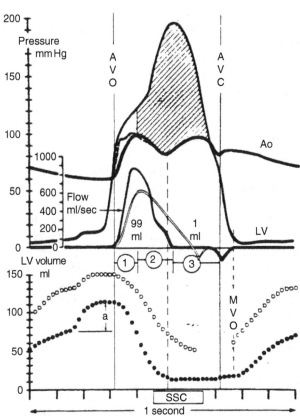

Figure 11.8 Dynamic gradient in hypertrophic cardiomyopathy. Ao = aorta; LV = left ventricle; MVO = mitral valve opening; AVC = aortic valve closure; AVO = aortic valve opening; a = atrial contribution to ventricular filling; SSC = onset of septal anterior leaflet motion and septal contact. Numbers in circles 1, 2, and 3 identify the three phases of ejection from the left ventricle and discrete alterations in pressure and waveform due to motion and obstruction with intraventricular pressure gradient development. See text for details. *Source:* Criley 1985 [9]. Reproduced with permission of Wolters Kluwer Health, Inc.

assessment of aortic valve stenosis. While acceptable in most circumstances, a pigtail catheter with shaft side holes should be replaced by an end hole or Halo (out-of-plane pigtail) catheter, because pigtail catheters have shaft side holes which may be positioned above the intra-cavitary obstruction, producing an erroneously low LVOT gradient. A Halo catheter with no shaft side holes is preferred. The most accurate hemodynamic assessment of LVOT obstruction uses a transseptal approach, with a balloon-tipped catheter placed at the left ventricular inflow region and a pigtail catheter in the ascending aorta, for simultaneous measurement of the LVOT gradient. The transseptal approach helps to avoid catheter entrapment, which can be confused with left ventricular pressure of LVOT obstruction. Use of an 8 F Mullins sheath for transseptal access also enables the recording of left atrial pressure via the side arm for assessment of concomitant diastolic dysfunction.

The dynamic LVOT gradient of HOCM is illustrated in a case of a 72-year-old man who presented with a history of increasing fatigue, vague chest pain, and mild shortness of breath over the last 6–12 months. The patient had mild left ventricular hypertrophy on ECG and an intermittent systolic ejection-type murmur, and the ECG revealed a hypertrophied left ventricle without a resting LVOT gradient. Left ventricular and simultaneous aortic pressures showed (Figure 11.6) no resting left ventricular–aortic gradient, but during bigeminy on the post-extra-systolic beat, a marked systolic gradient occurred. A diminution in the aortic pulse pressure on the beat following the extra-systolic beat is a hallmark finding of hypertrophic cardiomyopathy (Brockenbrough–Braunwald–Morrow sign) [12]. When the rhythm returns to normal sinus (right side of the tracing), the intraventricular gradient is no longer evident. Provoking the intraventricular gradient with extra-systolic beats may be easily obtained evidence of obstructive hypertrophic myopathy in some patients.

Brockenbrough, Braunwald, and Morrow first described the hemodynamic characteristics of patients with hypertrophic cardiomyopathies in 1961 [12], revealing striking differences between valvular aortic stenosis and discrete subvalvular stenosis. In patients with aortic stenosis, an increase in arterial pulse pressure accompanies a rise in peak left ventricular systolic pressure following premature ventricular contractions. In contrast, in patients with hypertrophic subaortic stenosis, premature ventricular contractions are followed by narrowing of the arterial pulse pressure in association with increasing left ventricular systolic pressure, the Brockenbrough–Braunwald–Morrow sign. A characteristic change in left ventricular–aortic gradient with an alteration of the aortic pressure contour reflects early forceful left ventricular ejection (spike and dome pattern), and can also be elicited during the Valsalva maneuver in these patients.

Although failure of the pulse pressure to increase in the post-PVC beat is often characteristic of hypertrophic cardiomyopathy, left ventricular ejection time may be a more sensitive and more specific finding [13]. Comparison of post-PVC hemodynamics for aortic stenosis and HOCM and the effect of loss of atrial contraction are illustrated in Figures 11.9–11.12.

Preload Alterations and Intraventricular Gradients

A 47-year-old woman was admitted with a recent history of increasing dyspnea. Left ventricular hypertrophy was documented by electrocardiography and echocardiography. No LV outflow tract flow disturbances were identified on Doppler echocardiogram. Simultaneous aortic and left ventricular pressures (Figure 11.13) showed a post-premature ventricular contraction without an intraventricular gradient. To provoke an intraventricular gradient, several maneuvers which alter preload were performed. During the Valsalva maneuver, intrathoracic pressure increases the left ventricular diastolic pressure and (after beat #7), the post-extra-systolic beats produce large intraventricular gradients and reduced aortic pulse pressure (see discussion of Brockenbrough–Braunwald–Morrow sign above). The intraventricular gradient is significantly reduced on release of the Valsalva maneuver (beat #3, from right). In this case, premature ventricular contraction alone did not elicit an intraventricular gradient (beat #2, from left). After Valsalva, premature ventricular contractions provoked an intraventricular gradient, establishing the diagnosis of obstructive hypertrophic myopathy.

In the same patient, the hemodynamic response to nitroglycerin was also examined (Figure 11.14). Left ventricular–aortic pressures after nitroglycerin now demonstrated reduced systolic pressure and a small resting gradient (approximately 10 mm Hg) not seen with Valsalva alone (Figure 11.13). Systolic aortic and left ventricular pressures before nitroglycerin (Figure 11.13) averaged around 140 mm Hg; after nitroglycerin, the left ventricular systolic pressure is 100 mm Hg and aortic pressure 90 mm Hg. A Valsalva maneuver was then performed. During the initial phases of the Valsalva maneuver, a run of four premature ventricular contractions produces a striking LVOT gradient. After Valsalva, the arterial pressure temporarily rises above resting levels. Later premature ventricular contractions also demonstrate an intraventricular gradient with nitroglycerin. Sustained preload reduction with nitroglycerin or transient reduction with Valsalva maneuver can elicit important changes in intraventricular gradients in these patients.

The Valsalva maneuver increases the intraventricular gradient by the progressive reduction in stroke volume.

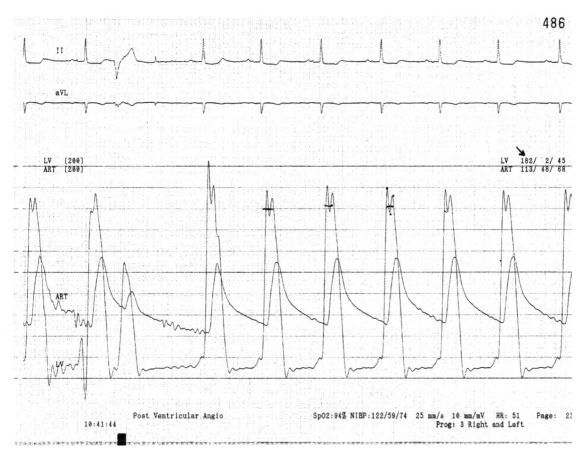

Figure 11.9 Aortic stenosis is characterized by an increased gradient, delayed aortic pressure upstroke, and normal or widened pulse pressure (above).

Increasing intrathoracic pressure reduces venous return and LV filling and progressively increases the magnitude of the pressure gradient. A reflex increase in contractility during the Valsalva maneuver does not appear to contribute to this gradient change, since increases in heart rate and peripheral vascular resistance occur only at the end of the Valsalva maneuver. The Valsalva maneuver reduces inflow and preload to the left ventricular chamber.

Nitroglycerin increases pressure gradients in HOCM, but decreases left ventricular–aortic pressure gradients in patients with valvular aortic stenosis [12, 14]. In HOCM a reduction in venous return to the heart decreases left ventricular filling and left ventricular outflow, increasing the intraventricular gradient.

Intraventricular pressure gradients can be noted in patients both with and without asymmetric and symmetric myocardial hypertrophy, and in those without hypertrophy in whom angiographic left ventricular cavity obliteration is observed. The post-extra-systolic beat potentiation phenomenon may also be observed in patients with symmetric as well as asymmetric septal hypertrophy, indicating that cavity obliteration by itself may have a hemodynamic significance. This contraction abnormality, the hyperejection of blood from the left ventricle, is characteristic of hypertrophic diseased states, and it may be observed in patients with hypertension, aortic stenosis, and symmetric hypertrophy related to pathophysiologic pressure overload of ventricular function [14].

Dynamic Left Ventricular Outflow Tract Gradients from Other Causes

Dynamic LVOT gradients may be present in normal or hypertrophied ventricles without myopathy in which inotropic, hypovolemic, or vasodilator provocations occur [9, 10, 15]. The gradient may result from mid-cavity obstruction, mitral anterior leaflet–septal opposition, or catheter entrapment in the apical portion of the left ventricle. Three phases characterize the dynamic gradients in patients with hypertrophic myopathy. Phase 1 occurs early in systole, in which the impulse gradient is larger than normal since peak flow and acceleration velocity are markedly enhanced. Phase 2 is characterized by an increasing left ventricular–aortic gradient with a

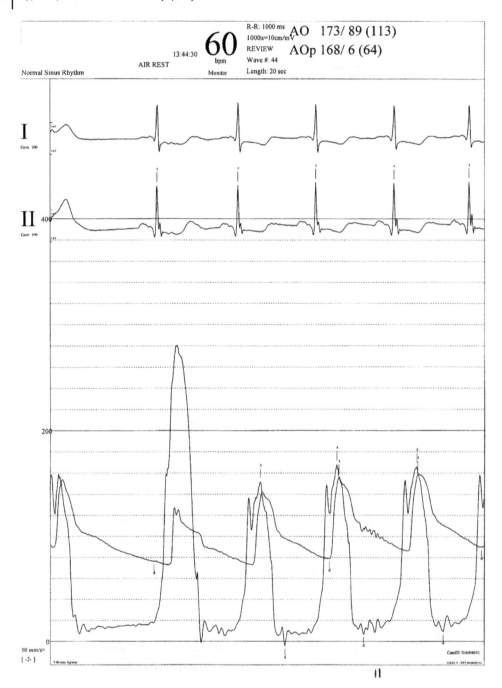

Figure 11.10 Hypertrophic obstructive cardiomyopathy is characterized by an increased gradient, rapid aortic pressure upstroke, and reduced pulse pressure (above) and a marked change in the configuration of the aortic pressure, with a sharp spike and delay pressure (dome) of impaired ejection from the ventricle.

decline in aortic flow to zero. The pressure gradient achieves its maximal dimension during phase 2. Left ventricular ejection ends as the ventricle realizes the smallest volume and a supernormal ejection fraction. In phase 3, aortic outflow has ceased. The ventricle is iso-volumetric at this point. A persistent decline in the pressure gradient occurs as the left ventricle relaxes and pressure falls. There is a secondary rise in outflow tract

and aortic pressures at this time (accounting for the dome of the spike and dome of arterial pressure).

Dynamic LVOT obstruction can also be seen without hypertrophic cardiomyopathy, especially in situations with decreased left ventricular filling and increased contractility [16–19]. A hemodynamically significant LVOT obstruction was observed during cardiac tamponade without hypertrophic myopathy, an association not previously

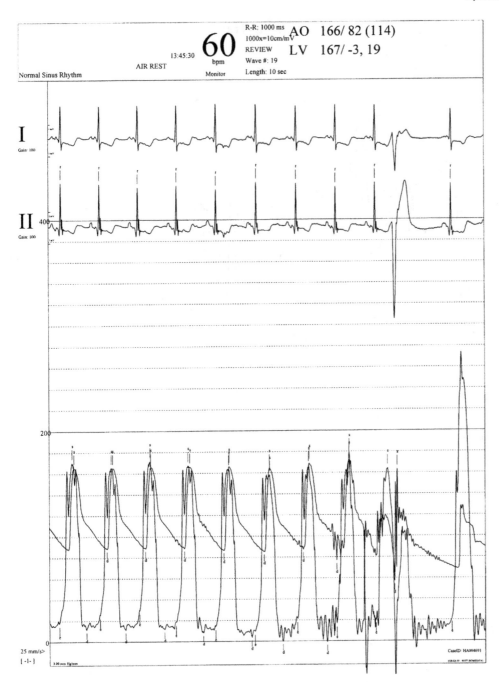

Figure 11.11 Post-premature ventricular contraction Brockenbrough–Braunwald–Morrow sign on last beat at right side of tracing. Note that the scale is 0–400 mm Hg. The arterial pressure wave on this beat shows the spike and dome waveform which is classic for hypertrophic obstructive cardiomyopathy.

described [20, 21]. A 64-year-old woman underwent successful left anterior descending coronary angioplasty for unstable angina five days after acute anterior myocardial infarction. Eighteen hours after angioplasty, hypotension, nausea, and vomiting with ST segment elevation were noted. Dobutamine, dopamine, levophed, and intubation were needed to maintain a systolic blood pressure of 80 mm Hg in the presence of a significant pericardial effusion. Coronary angiography revealed the left anterior descending angioplasty site to be intact. Simultaneous aortic (femoral artery) and left ventricular pressures are shown on Figure 11.15a, demonstrating a subaortic–left ventricular gradient prior to pericardiocentesis. The intraventricular gradient was documented on multiple catheter pullbacks. Akinesis of the apical septum was observed on ventriculography and marked systolic obstruction of the

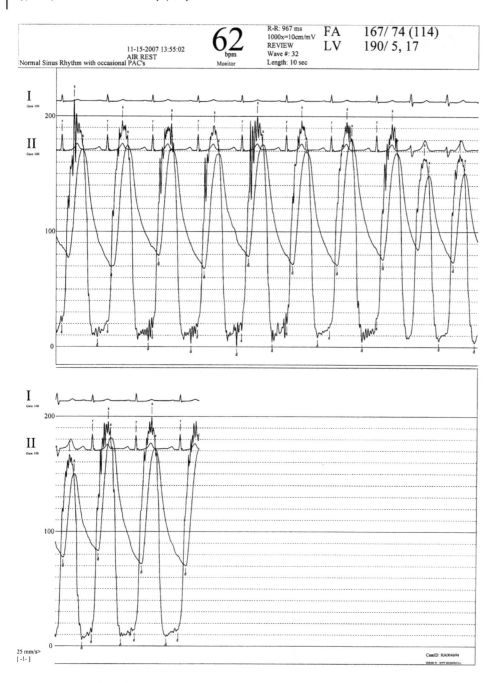

Figure 11.12 The loss of atrial filling ("kick") to cardiac output in patients with hypertrophic obstructive cardiomyopathy or any restrictive type of cardiomyopathy is reflected by loss of arterial pressure, as shown above by transition from normal sinus rhythm to junction rhythm, with loss of arterial and LV pressure by about 20–25 mm Hg. This can be disabling in some patients with marginal cardiac output.

outflow tract was documented, with approximation of the septum and anterior mitral valve leaflet (Figure 11.15b and 11.15b). There was no left ventricular septal or left ventricular free-wall hypertrophy. After pericardiocentesis, echocardiography confirmed absence of pericardial effusion and resolution of systolic anterior mitral leaflet motion, with normalization of aortic flow velocity. The intraventricular gradient also disappeared (Figure 11.15d).

Dynamic LVOT obstruction without hypertrophic myopathy after acute myocardial infarction with pericardial effusion was due to a marked decline in left ventricular volume as a result of marked underfilling of the ventricle, increased catecholamines during tamponade, and additional inotropic effects of intravenous pharmacologic pressure support agents, all contributing to the intraventricular gradient by increasing contractility while decreasing systolic

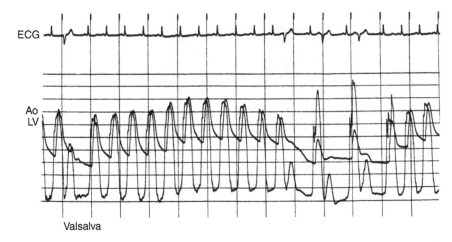

Valsalva

Figure 11.13 Simultaneous aortic (Ao) and left ventricular (LV) pressures (0–200 mm Hg scale) during Valsalva maneuver. Note the influence of premature ventricular contractions before and during the maneuver. See text for details.

Figure 11.14 Simultaneous aortic (Ao) and left ventricular (LV) pressures (0–200 mm Hg scale) during nitroglycerin and Valsalva maneuver (same patient as in Figure 11.13). Note the influence of premature ventricular contractions. See text for details.

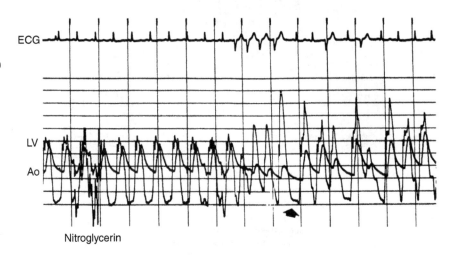

Nitroglycerin

volume. Pericardial tamponade was not previously known with the development of outflow tract obstruction in patients without hypertrophic myopathy, suggesting that systolic anterior motion of the mitral leaflet alone may contribute to some degree of intracavitary dynamic pressure development. This unusual case highlights the importance of understanding cardiac hemodynamics for the treatment of such complicated patients.

Intramyocardial Pressure as a Cause of Intraventricular Pressure Gradient

An intraventricular pressure gradient may also be encountered in some patients if the catheter becomes entrapped or embedded in the cardiac muscle. In late systole, a high left ventricular pressure would be recorded, reflecting subendocardial, intramyocardial tissue pressure. An entrapped catheter does not eject blood or permit blood sampling through its lumen during

systole. The initial inflow tract pressure as well as other intracavitary pressures would be equal to aortic systolic pressure. This type of pressure artifact must be identified before attributing intraventricular pressures to hypertrophic cardiomyopathy. The characteristic intramyocardial pressure usually has a very late-peaking pressure which is maximal at the aortic pressure of the dichrotic notch. Catheter entrapment, producing this artifact, is most commonly present when using end hole catheters deeply embedded from the transseptal or transvalvular aortic approach [22, 23].

Left Ventricular Diastolic Waveform Abnormalities: Relaxation Impairment

The diastolic left ventricular waveform in Figure 11.5 shows a large A wave and high left ventricular end-diastolic pressure. Beside increased "stiffness" (i.e., low compliance), other abnormalities of left ventricular diastolic

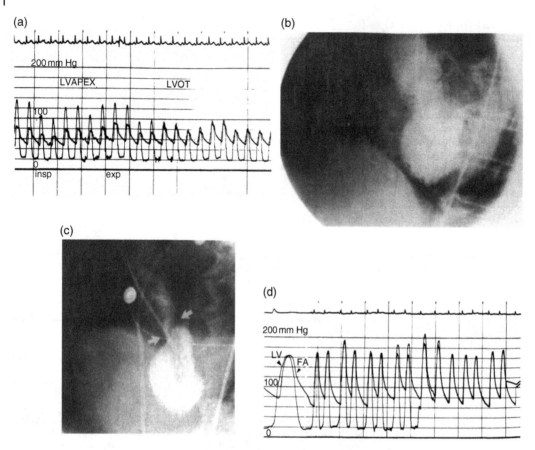

Figure 11.15 (a) Simultaneous femoral arterial (FC) and left ventricular (LV) pressures from the left ventricular apex and outflow tract document the subvalvular aortic gradient. The femoral arterial pressure showed pulsus paradoxus, with a decrease in systolic pressure and narrowing of the pulse pressure during inspiration. (b, c) End-systolic frames from the left anterior oblique cranial left ventrilculograms before percutaneous transluminal coronary angioplasty (PTCA, b) and during tamponade (c). A significant narrowing of the left ventricular outflow tract between the upper septum and the anterior mitral leaflet is clearly seen in c (arrows). The distal part of the septum was akinetic. (d) Immediately after pericardiocentesis, the simultaneous FA and LV pressures indicate no pressure gradient.

pressure have been described in these patients. For example, in Figure 11.14 (black arrow), the diastolic left ventricular pressure after the fourth premature ventricular contraction has an abnormal diastolic relaxation pattern. This waveform change should not be confused with artifact from pigtail catheter malposition partly in the aorta (the last two beats of Figure 11.14). (The effect of pigtail catheter side holes positioned slightly outside the aortic valve markedly elevates early left ventricular diastole. Normally, left ventricular pressure is at its lowest level in early diastole. Nonetheless, the systolic aortic–left ventricular gradient can still be appreciated. A malposition of the pigtail catheter side holes usually reduces the aortic–left ventricular gradient.)

A normal ventricle should have a rising left ventricular pressure across the entire diastolic period. The characteristic abnormality in hypertrophic myopathy of the left ventricular diastolic pressure, decreasing slowly in mid-diastole (Figure 11.14, black arrow), has been reported to be due to abnormal left ventricular relaxation [24].

Although uncommon even for patients with hypertrophic cardiomyopathy, left ventricular diastolic pressure may continue to decline over the course of diastole, an abnormal relaxation pattern which may be abolished by calcium channel blockers [15]. In the patient described in Figure 11.14 in whom an intraventricular gradient was provoked during nitroglycerin, Valsalva, and extra-systoles, the left ventricular diastolic pressure contour following a premature ventricular contraction and long pause (Figure 11.14, black arrow) can be seen to decline, suggesting intermittent abnormal relaxation on several of these post-systolic beats.

Although hypertrophic muscle may have an extraordinarily vigorous contraction, ventricular relaxation and compliance characteristics are markedly impaired. Consider the hemodynamics in a 75-year-old man with a hypertrophic cardiomyopathy (nonobstructive type) with no provocable gradient (Figure 11.16). Simultaneous left ventricular and aortic pressures were measured during an episode of paced rhythm in which

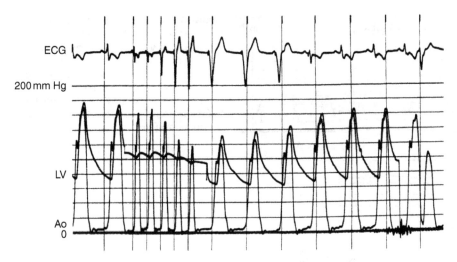

Figure 11.16 Simultaneous left ventricular (LV) and aortic (Ao) pressures (0–200 mm Hg scale) in an elderly patient with hypertrophic cardiomyopathy and no resting intraventricular gradient, who spontaneously goes into pacemaker rhythm. The contribution of atrial activity in a noncompliant left ventricle is evident by the marked drop in arterial pressure. See text for details.

atrial synchrony was lost. This arrhythmia resulted in a 20–25% drop in systolic aortic pressure, from 175 to 130 mm Hg, due to loss of the atrial contribution to left ventricular filling.

Hemodynamics of Dual-Chamber Pacing and Valsalva Maneuver in a Patient with Hypertrophic Obstructive Cardiomyopathy

Hypertrophic cardiomyopathy may present with disabling symptoms of exertional dyspnea, angina, and syncope. These symptoms have been variably ascribed to the associated obstructive left ventricular gradient, resulting in high-velocity left ventricular outflow, mitral regurgitation, and diastolic left ventricular dysfunction [25, 26]. Although the treatment for hypertrophic myopathy includes beta adrenergic and calcium channel blocking agents [27], some patients with medically refractory symptomatology may benefit from septal myectomy [28]. Past studies have suggested dual-chamber pacing as an alternative therapy [29–31]. A decrease in left ventricular outflow gradient and symptoms has been reported after implantation of a permanent dual-chamber pacemaker, thought to be due to uncoordinated activation of septal contraction from pacing at the right ventricular apex [32]. The effects have not been uniformly beneficial, and issues regarding diastolic dysfunction have suggested that AV sequential pacing may be superior to right ventricular pacing [29–31].

To demonstrate the effects of AV pacing in a patient with HCOM, left ventricular outflow hemodynamics were recorded at rest, during provocative maneuvers such as Valsalva and premature ventricular contractions and during AV sequential pacing, in a 36-year-old woman with progressive exertional dyspnea, lightheadedness, chest pain and a documented episode of syncope one month prior to evaluation. Echocardiography revealed marked asymmetric septal hypertrophy (intraventricular septum markedly thickened at 3.5 cm), with a systolic left ventricular outflow tract gradient at rest estimated at 64 mm Hg by Doppler. On physical examination, the S1 and S2 heart sounds were normal, with a III/VI late-peaking crescendo/decrescendo systolic murmur along the left sternal border radiating to the apex, which increased with standing and Valsalva maneuver and decreased with squatting. The electrocardiogram showed normal sinus rhythm and left ventricular hypertrophy.

Resting hemodynamics (Figure 11.17) demonstrated a mean right atrial pressure of 3 mm Hg, right ventricular pressure of 24/4 mm Hg, pulmonary artery pressure of 24/10 mm Hg with a mean of 14 mm Hg, and a mean pulmonary capillary wedge pressure of 8 mm Hg. Aortic pressure was 110/70 mm Hg, with a waveform that demonstrated two systolic peaks, characterizing pulsus bisferiens. Simultaneous left ventricular and aortic pressures (Figure 11.18) were 156/18 mm Hg and 120/70 mm Hg, respectively. There was a 34 mm Hg resting intraventricular pressure gradient. Left ventricular systolic pressure increased to 190 mm Hg and aortic pressure fell to 90/50 mm Hg, with the left ventricular outflow tract gradient increasing to 100 mm Hg post premature ventricular contraction. The left ventricular outflow tract gradient also increased to ~80 mm Hg during Valsalva maneuver within the first several beats of the strain phase (Figure 11.19). Following these maneuvers, atrial and ventricular pacemakers were placed in the right heart chambers. During AV pacing at 85 beats/min with an AV delay of 75 msec (Figure 11.20), the left ventricular

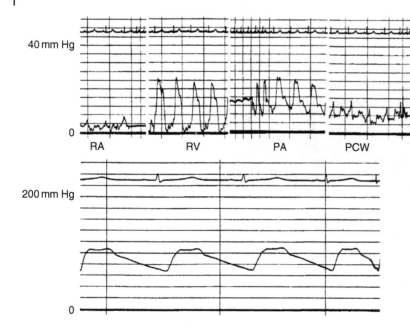

Figure 11.17 Hemodynamics at rest. Right-heart hemodynamics show right atrial (RA) pressure, right ventricular (RV) pressure, pulmonary artery (PA) pressure, and pulmonary capillary wedge (PCW) pressure on a 0–40 mmHg scale, and aortic (Ao) pressure on a 0–200 mm Hg scale. Note the bisferiens arterial pulse at rest on the aortic pressure waveform.

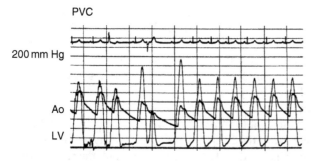

Figure 11.18 Left ventricular (LV) and aortic (Ao) pressures (0–200 mm Hg scale) during premature ventricular contractions (PVC).

Left ventriculography demonstrated normal systolic function with mid-chamber obliteration and ejection fraction greater than 70%. The coronary arteries were normal. The patient was treated with metoprolol without improvement and was switched to a calcium channel blocker. She remained symptomatic with frequent episodes of chest discomfort, lightheadedness, and near syncope. The event monitor excluded ventricular arrhythmias as playing any role in her symptomatology.

In contrast to the hemodynamic responses in the case presented above, Steely and colleagues [33] have provided an example of a different response to dual-chamber pacing in a 58-year-old woman with exertional dyspnea and chest discomfort ascribed to hypertrophic cardiomyopathy. The resting left ventricular outflow gradient was minimal, with left ventricular pressure at rest of 150/10 mm Hg and aortic pressure 156/66 mm Hg. With Valsalva maneuver, a significant increase in left ventricular outflow gradient was noted (Figure 11.21, left). PVCs provoked a further decrease in pulse pressure and an increase in the post-extra-systolic gradient, demonstrating the Brockenbrough–Braunwald–Morrow

pressure fell slightly (150/14 mm Hg), but with a concomitant fall in aortic pressure (120/70 to 105/75 mm Hg). The left ventricular outflow tract gradient remained ~50 mm Hg. At a paced heart rate of 100 beats/min with an AV delay of 75 msec, hemodynamics were largely unaffected, with the left ventricular outflow tract gradient remaining at 50–60 mm Hg. With an increase of the AV delay to 100 msec at the paced rate of 100 beats/min, findings were unchanged.

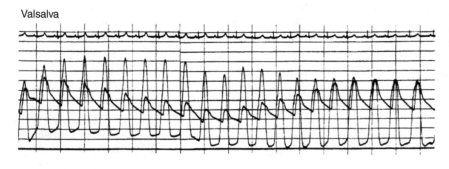

Figure 11.19 Left ventricular (LV) and aortic (Ao) pressures (0–200 mm Hg scale) during Valsalva maneuver.

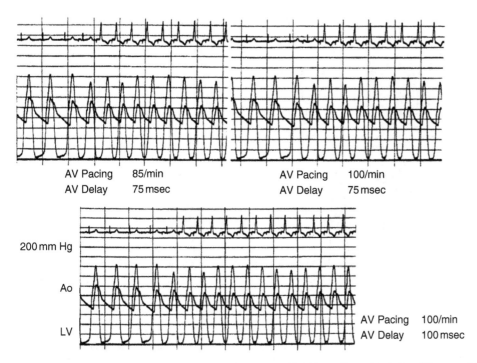

Figure 11.20 Left ventricular (LV) and aortic (Ao) pressures (0–200 mm Hg scale) during AV sequential pacing at 85 and 100 beats/min with AV delay 75 and 100 msec.

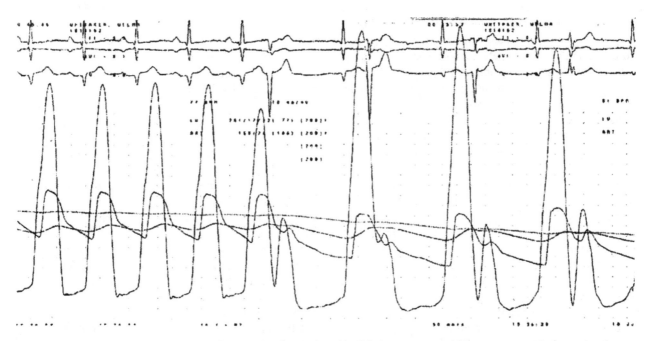

Figure 11.21 Increase in left ventricular outflow tract gradient induced by Valsalva maneuver with premature ventricular contractions inducing an increase in gradient and decrease in pulse pressure. Pressure scale is 0–200 mm Hg. *Source:* Steely 1997 [33]. Reproduced with permission of John Wiley & Sons.

sign. Temporary dual-chamber atrial and ventricular pacing was performed, which reduced the left ventricular and aortic pressures and eliminated the LVOT gradient during Valsalva maneuver (Figure 11.22).

These cases demonstrate alterations in left ventricular outflow tract gradient in patients with hypertrophic cardiomyopathy during Valsalva, PVC, and AV sequential pacing maneuvers. The decrease in left ventricular outflow gradient and hypertrophic obstructive cardiomyopathy with pacemaker therapy has been proposed to be due to three mechanisms: (i) a decrease in paradoxical septal motion; (ii) late activation of septal contraction

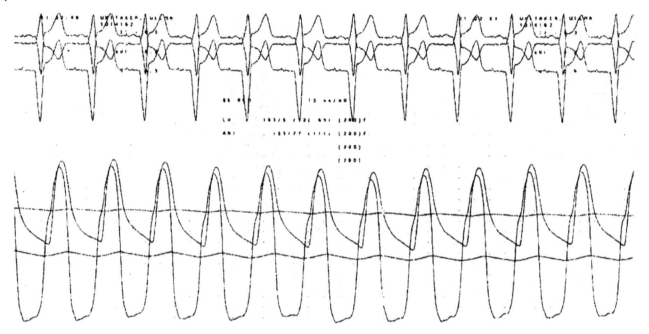

Figure 11.22 Dual-chamber atrioventricular pacemaker hemodynamics demonstrating abolishment of left ventricular outflow tract gradient during Valsalva maneuver. Pressure scale is 0–200 mm Hg. *Source:* Steely 1997 [33]. Reproduced with permission of John Wiley & Sons.

due to right ventricular pacing; and (iii) decrease in left ventricular global contractility. Nishimura *et al.* [31] reported the effects of dual-chamber pacing on systolic and diastolic function in patients with cardiomyopathy. In 29 patients with hypertrophic cardiomyopathy, high-fidelity pressure measurements of left ventricular outflow and left atrial pressures, ascending aortic pressure, cardiac output, and Doppler mitral flow velocity curves were obtained to evaluate cardiac function. During AV sequential pacing with an AV delay of 60 msec, there was significant decrease in cardiac output, positive dP/dt, and increase in mean left atrial pressure. There was also a prolongation of Tau, the time constant of left ventricular relaxation. During AV sequential pacing with an optimal AV delay (identified as the longest AV interval with pre-excitation), deterioration in both systolic and diastolic function variables occurred with lesser magnitude than during pacing with the shortest AV intervals. In 21 patients with and 8 patients without resting left ventricular outflow obstruction, this alteration of systolic and diastolic function was characterized by a modest decrease in left ventricular outflow tract gradient from 73 ± 45 to 61 ± 41 mm Hg *(P < 0.03)*, with dual-chamber pacing at the optimal AV delay compared to sinus rhythm. The investigators [31] concluded that the acute effect of pacing the right atrium and ventricle may be detrimental to both systolic and diastolic left ventricular function, particularly at the shorter AV intervals, and that further randomized studies to identify the benefits of dual-chamber pacing were required.

Previous studies [29, 30] have demonstrated a reduction in the left ventricular outflow gradient in patients with obstructive hypertrophic myopathy undergoing dual-chamber pacing. The hypertrophied septum projecting into the left ventricular outflow tract produced high-velocity blood flow and resultant anterior motion of the mitral valve, which were deemed responsible for the obstruction. With altered contraction of the septum, a reduction in the displacement of the mitral valve apparatus as well as an improved cross-sectional area of the outflow tract was identified. A uniform response of the left ventricular outflow tract gradient to dual-chamber pacing was not present. Although a statistically significant decrease in gradient was noted with dual-chamber pacing, some patients had no change, where others had a significant reduction. The short AV intervals may have contributed to inadequate filling of the left ventricle from ineffective atrial contraction, and thus may account for this lack of efficacy in some patients.

There remains a question as to whether the acute change in left ventricular outflow tract gradient in patients with hypertrophic obstructive cardiomyopathy can be used as a reliable indicator of a response to therapy [34]. Since the LVOT gradient is dependent on contractility as well as loading conditions, alterations in either of these two variables may produce a variation in the outflow tract gradient in the absence of mechanical intervention. The abnormal ventricular relaxation, typical of patients with HOCM, contributes to increased filling pressures. Whereas diastolic function can be altered by dual-chamber pacing, left atrial pressure may elevate further during pacing at short AV intervals [31]. The increase in left atrial pressure was probably related to both ventricular relaxation as well as interruption of the optimal AV synchrony for left ventricular emptying. Nishimura *et al.* [31] reported that the mean Tau reflections of relaxation for all patients was longer during dual-chamber pacing than normal sinus rhythm, suggesting a potentially detrimental effect of pacing on left ventricular diastolic function and relaxation. Pacing at short AV intervals results in the most marked impairment of left ventricular relaxation and is related to a primary decrease in systolic contraction.

Others have suggested that there is a difference in the hemodynamic change between acute and chronic DDD pacing [30]. Most of the subjective and objective improvement as a result of DDD pacing probably is related to myocardial, hemodynamic, and electric adaptive changes after chronic therapy. A considerable difference was noted in LVOT gradients during cardiac catheterization studies at 3 and 16 months after pacemaker implantation, attributed to myocardial adaptive changes [30]. Maron [34] stated in an editorial regarding the use of dual-chamber pacing that a continued examination of this modality for hypertrophic cardiomyopathy is warranted, especially in patients with both marked obstruction to left ventricular outflow and symptoms of congestive heart failure who are refractory to medical therapy. This subset of patients probably comprised only 5–10% of all patients with this clinical syndrome. Caution must be exercised in applying dual-chamber pacing as a treatment for the complex disease characterized by an abnormally hypertrophied, noncompliant left ventricle. Maron [34] also noted that pacing has no defined role in diminishing the risk for sudden cardiac death or in relieving symptoms of patients with nonobstructive hypertrophic myopathy. Until the uncertainty regarding the role of the efficacy of DDD pacing is resolved, clinicians should be aware of potentially deleterious effects or a lack of clinical benefit that may occur with DDD pacing in a patient with hypertrophic obstructive cardiomyopathy. However, some patient subgroups may derive substantial benefit from this technique and thus further studies are warranted.

As excellently reviewed by Criley and Segal [9] and Wigle [11, 15, 35], the spectrum of hypertrophic cardiomyopathy with its attendant different hemodynamic presentations, morbidity and mortality and propensity for sudden death may be attributable to the derangement of cellular architecture. Whether obstruction occurs or is a functional result of ejection is related to the magnitude of myocardial muscle hyperdevelopment. Neither an intraventricular pressure gradient nor systolic anterior mitral valve motion is equated with the presence of ventricular obstruction. Sorraja *et al.* [36] report the effect of mitral clipping to reduce mitral valve regurgitation and

reducing the LVOT gradient in HOCM, a procedure which strongly supports the mitral valve hypothesis in the genesis of the LVOT obstruction.

Hemodynamic Effects of Alcohol-Induced Septal Infarction for Hypertrophic Obstructive Cardiomyopathy

Patients with HOCM may demonstrate symptoms due to the low cardiac output resulting from outflow obstruction of hyperdynamic left ventricular contraction. Unlike patients with ischemic cardiomyopathy, treating these symptoms often requires paradoxical therapy directed at reducing the adverse effects of the hypercontractile myocardium. Although beneficial in many types of ischemic heart disease or congestive heart failure, digitalis, sympathomimetic amines, and preload-reducing pharmacologic therapy are detrimental in patients with hypertrophic myopathy, often exacerbating symptoms. Therapy that reduces myocardial contractility, such as beta-adrenergic blockers, calcium channel blockers, and other negative inotropic agents, has demonstrated symptomatic benefit in the HOCM patient. When medical therapy fails, mechanically altering the sequence or degree of left ventricular contraction by DDD pacing or surgically reducing the hypertrophied muscle segment in the outflow tract has been advocated. Nonsurgical septal mass reduction by controlled septal infarction using alcohol (called transluminal alcohol septal ablation for HOCM, TASH) has been reported with good success and durable late outcomes for the symptomatic patient with HOCM [37–40].

HOCM and TASH

A 68-year-old man with HOCM diagnosed 7 years ago had increasing dyspnea and near syncope. Persistent dyspnea and near syncope on minimal exertion occurred daily, despite treatment with multiple negative inotropic medications. Two-dimensional and Doppler echocardiography demonstrated a substantial intraventricular pressure gradient and severe mitral regurgitation with an enlarged left atrium. The intraventricular septum was 2.2 cm thick at the level of the mitral valve. Cardiac catheterization demonstrated a significant resting intraventricular gradient of 60 mm Hg with normal coronary arteries, and normal right heart hemodynamics prompted the patient to elect the alcohol septal ablation procedure.

The TASH methodology was as follows. The right and left femoral arteries and veins were cannulated using 6 F and 8 F sheaths, respectively. A 5 F (Halo Angiodynamics, Inc., Minneapolis, MN) angiographic catheter was inserted into the left ventricle. A 5 F balloon-tipped pacemaker was inserted through the right femoral vein to the right ventricle. A 6 F multipurpose catheter was also positioned in the right ventricle from the left femoral vein. An 8 F JL4 coronary guide catheter was inserted through the left femoral artery.

Following positioning of the catheters, coronary arteriography identified a single large septal artery from the proximal left anterior descending artery (Figure 11.23, patient J.H.). Prior to septal ablation, weight-adjusted intravenous heparin (100 U/kg) and Demerol 50 mg IV were given. The first large septal artery was cannulated using a large double 45° bend on a 0.014″ angioplasty guidewire over which a short angioplasty balloon (2.5 × 10 mm) was completely advanced into the first septal artery. The septal artery balloon catheter was inflated and radiographic

contrast was instilled into the occluding balloon to demonstrate the correct positioning of the balloon catheter without contrast reflux (Figure 11.23, top middle). Simultaneous two-dimensional transthoracic echocardiography was performed. For contrast opacification of the hypertrophied septum, Optison (Mallinckrodt, St. Louis, MO) echo contrast (3 cc) was diluted 1:10 and instilled via the septal balloon lumen. The echo contrast opacified the protruding septum at the site of the highest velocity in the left ventricular outflow tract. Following echocardiographic confirmation of correct septal branch occlusion, 3 cc of 98% dehydrated alcohol was delivered slowly into the septal artery over 5 min, followed by a 5-min waiting period.

Hemodynamics were continuously measured before, during, and after alcohol septal ablation (Figure 11.24).

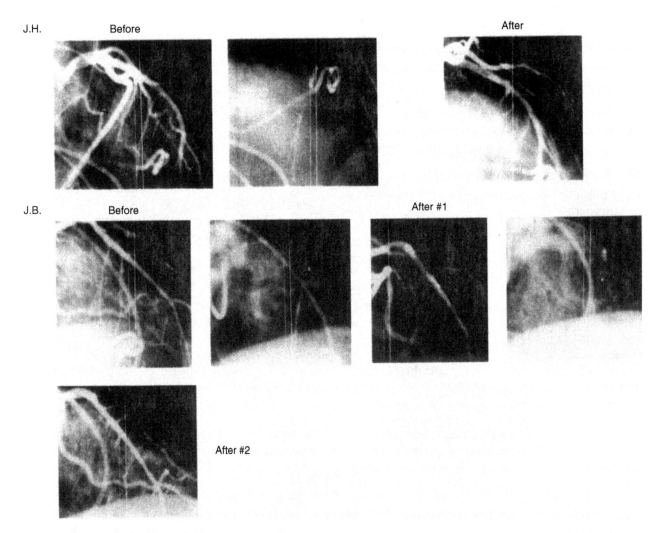

Figure 11.23 (Top) Patient #1, J.H. Angiographic frames showing first large septal artery (left), septal balloon occlusion (middle), and occluded septal artery after procedure (right). (Middle) Patient #2, J.B. Angiography of two large septal arteries (middle left) and sequential balloon occlusion and alcohol ablation (middle left, right, and far right). (Bottom) Angiogram of part 2 showing two occluded septal arteries.

(a)

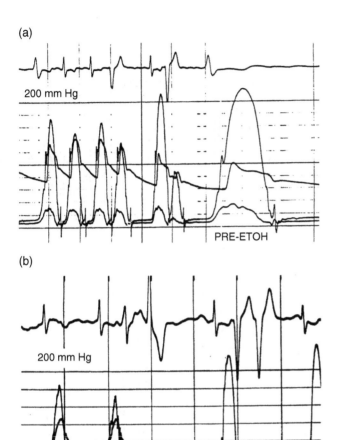

PRE-ETOH

(b)

Figure 11.24 (a) Left ventricular (LV), aortic (Ao), and right ventricular (RV) pressures on a 0–200 mm Hg scale in patient #1 before alcohol septal ablation. Note the large post-premature ventricular contraction (PVC) gradient of 120 mm Hg peak to peak with a spike and dome configuration of the aortic pressure wave on the beat at the far right at a fast recording speed. (b) Left ventricular (LV), aortic (Ao), and right ventricular (RV) pressures on a 0–200 mm Hg scale demonstrating the effect of a couplet on the post-PVC LV outflow tract gradient before septal ablation.

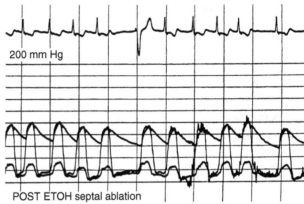

POST ETOH septal ablation

Figure 11.25 Hemodynamics following alcohol (ETOH) septal ablation in patient #1. Left ventricular (LV), aortic (Ao), and right ventricular (RV) pressures now show a 0 mm Hg gradient at rest, with loss of the spike and dome configuration of the aortic pressure. There is no post-premature ventricular contraction provocation of LV outflow tract gradient. Also note that the rhythm is not paced.

After the 5-min period following alcohol administration, the occluding balloon catheter was deflated and withdrawn. The patient had a junctional escape rhythm requiring temporary pacing. The classic spike and dome configuration of the arterial pressure (Figure 11.24a), especially prominent on the potentiated post-PVC beats, was eliminated, as were the potentiated PVC gradients and the Brockenbrough–Braunwald–Morrow sign of reduced arterial pulse pressure after PVC. The junctional rhythm and, to some degree, the infarcted septal activity likely accounted for the reduction in arterial pressure from 140/78 to 100/76 mm Hg. There was no significant change in the left ventricular end-diastolic pressure (28 to 32 mm Hg, pre- vs. post-alcohol). Note the significant reduction of the resting left ventricular outflow tract gradient and loss of the PVC provocable gradient after septal ablation (Figure 11.25). There was no significant change in right ventricular pressures after septal infarction. Coronary arteriography and coronary flow reserve were repeated (Table 11.1). The temporary pacemaker and the vascular sheaths were secured in place. The patient was transferred to the coronary care unit for observation. The peak creatine phosphokinase (CPK) was approximately 2,000 units, with MB fraction of 53 units. The electrocardiogram showed minimal ST elevation in leads V1 and V2 at the end of 18 hours. The patient had no requirement for pacing and the pacemaker was removed.

With elimination of the left ventricular outflow tract gradient (Figure 11.26), the patient saw dramatic symptomatic improvement within hours after the procedure and by the next morning was noted to be markedly improved. That afternoon the patient could, for the first time, walk the hallway without symptoms. He has been stable for six months.

HOCM, TASH, and Valsalva maneuver

A 60-year-old male had dyspnea on exertional with near syncope, and frequently occurring atypical chest pain. An echocardiogram demonstrated severe left ventricular hypertrophy, an abnormal left ventricular outflow tract

Table 11.1 Hemodynamic data before and after alcohol septal ablation (TASH).

Site	Before TASH	After TASH
Left ventricular pressure, mm Hg	124/15/36	116/17/21
Aortic pressure, mm Hg	115/69/88	129/70/92
PVC gradient, mm Hg	27	4
Heart rate, beats/min	88	86

PVC = premature ventricular contraction.

J.B.

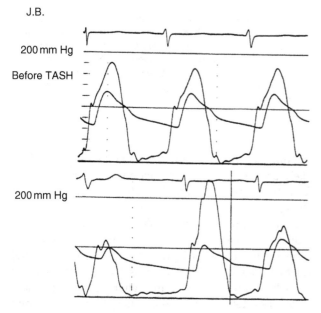

Figure 11.26 Hemodynamic tracing in patient #2 before septal ablation. There is an 0 mm Hg resting left ventricular outflow tract gradient (top) and 130 mm Hg post-premature ventricular contraction gradient between the aortic and left ventricular pressures (lower, beat #2). Note the spike and dome configuration of the aortic pressure waveform.

velocity and contour consistent with HOCM, and moderate, eccentric mitral regurgitation. Electrocardiogram showed normal sinus rhythm with severe left ventricular hypertrophy.

After discussion of the alternative therapies for HOCM, the patient and family elected to participate in the alcohol septal ablation protocol. At cardiac catheterization, the left ventricular outflow tract gradient was 60 mm Hg at rest and 130 mm Hg with provocable maneuvers (Figure 11.27). The arterial waveform showed classic features of the spike and dome pattern and the Brockenbrough–Braunwald–Morrow sign after a PVC. During the Valsalva maneuver with a PVC, a left ventricular outflow tract gradient was 110 mm Hg, which

J.B

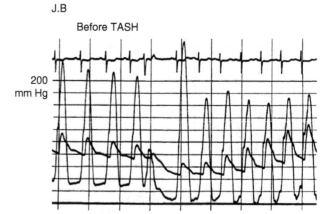

Figure 11.27 Hemodynamics in patient #2 during Valsalva maneuver. The left ventricular (LV) outflow tract gradient increases to 120 mm Hg, with a post-PVC gradient of 160 mm Hg and dramatic Brockenbrough–Braunwald–Morrow sign.

increased to nearly 200 mm Hg with a PVC (Figure 11.28). The arterial pressure on this beat was 62/48 mm Hg. Following positioning of left ventricular and pacing catheters, coronary arteriography demonstrated normal arteries and two large septal arteries (Figure 11.23, patient J.B., left panel). Weight-adjusted 40 u/kg intravenous heparin was administered. Left anterior descending coronary flow reserve was also measured as in the first patient. A 2.0 x 9.0 mm balloon was positioned into the first septal artery branch. Radiographic contrast, given through the occluded balloon catheter, demonstrated the totally occlusive positioning of the balloon catheter in the first septal artery (Figure 11.23, middle panels). Echo contrast (3 cc Optison, diluted 1:10) opacified only the top part of the obstructing septal muscle. Following echo contrast imaging, 3 cc of 98% dehydrated alcohol was delivered into the first septal artery over 5 min with a 5-min waiting period following alcohol administration, observing hemodynamics continuously. Following the waiting period, the balloon catheter was withdrawn, and coronary arteriography and coronary flow reserve of the left anterior descending coronary artery were repeated. Because of a residual 40 mm Hg provocable left ventricular outflow tract gradient, the septal occlusion and ablation procedure was repeated in the second septal artery (Figure 11.23, lower panel). After the two septal arteries were ablated, the left ventricular outflow tract gradient was < 10 mm Hg at rest without a PVC provocable gradient. During Valsalva and PVCs, the largest resting gradient was 30 mm Hg without PVC augmentation (Figure 11.28). Only at maximal Valsalva (Figure 11.29, bottom, beat #7) was the arterial spike and dome waveform demonstrated. The paced rhythm was associated with complete heart block and A–V dissociation. A waves

Figure 11.28 Hemodynamics following alcohol septal ablation (TASH) in patient #2. The rhythm is paced. There is no significant resting or post-PVC tract gradient (top and bottom right). During Valsalva maneuver (bottom middle), there is a minimal 20 mm Hg increase in the resting gradient.

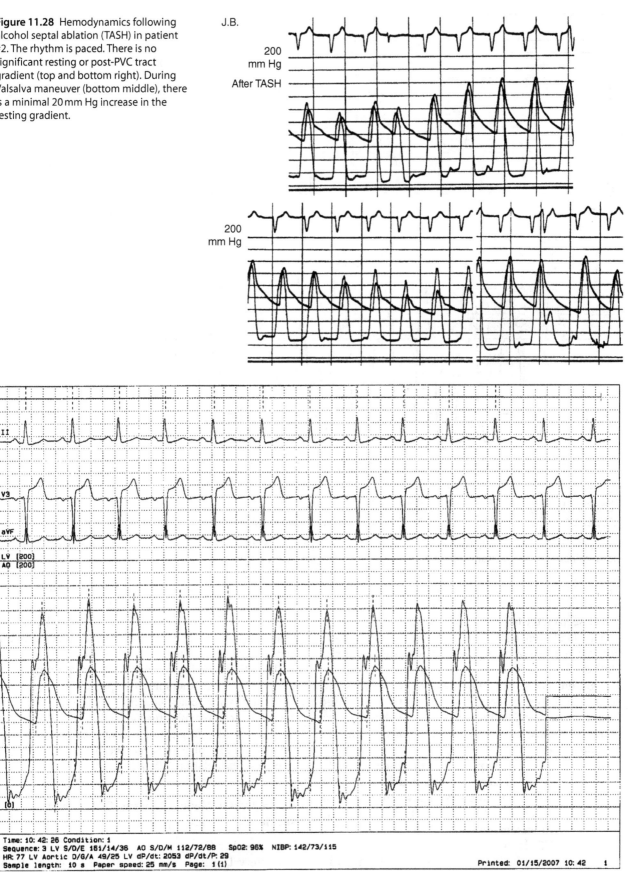

Time: 10:42:26 Condition: 1
Sequence: 3 LV S/D/E 161/14/36 AO S/D/M 112/72/88 SpO2: 96% NIBP: 142/73/115
HR: 77 LV Aortic D/G/A 49/25 LV dP/dt: 2053 dP/dt/P: 29
Sample length: 10 s Paper speed: 25 mm/s Page: 1 (1)
Printed: 01/15/2007 10:42 1

Figure 11.29 Left ventricular pressure with femoral artery sheath pressure. Note the dampening of the femoral artery sheath and the delay in time. Left ventricular end-diastolic pressure is approximately 30 mm Hg with a prominent A wave. The rapid upslope of the aortic pressure is still demonstrated in the femoral artery. Compare to Figure 11.30.

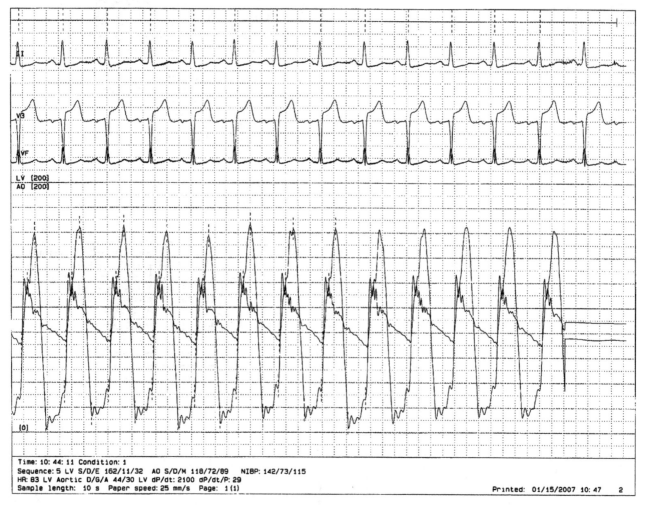

Figure 11.30 Left ventricular (LV) and central aortic pressure using a pigtail catheter positioned in the LV. A spike and dome pattern is clearly evident on the central aortic pressure in contrast to the femoral artery pressure.

can be seen on the left ventricular diastolic pressure wave (Figure 11.30, top, beats #5–7 and 9). It is interesting to note the increased arterial pressure (130/70 to 150/80 mm Hg) after septal ablation.

Regarding coronary flow reserve, coronary flow reserve in the left anterior descending artery increased from 1.5 before to 2.7 after septal ablation. Systolic flow reversal demonstrated prior to septal ablation was not seen afterward.

At the conclusion of the procedure, the vascular sheaths and temporary pacemaker were secured in place. The patient was transferred to the coronary care unit. Peak CPK was approximately 1,800 units with MB fraction of 59. The electrocardiogram showed junctional rhythm with minor ST elevation in leads V1 and V2. After 48 hours, the patient had persistent junctional bradycardia and episodes of complete heart block, for which he

received a DDD pacemaker. He was discharged asymptomatic on hospital day 5. A summary of the hemodynamic and echocardiographic data is shown in Table 11.1.

The pathophysiology of hypertrophic cardiomyopathy suggests that four therapeutic approaches may provide important symptomatic benefit. These methods include negative inotropic pharmacologic therapy [27], DDD pacing [29–31], surgical septal myomectomy with or without mitral valve replacement, and, most recently, alcohol septal ablation [39–41].

Alternatives to Medical Therapy: DDD Pacing and Surgical Myectomy

Dual-chamber (DDD) pacing shortens the AV conduction interval, altering the left ventricular depolarization and contraction sequence. The alteration of contractile events minimizes the obstructing septal contraction, reducing the narrowing of the left ventricular outflow tract. DDD pacing, in some cases, provides substantial hemodynamic benefit [42, 43]. The duration of symptomatic benefit of dual-chamber pacing has been reported to extend over a 5-year follow-up period [44].

Although dual-chamber pacing has been shown to reduce left ventricular outflow obstruction, diminish mitral regurgitation, and improve exercise performance, several reports of DDD pacing indicate that the acute and early cardiac changes may not be maintained over the long term. Prolonged pacing alters the electrical and hemodynamic properties of the myocardium [45]. Long-term DDD pacing results in adaptive left ventricular changes, reduction in left ventricular pressure, and late left ventricular remodeling. These alterations are associated with reduced angina and improved myocardial perfusion by stress imaging, with reduction in left ventricular cavity dilatation [29–31]. Although the adaptive changes contribute to the success of dual-chamber pacemaker therapy for HOCM, the correlation between acute and chronic effects does not permit identification of an individual patient who may receive benefit from this mode of therapy. Dual-chamber pacing may not relieve left ventricular outflow tract obstruction due to the dependence on AV delay and ventricular capture potentially interfering with left atrial emptying. Of HOCM patients so treated, 60% also require drug therapy for continued symptoms at rest. DDD pacing has been used in patients who fail medical therapy. DDD pacing is ineffective in patients with atrial arrhythmias. Left ventricular myomectomy may be recommended in patients failing DDD therapy or in those needing other cardiac procedures such as coronary artery bypass surgery or valve replacement [30].

Although effective in enlarging the left ventricular outflow tract and altering the left ventricular contractile sequence, septal myectomy is a complicated, open-chest surgical procedure with a mortality risk approaching 5% and a high incidence of intraventricular conduction block requiring a permanent pacemaker [28, 46, 47]. Additionally, in some patients the development of severe mitral regurgitation due to HOCM has required mitral valve replacement, a difficult and at times suboptimal therapy because of the reduced left ventricular cavity dimensions, which may interfere with prosthetic valve occluder motion. The long-term anticoagulation and its late prosthetic valve dysfunction make this an option of last resort.

The most recent technique, the induced septal infarction of the subaortic portion of the intraventricular septum by balloon occlusion with instillation of alcohol, as in our two patients, has been demonstrated to be a hemodynamically effective method of reducing left ventricular outflow tract obstruction. This procedure was first performed in 1995 by Sigwart [37], who noted that a brief septal artery balloon occlusion caused transient reduction in the outflow pressure gradient, and that localized septal infarction with ethanol in three patients was effective over a longer follow-up.

In 1997, the clinical outcome of the first series of patients undergoing nonsurgical septal reduction for HOCM was reported by Knight *et al.* [38]. Eighteen patients underwent selective intraseptal alcohol injection to reduce left ventricular outflow obstruction. Doppler echo evaluation of left ventricular outflow gradients was performed before the procedure on the first postoperative day and at three-month follow-up. Exercise testing and degree of symptom reduction three months after the procedure were also evaluated. Following the procedure, there was a significant reduction in the mean left ventricular outflow obstruction gradient (67 to 25 mm Hg; $P < 0.0006$). At three months, the left ventricular outflow tract gradient stabilized at 22 mm Hg. The reduction in left ventricular outflow obstruction was associated with marked improvement in symptoms, but an insignificant increase in exercise capacity in 10 patients of 25% time to symptoms. Left ventricular dimensions were not altered by alcohol septal ablation.

The complications in the first 18 patients included chest discomfort lasting from 1 to 2 min, which was treated with intravenous opiate analgesia. Four patients had complete heart block, which was temporary in all four cases. Two patients had ventricular arrhythmias, one secondary to severe bradycardia during sheath removal. Ventricular tachycardia occurred in one patient as a consequence of alcohol leakage down the main lumen of the left anterior descending artery, causing transient impairment of flow, marked ST elevation, and a large cardiac enzyme release. Arterial patency was restored by the following day without any long-term adverse events. The left ventricle appeared normal at follow-up. This complication was attributed to inadequate balloon occlusion of the first septal artery. This event led the investigators to caution operators that the balloon should not be positioned too proximally and should be of adequate size to prevent leakage. Injection of contrast into the septal artery through the balloon will ensure appropriate sealing of the septal artery prior to alcohol instillation, thus eliminating this complication.

In 1998, Seggewiss *et al.* [39] presented the acute and three-month follow-up results of alcohol septal ablation in 25 patients. The mean age was 55 ± 15 years and 1.4 ± 0.6 septal branches were occluded with 4.1 ± 2.6 mL of 96% alcohol. Three-month follow-up of the left ventricular outflow tract gradient in 22 of 25 patients demonstrated a reduction from 62 ± 30 mm Hg (range 4–152 mm Hg) to 19 ± 21 mm Hg (range 0–74 mm Hg). The post-extra-systolic pressure gradient reduction was 141 ± 45 to 61 ± 40 mm Hg. Maximal CPK enzyme increase was 780 ± 436 units after 11 hours. In 13 of 25 patients, trifascicular block was present for 5 min to 8 days. Temporary and permanent pacing was required in 8 and 5 patients, respectively. One patient, an 86-year-old woman, died 8 days after alcohol septal ablation from ventricular fibrillation. This patient was taking beta-sympathomimetics for chronic obstructive pulmonary disease. On average, patients were discharged 11 days (range 5–24 days) after the procedure. At three-month follow-up, there were no late complications. Twenty-one patients decreased their New York Heart Association functional class from 3.01 ± 1.0 to 1.4 ± 1.1. A further reduction in left ventricular outflow tract gradient occurred in 14 patients.

TASH is alternative to myomectomy for selected patients with HOCM. Caution should still be used in the decision to proceed with TASH, however. Fananapazir and McAreavey [48] have reviewed therapeutic options in patients with HOCM and severe drug refractory symptoms. They note that patients with HOCM remain prone to arrhythmias and sudden death, independent of the presence or degree of relief of left ventricular outflow tract obstruction. It has also been noted that hypertrophic left ventricular outflow tract obstruction is a highly variable condition [49] and may be induced by alterations of preload and intrathoracic pressures (cough, Valsalva maneuver). Functional mitral regurgitation due to increasing and adverse hemodynamic effects of systolic anterior motion of the mitral valve with increasing left ventricular outflow tract obstruction may also be the cause of disabling symptoms. Mid left ventricular cavity obstruction or complex forms of HOCM involving the apex, left ventricular, or right ventricular outflow tract may represent additional contributions to the symptoms and adverse outcome [50, 51]. Mechanically treating or chemically infarcting a hypertrophic septum may not necessarily alter impaired left ventricular diastolic and systolic function, subendocardial myocardial ischemia, or arrhythmias, all of which may co-exist and result in the symptomatic incapacitation that has been attributed to the obstructive component of HOCM alone.

Nonetheless, in many cases of HOCM, left ventricular outflow obstruction appears linked to symptomatic status. Therapies that reduce intraventricular pressure gradients appear to improve myocardial perfusion and reduce clinical symptoms [52, 53]. As shown in the two case examples, septal ablation using ethanol infused into one or more of the septal perforators at the site of outflow obstruction produces significant reduction in left ventricular pressure and can improve clinical symptoms.

Complications of Alcohol Septal Ablation

Several authorities have expressed concern over the potential early and late complications of alcohol septal ablation [42–45, 47, 48]. Alcohol-induced septal infarction is a controlled myocardial infarction with its attendant complications, which may include conduction abnormalities, some requiring permanent pacemaker implantation in approximately 20–30% of patients [38, 39]. Ventricular arrhythmias and sudden death have been noted. Late complications of the procedure remain unknown. Conduction abnormalities resulting from septal infarction may increase the propensity for late complete heart block. Ventricular arrhythmias in patients with HOCM secondary to myocardial fiber disarray and fibrosis may be exacerbated by a segmentally infarcted myocardium, leading to sustained ventricular arrhythmia or foci of arrhythmogenic ventricular myocardium.

Induced septal infarction may theoretically aggravate left ventricular dysfunction in the late course. Left ventricular hypertrophy eventually results in left ventricular remodeling with impairment of contractility, despite an increased left ventricular wall thickness. Low wall stress and small left ventricular volume, although associated with a hypercontractile left ventricle, may obscure impaired systolic left ventricular function. In the late phase, alteration of myocytes, generation of fibrosis, myocardial cellular energy depletion, and diastolic dysfunction ultimately result in cardiac failure with left ventricular thinning. Whether the reduction in left ventricular pressure gradient at the time of septal ablation results in reduced left ventricular filling and improved myocardial perfusion with a delay of adverse events associated with left ventricular remodeling remains to be seen.

Case Study in Alcohol Septal Ablation for Hypertrophic Cardiomyopathy (Courtesy of Ted Feldman, MD, Evanston Hospital, Evanston, IL)

A 50-year-old man with HOCM had dyspnea on exertion (New York Heart Association Class III) on maximal medical management. He has reported orthopnea and has been sleeping on a reclining chair for the last 2–3 years. Dizziness and lightheadedness with positional changes occur commonly, although he has not been hospitalized for heart failure. He had been treated for hypertension, hyperlipidemia, benign prostatic hypertrophy, and depression. He was symptomatic with hypotension when metoprolol exceeded 100 mg in 24 hours.

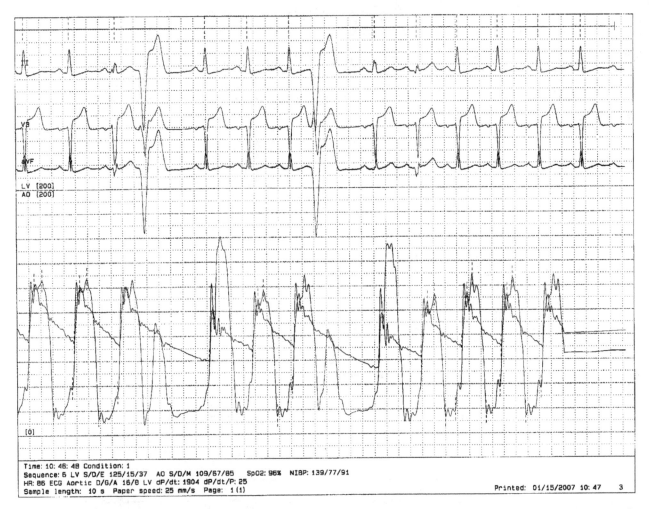

Time: 10: 46: 48 Condition: 1
Sequence: 6 LV S/D/E 125/15/37 AO S/D/M 109/67/85   SpO2: 96% NIBP: 139/77/91
HR: 86 ECG Aortic D/G/A 16/8 LV dP/dt: 1904 dP/dt/P: 25
Sample length: 10 s Paper speed: 25 mm/s Page: 1 (1)   Printed: 01/15/2007 10: 47   3

Figure 11.31 Demonstration of left ventricular outflow tract gradient as being quite a variable number with post-PVC augmentation of the gradient to approximately 60–70 mm Hg. This reproducible provocation of the left ventricular outflow tract gradient is quite evident on this tracing.

Echocardiography demonstrated peak left ventricular outflow tract gradient of 71 mm Hg with asymmetric septal hypertrophy and systolic anterior wall motion of the mitral valve. Cardiac catheterization with alcohol septal ablation for left ventricular outflow tract obstruction was performed using the right femoral artery with a 6 F vascular sheath, right femoral vein with a 6 F vascular sheath, and left femoral artery with a 5 F arterial sheath. Left-heart pressures were recorded using a 5 F pigtail catheter to the left ventricle and a 6 F pigtail catheter in the aorta from the right femoral artery. The left ventricular aortic gradient is demonstrated on Figures 11.31–11.34 and had a post-PVC Brockenbrough–Braunwald–Morrow sign.

Selective coronary arteriography was performed followed by coronary angioplasty balloon placement of 2 × 9 mm over the wire balloon into the second septal branch. After septal balloon occlusion, contrast cinefluoroscopy and contrast bubble imaging by echo demonstrated that the septum was supplied by this vessel. Then 1.5 mL of

100% ethanol was injected through the balloon catheter and the alcohol remained in place for 5 min. A significant reduction in the LV–Ao gradient was noted, with no gradient in the post-PVC augmented peak. Fluoroscopy confirmed that the septal branch had been ablated and that on echocardiography in the catheterization laboratory, there was akinesis of the proximal septum. No AV block was identified. At the conclusion of the procedure, the right femoral sheath was removed and closed with 6 F Perclose device; the left femoral sheath was removed using manual compression and a pacing wire via the right femoral vein was sutured and remained in place for 24 hours. There were no subsequent results of conduction delay and the patient symptomatically improved over time.

Left ventricular pressure with femoral artery sheath pressure is shown on Figure 11.30. Note the dampening of the femoral artery sheath and the delay in time. Left ventricular end-diastolic pressure is approximately

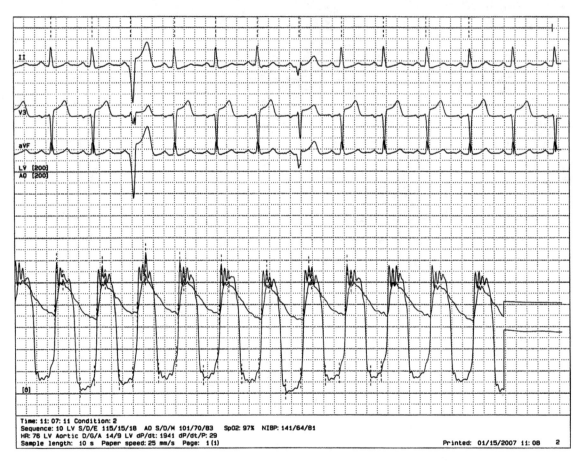

Figure 11.32 Electrocardiogram following alcohol septal ablation showing ST segment elevation in lead V3 with incomplete right bundle branch pattern.

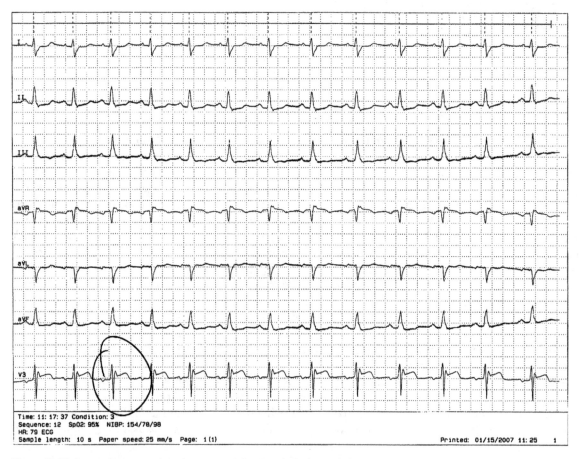

Figure 11.33 Femoral artery and aortic pressure following alcohol septal ablation shows no augmentation of gradient or PVC.

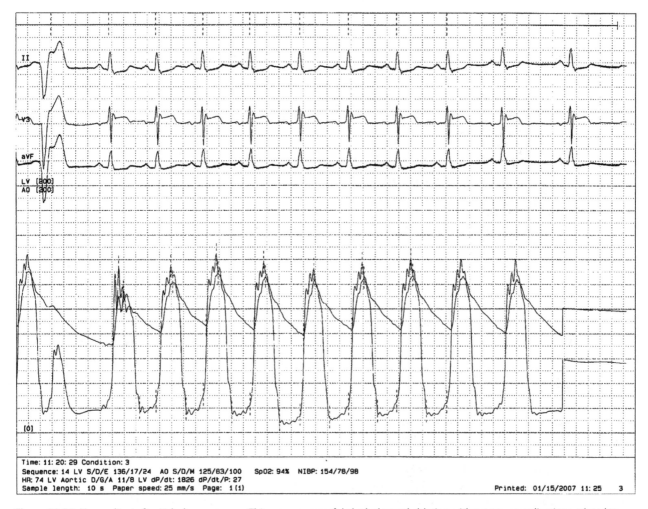

Figure 11.34 No gradient after Valsalva maneuver. This was a successful alcohol septal ablation without any complications related to alcohol induction of the incomplete right branch block and minor ST segment elevation in lead V3.

30 mm Hg with a prominent A wave. The rapid upslope of the aortic pressure is still demonstrated in the femoral artery. The left ventricular outflow tract gradient can be quite variable, with post-PVC augmentation of the gradient to approximately 60–70 mm Hg (Figure 11.31). This reproducible provocation of the left ventricular outflow tract gradient is quite evident on this tracing. TASH produces electrocardiographic tracings following alcohol septal ablation. Figure 11.32 shows ST segment elevation in lead V3 with incomplete right bundle branch pattern.

Left ventricular and aortic pressures after alcohol septal ablation show no gradient with post-PVC beat (Figure 11.33) or during Valsalva maneuver (Figure 11.34). This was a successful alcohol septal ablation without any complications related to alcohol induction of the incomplete right branch block and minor ST segment elevation in lead V3.

Key Points

1) Alcohol septal ablation for hypertrophic obstructive cardiomyopathy (HOCM) requires that patients have symptoms related to the left ventricular outflow tract gradient and that they are refractory to maximal medical therapy.
2) Contraindications to transluminal ablation of septal hypertrophy (TASH) include inadequate septal thickness (<18 mm), intrinsic mitral valve disease, or right bundle branch block.
3) Relative contraindications may include significant left ventricular dysfunction or right bundle branch block.
4) Alcohol septal ablation for HOCM demonstrates significant immediate hemodynamic and clinical benefit.
5) Long-term observations in large patient series appear to demonstrate the durable therapeutic effect of this technique.

References

1 Kern M, Deligonul U. Intraventricular pressure gradients. *Cathet Cardiovasc Diagn* 22:145–152, 1992.

2 Kern M, Puri S, Donohue T, Bach R. Hemodynamics of dual-chamber pacing and Valsalva maneuver in a patient with hypertrophic obstructive cardiomyopathy. *Cathet Cardiovasc Diagn* 44:438–442, 1998.

3 Kern M, Rajjoub H, Bach R. Hemodynamic effects of alcohol-induced septal infarction for hypertrophic obstructive cardiomyopathy. *Cathet Cardiovasc Diagn* 47:221–228, 1999.

4 Geske JB, Sorajja P, Ommen SR, Nishimura RA. Left ventricular outflow tract gradient variability in hypertrophic cardiomyopathy. *Clin Cardiol* 32(7): 397–402, 2009.

5 Sorajja P, Ommen SR, Holmes DR Jr, Dearani JA, Rihal CS, Gersh BJ, Lennon RJ, Nishimura RA. Survival after alcohol septal ablation for obstructive hypertrophic cardiomyopathy. *Circulation* 126(20):2374–2380, 2012.

6 Maron BJ, Bonow RO, Cannon RO III, Leon MB, Epstein SE. Hypertrophic cardiomyopathy: Interrelations of clinical manifestations, pathophysiology, and therapy (2). *N Engl J Med* 316(14):844–852, 1987.

7 Wigle ED, Rakowski H, Kimball BP, Williams WG. Hypertrophic cardiomyopathy: Clinical spectrum and treatment. *Circulation* 92(7):1680–1692, 1995.

8 Maron MS, Olivotto I, Betocchi S, Casey SA, Lesser JR, Losi MA, Cecchi F, Maron BJ. Effect of left ventricular outflow tract obstruction on clinical outcome in hypertrophic cardiomyopathy. *N Engl J Med* 348(4):295–303, 2003.

9 White RI, Criley M, Lewis KB, Ross RS. Experimental production of intracavity pressure differences. *Am J Cardiol* 19:806–817, 1967.

10 Criley JM, Siegel RJ. Has "obstruction" hindered our understanding of hypertrophic cardiomyopathy? *Circulation* 72:1148–1154, 1985.

11 Wigle ED. Hypertrophic cardiomyopathy: A 1987 viewpoint. *Circulation* 2:311–322, 1987.

12 Brockenbrough EC, Braunwald E, Morrow AG. A hemodynamic technique for the detection of hypertrophic subaortic stenosis. *Circulation* 23:189–194, 1961.

13 White CW, Zimmerman TJ. Prolonged left ventricular ejection time in the post-premature beat: A sensitive sign of idiopathic hypertrophic subaortic stenosis. *Circulation* 52:306–312, 1975.

14 Raizner AE, Chahine RA, Ishimori T, Awdeh M. Clinical correlates of left ventricular cavity obliteration. *Am J Cardiol* 40:303–309, 1977.

15 Wigle ED, Marquis Y, Auger P. Muscular subaortic stenosis: Initial left ventricular inflow tract pressure in the assessment of intraventricular pressure differences in man. *Circulation* 35: 1100–1117, 1967.

16 Come PC, Bulkley BH, Goodman ZD, Hutchins GM, Pitt B, Fortuin NJ. Hypercontractile cardiac states simulating hypertrophic cardiomyopathy. *Circulation* 55:901–908, 1977.

17 Agarwal S, Tuzcu EM, Desai MY, Smedira N, Lever HM, Lytle BW, Kapadia SR. Updated meta-analysis of septal alcohol ablation versus myectomy for hypertrophic cardiomyopathy. *J Am Coll Cardiol* 55(8):823–834, 2010.

18 Erdin RA Jr, Abdulla AM, Stefadouros MA. Hypercontractile cardiac state mimicking hypertrophic subaortic stenosis. *Cathet Cardiovasc Diagn* 7: 71–77, 1981.

19 Alam M, Dokainish H, Lakkis NM. Hypertrophic obstructive cardiomyopathy—alcohol septal ablation vs. myectomy: A meta-analysis. *Eur Heart J* 30(9):1080–1087, 2009.

20 Deligonul U, Uppstrom E, Penick D, Seacord L, Kern MJ. Dynamic left ventricular outflow tract obstruction induced by pericardial tamponade during acute anterior myocardial infarction. *Am Heart J* 121:190–194, 1991.

21 Leonardi RA, Kransdorf EP, Simel DL, Wang A. Meta-analyses of septal reduction therapies for obstructive hypertrophic cardiomyopathy: Comparative rates of overall mortality and sudden cardiac death after treatment. *Circ Cardiovasc Interv* 3(2):97–104, 2010.

22 Pasipoularides A. Clinical assessment of ventricular ejection dynamics with and without outflow obstruction. *J Am Coll Cardiol* 15:859–882, 1990.

23 Nagueh SF, Groves BM, Schwartz L, Smith KM, Wang A, Bach RG, Nielsen C, Leya F, Buergler JM, Rowe SK *et al.* Alcohol septal ablation for the treatment of hypertrophic obstructive cardiomyopathy: A multicenter North American registry. *J Am Coll Cardiol* 58(22):2322–2328, 2011.

24 Lorell BH, Paulus WJ, Grossman W, Wynne J, Cohn PF, Braunwald E. Improved diastolic function and systolic performance in hypertrophic cardiomyopathy after nifedipine. *N Engl J Med* 303:801–803, 1980.

25 Ross J Jr, Braunwald E, Gault JH, Mason DT, Morrow AG. The mechanism of the intraventricular pressure gradient in idiopathic hypertrophic subaortic stenosis. *Circulation* 34:558–578, 1966.

26 Murgo JP, Alter BR, Darethy JR, Altobelli SA, McGranahan GM Jr. Dynamics of left ventricular ejection in obstructive and non-obstructive hypertrophic cardiomyopathy. *J Clin Invest* 66:1369–1382, 1980.

27 Wigle ED, Rakowski H, Kimball BP, Williams WG. Hypertrophic cardiomyopathy: Clinical spectrum and treatment. *Circulation* 92(7):1680–1692, 1995.

28 Krajcer Z, Leachman RD, Cooley DA, Coronado R. Septal myotomy-myomectomy versus mitral valve replacement in hypertrophic cardiomyopathy: Ten-year

follow-up in 185 patients. *Circulation* 80 [suppl 1]:157–164, 1989.

29 Jeanrenaud X, Goy JJ, Kappenberger L. Effects of dual-chamber pacing in hypertrophic obstructive cardiomyopathy. *Eur Heart J* 339:1318–1323, 1992.

30 Fananapazir L, Cannon RO III, Tripodi D, Panza JA. Impact of dual-chamber permanent pacing in patients with obstructive hypertrophic cardiomyopathy with symptoms refractory to verapamil and beta-adrenergic blocker therapy. *Circulation* 85:2149–2161, 1992.

31 Nishimura RA, Hayes DL, IIstrup DM, Holmes DR Jr, Tajik AJ. Effect of dual-chamber pacing on systolic and diastolic function in patients with hypertrophic cardiomyopathy: Acute Doppler echocardiographic and catheterization hemodynamic study. *J Am Coll Cardiol* 27:421–430, 1996.

32 McDonald KM, Maurer B. Permanent pacing as treatment for hypertrophic cardiomyopathy. *Am J Cardiol* 68:108–110, 1991.

33 Steely D, Javier N, Bissett JK, Talley JD. It fits! (Intelligence transfer: From images to solutions): Pacemaker therapy in patients with hypertrophic obstructive cardiomyopathy. *J Interv Cardiol* 10:385–386, 1997.

34 Maron BJ. Appraisal of dual-chamber pacing therapy in hypertrophic cardiomyopathy: Too soon for a rush to judgment? *J Am Coll Cardiol* 27:431–432, 1996.

35 Wigle ED, Sasson Z, Henderson MA, Ruddy TD, Fulop J, Rakowski H, Williams WG. Hypertrophic cardiomyopathy: The importance of the site and the extent of hypertrophy: A review. *Prog Cardiovasc Dis* 28:1–83, 1985.

36 Sorajja P, Pedersen WA, Bae R, Lesser JR, Jay D, Lin D, Harris K, Maron BJ. First experience with percutaneous mitral valve plication as primary therapy for symptomatic obstructive hypertrophic cardiomyopathy. *J Am Coll Cardiol* 67:2811–2818, 2016.

37 Sigwart U. Non-surgical myocardial reduction for hypertrophic obstructive cardiomyopathy. *Lancet* 346:211–214, 1995.

38 Knight C, Kurbaan AS, Seggewiss H, Henein M, Gunning M, Harrington D, Fassbender D, Gleichmann U, Sigwart U. Nonsurgical septal reduction for hypertrophic obstructive cardiomyopathy: Outcome in the first series of patients. *Circulation* 95:2075–2081, 1997.

39 Seggewiss H, Gleichmann U, Faber L, Fassbender D, Schmidt HK, Strick S. Percutaneous transluminal septal myocardial ablation in hypertrophic obstructive cardiomyopathy: Acute results and 3-month follow-up in 25 patients. *J Am Coll Cardiol* 31:252–258, 1998.

40 Oakley CM. Non-surgical ablation of the ventricular septum for the treatment of hypertrophic cardiomyopathy. *Lancet* 346:1624, 1995.

41 Braunwald E. Induced septal infarction: A new therapeutic strategy for hypertrophic obstructive cardiomyopathy. *Circulation* 95:1981–1982, 1997.

42 Fananapazir L, Epstein ND, Panza A, Curiel R, Tripodi D, McAreavey D. Long-term results of dual chamber (DDD) pacing in obstructive hypertrophic cardiomyopathy: Evidence for progressive symptomatic and hemodynamic improvement and reduction of left ventricular hypertrophy. *Circulation* 90:2731–2742, 1994.

43 Simon JP, Sadoul N, de Chillou C, *et al*. Long-term dual chamber pacing improves hemodynamic function in patients with obstructive hypertrophic cardiomyopathy. PACE (Abstract) 18:1769, 1995.

44 Sadoul N, Simon J-P, Bruntz J-F, Isaaz K, de Chillou C, Beurrier D, Dodinot B, Aliot E. Long-term dual chamber pacing reduces left ventricular mass in patients with obstructive hypertrophic cardiomyopathy. *J Am Coll Cardiol* 21:94A, 1993.

45 McAreavey D, Fananapazir L. Altered cardiac hemodynamic and electrical state in normal sinus rhythm following chronic dual chamber pacing for relief of left ventricular outflow obstruction in hypertrophic cardiomyopathy. *Am J Cardiol* 70:651–656, 1992.

46 Mohr R, Schaff HV, Danielson GK, Puga FJ, Pluth JR, Tajik AI. The outcome of surgical treatment of hypertrophic obstructive cardiomyopathy: Experience over 15 years. *J Thorac Cardiovasc Surg* 97:666–674, 1989.

47 Morrow AG, Reitz BA, Epstein SE, Henry WL, Conkle DM, Itscoitz SB, Redwood DR. Operative treatment in hypertrophic subaortic stenosis: Techniques and the results of pre- and postoperative assessment in 83 patients. *Circulation* 52:88–102, 1975.

48 Fananapazir L, McAreavey D. Therapeutic options in patients with obstructive hypertrophic cardiomyopathy and severe drug refractory symptoms. *J Am Coll Cardiol* 31:259–264, 1998.

49 Kizilbash AM, Heinle SK, Grayburn PA. Spontaneous variability of left ventricular outflow tract gradient in hypertrophic obstructive cardiomyopathy. *Circulation* 97:461–466, 1998.

50 Spirito P, Chiarella F, Carratino L, Berisso MZ, Bellotti P, Vecchio C. Clinical course and prognosis of hypertrophic cardiomyopathy in an out-patient population. *N Engl J Med* 320:749–755, 1989.

51 Maron BJ, Bonow RO, Cannon RO, Leon MB, Epstein SE. Hypertrophic cardiomyopathy: Interrelations of clinical manifestations, pathophysiology, and therapy. *N Engl J Med* 316:780, 789, 844–852, 1987.

52 McCully RB, Nishimura RA, Tajik AJ, Schaff HV, Danielson GK. Extent of clinical improvement after surgical treatment of hypertrophic obstructive cardiomyopathy. *Circulation* 94:467–471, 1996.

53 Heric B, Lytle BW, Miller DP, Rosenkranz ER, Lever HM, Cosgrove DM. Surgical management of hypertrophic obstructive cardiomyopathy: Early and late results. *J Thorac Cardiovasc Surg* 110:195–208, 1995.

Part Three

Constriction and Tamponade

12

Introduction to Pericardial Disease

James A. Goldstein

An appreciation of normal pericardial anatomy and function serves as the foundation for understanding the complex hemodynamics of cardiac tamponade (CT) versus constrictive pericarditis (CP), and the still challenging problem of differentiating CP from restrictive cardiomyopathy (RCM).

Pericardial Anatomy

Although the pericardium is usually described as a single sac, anatomically it actually consists of two sacs intimately connected with one another, but totally different in structure [1]. The outer sac, the fibrous pericardium, forms a flask-shaped enclosure, the neck of which is closed by its fusion with the external coats of the great vessels, and its base attached to the central tendon and muscular fibers of the diaphragm, which serves to anchor and protect the heart; its construction of dense connective tissue renders it strong and relatively nondistensible (Figure 12.1). The serous pericardium is a second closed sac, composed of outer parietal and inner visceral layers. The parietal layer lines the inner surface of the fibrous pericardium to which it adheres, whereas the visceral layer envelops the epicardial surface of the heart, separated from it only by a layer of epicardial fat that contains the coronary vessels. Between the parietal and visceral layers, the pericardial cavity contains a thin film of pericardial fluid (approximately 20 mL) which physiologically resembles an ultrafiltrate of plasma. Both of these layers function in lubricating the heart to prevent friction during cardiac motion.

The pericardium which covers the great vessels is arranged in the form of two tubes. The aorta and pulmonary artery are enclosed in one, the arterial mesocardium. The superior vena cava (SVC) and inferior vena cava (IVC) and the pulmonary veins are enclosed in a second tube, the venous mesocardium, the attachment of which to the parietal layer forms an inverted U. The cul-de-sac enclosed between the limbs of the U lies behind the left atrium and is the oblique sinus. The passage between the venous and arterial mesocardia—that is, between aorta and pulmonary artery in front and the atria posteriorly—is termed the transverse sinus.

Pericardial Functions

Although an intact pericardium is not critical to maintenance of cardiovascular function, it has potentially important subsidiary functions [1]. These include (i) limitation of intrathoracic cardiac motion; (ii) balancing right and left ventricular output through diastolic and systolic interactions; (iii) buffering of positional changes in chamber filling and therefore output; (iv) suction filling; (v) limitation of acute dilatation; (vi) lubricant effects that minimize friction between cardiac chambers and surrounding structures; and (vii) lymphatic/immunological functions, mediated in part through anatomic barriers that help prevent the spread of infection from contiguous structures, especially the lung.

Compliance Properties of the Normal Pericardium

The pericardium is a "chamber" and therefore exhibits compliance properties whereby intrapericardial volume exerts intrapericardial pressure (IPP). Normally, IPP closely tracks intrapleural and right atrial (RA) pressures. The pericardium acts as a hydrostatic system, equally distributing hydrostatic forces over the surface of the cardiac chambers; this favors equality of end-diastolic transmural pressures throughout the ventricles and therefore uniform stretch of muscle fibers (thereby tending to balance preload), which permits the Frank–Starling mechanism to operate uniformly at all intraventricular pressures. The presence of the pericardium also constantly compensates for changes in inertial and

Hemodynamic Rounds: Interpretation of Cardiac Pathophysiology from Pressure Waveform Analysis, Fourth Edition.
Edited by Morton J. Kern, Michael J. Lim, and James A. Goldstein.
© 2018 John Wiley & Sons Ltd. Published 2018 by John Wiley & Sons Ltd.

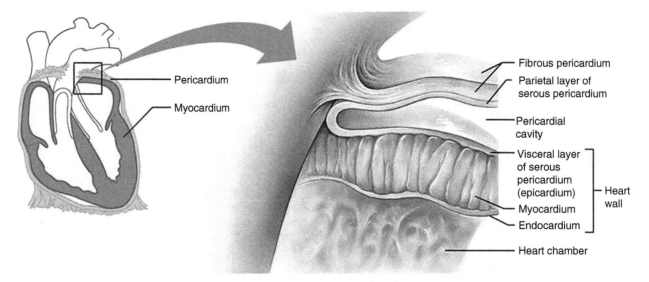

Figure 12.1 Pericardial anatomy: the pericardium consists of two sacs intimately connected. The outer fibrous pericardium constructed of dense connective tissue renders it relatively nondistensible. The serous pericardium is composed of outer parietal and inner visceral layers. The parietal layer lines the inner surface of the fibrous pericardium to which it adheres, whereas the visceral layer envelops the epicardial surface of the heart. *Source:* Reproduced with permission of Anatomy & Psychology 2016.

gravitational forces by distributing them evenly around the heart, providing a mutually restrictive intrapericardial chamber which favors balanced output from both ventricles when this is integrated over several cardiac cycles. It may be speculated that the presence of the parietal pericardium helps maintain a functionally optimal cardiac shape, since after pericardiectomy the heart tends to be more spherical.

The pericardium must accommodate not only its own fluid, but also the volume of all four cardiac chambers. Thus the compliance characteristics of the pericardium are an aggregate reflection of the intrinsic compliance of the pericardial layers (predominantly the stiff parietal layer), the volume of the pericardial space itself, and the combined volume of the cardiac chambers contained within the pericardium. Therefore, IPP reflects the total intrapericardial volume (chamber volumes plus fluid, clots, or masses in the pericardial space) relative to the compliance of the pericardial layers. Normally, the pericardium has a small capacitance reserve volume that allows for a modest amount of chamber dilatation, or fluid accumulation. Initial increments in intrapericardial volume (150–250 mL) result in trivial increases in IPP [2–5]. However, owing to the inelastic nature of the fibrous parietal layer, acutely the pericardial sac is stiff and noncompliant and once this capacitance has been exceeded, further increases in intrapericardial volume result in steep increments in IPP, inscribing a characteristic "J" shape to the pericardial compliance curve, whose ascending inflection point reflects the point at which the pericardium has reached its capacitance (Figure 12.2). Although the fibrous pericardial layer has the capacity to stretch and become more compliant over time in response to chronic effusion accumulation (e.g., neoplastic effusions), ultimately it also reaches the limits of its capacitance and demonstrates a similar "J" shape, albeit with the inflection point occurring at a larger intrapericardial volume (Figure 12.2).

Elevated Pericardial Pressure Intensifies Diastolic Ventricular Interactions

Pressure or volume overload of one ventricle influences the filling and compliance of the contralateral chamber through diastolic ventricular interactions mediated by the interventricular septum and augmented by the pericardium. Because the pericardium is acutely noncompliant, conditions that cause pericardial crowding elevate intrapericardial pressure (IPP), which may be the mediator of adverse cardiac compressive effects. Elevated IPP more tightly couples the two ventricles and intensifies these interactions. Elevated IPP may result from primary disease of the pericardium itself (fluid accumulation in tamponade or stiffened layers in CP) or from abrupt chamber dilatation (e.g., acute right ventricular [RV] dilatation from RV infarction or acute massive/submassive pulmonary embolus). Regardless of the mechanism leading to increased IPP, the resultant pericardial constraint exerts adverse effects on cardiac filling and output. Elevated IPP, whether from effusion or abrupt chamber dilatation, exerts adverse hemodynamic effects by limiting chamber filling through compressive effects, disproportionately on the thinner, lower-pressure right heart [6–9], wherein only limited filling can be achieved

Figure 12.2 Mechanism of tamponade pericardium and pressure–volume curves. (a) diagrams of heart with empty and filled pericardium, (b) pressure-volume curves of acute and chronic pericardial effusion.

(a)

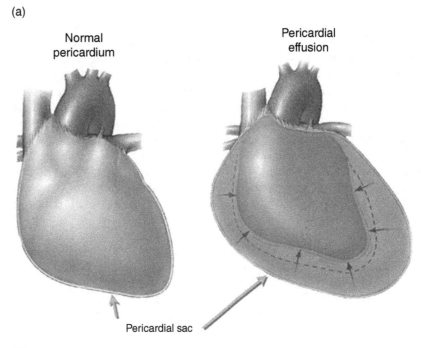

Normal pericardium

Pericardial effusion

Pericardial sac

(b)

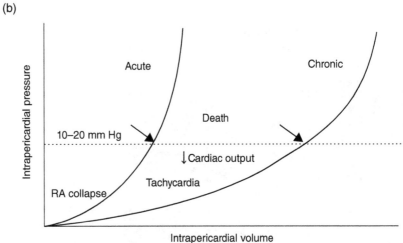

and this at elevated pressures, resulting in combined backward congestion (diastolic failure) together with preload reductions that limit forward output (systolic limitations).

Cardiac Tamponade

Cardiac tamponade is a life-threatening hemodynamic condition resulting from pericardial effusion that increases IPP sufficiently to externally compress and restrict cardiac chamber filling. Compression of the heart and prevention of adequate ventricular filling reduce stroke volume, cardiac output, and blood pressure. At its most severe stage, elevated IPP oppresses

and inundates the chambers, severely limiting their filling and, without intervention, rapidly progressing to cardiogenic shock and death. Tamponade may develop during viral infections, as a complication of cardiac catheterization or interventional procedures [10], after myocardial infarction, after open-heart surgery, or in patients with cancer or connective tissue diseases.

Pathophysiology of Cardiac Tamponade

Fluid accumulating in the pericardial space produces an elevation of pericardial pressure. Hemodynamic consequences reflect the volume of the effusion, rapidity of its accumulation, compliance of the pericardium and myocardium, cardiac compensatory mechanisms (contractility and heart rate), and total blood volume (Figure 12.2). Increased IPP acts as an external resistance to filling of the cardiac chambers. As IPP increases beyond 8–10 mm Hg, thus exceeding normal filling pressure, the atria and ventricles are deprived of preload, thereby limiting chamber filling and cardiac output. Hemodynamically significant effusions compress the cardiac chambers, particularly the thinner, more compliant right-heart chambers, throughout diastole. As the ventricles begin to relax at the end of systole, they are initially constrained by the elevated IPP, with further increases in restraint as pericardial volume is increased by progressive ventricular filling, resulting in a pattern of progressive pan-diastolic resistance. Although chamber volumes are markedly decreased, evident by echocardiography as diminished chamber volumes with chamber compression (Figure 12.3), filling pressures are markedly increased. As IPP increases, venous pressure is increased to maintain cardiac filling and prevent collapse of the cardiac chambers. Although the measured filling pressures by physical examination and invasive hemodynamic assessment are increased, echocardiography demonstrates that chamber volumes are remarkably reduced. This disparity between measured filling pressure and true preload or distending (transmural)

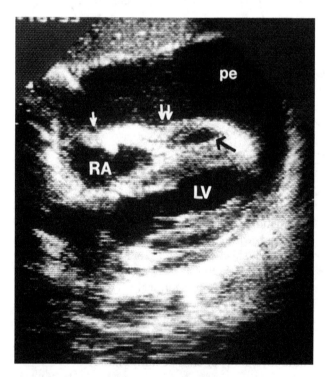

Figure 12.3 Severe cardiac tamponade. Echocardiogram demonstrating large pericardial effusion (pe) compressing the right atrium (RA, single white arrow) and the right ventricle (RV) free wall (double single white arrows), and nearly obliterating the severely preload-deprived RV cavity (black arrow). LV = left ventricle.

pressure is a reflection of the fact that fluid-filled catheters measure pressure, not volume. Measured pressure reflects the actual volume exerting transmural descending pressure plus the IPP and also the effect of chamber and compliance itself. Thus, in any cardiac condition, the actual measured filling pressure only reflects true preload assuming that chamber compliance, the pericardial space, and the pericardial layers are otherwise normal. For example, if effusion has elevated IPP to 15 mm Hg and the estimated jugular venous pressure (JVP) or measured right atrial (RA) pressure is 17 mm Hg, the true distending (or transmural) filling pressure is only 2 mm Hg, reflecting the hypovolemic predicament of the cardiac chambers despite elevated neck veins.

As described earlier, pericardial fluid accumulation is tolerated with compliance until pericardial reserve volume is reached, at which point there is a sharp increase in the slope of IPP (even sharper if pericardial layers are abnormal because of inflammation or fibrosis). Thus, acutely developing effusions of even 300–400 mL (e.g., related to pacemaker-induced chamber perforation) can abruptly elevate IPP and induce tamponade. However, given time, the pericardium can stretch and exhibit compliance. Accordingly, slow accumulation of fluid (even in amounts greater than 1 L associated with neoplasms) may be tolerated with little or no hemodynamic compromise. At some point, however, even chronic effusions can accumulate sufficiently to encroach on the limits of pericardial compliance. Then, even small increments in intrapericardial volume sharply increase IPP and compromise hemodynamics.

Hemodynamics of Cardiac Tamponade

These hemodynamic effects are reflected as elevated RA pressure with a prominent systolic X descent and a blunted diastolic Y descent (Figures 12.4–12.6). This pattern is due to rapid filling of the right atrium from a high-pressure venous system during ventricular systole, when there is "spare room" in the intrapericardial space, and to restricted filling of the ventricles during diastole owing to the compressive effects of elevated IPP. The Y descent is blunted, reflecting impaired emptying of the right atrium attributable to the pan-diastolic resistance to RV filling; the RA A wave is augmented, reflecting enhanced atrial contraction into the stiff noncompliant right ventricle. The prominent X descent can be considered as two components, a sharp early X descent reflecting enhanced atrial relaxation associated with augmented atrial contraction, with the latter portion of the X descent sharp as well, reflecting systolic intrapericardial depressurization as the ventricles empty during systole, thereby reducing intrapericardial volume; in fact, the sharp latter portion of the X descent reflects the fact that this is the

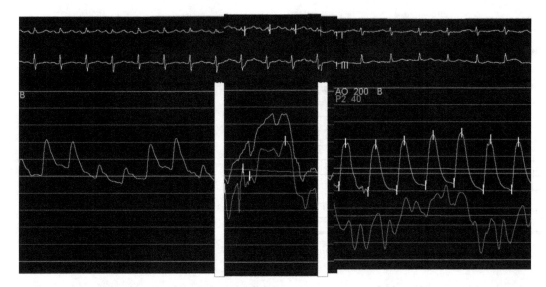

Figure 12.4 Hemodynamic findings in cardiac tamponade. (Left) Aortic pressure (0–200 mm Hg scale) before pericardiocentesis in patient with clinical and echocardiographic findings of tamponade. (Middle) Right atrial and pericardial pressures (0–40 mm Hg scale) before pericardiocentesis. (Right) Aortic pressure (0–200 mm Hg scale) and pericardial pressure (0–40 mm Hg scale) after pericardiocentesis. Note restoration of arterial pulse with loss of marked respiratory variance (pulsus paradoxus) and reduction of pericardial pressure from 22 to 12 mm Hg. (*See insert for color representation of the figure.*)

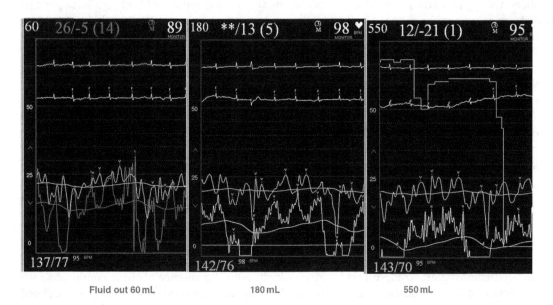

Figure 12.5 Hemodynamic tracings during pericardiocentesis in a patient with shortness of breath and pericardial effusion. The presumed cause of dyspnea was tamponade. (Left) Baseline hemodynamics. Right atrial (RA) pressure is yellow tracing. (Middle) RA and pericardial pressure after 180 mL removed. (Right) Pressures after 550 mL fluid removed from pericardium. However, the relief of pericardial pressure by pericardiocentesis demonstrated no change in RA pressure. No cardiac tamponade is present. The diagnosis is effusive constrictive pericardial disease with left ventricular dysfunction. (*See insert for color representation of the figure.*)

only period in which the pericardium is "relatively" empty, at which time atrial filling has the best chance of being accommodated within the crowded pericardium.

The intracardiac volumes are decreased on both sides of the heart, but the diastolic filling pressures are elevated and equalized throughout the cardiac chambers, reflecting the common effects of the elevated IPP as well as intensification of ventricular interactions between right and left heart. This equalization pattern may be altered if the effusion is loculated or nonconcentric and pericardial resistance not equally distributed to all cardiac chambers, and by intrinsic cardiopulmonary disease, in which the pulmonary artery (PA) diastolic pressure is elevated out of proportion to the wedge

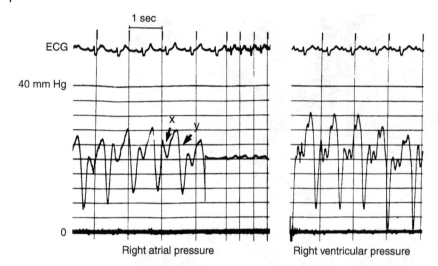

pressure, no doubt reflecting the patient's lung disease and elevated pulmonary resistance. Similarly, patients with intrinsic left ventricular disease may suffer hemodynamic compromise from a pericardial effusion, though the left ventricular filling pressure is greater than that of the right-heart chambers. Owing to marked reductions in intracardiac preload, stroke volume is reduced and ultimately results in elicitation of neuro-hormonal compensatory responses to maintain output and blood pressure through increased sympathetic and catecholamine stimulation, leading to increased contractility, tachycardia, and vasoconstriction. Most importantly, sinus tachycardia reflects exhaustion of compensatory mechanisms and not only signals the presence of a hemodynamically important effusion, but may herald impending hemodynamic collapse.

Pulsus Paradoxus in Cardiac Tamponade

Cardiac tamponade induces pulsus paradoxus (also known as paradoxical pulse), defined as an inspiratory decrease in systolic blood pressure greater than 10 mm Hg, an ominous sign of hemodynamic compromise induced by complex respiratory effects on cardiac filling [11–13]. The term was coined in 1873 by William Kussmaul [14], who described a "pulse simultaneously slight and irregular, disappearing during inspiration and returning upon expiration" despite the continued presence of the cardiac impulse during both respiratory phases. Hemodynamically significant effusion crowds the intrapericardial space, the resultant increased IPP tightly coupling the two ventricles. Under these conditions, increased filling on one side of the heart results in a concomitant decrement in filling on the contralateral chamber. In tamponade, despite markedly elevated intracardiac and systemic venous filling pressures, negative intrathoracic pressure (ITP) is transmitted through the

pericardial fluid, and therefore inspiratory augmentation of venous return is intact. The result is that inspiratory preload expansion of the right heart competes for space within the crowded tense pericardial space, thereby compressing the LV through ventricular interaction across the septum and reducing LV filling. Since pericardial pressure approximates LV diastolic pressure in severe tamponade, inspiration induces a larger decrement in wedge pressure than LV pressure, reducing the gradient for LV filling (evident as decrement in mitral valve flow). Together these inspiratory effects result in reduced LV preload, stroke volume, and cardiac output, manifest as pulsus paradoxus. At moderate levels of cardiac tamponade, these can be measured as a drop in aortic systolic pressure of > 15 mm Hg; at the end stage of hemodynamic embarrassment, the pulse can be felt to disappear in muscular arteries by palpation.

It is important to consider the conditions that must exist for pulsus paradoxus, including pericardial resistance that affects both ventricles and intact atrial and ventricular septa, as well as spontaneous generation of negative intrathoracic pressure with respiration. Accordingly, with the absence of these conditions such as may be seen in asymmetric tamponade (e.g., loculated effusions or compressive hematomas), patients on mechanical ventilation or those with atrial-ventricular septal defects should not be expected to manifest paradoxical pulse despite the presence of hemodynamically embarrassing infusions. It is also important to note that other mechanisms may contribute to paradoxical pulse beyond intraventricular competition for preload, including inspiratory effects on pulmonary venous pooling and differential effects on LV and aortic pressure, as may be seen in chronic obstructive pulmonary disease (COPD). Therefore, paradoxical pulse is not pathognomonic for cardiac tamponade, as other conditions may result in exaggerated respiratory oscillations, including intrapericardial crowding due to abrupt RV dilatation (e.g., acute RV infarction or massive pulmonary embolus), as well as marked ITP swings associated with severe reactive airway disease and tension pneumothorax. The phenomenon may be difficult to detect when the patient is extremely tachycardiac, or has an irregular rhythm such as on an atrial fibrillation ventilator. Pulsus paradoxus may be absent in patients on ventilators who lose inspiratory variation in negative intrathoracic pressures. In addition, pulsus paradoxus may be absent in patients with intracardiac communication such as atrial septal defects (ASDs), and post-surgical cardiac tamponade with localized cardiac hematoma or collections of clot (and loculated fluid). In some patients, however, the presence of a large pericardial effusion does not always mean that hypotension or dyspnea is due to pericardial tamponade. The hemodynamics of patient with large pericardial effusion but no echocardiographic findings of tamponade are shown in Figure 12.5. On removal of pericardial fluid, it can be seen that despite the drop in pericardial pressure, RA pressure remained elevated with marked X and Y descents, consistent with effusive-constrictive pericardial disease and not tamponade.

Both tamponade and pericardial constriction may be associated with a paradoxical pulse >10 mm Hg reduction in arterial pressure during inspiration (Figure 12.4), low cardiac output, tachycardia, and hypotension. Cardiac tamponade and constrictive pericarditis have important pathophysiologic differences (discussed in detail in Chapter 13). Briefly, in constriction, early diastolic filling is very rapid, as the ventricle rapidly recoils after ejection. This results in the characteristic brisk Y descent that is almost universally observed. In contrast, elevated pericardial pressure in cardiac tamponade limits filling throughout all of diastole, and the Y descent is characteristically blunted. Figure 12.4 illustrates the hemodynamics of cardiac tamponade and its relief after pericardiocentesis.

Echocardiography in Cardiac Tamponade

Echocardiography has revolutionized the evaluation and management of cardiac tamponade. This simple-to-apply technique easily detects the presence and magnitude of pericardial effusion and the effects of the effusion on cardiac filling, and serves to guide therapeutic pericardiocentesis. It must be emphasized that the magnitude of the fluid by itself does not determine its hemodynamic significance, for, as described earlier, a modest effusion accumulating acutely may induce hemodynamic embarrassment, whereas a chronically developing large effusion may be accommodated by pericardial compliance and not embarrass cardiac function. The key is to link the anatomic presence of the effusion with its effects on cardiac filling, both by evidence of chamber preload

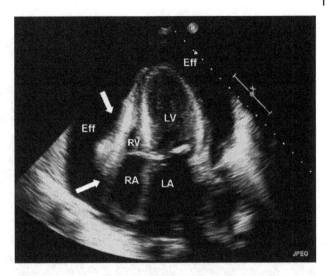

Figure 12.7 Echocardiographic frame of patient with cardiac tamponade. Pericardial tamponade with right-sided collapse. Eff = effusion; LA = left atrium; LV = left ventricle; RA = right atrium; RV = right ventricle.

deprivation and collapse as well as by exaggerated respiratory variations measured by Doppler. When IPP exceeds filling pressure, chamber compression becomes evident (Figure 12.7). This is most notable and seen earliest on the right-heart chambers, which are lower pressure and therefore more easily affected [6–9]. Signs of compression occur first in the RA, in which collapse persisting over more than one-third of the cardiac cycle is highly sensitive and specific for cardiac tamponade. In early cases of tamponade, RV compression is seen early in diastole when the chamber is less filled, and may become less apparent at the end of diastole. RV diastolic collapse is less sensitive but quite specific (RV is less compressible than RA). Conversely, RV collapse may not manifest when the RV is hypertrophied. The greater the magnitude of IPP elevation, the "drier" or volume deprived the ventricles appear. In severe tamponade, the heart may appear to swing within the pericardial fluid on a beat-to-beat basis, a phenomenon correlating with electrical alternans on ECG and an ominous sign of profound and often end-stage hemodynamic compromise. Doppler echocardiography has further refined delineation of the hemodynamic impact of any given pericardial effusion [11]. Analogous to the pathophysiology of pulsus paradoxus in tamponade, Doppler can detect exaggerated respiratory variation characterized by inspiratory increase of tricuspid flow velocity with concomitant decrement of more than 25% in mitral flow velocity, reflecting the increased ventricular interdependence induced by pericardial crowding (Figure 12.8). This parameter is particularly helpful when the pericardial effusion is detected by echocardiography, but its hemodynamic significance is clinically uncertain; exaggerated respiratory tricuspid and mitral flow velocities may be a powerful arbiter.

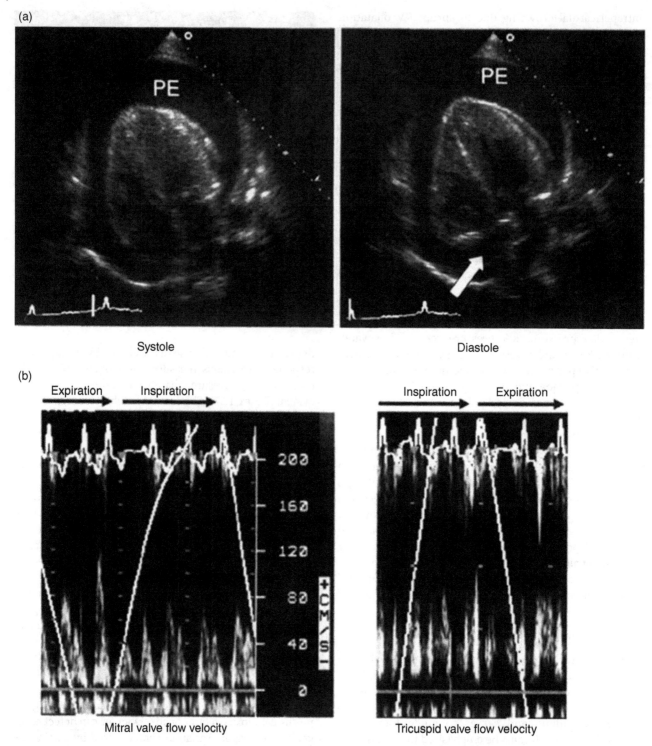

Figure 12.8 Cardiac tamponade. (a) Two-dimensional echocardiogram demonstrating large pericardial effusion (PE). (b) Doppler flow velocities demonstrate marked respiratory variation (>25%) in the Doppler signal, with inspiratory increase in tricuspid flow and concomitant decrease in mitral flow, the mechanism underlying intrapericardial competition resulting in pulsus paradoxus. The opposite changes occur with expiration. *Source:* Little 2006 [15]. Reproduced with permission of Wolters Kluwer Health, Inc.

The Three Phases of Cardiac Tamponade

Cardiac tamponade was initially thought to be an all or none phenomenon, with hypotension and decreased cardiac output as a result of fluid accumulation reaching a critical level impairing ventricular filling. The all or none hypothesis stated that increased pericardial pressure produced equilibration with right ventricular pressure and thus limited ventricular filling and cardiac output. Early in the course of effusion, cardiac pressures remain unchanged. With increasing fluid, both the pericardial and right ventricular filling pressures increase together, eventually equilibrating with left ventricular pressure. At this point, elevated right ventricular pressure without depression of cardiac output or pulsus paradoxus may be evident. Reddy *et al.* [3] described this intermediate presentation as right-heart tamponade. With continued fluid accumulation, pericardial, right ventricular, and left ventricular filling pressures increase and equilibrate, decreasing cardiac output and producing pulsus paradoxus. Thus, three phases of cardiac tamponade can be readily appreciated.

Reddy *et al.* [4] have subsequently modified their earlier observations (Figure 12.9). Phase I cardiac tamponade occurs when intrapericardial pressure is less than right ventricular and pulmonary capillary wedge (left ventricular filling) pressures. A characteristic hemodynamic response on pericardiocentesis in phase I patients decreases pericardial and right atrial pressures, with minimal change in the inspiratory decrease in arterial systolic pressure and no change in cardiac output. Phase II cardiac tamponade occurs when intrapericardial pressure equilibrates with right ventricular but not pulmonary capillary wedge pressure. Pericardiocentesis in phase II decreases pericardial, right atrial, and, to some

extent, pulmonary capillary wedge pressures with a larger change in the inspiratory decrease in arterial pressure (paradox) and a modest increase in cardiac output. Classical phase III cardiac tamponade is observed when intrapericardial pressure equilibrates with right ventricular and pulmonary capillary wedge (left ventricular filling) pressures. Pericardiocentesis in phase III decreases pericardial, right atrial, and pulmonary capillary wedge pressures with normalization of the exaggerated inspiratory decrease in arterial systolic pressure and a pronounced increase in cardiac output. The changes after pericardiocentesis indicate that pericardial effusion and tamponade physiology exhibits the greatest abnormalities in phase III, and is associated with significant abnormalities of pressure and flow in phase II and with only pressure alterations in phase I. As Reddy *et al.* [4] conclude, cardiac tamponade is not an all or none phenomenon. The severity of hemodynamic derangement rather than its mere presence should be assessed in patients with pericardial effusion. Echocardiography has significantly improved our ability to assess the hemodynamic phases of cardiac tamponade. As described in the above discussion of the hemodynamic spectrum, many patients with moderate pericardial effusion may have only minimal hemodynamic compromise, with systolic pressures over 100 mm Hg and at least half having a cardiac index of over 2.3 L/min/m^2 [9]. Pericardiocentesis in these patients resulted in hemodynamic improvement, but did not alleviate symptoms of dyspnea or modify tachycardia. Subtle or early evidence of hemodynamic compromise was obtained in distinction to the classic reports of cardiac tamponade in decades past, where only phase III patients with severe hemodynamic compromise were recognized.

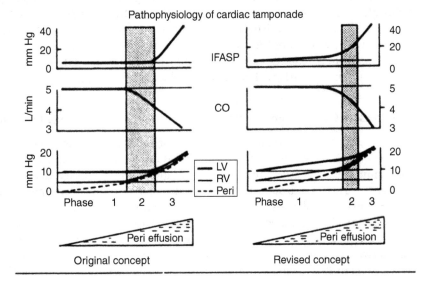

Figure 12.9 Concepts of the three phases of cardiac tamponade. The previous concept on the left has been modified by including data and theories of ventricular compliance on the right. Hemodynamic changes of pericardial pressure (peri), right ventricular (RV) and left ventricular (LV) pressure, and inspiratory increase in arterial systolic pressure (IFASP) and cardiac output (CO) are demonstrated with increasing pericardial effusion for a given patient. The height of the triangle from left to right is the amount of pericardial effusion accumulating. Phase II is represented by the stippled bar. See text for details. *Source:* Leimgruber 1989 [8]. Reproduced with permission of Wolters Kluwer Health, Inc.

Atypical Pericardial Compression Syndromes

Regional Tamponade

Classic cardiac tamponade results when a free-flowing effusion concentrically encompasses all of the cardiac chambers. Regional tamponade occurs when loculated eccentric effusions or localized hematoma produce selective chamber compression [16]. The effusion contents may vary from serous fluid to frank clot; its consistency and physical properties may evolve over time from fully compressible fluid to inelastic organized hematoma. Postoperative adherence of anterior structures (RV, RA, and pericardium) to the anterior chest wall and the adhesions that develop promote regional posterior-lateral effusions, for there is little room for fluid collection anteriorly. Not surprisingly, loculated effusions now most commonly develop due to fluid constrained within pockets bordered by pericardial adhesions post pericardiotomy. Regional compressing hematomas also occur most commonly in postsurgical patients and post myocardial infarction (MI), where they may reflect contained perforation or hemorrhagic transformation of a benign effusion by anti-coagulants. Regional tamponade results in atypical hemodynamic findings, as only the compressed chambers will manifest altered diastolic properties. Thus, although low-output hypotension may develop from severe under-filling of a single selectively compressed chamber (RA, RV, LA, or LV), equalization of diastolic filling pressures is lacking and pulsus paradoxus absent. However, loculated effusion can also induce classic tamponade though tightening of the uninvolved pericardium. Because the hemodynamics may be atypical, regional tamponade should be suspected in any patients who develop unexplained low-output hypotension following MI or cardiac surgery. Although standard two-dimensional echocardiography may be sufficient to establish the diagnosis in some cases, in others with posterior or LA compression, transesophageal echo or magnetic resonance imaging (MRI) scanning may provide superior delineation of all chambers.

Low-Pressure Cardiac Tamponade

Low-pressure cardiac tamponade is a form of cardiac tamponade with low pericardial pressure, resulting in the compromise of cardiac function despite low filling pressures. This syndrome is poorly characterized because only isolated cases have been reported. Sagrista-Sauleda *et al.* [17] examined 1,429 patients with pericarditis, of whom 279 had combined pericardiocentesis and catheterization. Low-pressure cardiac tamponade criteria were met in 29 patients, as opposed to the 114 patients

in this group with classic tamponade. Patients with low-pressure tamponade as a typical sign of tamponade were less frequent, but the rate of constitutional symptoms, use of diuretics, and echocardiographic findings of tamponade were similar. Low-pressure tamponade showed a significant increase in cardiac output after pericardiocentesis, but less severe cardiac tamponade beforehand. Prognosis was related to underlying cardiac disease. Low-pressure tamponade was identified in 20% of patients with catheter-based criteria and clinical recognition of low-pressure tamponade may be difficult. Typical clinical findings supporting low-pressure tamponade were associated with a slightly higher heart rate, but acute clinical tamponade, jugular venous distension, and pulsus paradoxus were lower in the low-pressure tamponade group. There were no differences in echocardiographic findings nor any origins of the pericardial disease. Hemodynamic differences between low-pressure tamponade and high-pressure tamponade were noted in heart rate, intracardiac pressure being lower, right atrial pressure being lower, and left ventricular end-diastolic pressure (LVEDP) being lower before treatment. A compensatory increase in venous pressure may be attenuated because of hypovolemia and thus cardiac output may be compromised in the presence of low ventricular filling pressures equilibrated with intrapericardial pressure, defining the syndrome of low-pressure tamponade. A subgroup of patients with equilibration of pericardial and ventricular pressures of less than 10 mm Hg may experience a significant increase in cardiac output after pericardiocentesis. Intrapericardial pressure closely follows changes in right atrial pressure and volume during the cardiac cycle. Pressure changes within the pericardium reflect the volume of fluid, as influenced by myocardial chamber size during filling and emptying. The pericardial pressure waves generally parallel right atrial pressure when early tamponade is present, but distinctly different waveforms are seen in patients without cardiac tamponade. Low-pressure tamponade thus should be expected with pericardial effusion, pulsus paradoxus, and hypotension, with findings on echocardiography of tamponade despite having a low to normal RA pressure.

Effusive-Constrictive Pericarditis

Effusive-constrictive pericarditis is a form of subacute constriction characterized by effusion into a free pericardial space associated with constriction of the visceral pericardium [18]. Effusion contents may vary from serous fluid to frank clot; its consistency and physical properties may evolve over time from fully compressible fluid to inelastic organized hematoma; and the effusion may be concentric, regional, or loculated. Furthermore, over time the effusion contents may organize and the inflamed pericardial layers may become stiffened. This dynamic spectrum of physical properties interacts with changes in the intrinsic properties of the healing pericardium, giving rise to a spectrum of hemodynamic patterns from pure tamponade through effusive-constrictive physiology to pure constriction. Effusive-constrictive pericarditis is characterized by mixed clinical and hemodynamic findings. In some cases a constrictive pericarditis underlies a free-flowing effusion. In patients with scarred rigid visceral and parietal pericardial layers, tamponade can occur with relatively modest fluid accumulation. The effusive-constrictive nature of the physiology may only be fully revealed when pericardiocentesis fails to completely reduce diastolic pressures.

Hancock suggested three types of compressive pericardial effects: tamponade, subacute "elastic" constriction, and chronic "rigid" constriction [18]. Effusive-constrictive pericarditis, one of the types of subacute elastic constrictive processes, is characterized by effusion into a free pericardial space associated with constriction of the heart by the visceral pericardium. Effusive-constrictive pericarditis has been described and attributed to hemopericardium and serosal injury. It is most commonly seen post pericardiotomy, but can be seen with any postinflammatory pericarditis from infection, irradiation, or uremia. Effusive-constrictive disease results in a hybridized hemodynamic state with patterns that are intermediate between those of tamponade and constriction. The physical examination and hemodynamic findings before pericardiocentesis resemble those of tamponade, with the characteristics of constriction revealed after pericardial drainage results in only partial relief of the hemodynamic abnormalities. Prior to pericardiocentesis, effusive-constrictive disease looks hemodynamically more like tamponade than constriction, with elevated equalized filling pressures and a prominent paradoxical pulse, but in contrast to classical tamponade the Y descent may be preserved and a Kussmaul's sign present, which may be indicators that a constrictive physiological component exists. The co-existent condition of fibroelastic visceral constriction is confirmed when pericardiocentesis results in relief of pulsus paradoxus but incomplete resolution of elevated filling pressures, with hemodynamics developing more prominent atrial Y descents and the ventricular "dip and plateau" characteristic of constriction. It is important to emphasize that effusive-constrictive disease does not inexorably progress to chronic constriction. In some cases the disease is transitory, reflecting the dynamic healing changes ongoing within the inflamed pericardial sac. Thus, patients requiring pericardiocentesis for clinical relief of the effusion component should subsequently be treated with anti-inflammatory agents and followed clinically, as some cases will resolve without a requirement for surgical intervention.

Assessment and Management of Pericardial Effusions: Clinical Algorithms

Cardiac tamponade is a potentially life-threatening emergency that responds dramatically to properly performed and optimally timed pericardial drainage and decompensation. The most critical initial step in management is establishing the magnitude of hemodynamic compromise through integration of symptomatic manifestations, signs of physical examination, echocardiographic features, and hemodynamic characteristics. Regardless of the circumstances, the hemodynamic impact of effusions can be categorized as follows.

Hemodynamically Unimportant Effusions

The earliest hemodynamic manifestation of elevated IPP is reflected in RA and JVP pressure. Therefore, if an effusion is present by ultrasound, the key feature of the physical examination is the presence or absence of JVP elevation (normal JVP < 5–7 mm Hg). Accordingly, in patients with a hemodynamically insignificant effusion, the neck veins are flat and the blood pressure, heart rate, and respiratory rate normal; clinical stigmata of impaired perfusion are absent, as is dyspnea. On ultrasound the effusion could in fact be large, but there will be no evidence of chamber compression or exaggerated respiratory variation in transvalvular flows.

Management

These patients do not need pericardiocentesis. Attention should be focused on diagnosis of the etiology. Monitoring of effusion size by echocardiography and daily evaluation for elevating JVP and paradoxical pulse are essential.

Hemodynamically Significant but Compensated Effusion

An early hemodynamically significant effusion will result in elevated JVP (8–12 mm Hg), with a sharp X but blunted Y descent. Echocardiography shows effusion with mild compression of the RA and/or RV free wall. Doppler documents exaggerate respiratory variation of transvalvular flows and therefore pathological pulsus paradoxus may be present (>12–15 but < 20 mm Hg). When the effusion is modest in hemodynamic significance, it will be fully compensated without elicitation of significant neuro-hormonal stimulation. Therefore, there is neither tachycardia nor hypotension, perfusion is not compromised, and dyspnea is absent.

Management

These patients need pericardiocentesis, not urgently but preferably "before the sun goes down," as bleeding may rapidly push the pericardium up its steep "J-shaped" compliance curve and lead to more severe hemodynamic compromise.

Hemodynamically Severe Effusion with Compensatory Mechanisms Maximally Activated

As the effusion becomes more hemodynamically embarrassing, neuro-hormonal compensatory systems will be more intensely activated to try to maintain cardiac output and blood pressure in the face of markedly reduced chamber preload. Accordingly, those patients will have markedly elevated JVP (>15 mm Hg) and will begin to manifest signs of intense neuro-hormonal stimulation, including tachycardia. Patients may be short of breath owing to impaired cardiac compliance (although interestingly, the lungs are almost always clear despite elevated wedge pressure) and the respiratory rate may be elevated. Systemic vascular resistance will be increased as vasoconstriction attempts to compensate for low output to maintain blood pressure, and therefore perfusion may be compromised, although the patients will not yet be hypotensive. However, such patients will manifest prominent paradoxical pulse (>20 mm Hg) and ultrasound typically reveals dramatic chamber collapse of the IVC, RA, and right ventricle, with marked reduction of LV preload and prominent respiratory flow variations.

Management

These patients need urgent pericardiocentesis. Gentle fluids should be given while preparing to transfer the patient to the catheterization laboratory or coronary care unit (CCU) for echocardiographically guided pericardial drainage. Vasopressors can be administered for borderline blood pressure.

Hemodynamically Severe Effusion, Decompensated

In the most hemodynamically extreme decompensated state, the compensatory mechanisms are overwhelmed and patients manifest a striking elevation of JVP (>20 mm Hg), tachypnea, and dramatic palpable paradox (pulse in the muscular arteries may frankly disappear during inspiration). Despite pronounced sinus tachycardia, hypotension is striking and compromise of perfusion

is evident clinically, often by altered mental status and low urine output. Ultrasound shows prominent effusion with profound chamber collapse. However, of note is that modest effusions that accumulate rapidly may produce such profound hemodynamic effects. The heart may be swinging in the pericardium, giving rise to electrical alternans affecting all components of the ECG waveform (P, QRS, and T waves).

Management

These patients need emergency pericardiocentesis. Vasopressors and fluid should be given while preparing to perform bedside pericardial drainage, without echocardiographic guidance if the patients is in extremis. This intervention can be life-saving. Waiting to transfer to the catheterization laboratory or CCU is generally unwise and not feasible, unless the blood pressure rapidly stabilizes with the above measures.

Pericardiocentesis

Historically, pericardiocentesis was performed "blind," employing a two-ended alligator clamp connecting the needle to the V_1 lead of the electrocardiogram. Now, routine utilization of echocardiographic guidance for percutaneous pericardial drainage is associated with excellent procedural success, with minimal patient discomfort and low risk, and has rendered "blind" needle pericardiocentesis outmoded, except in an emergency when there is no other option. Two-dimensional echo guidance can help track needle placement in the pericardium and thus avoid laceration of critical and vulnerable structures such as the right ventricle and coronary arteries. Echo contrast visualization of the pericardium by injection of agitated saline through the pericardiocentesis needle can further help establish proper needle placement and insure subsequent safe insertion of a J-tipped guidewire, over which is placed a multiple side holed catheter for pericardial drainage. Hemodynamic monitoring during pericardiocentesis has proven to be extremely informative and effective in confirming intrapericardial hemodynamics and, along with echocardiography, insuring optimal decompression.

Successful pericardiocentesis can be documented by improvement in the hemodynamics with four specific indicators: (i) reduction of IPP to levels of 0 ± 3 mm Hg; (ii) return of RA pressure to near normal levels with separation between right and left ventricular diastolic filling pressures; (ii) increase in cardiac output; and (iv) restoration of normal inspiratory response of the RA and arterial pressures, with disappearance of the pulsus paradoxus. The presence of persistent elevation and (near) equilibration of right and left ventricular diastolic pressures, as we will see, suggests a continued constricting pericardial process (e.g., effusive-constrictive pericarditis). In many instances, post-pericardiocentesis management includes suturing of the pericardial catheter to the skin and attaching the catheter to a closed drainage system. The installation of carbon dioxide or air into the pericardial space to outline the pericardium at the end of the procedure is not advocated. The catheter should be removed within 24–48 hours to reduce the risk of infection. Assessment of pericardial fluid drainage and serial echocardiography at 12–24-hour intervals will identify whether pericardial fluid reaccumulation is rapid and may require more definitive drainage by a surgical pericardial window.

Case: Pericardial Fluid after Cardiac Transplantation and Early Tamponade

A 53-year-old woman underwent orthotopic cardiac transplantation for dilated cardiomyopathy. The postoperative course was uncomplicated. Medications at the time of discharge included cyclosporin, azathioprine, and steroids. On the fourth hospital day, a moderate pericardial effusion without echocardiographic evidence of hemodynamic compromise was noted. Over the next week, increasing jugular venous distension, hepatomegaly, and increasing abdominal girth with clear lung fields prompted a repeat echocardiogram, which showed right ventricular enlargement, normal systolic left ventricular function, and larger anterior and posterior pericardial effusions without echocardiographic signs of tamponade [2]. Cardiac catheterization was then performed during routine endomyocardial biopsy from the femoral approach. During the right-heart catheterization, mean right atrial pressure of 20 mm Hg, pulmonary artery diastolic pressure of 20 mm Hg, and mean pulmonary capillary wedge pressure of 18 mm Hg were recorded, with equalization of left and right ventricular diastolic pressures (Figure 12.6). Note the prominent Y descent on the right atrial tracing and the dip and plateau configuration of the right ventricular pressure (Figure 12.6). Left ventricular and pulmonary capillary wedge pressures were also mildly elevated and equilibrated (Figure 12.10). No biopsy evidence of transplant rejection was found. Because pericardial effusion and abnormal hemodynamics of this type have been described early after cardiac transplant [3, 4], diuretics, nitrates, and isoproterenol were prescribed, but without effect on jugular venous distension or dyspnea on minimal exertion. One week later, the patient was dyspneic with a systolic blood pressure of 85 mm Hg and a pulsus paradoxus (>10 mm Hg) not previously observed (Figure 12.11). Equilibration of right atrial and pulmonary artery pressures was present. Urgent pericardiocentesis was performed.

Before assessing the results of the pericardiocentesis, consider the following issues. Based on the right atrial waveforms, does this patient more likely have pericardial constriction, early tamponade, or both? Does equilibration of right and left ventricular pressures favor constriction or tamponade? Finally, based on hypotension with newly observed pulsus paradoxus, does one delay pericardiocentesis until after confirmation by echocardiography?

Pericardiocentesis was performed from the sub-xyphoid approach with hemodynamic monitoring. Pericardial pressure was initially measured through the long 18-gauge pericardial needle. After passing the J-tipped guidewire and an 8 F dilator, a multiple side hole catheter was advanced into the pericardial space for fluid drainage and pressure measurement. A balloon-tipped catheter measured pressures in the right heart. A 5 F sheath was placed in the femoral artery.

Hemodynamic data at the time of pericardiocentesis (Figure 12.12) again showed equalization of diastolic pressures, with a mean right atrial pressure of 26 mm Hg and a dip and plateau configuration of the right ventricular tracing, as in Figure 12.10. Arterial pressure was 85/58 mm Hg. A two-dimensional echocardiogram, performed at the bedside, confirmed the larger pericardial effusion and moderate depression of both right and left ventricular systolic function. Right atrial and right ventricular diastolic collapse, although present, was not striking.

Surprisingly, intrapericardial pressure was elevated to only 10 mm Hg (Figure 12.12). After removal of 250 cc of serosanguinous pericardial fluid, the pericardial pressure fell to zero with no change in right atrial or systemic pressure, or cardiac output. Note the absence of waveform alteration of right atrial pressure and persistence of hypotension with pulsus paradoxus after pericardiocentesis.

A presumptive diagnosis of cardiac allograft rejection was confirmed by biopsy. Treatment of allograft rejection permitted the patient to be discharged with resolution of the symptoms and hemodynamic abnormalities. Repeat right-heart catheterization two months later showed only mild elevation of right-heart pressures without diastolic pressure equalization.

This patient initially demonstrated hemodynamics of constrictive physiology in association with a pericardial effusion. Later development of hypotension and pulsus paradoxus suggested early cardiac tamponade. Most surprising was the fact that pericardial pressure was significantly lower than right atrial pressure, and hence pericardiocentesis did not alter the systemic hemodynamic response. With treatment of allograft rejection,

(a)

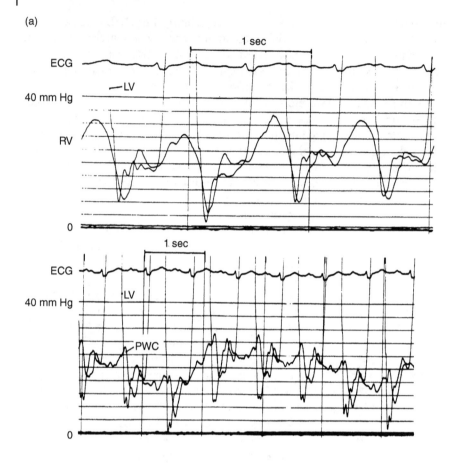

(b)

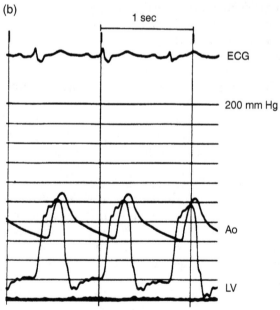

Figure 12.10 (a, top) Left (LV) and right ventricular (RV) pressure waves (0–40 mm Hg full scale). (Bottom) LV and pulmonary capillary wedge pressure (PCW) demonstrating diastolic equalization in a patient with pericardial effusion after cardiac tamponade. See text for details. *Source:* Kern 1992 [19]. Reproduced with permission of John Wiley & Sons. (b) Aortic (Ao) and left ventricular (LV) pressures prior to hemodynamic compromise in a patient with pericardial effusion. Note the pattern of left ventricular filling with early but moderate diastolic dip with a plateau phase over the second two-thirds of the diastolic filling period. Arterial pressure is satisfactory despite symptoms of dyspnea at this time.

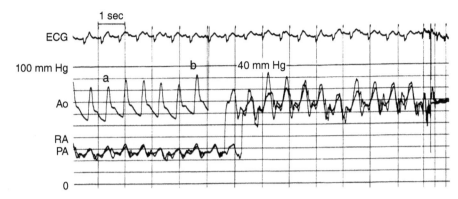

Figure 12.11 Hemodynamics after an episode of hypotension with echocardiographic signs of hemodynamic compromise. Arterial (Ao), right atrial (RA), and pulmonary artery (PA) pressures are shown on a 0–100 mm Hg scale (left) and a 0–40 mm Hg (right). Note the change in inspiratory systolic pressure (a to b) during a respiratory phase without alteration of the right atrial or pulmonary artery pressures. Equilibration of right atrial and pulmonary artery pressures is striking, as shown on the right side of the panel.

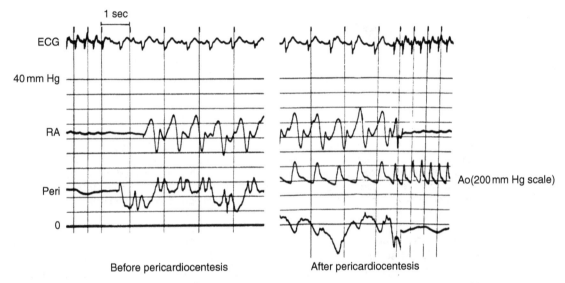

Figure 12.12 Right atrial (RA) and intrapericardial pressure (peri) before (left) and after (right) pericardiocentesis (0–40 mm Hg scale). Note absence of change in RA waveform and low arterial pressure after pericardial fluid removed. See text for details. *Source:* Kern 1992 [19]. Reproduced with permission of John Wiley & Sons.

the hemodynamics reverted toward normal. Restrictive physiology was the true pathophysiologic explanation of the hemodynamics [20].

Case: Pulsus Paradoxus

A 68-year-old man with chronic renal failure on dialysis presented with increasing shortness of breath and dyspnea over two months. His cardiac silhouette on chest X-ray was reported to be enlarged compared to previous film. A marked inspiratory decline in arterial pressure was noted by the referring physician. The patient was being treated for persistent hypertension and had recently had cardiac catheterization for a chest pain syndrome, which showed normal coronary arteries and moderately

diminished left ventricular function. Echocardiography revealed a large pericardial effusion with right-heart chamber collapse in diastole. Pericardiocentesis was performed with the technique used in patient #1. Arterial pressure (Figure 12.13) varied from 180/120 mm Hg to 145/95 mm Hg over a single respiratory cycle. The inspiratory decline in arterial pressure was 40 mm Hg. Corresponding with the labored inspiration was the marked increase and decrease in the matching right atrial and pericardial pressures. Of note is the abbreviated Y descent on the right atrial tracing. The inspiratory increase in right atrial and intrapericardial pressures was also abnormal.

Compare the right atrial pressure wave to that obtained in patient #1 prior to pericardiocentesis. Several differences can be seen. The inspiratory increase in right atrial

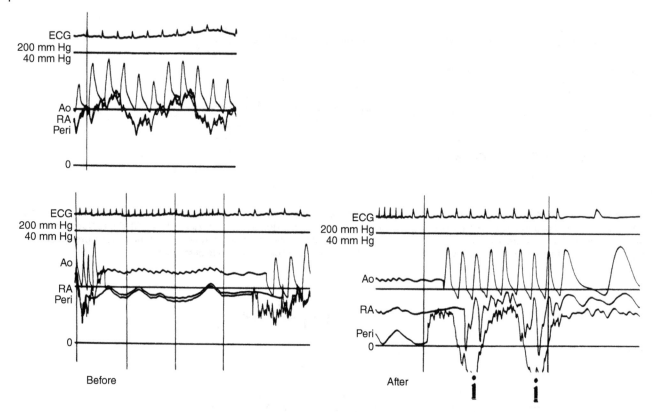

Figure 12.13 Hemodynamics in a patient with large pericardial effusion and dyspnea. Ao = aortic pressure; RA = right atrial pressure; Peri = pericardial pressure. Top panel shows initial hemodynamics with inspiratory alterations in arterial pressure and right atrial and pericardial pressures. Mean right atrial and pericardial pressures shown on the lower panel before pericardiocentesis demonstrate a marked inspiratory increase in these waveforms. After pericardiocentesis (right side, lower panel), pericardial and right atrial pressures are reduced; i shows influence of normal inspiration on right atrial and pericardial pressure waveforms. See text for details.

(and pericardial) pressures is not as prominent. The striking Y descent is absent in patient #2. The severity of pulsus paradoxus is also greater in patient #2. Pericardial catheter drainage removed 450 cc of serosanguinous fluid, reducing the pericardial pressure to 2–3 mm Hg and the right atrial pressure from a mean of 18 mm Hg to a mean of 10 mm Hg (Figure 12.13, lower right). Release of pericardial pressure changed the right atrial pressure waveform toward normal, with restoration of the X and Y filling patterns, especially prominent during inspiration. The A and V waves with the corresponding X and Y descents are altered to various degrees depending on the type of pericardial physiology present (Table 12.1).

This patient example demonstrates the remarkable feature of extreme pulsus paradoxus that can occur in the absence of classical tamponade (hypotension, narrow pulse pressure, low cardiac output, and tachycardia). The resolution of pulsus paradoxus, evident after pericardiocentesis, corresponded to improvement in dyspnea with slowing of the heart rate. Incidentally, the pulmonary artery oxygen saturation, obtained with an oximetric catheter before pericardiocentesis, had risen from 48% to 72%, demonstrating a marked increase

in cardiac output. This patient in phase II cardiac tamponade had a clear symptomatic and hemodynamic indication for a therapeutic pericardial drainage due to uremic pericarditis. Note that the right atrial pressure did not normalize (8 mm Hg). The failure to normalize right atrial pressure suggests a continuing restrictive or occult effusive constrictive physiology.

Pulsus paradoxus occurs to varying degrees depending on the equilibration of pericardial and ventricular filling pressures, as determined by venous return. In phase I, a compensatory increase in venous pressure usually maintains ventricular volume close to basal levels. Right and left ventricular pressures are generally higher than pericardial pressure, and thus the inspiratory decrease in arterial pressure may be exaggerated but rarely reaches the diagnostic level. In phase II, pericardial pressure increases more than ventricular filling pressures, equilibrating first with the right and then with the left ventricular pressure. Venous pressures may compensate by increasing venous return, but with inadequate ventricular filling to maintain baseline cardiac output. The inspiratory decrease in arterial systemic pressure is further exaggerated beyond that observed in phase I and

Table 12.1 Clinical and hemodynamic findings in compressive pericardial disease.

	Tamponade	Subacute constriction	Chronic constriction
Etiology	Idiopathic Neoplasm Trauma	Idiopathic Uremic Radiation malignancy Collagen vascular disease Infectious (e.g., tuberculosis)	Idiopathic Infectious (e.g., tuberculosis)
Pulsus paradoxus (>10 mm Hg)	Marked	Moderately prominent	Usually slight
Right atrial pressure waveforms[a]	X, Xy	Xy, XY	XY, xY
LV–RV equilibration	∫	±	+
RA = PCW	∫	±	+
CXR pericardial calcification	–	±	+
Cardiomegaly	∫	±	+

[a] X = large or prominent; x = diminished or absent; ± = occasionally present; + = present; – = absent.
∫ = depending on which phase of cardiac tamponade.
CXR = chest X=ray; LV = left ventricular; PCW = pulmonary capillary wedge; RA = right atrial; RV = right ventricular.

reaches a diagnostic level for pulsus paradoxus in some but not all patients, depending on ventricular compliance. In phase III, increased pericardial pressure equilibrates with right and left ventricular pressures and initiates severe hemodynamic compromise. Cardiac output declines markedly and pulsus paradoxus may often exceed a > 20 mm Hg inspiratory decline in pressure.

The hemodynamic findings typically associated with cardiac tamponade, subacute (elastic) pericardial constriction, or chronic (rigid) pericardial constriction are compared on Table 12.1. As noted in patient #1, the prominent Y descent favors a more constrictive pericarditis, whereas in patient #2 with cardiac tamponade, the X is prominent with a blunted Y descent. The elevation and equilibration of the ventricular diastolic pressures may be seen in all three conditions and do not distinguish one from the other. In the restriction to diastolic filling, the dip and plateau is more prominent with the constrictive physiology than with tamponade, but may be seen with either depending on the hemodynamic phase in the spectrum of cardiac tamponade.

Case: Malignant Tamponade

A 52-year-old bisexual man with hepatitis B and AIDS presented to the emergency department with a one-week history of progressive dyspnea, chills, night sweats, and increased abdominal girth. His medications on admission included clarithromycin, didanosine, stavudine, nelfinavir, acyclovir, and Septra DS. Six months prior to admission, he had had a negative intradermal purified protein derivative (PPD) test. On physical examination he was dyspneic. Blood pressure was 160/100 mm Hg, pulse 100 beats/min, and respiratory rate 24 breaths/min. There was jugular venous pulsation at the angle of the jaw and bilateral submandibular lymphadenopathy. The lungs were clear. The heart sounds were distant, without gallop or rub. There was shifting abdominal dullness and bilateral inguinal lymphadenopathy. The lower extremities were without edema. The admission electrocardiogram revealed sinus tachycardia and low-voltage QRS. The admission chest radiograph showed cardiomegaly and a possible mediastinal mass. Creatinine was 1.2 mg/dL, total leukocyte count 3200 cells/μL, and serum LDH 1532 U/L. Computerized tomography of the chest revealed bilateral axillary, mediastinal, deep pelvic, and inguinal adenopathy, a large pericardial effusion, bilateral pleural effusions, and ascites. A transthoracic echocardiogram confirmed the presence of a large pericardial effusion with right atrial and ventricular collapse. There was marked respiratory variation in the aortic and mitral valve velocities.

The patient was taken to the cardiac catheterization laboratory and underwent pericardiocentesis. Initial hemodynamics prior to pericardiocentesis showed that the arterial pressure was 120/80 mm Hg, but was associated with > 80 mm Hg pulsus paradoxus, with complete loss of femoral arterial upstroke periodically during inspiration (Figure 12.14). Mean right atrial pressure was 40 mm Hg, with striking respiratory variation and obliteration of phasic waveforms (Figure 12.15). Pulmonary artery and right ventricular systolic pressures matched peak expiratory right atrial pressure. The mean pulmonary artery wedge, right atrial, and mean intrapericardial pressures were elevated and equal. Right ventricular pressure was 62/20 mm Hg, pulmonary artery pressure 64/40 mm Hg, mean pulmonary artery pressure 48 mm Hg,

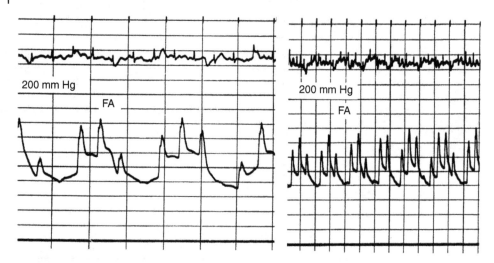

Figure 12.14 Aortic (FA) pressure on a 0–200 mm Hg scale, demonstrating marked pulsus paradoxus and obliteration of the aortic pulse during inspiration. (Left) Pressure waveform at 25 mm/sec. (Right) Pressure waveform at 10 mm/sec. Note the cyclical variation and marked respiratory difference between systolic pressures during the inspiratory cycle.

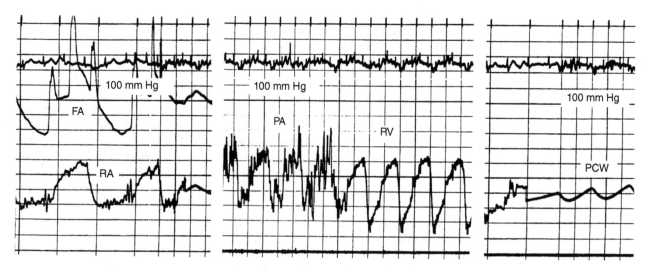

Figure 12.15 (Left) Aortic (FA) and right atrial (RA) pressure on a 0–100 mm Hg scale. Mean right atrial pressure is approximately 40 mm Hg, with obliteration of phasic waveforms of A and V waves. Note the marked inspiratory and expiratory variation of the right atrial pressure. (Middle) Pulmonary artery (PA) and right ventricular (RV) pressures during catheter pullback, demonstrating the high filling pressures of right ventricular pressure. (Right) Mean pulmonary capillary wedge (PCW) pressure of 40 mm Hg on a 0–100 mm Hg scale.

mean pulmonary capillary wedge pressure 40 mm Hg, mean pericardial pressure 40 mm Hg, and arterial pressure 160/100 mm Hg. After removal of 420 cc hemorrhagic pericardial fluid, the hemodynamics were repeated, with a decrease in mean right atrial pressure to 22 mm Hg, mean pulmonary artery capillary wedge pressure to 24 mm Hg, pulmonary artery pressure to 58/28 mm Hg, mean pulmonary artery pressure to 38 mm Hg, and mean pericardial pressure to 14–16 mm Hg. Following removal of a total of 1450 mL of pericardial fluid, mean right atrial pressure declined to 22 mm Hg, with reinstitution of phasic waveforms and a prominent Y descent. Mean intrapericardial pressure was 16 mm Hg, with no evidence of residual pericardial fluid

(Figure 12.16). After pericardiocentesis, pulsus paradoxus was alleviated, with a return of near normal right ventricular pressure (Figure 12.17). The patient tolerated the procedure well. Pericardial fluid analysis revealed a lactate dehydrogenase (LDH) concentration of 17,760 U/L, and a total leukocyte count of 200 cells/μL. Microscopic examination revealed lymphocytosis without evidence of opportunistic infection, and flow cytometric analysis revealed 76% of cells within the monocyte region expressing a monoclonal B-cell immunophenotype. These data, along with cytomorphological examination, were diagnostic of involvement of the pericardial fluid by malignant lymphoma, non-Hodgkin's, small non-cleaved cell (Burkitt's lymphoma).

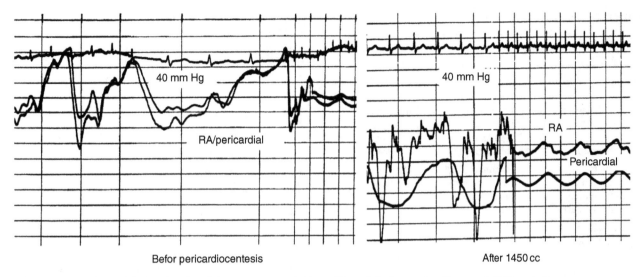

Befor pericardiocentesis   After 1450 cc

Figure 12.16 Right atrial (RA) and pericardial pressures on a 0–40 mm Hg scale before pericardiocentesis (left) and after pericardiocentesis (right). Note the reduction in right atrial and pericardial pressure with return of some A wave, and the phasic nature of the right atrial pressure. Mean right atrial pressure is 22 mm Hg and pericardial pressure 14 mm Hg.

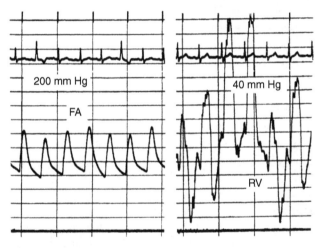

Figure 12.17 (Left) Femoral artery (FA) pressure after pericardiocentesis. (Right) Right ventricular (RV) pressure after pericardiocentesis. Note the absence of pulsus paradoxus, the regularization of the arterial pressure waveform, and the return of the right ventricular end-diastolic pressure notch, consistent with right atrial pressure.

In this case, the striking pulsus paradoxus obliterated the arterial waveform at end inspiration, a phenomenon rarely observed [4, 11, 18, 21]. The "group beating" changing over the respiratory cycle can be appreciated with the arterial pressure recorded at a slower paper speed (Figure 12.14, right). The presentation of tamponade-related hypotension was modified by the large respiratory variation, resulting in a mean arterial pressure of approximately 80 mm Hg. The narrow pulse pressure and tachycardia were consistent with a reduced cardiac output of the compromised left ventricle. The marked elevation and equilibration of the right-heart pressures were also

noteworthy. The right ventricular, pulmonary artery, and systolic pressures were only slightly higher than the expiratory mean right atrial pressure, consistent with severe tamponade physiology. The right atrial waveform was also unusual in the dramatic obliteration of its phasic components, a feature which improved on relief of the tamponade. The final right atrial and pericardial pressures remained elevated but separate, despite complete pericardial drainage. These postprocedural hemodynamics are not unusual for effusive-constrictive pericardial effusions [18]. The finding of malignant (neoplastic) pericardial tamponade, an unusual complication of AIDS-related malignant lymphoma, was a sentinel sign for the diagnosis of this entity. Furthermore, the hemodynamic features associated with pericardial tamponade were also remarkable for the severity of pulsus paradoxus and elevated and equilibrated right-heart pressures.

Discussion: Malignant Pericardial Effusions

Malignant pericardial effusion is a life-threatening complication of an end-stage disease; the prognosis typically dismal related to the underlying metastatic carcinoma (e.g., lung, breast). In patients with cancer, autopsy series reveal that pericardial effusions are present in up to 20% of individuals. Primary tumors associated with pericardial effusions include lung (40%), breast (23%), lymphoma (11%), and leukemia (5%) [20]. Pericardial effusions are malignant in approximately 50% of cases, with nonmalignant causes being secondary to radiation-induced pericarditis and infections. A listing of tumors of the pericardium is provided in Table 12.2 and indicates the infrequency of Burkitt's type. General clinical

Table 12.2 Tumors of the pericardium.

Primary		Secondary
Benign	**Malignant**	
Pericardial (coelomic) cyst (15.49%) (pericardial diverticulum)	Mesothelioma (3.6%) (diffuse type or, rarely, solitary type)	Carcinomas of the lung Carcinomas of the breast
Angiomas (hemangioma, lymphangioma, vascular hamartoma)	Sarcomas (3%): angiosarcoma, fibrosarcoma, other	Malignant melanoma Leukemias
Mesothelioma (solitary type)	Teratoma	Other malignant neoplasms
Heterotopic tissue origin (bronchial cyst, dermoid cyst, teratoma [2.6%], thymoma, thyroid adenoma)		
Miscellaneous: lipoma, fibroma, leiomyoma, neurilemoma, neurofibrom		

Table 12.3 General clinical manifestations of cardiac (and pericardial) tumors.

Pericardial involvement

 Chest pain

 Pericarditis

 Pericardial effusion

 Abnormal cardiac silhouette on chest roentgenogram

 Arrhythmias, usually atrial

 Cardiac compression/constriction

 Cardiac tamponade

Myocardial involvement

 Arrhythmias, ventricular and atrial

 Electrocardiographic changes

 Abnormal cardiac silhouette on chest roentgenogram

  Generalized cardiac enlargement

  Localized cardiac enlargement

 Conduction disturbances and heart block

 Congestive heart failure

 Coronary involvement

  Angina pectoris

  Myocardial infarction

Intracavity tumor

 Cavity obliteration

 Valve obstruction and valve damage

 Embolic phenomena: systemic, neurological, coronary

 Constitutional manifestations

manifestations of cardiac tumors are listed in Table 12.3 and demonstrate the wide variety of pathologic involvement of this rare entity. The common presentations of dyspnea, cough, orthopnea, and chest pain are present in approximately 85%, 30%, 25%, and 20% of patients, respectively, with a paradoxic pulse associated with pericardial effusion in 45% of patients also noting tachypnea, tachycardia, hypotension, and peripheral edema. As in the case example, however, cardiac tamponade requires prompt treatment to eliminate dyspnea, congestion, and hypotension.

A malignant effusion is relatively easy to relive acutely, but challenging to pacify over time, since, given the underlying malignant nature of the effusion, recurrent effusions are problematic [22–27]. Thus, the underlying cancer that induces the effusion is virtually always the key factor influencing prognosis, which is usually poor; the dismal median survival of these patients supports a conservative approach to this problem. Therefore, relief of hemodynamically significant effusions is usually intended to achieve short-term palliation. In these cardio-oncology cases, good clinical judgment informed by detailed knowledge of the patient's overall condition allows prudent decisions. Although there is a lack of solid data to guide therapy, in those patients whose cancer and overall clinical condition are clearly end-stage, short-term palliative relief by simple pericardiocentesis is reasonable, and this simple intervention can be repeated for recurrent effusions over time. Catheter drainage of malignant pericardial effusions has been reported to control fluid reaccumulation for more than 30 days in over 90% of patients. Instillation of sclerosing agents has been disappointing [22–24], is painful, and has largely been abandoned. At present there is a lack of solid data to guide therapy in those with recalcitrant effusions. Surgical drainage is definitive and can usually be accomplished with a limited thoracotomy, but nevertheless the attendant surgical morbidity is unattractive in patients whose underlying disease is typically incurable and associated with high short-term mortality. Intractable effusions can also be treated by catheter balloon pericardiotomy [27]. However, this technique is associated with patient discomfort, is technically unfamiliar to most operators, and may lead to complications not seen with catheter drainage alone. Regardless, in experienced hands it is a reasonable alternative. Whether balloon pericardiotomy should be employed as a primary strategy or be reserved for recurrent effusions has not been established. Furthermore, there are no good comparisons versus surgical drainage. In summary, one

(a)

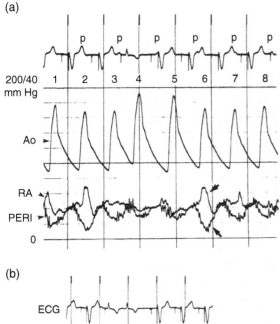

(b)

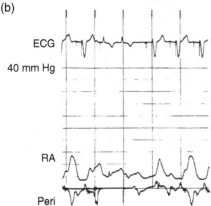

Figure 12.18 (a) Hemodynamic data during DDD pacing before pericardiocentesis. Ao = femoral artery pressure; RA = right atrial pressure; Peri = pericardial pressure; P = p waves. Scale is 0–200 mm Hg for arterial pressure and 0–40 mm Hg for right atrial and pericardial pressures. (b) Hemodynamic data after pericardiocentesis. See text for details. *Source:* Gudipati 1990 [28]. Reproduced with permission of Elsevier.

reasonable and practical approach is initially percardiocentesis (once or twice), with balloon pericardiotomy or surgical drainage reserved for multiple recurrences.

Case: Low-Pressure Tamponade

Examine the hemodynamic tracings of a 64-year-old woman admitted for elective pericardiocentesis because of increasing fatigue, with moderate pericardial effusion and early tamponade physiology (Figure 12.18). The patient had a DDD pacemaker which had intermittent failure to sense and capture the atrium, with periods of atrial ventricular dissociation. Pericardiocentesis was performed with hemodynamic monitoring and measurement of right atrial pressure with a 7 F balloon-tipped flotation catheter. Arterial pressure was measured with a

5 F sheath with fluid-filled catheter. As can be observed in Figure 12.18a, there was minimal pulsus paradoxus. The right atrial mean and pericardial mean pressures were both 9 mm Hg. The mean pulmonary capillary wedge pressure was 14 mm Hg. Of interest are the large negative pericardial pressure waves occurring during atrial ventricular dissociation. The decline in pericardial pressure is especially evident on beats #2 and 6. These negative waves occur during atrial systole against a closed tricuspid valve. Large atrial cannon waves are coupled with a negative mirror-image pericardial wave of a proportional size. The effect was most evident on the longest and largest cannon waves (compare beats #6 and 7). After pericardiocentesis (Figure 12.18b), the mean right atrial pressure was 6 mm Hg, with mean intrapericardial pressure of 0 mm Hg. Echocardiography revealed absence of pericardial fluid and no signs of tamponade physiology. Pericardial pressure continued to demonstrate large negative waves associated with right atrial cannon waves. Normally right atrial pressure and volume decrease after atrial systole and before ventricular systole, producing an X descent. As ventricular volume decreases during ejection, pericardial pressure decreases, increasing transmural (that is, right atrial–pericardial pressure gradient) pressure, resulting in venous influx into the right atrium during late ventricular systole (beginning the V wave). In A–V dissociation, atrial systole may occur during ventricular systole, resulting in a large venous cannon wave. The decrease in atrial volume produces a proportional decrease in intrapericardial pressure (a negative cannon wave), exaggerated by atrial and ventricular contraction and volume reduction at the same time. This unusual observation demonstrates the interesting pressure changes that occur normally within the pericardium. The clinical syndrome of this patient was attributed to loss of the atrial contribution to cardiac output rather than to pericardial fluid.

Key Points

1) Cardiac tamponade is a clinical syndrome characterized by a spectrum of hemodynamic abnormalities, but usually associated with an elevated venous pressure, exaggerated inspiratory fall in arterial pressure (pulsus paradoxus), and, as a late (phase III) event, arterial hypotension.

2) Echocardiographic evidence of right atrial and right ventricular collapse are useful signs differentiating hemodynamically insignificant pericardial effusion from tamponade.

3) The change in pressure waveforms after pericardial pressure reduction will reflect the atrial and ventricular filling related to myocardial compliance and occult pericardial disease.

References

1 Spodick D. *The Pericardium: A Comprehensive Textbook*. New York: Marcel Dekker, 1997.

2 Holmes DR, Nishimura R, Fountain R, Turi ZG. Iatrogenic pericardial effusion and tamponade in the percutaneous intracardiac intervention era. *J Am Coll Cardiol Intv* 2:705–717, 2009.

3 Reddy PS, Curtiss EI, O'Toole JD, Shaver JA. Cardiac tamponade: Hemodynamic observations in man. *Circulation* 58:265, 1978.

4 Reddy PS, Curtiss EI, Uretsky BF. Spectrum of hemodynamic changes in cardiac tamponade. *Am J Cardiol* 66:1487, 1990.

5 Spodick DH. Acute cardiac tamponade. *N Engl J Med* 349:684, 2003.

6 Gillam LD, Guyer DE, Gibson TC, King ME, Marshall JE, Weyman AE. Hydrodynamic compression of the right atrium: A new echocardiographic sign of cardiac tamponade. *Circulation* 68:294, 1983.

7 Reydel B, Spodick DH. Frequency and significance of chamber collapses during cardiac tamponade. *Am Heart J* 119:1160, 1990.

8 Leimgruber PP, Klopfenstein HS, Wann LS, Brooks HL. The hemodynamic derangement associated with right ventricular diastolic collapse in cardiac tamponade: An experimental echocardiographic study. *Circulation* 68:612, 1983.

9 Mercé J, Sagristà-Sauleda J, Permanyer-Miralda G, Evangelista A, Soler-Soler J. Correlation between clinical and Doppler echocardiographic findings in patients with moderate and large pericardial effusion: Implications for the diagnosis of cardiac tamponade. *Am Heart J* 138:759, 1999.

10 Holmes DR Jr, Nishimura R, Fountain R, Turi ZG. Iatrogenic pericardial effusion and tamponade in the percutaneous intracardiac intervention era. *JACC Cardiovasc Interv* 2:705–717, 2009.

11 Shabetai R, Fowler NO, Fenton JC, Masangkay M. Pulsus paradoxus. *J Clin Invest* 44:1882, 1965.

12 Curtiss EI, Reddy PS, Uretsky BF, Cecchetti AA. Pulsus paradoxus: Definition and relation to the severity of cardiac tamponade. *Am Heart J* 115:391–398, 1988.

13 Fitchett DH, Sniderman AD. Inspiratory reduction in left heart filling as a mechanism of pulsus paradoxus in cardiac tamponade. *Can J Cardiol* 6:348, 1990.

14 Bilchick KC, Wise RA. Paradoxical physical findings described by Kussmaul's sign. *Lancet* 359:1940–1942, 2002.

15 Little WC, Freeman GL. Pericardial disease. *Circulation* 113:1622–1632, 2006.

16 Torelli J, Marwick TH, Salcedo EE. Left atrial tamponade: Diagnosis by transesophageal echocardiography. *J Am Soc Echocardiogr* 4:413, 1991.

17 Sagristà-Sauleda J, Angel J, Sambola A, Alguersuari J, Permanyer-Miralda G, Soler-Soler J. Low-pressure cardiac tamponade: Clinical and hemodynamic profile. *Circulation* 114:945, 2006.

18 Hancock EW. Subacute effusive constrictive pericarditis. *Circulation* 43:183, 1971.

19 Kern MJ, Aguirre FV. Hemodynamic rounds: Interpretation of cardiac pathophysiology from pressure waveform analysis: Pericardial compressive hemodynamics, Part III. *Cathet Cardiovasc Diagn* 26:152–158, 1992.

20 Wilkes JD, Fidias P, Vaickus L, Perez RP. Malignancy-related pericardial effusion: 127 cases from the Roswell Park Cancer Institute. *Cancer* 76:1377–1387, 1995.

21 Ramsey HW, Sbar S, Elliott LP, Eliot RS. The differential diagnosis of restrictive myocardiopathy and chronic constrictive pericarditis with calcification: Value of coronary arteriography. *Am J Cardiol* 25:635–638, 1970.

22 Laham RJ, Cohen DJ, Kuntz RE, Baim DS, Lorell BH, Simons M. Pericardial effusion in patients with cancer: Outcome with contemporary management strategies. *Heart* 75:67–71, 1996.

23 Goldstein JA. "Cardio-oncology": Implications for interventionists. *Cath Cardiovasc Interv* 87:900–901, 2016.

24 Liu G, Crump M, Goss PE, Dancey J, Shepherd FA. Prospective comparison of the sclerosing agents doxycycline and bleomycin for the primary management of malignant pericardial effusion and cardiac tamponade. *J Clin Oncol* 14:3141–3147, 1996.

25 Goldstein JA. Balloon pericardiotomy for malignant effusion: First at bat or on-deck hitter? *Catheter Cardiovasc Interv* 71(4):508, 2008.

26 Gumrukcuoglu HA, Odabasi D, Akdag S, Ekim H. Management of cardiac tamponade: A comparative study between echo-guided pericardiocentesis and surgery—a report of 100 patients. *Cardiol Res Pract* 2011:197838, 2011.

27 Uramoto H, Hanagiri T. Video-assisted thoracoscopic pericardiectomy for malignant pericardial effusion. *Anticancer Res* 30:4691, 2010.

28 Gudipati CV, Deligonul U, Janosik D, Vandormael M, Kern MJ. Intrapericardial "negative" cannon waves during atrioventricular dissociation in large pericardial effusion. *Am Heart J* 119:964–965, 1990.

13

Restrictive Cardiomyopathy: Differentiating Constrictive Pericarditis and Restriction

James A. Goldstein

Restrictive cardiomyopathies (RCM) are indolent disabling diseases resulting from pathophysiologic processes that induce predominant diastolic chamber dysfunction with lesser impairment of systolic performance. RCM is characterized by ventricles with thick walls, small cavities with intact systolic function, and dilated atria (Figures 13.1 and 13.2). Progressive ventricular noncompliance results in impairment of diastolic filling, leading to the hemodynamic conundrum of low preload but high filling pressures (Figure 13.3). This pattern of diastolic dysfunction leads to elevated mean atrial pressures, resulting clinically in biventricular "backward failure," manifest as pulmonary venous congestion (dyspnea) as well as systemic venous pressure elevation (peripheral edema). Systolic function is preserved in most cases, depending on the underlying cause. Yet despite intact systolic function, the restrictive constraints on true ventricular preload limit stroke volume, thereby resulting in low cardiac output (fatigue) and ultimately hypoperfusion.

RCMs may be classified as arising from primary diseases of the myocardium (hypertrophy, infiltration, inflammation, or fibrosis) or the endomyocardial surfaces (inflammation and scarring). RCM can be further subcategorized based on the underlying pathophysiologic process (Figure 13.4), including hypertrophic (e.g., hypertension, heritable hypertrophic cardiomyopathy, aortic stenosis); deposition diseases, which encompass both infiltrative (e.g., amyloidosis) and storage (e.g., hemochromatosis) processes; inflammatory (e.g., hypereosinophilic syndrome); or primary/idiopathic (e.g., diabetic). However, from a clinical perspective, RCM is best viewed as a "syndrome" rather than a "disease" with a distinct etiology. That is, whereas the term RCM may commonly conjure the image of cardiac amyloidosis, an infiltrative disease inducing "classic" and dramatic clinical manifestations of RCM, far more prevalent is restrictive "pathophysiology," most commonly resulting from hypertrophic states (e.g., hypertension), which when advanced result in severe diastolic dysfunction and a clinical syndrome of RCM [2]. Regardless of the cause, restrictive pathophysiology is characterized by chamber diastolic dysfunction resulting in congestive manifestations; when it is severe, the noncompliant chamber restricts filling, leading to low stroke volume and cardiac output. Given the prevalence of hypertension in our increasing elderly and obese population, it is hardly surprising that restrictive pathophysiology is rampant and underlies the vast majority of cases of heart failure with preserved ejection fraction (HFPEF), a disease near-epidemic in the rapidly growing number of aged patients and those suffering the effects of the metabolic syndrome. Whatever the cause, it can be quite challenging to diurese the congested but stiff, under-filled left ventricle (LV). "Restriction" is also inherent to the pathophysiology of LV outflow obstruction syndromes, both in valvular aortic stenosis (AS) as well as familial hypertrophic cardiomyopathy. The presence of any obstruction further exacerbates the forward output limitations of the stiff, restricted, and hypertrophic LV. Restrictive physiology underlies the clinical entity of "low flow–low gradient AS" with preserved LV systolic function, wherein profound LV preload limitation reduces stroke volume, which contributes to low gradient despite significant obstruction [3]. Various myocardial diseases are characterized by thick ventricular walls (Figure 13.2), including those related to myocyte hypertrophy (congenital hypertrophic cardiomyopathy, or acquired hypertensive and valvular heart disease), as well as infiltrative diseases (e.g., amyloidosis, glycogen storage diseases, and hyperoxalosis). Coronary artery disease, especially in diabetics, can also mimic clinical RCM. Careful history, physical examination, serologic analyses, noninvasive testing particularly with cardiac magnetic resonance imaging (MRI), and coronary arteriography serve to exclude these conditions.

RCM and constrictive pericarditis (CP) are remarkably similar in their hemodynamic pathophysiology and clinical presentation; therefore, their clinical presentations,

Hemodynamic Rounds: Interpretation of Cardiac Pathophysiology from Pressure Waveform Analysis, Fourth Edition.
Edited by Morton J. Kern, Michael J. Lim, and James A. Goldstein.

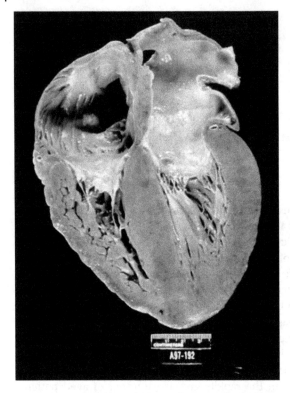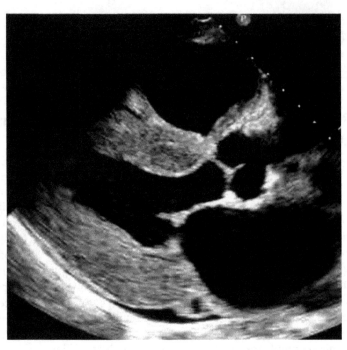

Figure 13.1 Amyloid restrictive cardiomyopathy. (Left) Gross specimen of heart shows thickened left ventricle (LV), septum, and right ventricular (RV) free wall, with dilated atria. *Source:* Falk 2005 [1]. Reproduced with permission of Wolters Kluwer Health, Inc. (Right) Echocardiogram in another patient with cardiac amyloid demonstrates the thick bright hyper-contractile LV myocardium, with corresponding small LV cavity and dilated left atrium.

appearance by echocardiography, and invasive hemodynamic patterns overlap [4–11], posing a diagnostic challenge (discussed in detail in Chapter 12). Radiation-induced cardiac disease deserves special attention, for in such cases the two processes may co-exist, owing to concomitant radiation-induced pericardial disease (pericarditis evolving to CP) and myocardial disease (myocarditis leading to diffuse interstitial myocardial fibrosis and RCM). Hemodynamically, the combination manifests a mixed constrictive and restrictive physiologic picture. The results of pericardiectomy are less satisfactory [12, 13] owing to more difficult surgical stripping and residual symptomatic RCM after pericardiectomy. For the interventionist, differentiating RCM from CP poses one of the more challenging clinical hemodynamic conundrums and deserves special consideration, since the two conditions share similar and overlapping hemodynamic pathophysiology.

Pathophysiology of Restrictive Cardiomyopathy

The pathognomonic feature of RCM is stiffness of the ventricular walls, which impairs diastolic filling, resulting in reduced ventricular preload (and therefore stroke volume) despite increased diastolic filling pressures. Echo-Doppler demonstrates small ventricles, dilated atria, and Doppler features of impaired diastolic function with impaired myocardial relaxation, increased early LV filling velocity, decreased atrial filling velocity, and decreased isovolumic relaxation time. In the early stages of RCM, systolic function is typically preserved, although deterioration in contractility may be observed as the disease progresses; the severity and patterns of dysfunction depend on the specific etiology and severity of the underlying disease entity. Despite preserved systolic ventricular function, impaired diastolic filling limits ventricular preload, thereby rendering the stiff heart limited in its ability to increase cardiac output with exercise, resulting in fatigability. Low output, combined with autonomic insufficiency characteristic of some RCMs (e.g., amyloidosis), renders patients susceptible to symptoms of orthostatic hypotension. Atrial dilation often leads to atrial fibrillation, which further exacerbates diastolic dysfunction due to high heart rate and loss of atrial contraction.

By invasive hemodynamic assessment, RCM is characterized by elevated ventricular diastolic pressures, often with a diastolic "dip and plateau" or "square root" pattern in either or both ventricles (Figure 13.5), a nonspecific indicator of stiff noncompliant chambers (and typically

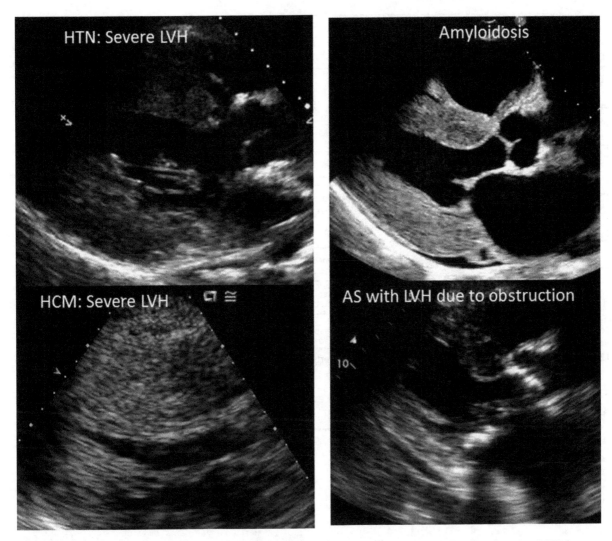

Figure 13.2 Panorama of thick hearts inducing restriction. Pathogenesis includes hypertrophy from hypertension (HTN), hypertrophic cardiomyopathy (HCM), aortic stenosis (AS), or infiltration (amyloidosis). All hearts are characterized by thick walls, and small cavities with intact LV systolic function. LVH = left ventricular hypertrophy.

Figure 13.3 Ventricular compliance curves in normal heart (green curve) and restrictive cardiomyopathy (RCM) due to amyloidosis (yellow curve). The pathognomonic feature of RCM is stiffness of the ventricular walls, which impairs diastolic filling, resulting in increased diastolic filling pressures despite reduced ventricular preload. LV = left ventricular.

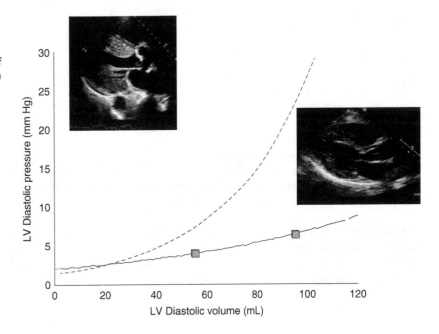

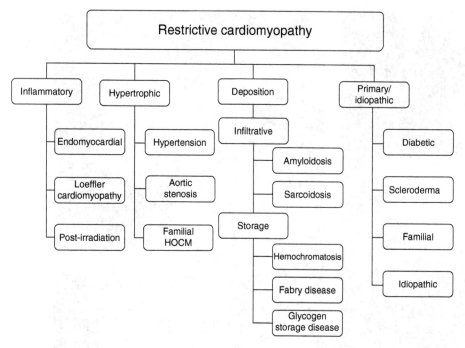

Figure 13.4 Classification of restrictive cardiomyopathy. HOCM = hypertrophic obstructive cardiomyopathy.

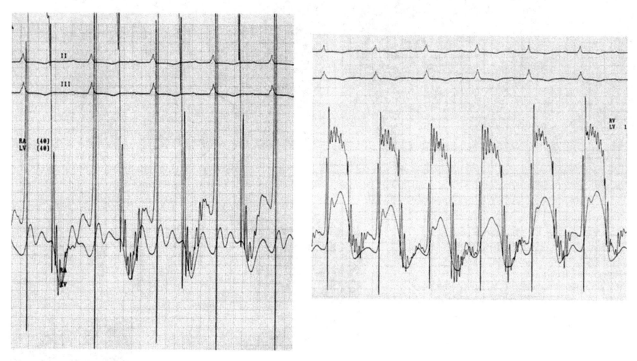

Figure 13.5 Classic "traditional" hemodynamic features of restrictive cardiomyopathy in patient with systemic amyloidosis. (Left) Simultaneous left ventricular (LV) and right atrial (RA) pressures documenting elevated and equalized diastolic filling pressures. Note the RA "M" pattern. (Right) Simultaneous LV and right ventricular (RV) pressures demonstrating equalized diastolic filling pressures, RV "dip and plateau," and "concordant" RV and LV systolic pressures.

seen in other conditions such as CP). Ventricular systolic function is typically preserved until the later stages of the underlying disease. Biatrial enlargement reflects ventricular noncompliance and may also result from primary atrial myocardial involvement by the disease process (e.g., amyloidosis). Atrial filling pressures are elevated, and the X and Y descents tend to be relatively blunted, giving rise to an "M" pattern (Figure 13.5); in cases in which the atria are primarily involved by the restrictive process (e.g., amyloidosis), the A wave may be depressed. In RCM, a pattern of "elevated and equalized" chamber diastolic filling pressures indicating pan-cardiac "stiffness" is typical, but since it is attributable to the myocardial process common to all the chambers, left-sided pressures are typically somewhat higher than right due to the greater intrinsic stiffness of the LV. This difference may be amplified by maneuvers that augment ventricular filling such as volume infusion, leg-raising, or post–premature ventricular contraction increased filling time. Disproportionate left-heart stiffness may also result in moderate pulmonary hypertension (a subtle distinguishing feature from CP).

Dynamic respiratory hemodynamics are blunted in RCM. In contrast to CP, in which the heart is isolated from the lungs and influences of intrathoracic pressure (ITP) on the cardiac chambers are "extrinsically" blunted, in RCM inspiratory changes in ITP are fully transmitted through the pericardium to the cardiac chambers. However, "intrinsic" myocardial noncompliance contributes to a relative lack of respiratory variation in cardiac filling, and therefore mitral and tricuspid flow velocity during respiration are typically decreased (Figure 13.6). Because of the lack of pericardial constraint and a relatively noncompliant interventricular septum, there is

minimal ventricular interdependence, and thus inspiratory effects on ventricular systolic pressures are concordant (i.e., there is little change in peak ventricular systolic pressures with respiration and they move in the same direction; Figure 13.5). This pattern is to be distinguished from the "discordant" pattern characteristic of CP, a finding which may serve to help differentiate the two conditions (Figure 13.7). As RCM progresses and right-sided chambers become less distensible, the respiratory swings in pressure diminish further. At its most severe, noncompliance to inflow results in "Kussmaul's sign," in which inspiratory augmentation of right-heart venous return is intact, but the increased preload cannot be accommodated by the stiff chambers, which "dam up" the return, thereby resulting in inspiratory elevation of right atrial (RA) and jugular venous pressures.

Differentiating Restrictive Cardiomyopathy from Constrictive Pericarditis

Differentiating RCM and CP poses one of the most challenging clinical–hemodynamic conundrums. These two conditions are remarkably similar in their hemodynamic

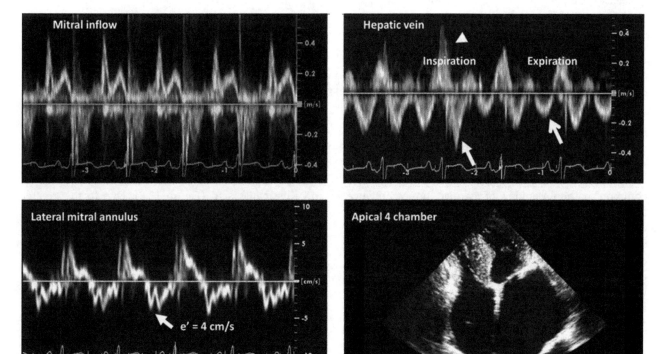

Figure 13.6 Doppler findings in restrictive cardiomyopathy. (Upper left) Pulsed-wave Doppler of the mitral inflow shows a restrictive pattern, with early diastolic mitral inflow Doppler velocity (E) greater than late velocity (A) and short deceleration time. (Upper right) Hepatic vein pulsed-wave Doppler shows increased inspiratory forward velocities (arrow), inspiratory diastolic flow reversals (arrowhead), and minimal expiratory diastolic flow reversals (rounded arrow). (Lower left) Lateral mitral annulus tissue Doppler demonstrates markedly reduced early diastolic velocity (e′). (Lower right) Apical 4-chamber 2-dimensional echocardiography reveals severe biatrial enlargement. *Source:* Geske 2016 [10]. Reproduced with permission of Elsevier.

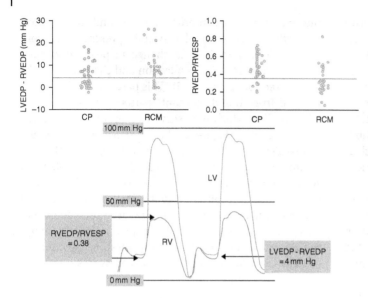

Figure 13.7 Differentiation of constriction and restriction by traditional hemodynamics. There have been a number of criteria proposed comparing left ventricular (LV) and right ventricular (RV) pressures at the time of cardiac catheterization in order to differentiate constrictive pericarditis (CP) from restrictive cardiomyopathy (RCM). These include the difference of left ventricular end-diastolic pressure (LVEDP) and right ventricular end-diastolic pressure (RVEDP); and the ratio of RVEDP to right ventricular end-systolic pressure (RVESP). Although there is a statistical difference when comparing the means of these criteria in a number of patients, the degree of overlap makes application to an individual case difficult. *Source:* Geske 2016 [10]. Reproduced with permission of Elsevier. (*See insert for color representation of the figure.*)

Table 13.1 Traditional hemodynamic criteria for diagnosing constrictive pericarditis.

	Constrictive Pericarditis	Restrictive Cardiomyopathy
End-diastolic pressure equalization	LVEDP – RVEDP ≤ 5 mm Hg	LVEDP – RVEDP > 5 mm Hg
Pulmonary artery pressure	PASP < 55 mm Hg	PASP > 55 mm Hg
High RVEDP	RVEDP/RVSP > 1/3	RVEDP/RVSP ≤ 1/3
Dip plateau morphology	LV rapid filling wave > 7 mm Hg	LV rapid filling wave ≤ 7 mm Hg
Kussmaul's sign	Lack of respiratory variation in mean RAP	Normal respiratory variation in mean RAP

LV, left ventricle; LVEDP – RVEDP, left and right ventricular end-diastolic pressure difference; PASP, pulmonary artery systolic pressure; RAP, right atrial pressure; RVEDP, right ventricular end-diastolic pressure; RVSP, right ventricular systolic pressure.

pathophysiology, impaired myocardial compliance being common to both conditions, although via disparate mechanisms ("intrinsic" myocardial inelasticity in RCM versus "extrinsic" pericardial constraint in CP). The common pathophysiology of cardiac noncompliance underlies their nearly identical clinical presentations, characterized by systemic and pulmonary congestion due to biventricular diastolic dysfunction with limited cardiac output, and they appear quite similar by echocardiography, with small ventricles, dilated atria, and intact systolic function. However, they are distinctly different entities in terms of clinical course, management, and prognosis. CP is "curable" through surgical pericardiectomy, whereas RCM is treated by palliative measures and is rarely if ever cured. Because of this important distinction, accurate differentiation is crucial.

The differentiation of CP from RCM has been discussed in detail in Chapter 12. Briefly, there is a substantial overlap in the hemodynamic features of CP and RCM (Table 13.1; Figure 13.7), which reflects greater similarities in pathophysiology rather than the true underlying pathologic differences. Both conditions are characterized by pan-cardiac diastolic dysfunction and thus the two conditions both manifest similar patterns of elevated equalized diastolic filling pressures, RV dip and plateau, and Kussmaul's sign (Figure 13.5). Due to the greater intrinsic stiffness of the LV, patients with RCM tend to have somewhat higher pulmonary artery (PA) pressures, thus the presence of mild to moderate pulmonary hypertension favors the diagnosis of RCM, but may occur in constriction due to pre-existent left-heart or intrinsic pulmonary disease. Atrial pressures are elevated, reflecting the corresponding noncompliance of the stiff ventricle they are trying to empty into. Hemodynamic challenges including rapid volume loading, leg elevation, or exercise to effect a disproportionate rise in LV diastolic pressure suggest RCM, but are not diagnostic. In aggregate, traditional hemodynamic criteria used in the cardiac catheterization laboratory for the diagnosis of CP include end-diastolic pressure equalization (LV end-diastolic pressure minus RV end-diastolic pressure less than or equal to 5 mm Hg), pulmonary artery pressure

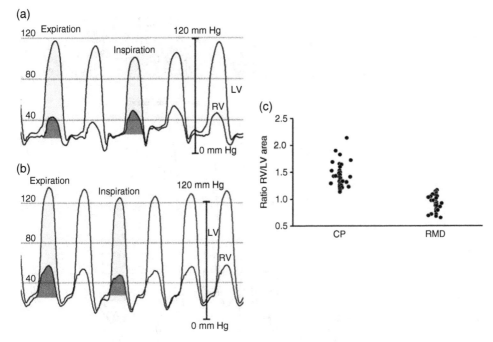

Figure 13.8 Left ventricular (LV) and right ventricular (RV) pressure traces in two patients with constriction (a) vs restriction (b) during respiration. Note that both patients have early rapid filling and elevation and end-equalization of the LV and RV pressures at end expiration. (a) Patient with surgically documented constrictive pericarditis (CP). During inspiration there is an increase in the area of the RV pressure curve (orange shaded area) compared with expiration. The area of the LV pressure curve (yellow shaded area) decreases during inspiration as compared with expiration. (b) Patient with restrictive cardiomyopathy (RMD) documented by endomyocardial biopsy. During inspiration there is a decrease in the area of the RV pressure curve (orange shaded area) as compared with expiration. The area of the LV pressure curve (yellow shaded area) is unchanged during inspiration as compared with expiration. (c) Scatter plot of the ratio of RV to LV areas comparing expiration and inspiration shows that patients with CP have consistently greater RV/LV systolic areas, indicative of ventricular interdependence. *Source:* Talreja 2008 [9]. Reproduced with permission of Elsevier. (*See insert for color representation of the figure.*)

less than 55 mm Hg, RV end-diastolic pressure divided by RV systolic pressure greater than 1/3, dip and plateau diastolic pressure morphology as reflected by the height of the left ventricular rapid filling wave (greater than 7 mm Hg), and Kussmaul's sign (lack of an inspiratory fall in mean RA pressure; Table 13.1; Figure 13.7).

In contrast, "dynamic" respiratory hemodynamic criteria have been shown to be reliable discriminators of CP versus RCM. In CP, the inelastic fibrocalcific pericardial shell isolates the heart from the lungs, and therefore respiratory changes in ITP are not fully transmitted to the cardiac chambers, resulting in dissociation of respiratory effects on ITP and intracardiac flows in the right heart versus the left heart. Further, increased pericardial resistance more tightly couples the two ventricles and increases their interdependence. In CP, inspiratory decrements in ITP reduce the transmitral pressure gradient and flow velocity, which diminishes LV filling and systolic pressure [4–11]. Because the total intrapericardial volume is fixed in CP, there is a reciprocal relation between left- and right-heart filling due to tight ventricular coupling. Therefore, the inspiratory decrease in LV filling allows a small relative increase in tricuspid inflow and RV filling as the intraventricular septum shifts. In

aggregate, these disparate effects on ventricular filling lead to opposite directional changes in ventricular systolic pressures, with inspiration inducing an increase in RV but a decrease in LV systolic pressure (Figure 13.8). This phenomenon, called "ventricular discordance," is indicative of enhanced ventricular interaction and constitutes a most reliable hemodynamic indicator of constriction [4–11].

In RCM, inspiratory changes in ITP are fully transmitted through the pericardium to the cardiac chambers. However, "intrinsic" myocardial noncompliance limits to accommodation of preload in general and markedly blunts augmentation with inspiration, leading to a relative lack of respiratory variation in cardiac filling, as documented by blunted Doppler mitral and tricuspid flow velocity during respiration (Figure 13.6). Because of the lack of pericardial constraint and a relatively noncompliant interventricular septum, there is minimal ventricular interdependence, and thus inspiratory effects on ventricular systolic pressures are "concordant"; that is, there is little change in peak RV and LV systolic pressures with respiration and they move in the same direction (Figures 13.5 and 13.8–13.11). These disparate respiratory patterns have high reliability to

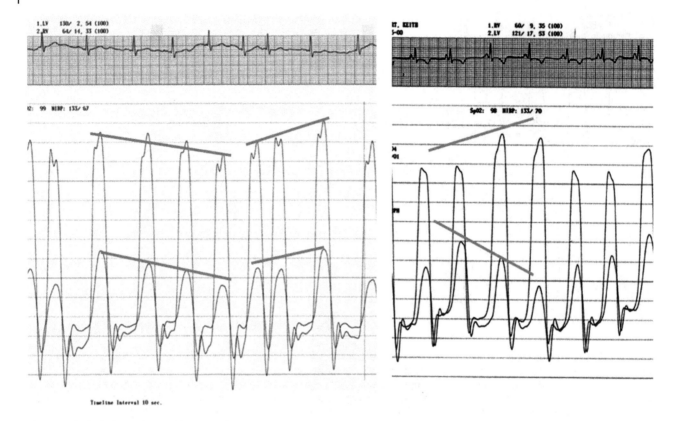

Figure 13.9 (Left) Restrictive cardiomyopathy shows concordant increases and decreases in left ventricular – right ventricular (LV–RV) systolic pressures during respiration. (Right) Discordant LV–RV systolic pressure during respiration in a patient with constrictive pericarditis.

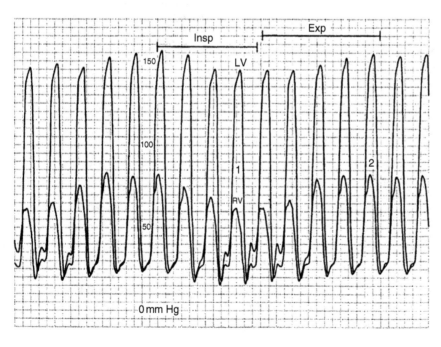

Figure 13.10 Simultaneous recordings of left ventricular (LV) and right ventricular (RV) pressures demonstrating absent ventricular interdependence. Note the concordance in left and right ventricular systolic pressures with respiration. With inspiration, the left ventricular systolic pressure decreased along with the right ventricular systolic pressure (beat #1 vs. 2). Exp = expiration; Insp = inspiration.

Figure 13.11 Simultaneous recordings of left ventricular (LV) and right ventricular (RV) pressures demonstrating absent ventricular interdependence. Note the concordance in left and right ventricular systolic pressures with respiration. With inspiration, the left ventricular systolic pressure decreased along with the right ventricular systolic pressure (beat #1 vs. 2). The nasal respirometer tracing is also shown. Exp = expiration; Insp = inspiration; LV.

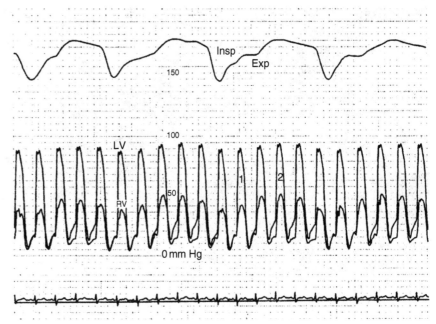

differentiate CP from RCM (see Figure 13.9). However, these "traditional" and "dynamic" hemodynamic criteria, both alone and in combination, are not sufficient to provide the basis for definitive diagnosis in an individual patient.

Role of Noninvasive Imaging to Differentiate Constrictive Periocarditis from Restrictive Cardiomyopathy

Traditional Imaging

The chest X-ray in CP may reveal pericardial calcification. In both conditions, the ECG is nonspecific but often reveals diffuse low voltage with nonspecific ST–T changes. Echocardiography shows small ventricles but enlarged atria in both conditions. Echo can be used to identify normal or increased LV wall thickness with generally normal LV chamber size (Figures 13.1 and 13.2). Echocardiographic imaging can eliminate alternative etiologies of diastolic dysfunction, such as systolic dysfunction, significant valvular dysfunction, pulmonary hypertension, and pericardial effusion with early tamponade physiology. Echocardiography may also establish a high likelihood of infiltrative disease, for instance amyloidosis by thick walls with bright hyper-contractile myocardial appearance (Figures 13.1 and 13.2). Doppler respiratory variation of the ventricular inflow velocities help differentiate CP from RCM, with hepatic venous flow usually reversed during expiration in CP but reversed during inspiration in RCM.

Advanced Cardiac Imaging

MRI and computed tomography (CT) have revolutionized the assessment and differentiation of CP from RCM [14–16]. It is imperative that any patient suspected of either entity should preferably undergo cardiac MRI (if feasible), which provides direct visualization of the pericardium (abnormal thickness and adherence to myocardium) and myocardium (inflammation, infiltration, and fibrosis; Figures 13.12 and 13.13). MRI provides insight regarding not only pericardial thickness, but also the dynamic nature of myocardial–pericardial interactions, specifically whether the pericardial layers are adherent to the heart and whether the heart slides normally in a smooth, independent pattern within the pericardium during cardiac motion. If MRI is not feasible (metallic devices etc.), CT can document increased pericardial thickness and calcification of the pericardium. MRI provides data regarding not only chamber size, wall thickness, and ventricular function, but also the presence or absence of myocardial infiltration, inflammation, or fibrosis, patterns that inform the diagnosis of specific forms of RCM. After establishing that the myocardium appears normal, the delineation of pericardial thickness provides a basis for a therapeutic algorithm to definitively delineate CP versus RCM (Figure 13.14). Documentation of a thickened pericardium adherent to the epicardium and lack of independent motion are sufficient to diagnose CP, although RCM and CP may co-exist (e.g., radiation induced). Optimally, advanced pericardial–myocardial imaging

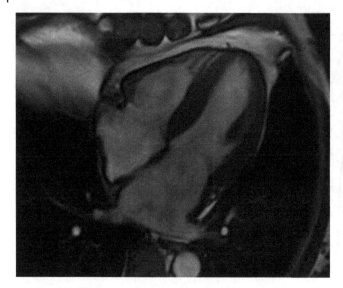
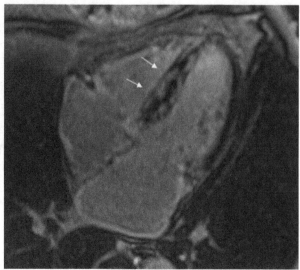

Figure 13.12 MRI in cardiac amyloidosis. (Left) Note thick left ventricle with small cavity and bi-atrial enlargement. (Right) Diffuse delayed enhancement typical of myocardial infiltrative disease (arrows).

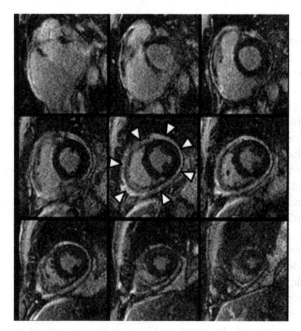
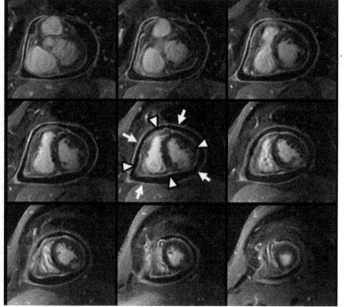

Figure 13.13 MRI in constrictive pericarditis and effusive constrictive disease. (Left) Pericardial enhancement (arrowheads) in the setting of fibrotic constrictive pericarditis. (Right) Delayed enhancement of visceral (arrowheads) and parietal pericardium (arrows) in effusive constrictive pericarditis and circumferential pericardial effusion. *Source:* Geske 2016 [10]. Reproduced with permission of Elsevier.

should be performed prior to invasive evaluation, such data allowing patients in whom CP is to be differentiated from RCM to undergo endomyocardial biopsy during the same procedure if the hemodynamic findings do not support the diagnosis of CP and the pre-procedure MRI/CT showed no morphologic derangements of the pericardium. Advanced pericardial imaging may also guide surgical pericardiectomy.

Case: Limitations of Traditional Hemodynamic Criteria

Consider the right- and left-heart hemodynamics (Figure 13.15) recorded in a patient with congestive heart failure one year following cardiac surgery. Mean RA pressure was elevated (12 mm Hg) with Kussmaul's sign during inspiration (Figure 13.15, upward arrow).

The RA Y descent was more prominent than the X descent. Simultaneous RA and RV pressures also demonstrated diastolic equilibration with early diastolic dip and matching of diastolic pressures. Because of the rapid heart rate, the plateau phase was not appreciated until a pause from an atrial premature beat was observed (Figure 13.15a, second beat from right, downward arrow). The LV and RV diastolic pressures appear equilibrated on the 0–100 mm Hg scale (Figure 13.15b, left), but the left ventricular pressure is 4–5 mm Hg higher than the right ventricular pressure on the higher 0–40 mm Hg scale (Figure 13.15b, right). The pressures track equally but are not superimposed. Because of the

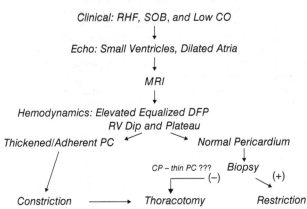

Constriction vs Restriction

Clinical: RHF, SOB, and Low CO
↓
Echo: Small Ventricles, Dilated Atria
↓
MRI
↓
Hemodynamics: Elevated Equalized DFP
RV Dip and Plateau

Thickened/Adherent PC ← → Normal Pericardium

CP – thin PC ??? Biopsy
(−) (+)

Constriction —→ Thoracotomy Restriction

Figure 13.14 Clinical algorithm to differentiate constrictive pericarditis (CP) from restrictive cardiomyopathy. CO = cardiac output; DFP = diastolic filling pressure; ECHO = echocardiography; MRI = magnetic resonance imaging; PC = pericardium; RHF = right-heart failure; RV = right ventricle; SOB = shortness of breath.

rapid heart rate, the diastolic period shows continued filling (i.e., increasing pressure). This patient had constrictive physiology, but a degree of RCM (due to earlier myocardial infarctions and fibrosis) could not be excluded from either the noninvasive or hemodynamic data. Of interest is that an RV systolic pulsus paradoxus is seen (Figure 13.15b, left). The more than 10% inspiratory decrease in systolic pressure is generally reflected in systemic pressure occurring when diastolic pressures are equilibrated with an elevated pericardial pressure [17]. RV filling in this patient was occurring against the stiffness of the pericardium, causing both ventricles to be filled to the same degree with equal back pressure. Respiratory changes in intrathoracic pressure alternately favor left and right ventricular filling, leading to a pulsus paradoxus. During inspiration, pulmonary venous pressure decreases below systemic venous pressure, whereas the reverse occurs during expiration [17–19]. Pulsus paradoxus is most commonly observed to occur in patients whose RV filling pressures are equilibrated with pericardial but not LV filling pressures [17, 18]. Ventricular septal interaction has been called upon to explain the complex mechanism of pulsus paradoxus in patients in whom only RV–pericardial equilibration occurs. In these patients, the right–left ventricular interaction appears to be exaggerated, as the ventricles are increasingly stiffened by pericardial effusion. It is critical to distinguish CP from the other restrictive diseases because of the excellent results of pericardiectomy. This case illustrates the difficulty in using traditional hemodynamic criteria alone in the cardiac catheterization laboratory to differentiate CP from RCM.

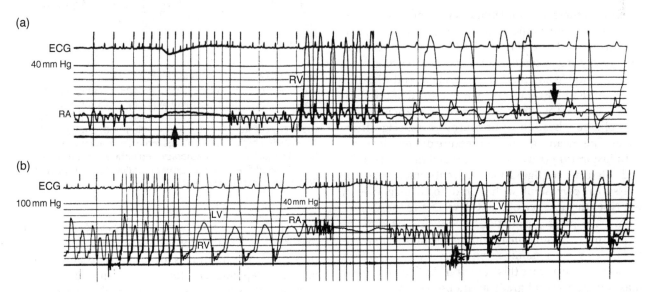

Figure 13.15 (a) Simultaneous right atrial (RA), right ventricular (RV, 0–40 mm Hg scale), and (b) left ventricular (LV) pressures (0–100 mm Hg scale) in a patient with shortness of breath one year following coronary artery bypass surgery. See text for details.

Constriction versus Restriction: Value of Dynamic Respiratory Hemodynamics

A 73-year-old physician from Iowa was referred for evaluation of dyspnea on exertion, edema, and weight gain. He had previously been healthy except for non-insulin-dependent diabetes mellitus. In the preceding year, he had developed progressive dyspnea on exertion, lower-extremity swelling, abdominal bloating, and weight gain. On examination, he was tachycardic with an irregular rhythm. The jugular venous pressure was elevated. There was evidence of bilateral pleural effusions, ascites, and extensive lower-extremity edema (graded 3/4). The chest X-ray showed bilateral pleural effusions and cardiomegaly. Comprehensive echocardiography (with respirometer assessment) revealed normal LV systolic function with an ejection fraction of 55%, a posterior pericardial effusion measuring 2.8 cm, severe tricuspid regurgitation, and pulmonary hypertension (estimated pulmonary artery systolic pressure of 70 mm Hg). No significant respiratory changes in mitral inflow (E wave) were noted. Systolic flow reversals were noted in the hepatic veins, consistent with severe tricuspid regurgitation. Interestingly, the reversals became exaggerated with expiration. A definitive diagnosis of constrictive pericarditis could not be made due to atrial fibrillation and tricuspid regurgitation. An ultrafast CT scan showed pleural and pericardial effusions; however, the actual pericardial thickness was difficult to measure due to the difficulty in separating the pericardium from the fluid. The impression was that the pericardial thickness was normal. Additionally, the ventricular morphology appeared normal and did not suggest tamponade or constriction.

In the catheterization laboratory, several of the traditional hemodynamic criteria for constrictive pericarditis were absent (Figures 13.10, 13.16, 13.17). The pulmonary artery systolic pressure (PASP) was greater than 55 mm Hg and the right ventricular end-diastolic pressure (RVEDP) was less than one-third of the right ventricular systolic pressure. However, there was end-diastolic equalization of pressures (5 mm Hg difference). The mean right atrial pressure did not decrease with inspiration (Kussmaul's sign) and there was a dip and plateau configuration of ventricular diastolic pressures, consistent with a traditional diagnosis of CP. Note the absence of the X descent and the V wave from tricuspid regurgitation. The diagnosis remains indeterminate using the traditional hemodynamic criteria. Using the dynamic respiratory criteria, however, it was quite clear that this patient had RCM. The early diastolic transmitral gradient did not vary with respiration, indicating normal transmission of intratho-

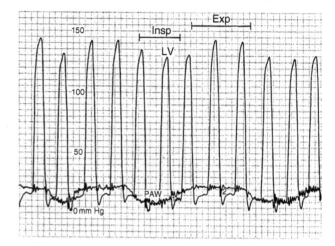

Figure 13.16 Simultaneous recordings of left ventricular and pulmonary capillary wedge pressures demonstrating what appears to be dissociation of intrathoracic and intracardiac pressures (beat #1 vs. 2). A fluid-filled catheter was used for obtaining the pulmonary capillary wedge pressure. Note the excessive oscillations from underdamping typical of fluid-filled catheter systems. The poor fidelity of these tracings makes interpretation problematic. Exp = expiration; Insp = inspiration; LV = left ventricle; PAW = pulmonary artery wedge.

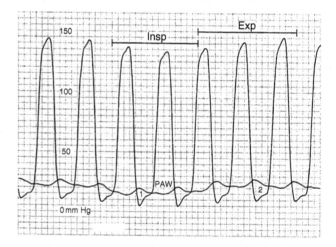

Figure 13.17 Simultaneous recordings of left ventricular and pulmonary capillary wedge pressures demonstrating lack of dissociation of intrathoracic and intracardiac pressures. Both tracings are from high-fidelity micro manometer catheters. Note the nearly constant early diastolic gradient with respiration (beat #1 vs. 2). The high-fidelity tracings more clearly demonstrate the lack of dissociation of intrathoracic and intracardiac pressures than the fluid-filled tracings. Exp = expiration; Insp = inspiration; PAW = pulmonary artery wedge.

racic pressures to intracardiac pressure (or lack of dissociation of the intrathoracic and intracardiac pressures). This finding is less sensitive than ventricular interdependence for diagnosing constrictive pericarditis [5, 20]. However, ventricular concordance is noted in the RV and LV systolic pressures. With inspiration, the LV systolic pressure decreased along with the right ventricular systolic pressure. RV endomyocardial biopsy revealed nonspecific changes and did not establish a specific disease entity. The patient's idiopathic RCM was treated with aggressive diuresis and afterload reduction. During the subsequent three years on medical therapy, he has done well without recurrent edema or ascites.

Case: RCM from Systemic Illness

A previously healthy 59-year-old male was referred for a one-year history of 25- to 30-pound weight loss, dysphagia, muscle weakness, dyspnea on exertion, and lower-extremity edema. Extensive prior evaluation had shown significant biventricular hypertrophy and bilateral pleural effusions. A complete gastroenterologic evaluation was negative. At Mayo Clinic, the physical examination was consistent with biventricular failure and bilateral pleural effusions. Skin fragility was also noted. An echocardiogram showed normal left ventricular size with borderline low function and an ejection fraction of 50%. The wall thickness was increased and the myocardial texture appeared typical of amyloid infiltration. There was a small to moderate-sized circumferential pericardial effusion measuring between 10 and 17 mm. The Doppler-derived pulmonary artery systolic pressure

was 55 mm Hg. The mitral inflow showed restrictive pattern, with an E/A ratio greater than 2 and a deceleration time of 150 milliseconds. Doppler of the pulmonary vein revealed predominant diastolic flow consistent with restrictive filling.

At catheterization, the coronary angiogram revealed mild atherosclerosis. Several of the traditional hemodynamic criteria for CP were present (Figures 13.11, 13.18, 13.19). There was severe elevation and near equalization of diastolic pressures. There was a dip and plateau configuration of ventricular diastolic pressures. The RA pressure had the typical "W" or "M" configuration and the mean right atrial pressure did not decrease with inspiration (Kussmaul's sign). The pulmonary artery systolic pressure was less than 50 mm Hg and the RVEDP was more than one-third of the RV systolic pressure. These criteria would suggest CP. Using the dynamic respiratory criteria, however, a diagnosis of RCM was made. There was ventricular concordance and no evidence of dissociation of the intrathoracic and intracardiac pressures. There was no change in early transmitral gradient with respiration. Additionally, a cardiac biopsy was positive amyloidosis on Congo red staining. Serum immunoelectrophoresis also revealed a monoclonal protein consistent with systemic amyloidosis. The patient was given chemotherapy and did respond to the regimen initially. However, he finally expired of intractable heart failure 26 months after the diagnosis.

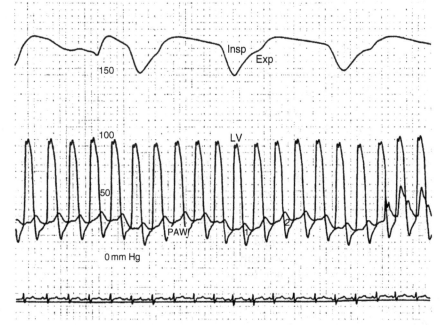

Figure 13.18 Simultaneous recordings of left ventricular (LV) and pulmonary capillary wedge pressures demonstrating lack of dissociation of intrathoracic and intracardiac pressures. Note the constant early diastolic gradient with respiration (beat #1 vs. 2). Both tracings are from high-fidelity micromanometer catheters. The nasal respirometer tracing is also shown. Exp = expiration; Insp = inspiration; PAW = pulmonary artery wedge.

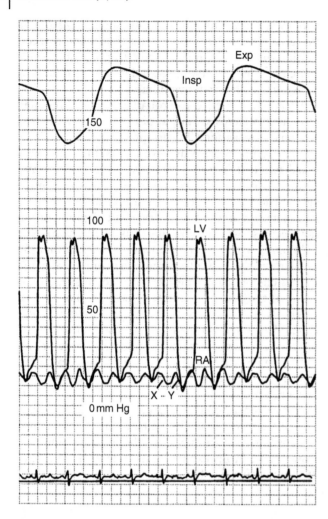

Figure 13.19 Simultaneous recordings of left ventricular (LV) and right atrial (RA) pressures. Note the marked "W" or "M" pattern in the right atrial pressure tracing, with prominent X and Y descents and no fall with inspiration (Kussmaul's sign). The nasal respirometer tracing is also shown. Exp = expiration; Insp = inspiration.

Case: Amyloidosis Suspected by Echocardiography, Affirmed by MRI, Confirmed by Hemodynamics, and Proven by Biopsy

A 65-year-old woman presented with three months of FC III fatigue and dyspnea on exertion, leg swelling, and increased abdominal girth. Physical examination showed BP = 100/65 mm Hg, respiratory rate = 18 breaths/min, heart rate of 90 beats/min, and afebrile. The extremities revealed 3+ edema to the mid-tibias bilaterally, the chest was clear to auscultation and percussion, jugular venous pressure (JVP) = 18 mm Hg with Kussmaul's sign, the carotids were intact, the precordium quiet, and auscultation revealed normal S1 and S2 without murmurs or gallops. The ECG showed sinus rhythm with diffuse

low voltage. The chest X-ray was unremarkable. Echocardiography showed small thick ventricles with intact ejection fraction and biatrial enlargement; the LV myocardium appeared bright and hyper-refractile (Figure 13.1). Laboratory studies showed normal blood counts and negative serum-free light chains. Prior to catheterization, cardiac MRI was performed, which confirmed small thick ventricles and a pattern of diffuse late gadolinium enhancement (Figure 13.12), consistent with infiltrative cardiomyopathy. Invasive hemodynamic assessment documented marked elevation of RA pressure with an "M" pattern, elevated RV diastolic pressure with a dip and plateau, and mild RV systolic hypertension (Figure 13.5). Simultaneous RV and LV pressure measurements showed elevated and equalized diastolic pressures and a respiratory pattern of "concordance" consistent with RCM. Endomyocardial biopsy was performed which confirmed cardiac amyloid, with immunohistochemical staining demonstrating the transthyretin (TTR) variant. The patient improved on diuretic therapy.

Algorithm to Differentiate Constriction from Restriction

Since the clinical presentation of these two entities is often similar, separating them on the basis of anatomic and physiologic derangements is essential and requires the use of techniques that visualize the cardiac chambers and the pericardium, in conjunction with hemodynamic modalities that delineate the physiologic manifestations of the anatomic abnormalities. Most importantly, the single distinctive feature differentiating CP from RCM is anatomic, not physiologic. In patients with CP, the pericardium is usually thickened and motion of the heart within the pericardium constrained, whereas in RCM patients, this is not the case. Therefore, anatomic documentation of pericardial thickness in patients with constrictive–restrictive physiology is highly valuable in differentiating these conditions (Figure 13.14). However, it must be emphasized that the finding of pericardial thickening should not be construed as the equivalent of a physiologic disorder, because a thickened pericardium does not necessarily constrict. For example, pericardial thickening can be present in patients without physiologic constriction, particularly with tuberculosis or after open-heart surgery. Conversely, there can be physiologic pericardial constriction with normal-appearing pericardium by advanced cardiac imaging modalities, in one study 18% of patients with surgically proven CP [21]. These observations emphasize that in patients in whom clinical, noninvasive imaging or invasive hemodynamic features indicate possible CP, the absence of thickened pericardium does not exclude CP and such patients should be considered for pericardiectomy, following a complete step-wise assessment to exclude RCM.

Importance of Advanced Imaging before Invasive Evaluation

In patients with a clinical presentation and echo-Doppler findings consistent with the differential diagnosis of CP vs. RCM, advanced cardiac imaging is essential to have in hand pre-procedure. Evaluation of the myocardium to exclude infiltration and inflammation and, most critically, assessment of pericardial thickness and adherence facilitate the most sophisticated and definitive invasive assessment. Employing this strategy, if hemodynamic findings are consistent with CP and pericardial imaging is confirmatory, surgical exploration and pericardiectomy are warranted. In contrast, if hemodynamics support RCM and the pericardium was normal by imaging, then endomyocardial biopsy can be performed at the time of cardiac catheterization in a search for disease entities that result in RCM (e.g., amyloidosis, hemochromatosis, scleroderma). Finally, it is important to emphasize that some patients with severe pericardial constriction proven at surgical exploration may have normal pericardial thickness by imaging techniques. Accordingly, in patients with severe clinical and hemodynamic manifestations, lack of increased pericardial thickness, and normal endomyocardial biopsy, thoracoscopy or minimally invasive exploratory thoracotomy with provisional planned pericardiectomy should be considered.

Key Points

1) RCM is characterized by ventricles with thick walls, small cavities with intact systolic function and dilated atria.
2) RCM has intact systolic function but the restrictive constraints on ventricular preload limit stroke volume, resulting in low cardiac output and ultimately hypoperfusion.
3) RCM but not constrictive pericarditis has biatrial enlargement reflecting ventricular non-compliance, possibily from primary atrial involvement by the underlying disease process (e.g., amyloidosis).
4) RCM is often associated with concordant dynamic respiratory responses of ventricular filling and LV and RV systolic pressures as opposed to the discordant association of LV/RV pressures in patients with constrictive physiology.
5) To improve identification of CP vs RCM, advanced cardiac imaging is essential. Evaluation of the myocardium to exclude infiltration and inflammation and most critical assessment of pericardial thickness and adherence will facilitate the most definitive invasive assessment.

Note

The author of this chapter has previously authored treatises on restrictive cardiomyopathy (referenced below) from which substantial portions of the present text have been derived.

References

1 Falk RH. Diagnosis and management of the cardiac amyloidoses. *Circulation* 112:2047–2060, 2005.
2 Goldstein JA. Restrictive cardiomyopathy. In M Crawford (ed.), *Current Diagnosis and Treatment: Cardiology*, 5th ed. New York: Lange/McGraw-Hill, 2016.
3 Jander N, Minners J, Holme I, Gerdts E, Boman K, Brudi P, *et al*. Outcome of patients with low-gradient "severe" aortic stenosis and preserved ejection fraction. *Circulation* 123:887–895, 2011.
4 Hatle LK, Appleton CP, Popp RL. Differentiation of constrictive pericarditis and restrictive cardiomyopathy by Doppler echocardiography. *Circulation* 79:357–370, 1989.
5 Vaitkus PT, Kussmaul WG. Constrictive pericarditis versus restrictive cardiomyopathy: A reappraisal and update of diagnostic criteria. *Am Heart J* 122:1431–1441, 1991.
6 Hurrell DG, Nishimura RA, Higano ST, Appleton CP, Danielson GK, Holmes DR, Jamil TA. Value of dynamic respiratory changes in left and right ventricular pressures for the diagnosis of constrictive pericarditis. *Circulation* 93:2007–2013, 1996.
7 Higano ST, Azrak E, Tahirkheli NK, Kern MJ. Hemodynamic rounds series II: Hemodynamics of constrictive physiology: Influence of respiratory dynamics on ventricular pressures. *Cather Cardiovasc Interv* 46:473–486, 1999.
8 Goldstein JA. Cardiac tamponade, constrictive pericarditis and restrictive cardiomyopathy. *Curr Prob Cardiol* 29:503–567, 2004.

9 Talreja DR, Nishimura RA, Oh JK, Holmes DR. Constrictive pericarditis in the modern era. *J Am Coll Cardiol* 51:315, 2008.

10 Geske JB, Anavekar NS, Nishimura RA, Oh JK, Gersh BJ. Differentiation of constriction and restriction: Complex cardiovascular hemodynamics. *J Am Coll Cardiol* 68:2329–2347, 2016.

11 Garcia MJ. Constrictive pericarditis versus restrictive cardiomyopathy? *J Am Coll Cardiol* 67:2061–2076, 2016.

12 Ling LH, Oh JK, Schaff HV, Danielson GK, Mahoney DW, Seward JB, Tajik AJ. Constrictive pericarditis in the modern era: Evolving clinical spectrum and impact on outcome after pericardiectomy. *Circulation* 100:1380, 1999.

13 Bertog SC, Thambidorai SK, Parakh K, Schoenhagen P, Ozduran V, Houghtaling PL, Lytle BW, Blackstone EH, Lauer MS, Klein AL. Constrictive pericarditis: Etiology and cause-specific survival after pericardiectomy. *J Am Coll Cardiol* 43:1445, 2004.

14 Verhaert D, Gabriel RS, Johnston D, Lytle BW, Desai MY, Klein AL. The role of multimodality imaging in the management of pericardial disease. *Circ Cardiovasc Imaging* 3:333, 2010.

15 Miller C, Dormand H, Clark D, Jones M, Bishop P, Schmitt M. Comprehensive characterization of constrictive pericarditis using multiparametric CMR. *J Am Coll Cardiol Img* 4:917–920, 2011.

16 Zurick AO, Bolen MA, Kwon DH, Tan CD, Popovic ZB, Rajeswaran J, Rodriguez ER, Flamm SD, Klein AL. Pericardial delayed hyperenhancement with CMR imaging in patients with constrictive pericarditis undergoing surgical pericardiectomy: A case series with histopathological correlation. *JACC Cardiovasc Img* 4:1180, 2011.

17 Reddy PS, Curtiss EI, O'Toole JD, Shaver JA. Cardiac tamponade: Hemodynamic observations in man. *Circulation* 58:265–272, 1978.

18 Reddy PS, Curtiss EI, Uretsky BF. Spectrum of hemodynamic changes in cardiac tamponade. *Am J Cardiol* 166:1487–1491, 1990.

19 Shabetai R, Fowler NO, Guntheroth WG. The hemodynamics of cardiac tamponade and constrictive pericarditis. *Am J Cardiol* 26:480–489, 1970.

20 Oh JK, Hade LK, Seward JB, Danielson GK, Schaff HV, Reeder GS, Tajik AJ. Diagnostic role of Doppler echocardiography in constrictive pericarditis. *J Am Coll Cardiol* 23:154–162, 1994.

21 Talreja DR, Edwards WD, Danielson GK, Schaff HV, Tajik AJ, Tazelaar HD, Breen JF, Oh JK. Constrictive pericarditis in 26 patients with histologically normal pericardial thickness. *Circulation* 108:1852, 2003.

14

Hemodynamic Manifestations of Ischemic Right-Heart Dysfunction

James A. Goldstein

Acute right coronary artery (RCA) occlusion proximal to the right ventricular (RV) branches compromises RV free wall (RVFW) perfusion, resulting in RV dysfunction in nearly 50% of patients with transmural inferior–posterior myocardial infarctions [1–6]. A spectrum of hemodynamic perturbations is manifest, with the pattern and severity dependent on the site of RCA occlusion and the extent of ischemic RV and right atrial (RA) involvement. In its most severe form, the clinical syndrome of predominant RV infarction (RVI) develops, characterized by right-heart failure with clear lung fields and hypotension. Hemodynamic evaluation in such patients typically reveals disproportionate elevation of right-sided filling pressures, equalization of right- and left-sided diastolic pressures, and low cardiac output despite intact left ventricular (LV) function [3–7] (Table 14.1).

Ischemic Right Ventricular Dysfunction

The RCA is the culprit vessel in nearly all cases with RV ischemic dysfunction [5–8], the vast majority of which show proximal high-grade occlusion compromising flow to the major RV branches, resulting in severe depression of RVFW motion, depressed RV ejection fraction, and RV dilatation, which reduces transpulmonary flow and results in diminished LV preload and decreased cardiac output despite preserved LV contractility (Figure 14.1). In contrast, patients without RVI tend to have more distal RCA lesions or circumflex culprits that spare RV branch perfusion. RVI results in characteristic hemodynamic derangements [5–12]. Acute RVI depresses global RV performance, with RV systolic dysfunction manifest in the RV waveform by a slow upstroke, diminished peak pressure, and delayed relaxation (Figures 14.2 and 14.3). RVFW ischemia also causes severe RV diastolic

dysfunction. Depressed RV systolic performance results in gross RV enlargement, and ischemia both impairs RV relaxation and renders the right ventricle intrinsically stiff. At the beginning of diastole, the right ventricle is dilated and its filling pressure is elevated, thereby imparting increased resistance to early filling. There is progressively increased impedance to inflow as the right ventricle fills and ascends a steep noncompliant diastolic pressure–volume curve. This progressive pan-diastolic resistance to RV filling is manifest in the RV waveform as a rapid rise in diastolic pressure to an elevated plateau, and in the right atrial (RA) waveform by elevated mean RA pressure and a blunted Y descent. Patients with RCA occlusion proximal to the RV branches but distal to the RA branches manifest RVI with enhanced RA contraction/relaxation, resulting in an augmented A wave and steep X descent ("W" pattern) in the RA trace (Figure 14.2). RCA occlusion proximal to the RA branches results in RA ischemia/infarction and depressed RA function manifest by a depressed "a" wave and X descent ("M" pattern) (Figure 14.3).

RV diastolic dysfunction adversely affects LV diastolic properties. Acute RV dilatation and elevated RV diastolic pressure shift the interventricular septum toward the volume-deprived left ventricle, thereby impairing LV compliance and further limiting LV filling (Figures 14.4). Abrupt RV dilatation within the noncompliant pericardium leads to elevated intrapericardial pressure (Figure 14.5). The resultant pericardial constraint further impairs both RV and LV compliance and filling, both directly and by intensifying the adverse effects of diastolic ventricular interactions. Furthermore, as both ventricles fill and compete for space within the crowded pericardium, the effects of pericardial constraint contribute to the pattern of progressive pan-diastolic impedance to RV filling, reflected hemodynamically by a blunted RA Y descent and RV dip and plateau pattern. LV and RV diastolic pressures are elevated and equalized.

Hemodynamic Rounds: Interpretation of Cardiac Pathophysiology from Pressure Waveform Analysis, Fourth Edition.
Edited by Morton J. Kern, Michael J. Lim, and James A. Goldstein.
© 2018 John Wiley & Sons Ltd. Published 2018 by John Wiley & Sons Ltd.

Table 14.1 Clinical hemodynamic profile of acute right ventricular infarction.

Clinical profile

Elevated jugular venous pressure

Clear lungs

Hypotension

Hemodynamic profile

Low-output hypotension

Disproportionate elevation RA–RV pressures

Equalization of diastolic pressures

RV "dip and plateau" (square root sign)

+ Kussmauls' sign and pulsus paradoxus

RA = right atrium; RV = right ventricle.

Determinants of Right Ventricular Performance with Acute Right Ventricular Dysfunction

Under conditions of acute RVFW dysfunction, RV performance is dependent on LV–septal contractile contributions transmitted via systolic ventricular interactions, mediated by the septum through both paradoxical septal motion and primary septal contributions [6–8, 11, 12]. In early isovolumic systole, unopposed LV–septal pressure generation creates a left to right transseptal pressure gradient, resulting in early systolic septal bulging into the RV cavity (Figure 14.4). This paradoxical motion not only contributes to early generation of RV systolic pressure, but also helps stretch the dyskinetic RVFW, a prerequisite to providing a stable buttress upon which later LV–septal thickening and shortening

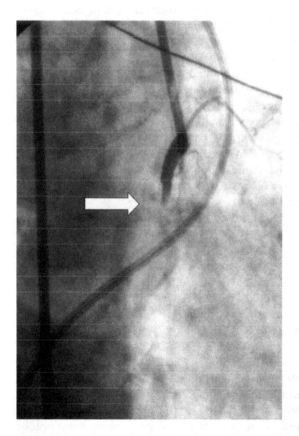

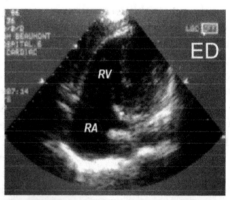

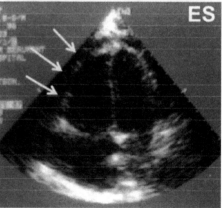

Figure 14.1 Angiogram from patient with proximal total right coronary artery occlusion (arrow) and no patent right ventricular (RV) branches. Two-dimensional echocardiogram in this patient demonstrates RV dilatation at end-diastole (ED) with normal left ventricle (LV) size. At end-systole (ES), the right ventricular free wall (RVFW) can be seen to be akinetic (arrows), with severe depression of RV global performance. Yellow arrow indicates proximal right coronary artery occlusion. Orange arrows illustrate RV free wall dyskinesis. *Source:* Bowers 1998 [7]. Reproduced with permission of The New England Journal of Medicine.

Figure 14.2 Hemodynamic recordings from right ventricular infarction (RVI) patient with right atrial (RA) "W" pattern. Peaks of RA wave formed by prominent A waves indicative of augmented atrial contraction, with most prominent RA descent just before T wave of ECG (panel a). Simultaneous RA and right ventricular (RV) pressures (panel b) demonstrate that this prominent descent coincides with peak RV systolic pressure (RVSP) and is therefore an X′ systolic descent, followed by a comparatively blunted Y descent. Peak RVSP is depressed, RV relaxation is prolonged, and there is a dip and rapid rise in RV diastolic pressure. Prominent RA A waves are reflected in the RV as an augmented end-diastolic pressure (EDP) rise (arrows). Simultaneous RA and RV waveforms confirm the timing of the A wave and X and Y descents (panel c). *Source:* Goldstein 1990 [5]. Reproduced with permission of Wolters Kluwer Health, Inc.

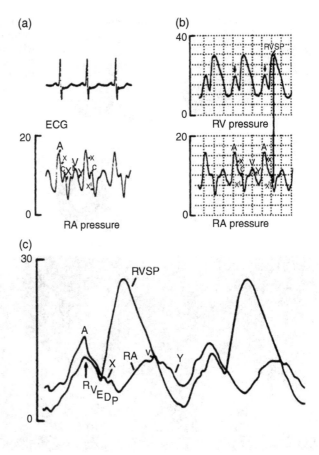

Figure 14.3 Hemodynamic recordings from right ventricular infarction (RVI) patient with right atrial (RA) "M" pattern. Tracings of simultaneous RA pressure and ECG (panel a) demonstrate markedly depressed A waves indicative of atrial ischemic dysfunction; most prominent negative deflection (X′) coincident with T wave suggesting a Y descent. However, timing of RA pressure with pulmonary artery systolic pressure (PASP) (panel b) demonstrates that this descent is coincident with peak PASP and therefore a systolic X′ descent. The Y descent is blunted. *Source:* Goldstein 1990 [5]. Reproduced with permission of Wolters Kluwer Health, Inc.

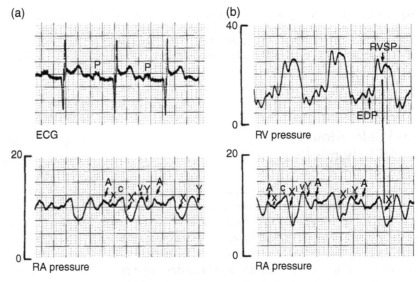

can generate peak RV pressure and effective pulmonary flow. These interactions result in a bifid RV systolic pressure waveform, with the initial peak correlating with early paradoxical septal bulging and the later peak with maximal LV–septal shortening and peak systolic pressure generation.

Depressed LV contractility exacerbates biventricular dysfunction, worsening hemodynamic compromise, whereas inotropic stimulation augments LV contractility directly, which then indirectly enhances RV performance via enhanced systolic ventricular interactions.

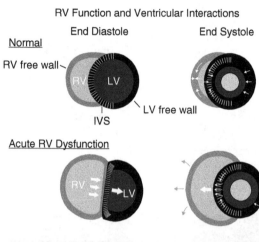

RV Function and Ventricular Interactions

Figure 14.4 Septal relationships in acute right ventricular infarction (RVI). Under normal conditions, intraventricular septum (IVS) is curved convex left to right at end-diastole, moving toward left ventricle (LV) at end-systole. In acute RVI, the right ventricle (RV) is dilated at end-diastole and the IVS flattened toward the volume-deprived LV. In systole, the IVS bulges paradoxically into the RV, stretching the dyskinetic RV free wall.

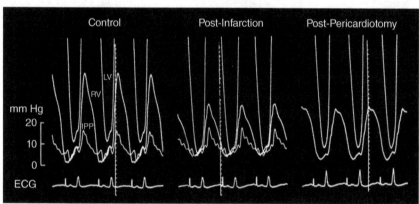

Figure 14.5 Pressure recordings from the experiment shown in Figure 14.4 during control, post-infarction, and post-pericardiotomy periods. Left ventricular (LV) pressure (high gain to illustrate diastolic pressure), right ventricular (RV), and intrapericardial pressure (IPP) zeroed at a common baseline. After RV infarction, RV systolic pressure decreased while RV diastolic pressure increased. IPP increased while LV diastolic pressure decreased. Diastolic pressures equalized after infarction but resolved after pericardiotomy. *Source:* Goldstein 1983 [10]. Reproduced with permission of Wolters Kluwer Health, Inc.

Compensatory Contributions of Augmented Right Atrial Contraction and Deleterious Effects of Right Atrial Ischemic Dysfunction

Under conditions of RVI, the strength of RA contraction is an important determinant of hemodynamic stability [5–8, 11, 12]. To appreciate the importance of RA function in patients with RVI, it is critical to appreciate normal atrial mechanics. The principles governing the mechanical behavior of atrial myocardium are similar to those operating in ventricular muscle. Thus, the strength of atrial contraction, reflected in the upstroke and peak amplitude of the RA "a" wave, is determined by the intrinsic atrial inotropic state, modulated by extrinsic neuro-humoral stimuli, and influenced by atrial preload (maximal atrial volume) and afterload (imposed by the tricuspid valve and right ventricle). Evaluation of the RA waveform provides insight into the status of RA function. Interpretation of the RA waveform may be facilitated by timing waveform components not only to the ECG, but also to mechanical

correlates from simultaneous RV or pulmonary artery pressures. The RA waveform components include:

1) The "a" wave, a positive deflection immediately following the P wave on the ECG and immediately preceding ventricular systole. The upstroke and amplitude of the a-wave reflect the strength of atrial contraction.

2) The X descent, a negative deflection following the "a" wave and coincident with the QRS complex and mechanical ventricular systole. The X descent reflects both atrial relaxation and systolic intrapericardial pressure changes.

3) The "c" wave, a positive wave coinciding with early RV pressure generation and tricuspid valve closure, just following the QRS complex. The "c" wave likely represents mild early tricuspid valve regurgitation. When present, the "c" wave separates the X descent into two components, the X portion prior to the "c" wave reflecting atrial relaxation; and the X′ descent following the "c" wave representing systolic intrapericardial depressurization.

4) (4) The "v" wave, a positive deflection during ventricular systole, reflecting passive atrial filling or, when exaggerated, tricuspid regurgitation.

5) The Y descent, a negative deflection following the "v" wave during ventricular diastole and just following the T wave, but prior to the subsequent P wave. The slope of the Y descent is an indicator, in part, of RV compliance.

Patients with RVI manifest one of two distinct RA waveform patterns that share in common a blunted Y descent reflecting pan-diastolic resistance to RV filling, but are differentiated by the status of RA contraction and relaxation, as reflected in the morphology of the "a" wave and X descent [5, 6, 11, 12]. Patients with RCA occlusion proximal to the RV branches but distal to the RA branches manifest RVI with enhanced RA contraction/relaxation, resulting in an augmented "a" wave and steep X descent ("W" pattern) in the RA trace (Figure 14.2). RCA occlusion proximal to the RA branches result in RA ischemia/infarction and depressed RA function, manifest by a depressed "a" wave and X descent ("M" pattern; Figure 14.3). These findings have prognostic and therapeutic impact. Patients with enhanced RA contraction have higher peak RV pressure, better cardiac output, and a more favorable therapeutic response to volume infusion and inotropic stimulation relative to those with depressed atrial function. However, when patients with augmented RA contraction lose this compensatory atrial kick due to atrioventricular asynchrony, more severe hemodynamic compromise results. Similarly, ischemic depression of atrial contractility is associated with more severe hemodynamic compromise.

Hemodynamic Impact of Rhythm Disorders and Reflexes Associated with Right Ventricular Infarction

High-grade atrioventricular (AV) block and bradycardia–hypotension without AV block commonly complicate inferior myocardial infarction, and have been attributed predominantly to the effects of AV nodal ischemia and cardio-inhibitory (Bezold–Jarisch) reflexes arising from stimulation of vagal afferents in the ischemic LV inferioposterior wall [13]. Reflex bradycardia–hypotension and AV block are far more common in patients with proximal RCA occlusion (Figure 14.6) inducing right-heart and LV inferior–posterior ischemia, compared to more distal occlusions compromising LV perfusion but sparing the RV branches without right-heart involvement [14], findings suggesting that the ischemic right heart may also be a trigger for cardio-inhibitory–vasodilator reflexes. Following successful thrombolysis or primary angioplasty of the acutely occluded RCA, transient but profound bradycardia–hypotension may paradoxically develop in a patient whose rhythm and blood pressure were stable during occlusion (Figure 14.7). Based on its abrupt and transient nature, reperfusion-induced bradycardia–hypotension appears to be reflex mediated and, based on recent findings, also appears to be more common with proximal versus distal RCA occlusions, suggesting a right-heart mechanism.

Impact of Reperfusion

Until recently, there were scant clinical data regarding the effects on ischemic RV myocardium of interventions designed to achieve reperfusion. In recent studies of experimental animals [15–17] and patients with RVI undergoing primary angioplasty [6], we have now documented that successful complete reperfusion of the main RCA and the major RV branches (Figure 14.8) leads to immediate improvement in and later complete recovery of RVFW function and consequently global RV performance (Figure 14.9). Most importantly, reperfusion-mediated recovery of RV performance is associated with excellent clinical outcome (Figure 14.10). In contrast, failure to restore flow to the major RV branches was associated with lack of recovery of RV performance and refractory hemodynamic compromise, leading to high in-hospital mortality, even if flow was restored in the main RCA. These findings emphasize the crucial relationship between reperfusion-mediated recovery of RV performance and clinical outcome. Importantly, these results support the concept that, under conditions of ischemia and reperfusion, the right ventricle is more resilient than the left ventricle, consistent with the notion that RV "infarction" is to a great extent a misnomer, for the acutely ischemic dysfunctional right ventricle appears to represent predominantly viable myocardium, which responds favorably to successful reperfusion, even late after the onset of occlusion.

Mechanical Complications Associated with Right Ventricular Infarction

Patients with acute RVI may suffer additional mechanical complications of acute infarction that may compound hemodynamic compromise and confound the clinical–hemodynamic picture. Ventricular septal rupture is a particularly disastrous complication, adding substantial overload stress to the ischemically dysfunctional right ventricle [18]. As in other post-infarction myonecrotic septal ruptures, acute left to right shunting reduces effective forward LV output, precipitates pulmonary edema, and elevates pulmonary pressures and resistance. In aggregate, these effects exacerbate the RV dysfunction and low output associated with RVI. Surgical repair is imperative, but may be technically difficult. Severe right-heart dilatation and diastolic pressure elevation associated with right-heart ischemia may stretch open a patent foramen ovale, precipitating acute right to left shunting manifest as systemic hypoxemia or paradoxic emboli, which may resolve as

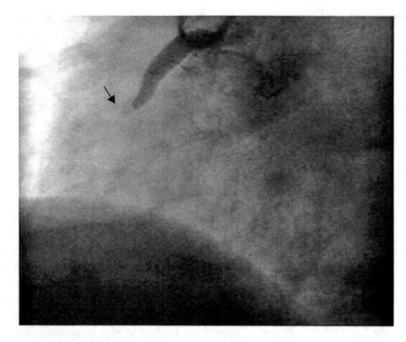

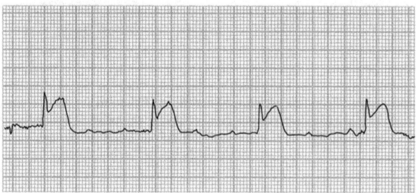

Figure 14.6 Patient with acute inferior myocardial infarction with right ventricular infarction attributable to proximal right coronary artery occlusion compromising flow to the right ventricular branches. The ECG shows complete (3°) heart block, which is typically vagal driven. *Source:* Goldstein 2005 [14]. Reproduced with permission of Wolters Kluwer Health, Inc.

right-heart pressures diminish with recovery of RV performance, although some may require closure. Severe tricuspid regurgitation may also complicate RVI developing as a result of primary papillary muscle ischemic dysfunction or rupture, as well as secondary functional regurgitation attributable to severe RV and tricuspid valve annular dilatation.

Right Ventricular Infarction Associated with Severe Left Ventricular Systolic Dysfunction

Despite the generally favorable prognosis for patients undergoing successful mechanical reperfusion, some patients with acute inferior myocardial infarction (IMI)–RVI still suffer refractory hemodynamic compromise associated with poor outcomes. Recent observations document that the status of LV function

is a key determinant of hemodynamic stability and survival in patients with acute RVI, for those with concomitant depressed LV systolic function (ejection fraction < 40%) are at risk for greater hemodynamic compromise and higher in-hospital mortality [19]. Given the profound influence of the status of LV systolic function on hemodynamics and outcome in all patients with acute ST-segment elevated myocardial infarction (STEMI), taken together with the fact that under conditions of acute RV ischemia RV systolic performance and systemic output are critically dependent on compensatory LV–septal contractile contributions, it is not surprising that depressed LV function is associated with more severe hemodynamic compromise. These findings support the concept that under conditions of acute ischemic RV dysfunction, biventricular performance and systemic hemodynamics are critically dependent on LV

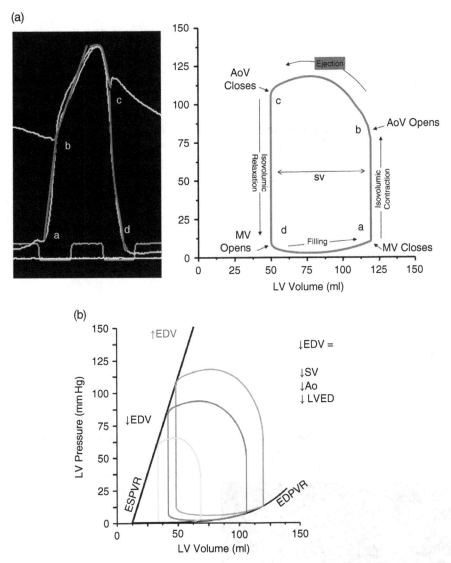

Figure 1.4 (a) The pressure–volume (PV) loop characterizes the changes in pressure flow over the course of one cardiac cycle. Left panel, the left ventricular (LV) and aortic pressure as measured during cardiac catheterization. Right panel, the PV loop derived from the hemodynamics of LV pressure and volume. Point a, LV end-diastolic pressure is followed by isovolumetric contraction ending at point b, the aortic valve (AoV) opening. Ejection continues until the repolarization of the LV produces a fall in LV ejection. LV pressure falls pasts point c, aortic valve closure, and continues to fall along the line of isovolumetric relaxation to point d, mitral valve (MV) opening. Changes in the shape of the PV loop demonstrate changes in contractility and cardiac output (stroke volume, SV). Load-independent LV contractility, also known as Emax, is defined as the maximal slope of the end-systolic pressure–volume (ESPV) point under various loading conditions, known as the ESPV relationship (ESPVR). Effective arterial elastance (Ea) is a measure of LV afterload and is defined as the ratio of end-systolic pressure and stroke volume. (b) The effect of changes in LV preload. Increasing the left ventricular end-diastolic pressure (LVEDP) along the line of the end-diastolic pressure–volume relationship (EDPVR). As volume is increased, LVEDP, SV, and aortic pressure increase. Courtesy of Dr. Daniel Burkhart, Columbia University, NY.

Hemodynamic Rounds: Interpretation of Cardiac Pathophysiology from Pressure Waveform Analysis, Fourth Edition.
Edited by Morton J. Kern, Michael J. Lim, and James A. Goldstein.
© 2018 John Wiley & Sons Ltd. Published 2018 by John Wiley & Sons Ltd.

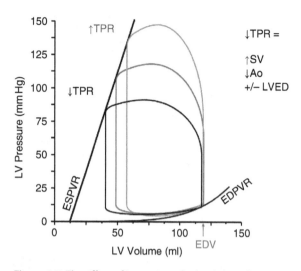

Figure 1.5 The effect of increasing afterload or total peripheral vascular resistance (TPR) decreases SV, increases aortic pressure, and minimally modifies LVEDP. Courtesy of Dr. Daniel Burkhart, Columbia University, NY.

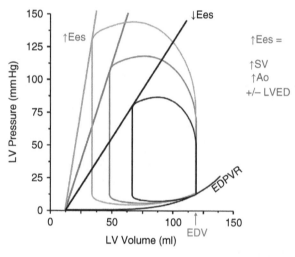

Figure 1.6 The effect of increasing contractility: the increasing slope of the line of end-systolic elastance (Ees) increases SV and aortic pressure, with minimal effect on LVEDP. Courtesy of Dr. Daniel Burkhart, Columbia University, NY.

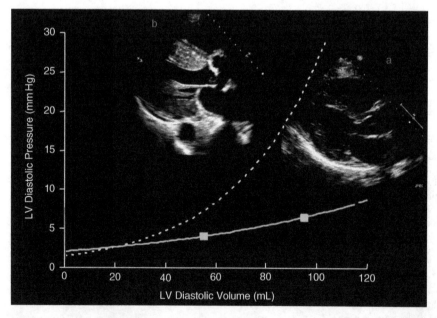

Figure 1.7 Left ventricular pressure–volume relationships demonstrating compliance curves in a normal LV (b) versus a thick stiff LV (a).

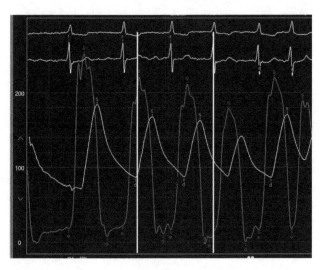

Figure 1.29 Left ventricular and aortic pressures measured from table-side transducers. The vertical yellow lines indicate left ventricular end diastolic pressure (LVEDP) and timing to ECG. Note the delay in aortic pressure due to pressure transmission from the femoral arterial sheath-side arm. The computer has placed "d" on aortic diastolic pressures and "e" on LVEDP. The "e" position varies, but is mostly close to the true LVEDP. Scale 0–200 mmHg.

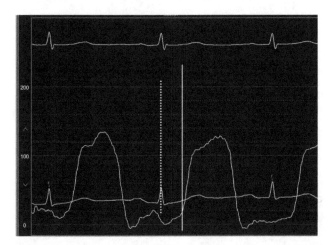

Figure 1.30 Left ventricular pressure recorded with an ACIST transducer, demonstrating delay in pressure relative to ECG. The R wave precedes the LVEDP by almost 100 msec. Manual selection of LVEDP is required.

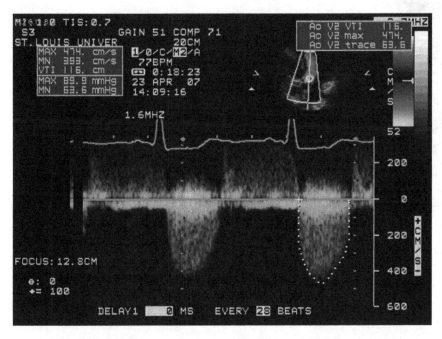

Figure 6.3 Continuous-wave Doppler recording of maximal aortic valve velocity. The dotted line represents the operator tracing of the velocity envelope. From this envelope, the maximal velocity was found to be 4.74 m/sec (474 cm/sec) and the gradients were found to be 89.9 mm Hg (peak) and 63.6 mm Hg (mean).

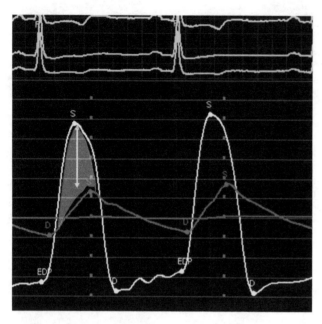

Figure 6.5 The best technique currently in routine practice to measure the aortic valve gradient is with a dual-lumen pigtail fluid-filled catheter. The left ventricular (LV) pressure is shown in yellow and the aortic (Ao) pressure in red. The LV–Ao gradient is shaded, with the arrow showing the peak-to-peak pressure measurement.

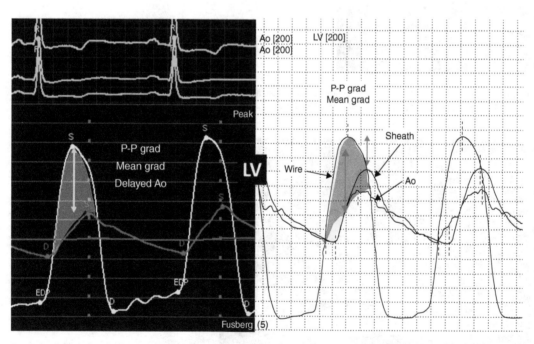

Figure 6.8 Simultaneous recording of the left ventricular (LV), femoral arterial (FA), and aortic (Ao) pressures in a patient with aortic stenosis on a 200 mm Hg scale. One can observe that the peak instantaneous pressure gradient occurs early in systole, as is typical with more severe valvular narrowing. Furthermore, when comparing the FA and Ao tracings, there is a similar systolic pressure but a larger difference in the diastolic pressure. This difference will overestimate the peak instantaneous and mean pressure gradients in this patient.

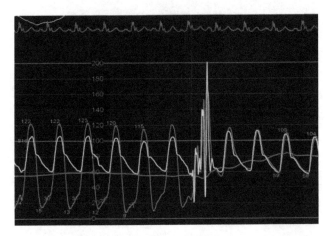

Figure 6.11 Left ventricular and aortic pressures during pullback. Peak-to-peak gradient is 45 mm Hg. Systolic pressures correspond on pullback, but disparity of diastolic pressure suggests sheath damping.

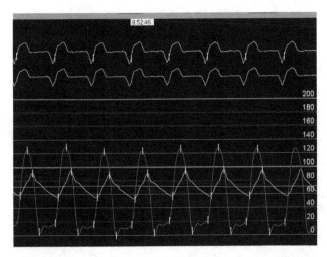

Figure 6.12 A 68-year-old man with low ejection fraction of 25% and cardiac output of 3.2 L/min. Peak-to-peak left ventricular–aortic pressure gradient was 25 mm Hg with an aortic valve area calculation of 0.7 cm^2.

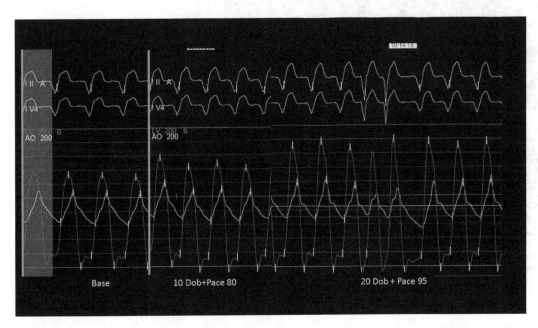

Figure 6.13 Hemodynamics during dobutamine infusion. Left panel is baseline, middle panel 10 mcg/min dobutamine infusion and paced rhythm 80 bpm. Right panel is 20 mcg/min infusion of dobutamine with pacing at 95 bpm. Hemodynamics at peak dobutamine show increased cardiac output of 4.2 L/min, peak-to-peak left ventricular (LV)–aortic (AO) pressure of 50 mm Hg, with a calculated aortic valve area of 0.6 cm^2. The valve area is fixed and the patient will likely benefit from aortic valve replacement or transcatheter aortic valve replacement.

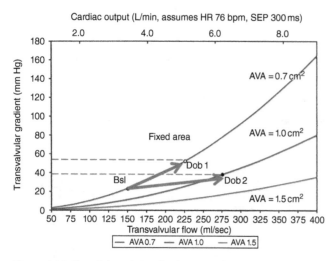

Figure 6.14 Plot of the relationship between mean gradient (y axis) and transvalvular flow (x axis, bottom) according to the Gorlin formula for three different values of aortic valve area (AVA): 0.7, 1.0, and 1.5 cm². Cardiac output (x axis, top) is also shown, assuming a heart rate of 75 bpm and systolic ejection period of 300 ms. At low transvalvular flows, mean gradient is low at all three valve areas. Two different responses to dobutamine challenge are illustrated for a hypothetical patient (Bsl) with a baseline flow of 150 mL/s, mean gradient of 25 mm Hg, and calculated AVA of 0.7 cm². In one scenario (Dob 1), flow increases to 225 mL/s, mean gradient increases to 52 mm Hg, and AVA remains at 0.7 cm², consistent with fixed aortic stenosis (AS). In the second scenario (Dob 2), flow increases to 275 mL/s, mean gradient increases to 50 mm Hg, and AVA increases to 1.0 cm². This patient has changed to a different curve, consistent with relative or pseudo-AS. HR = heart rate; SEP = systolic ejection period. *Source:* Grayburn 2006 [10]. Reproduced with permission of Wolters Kluwer Health, Inc.

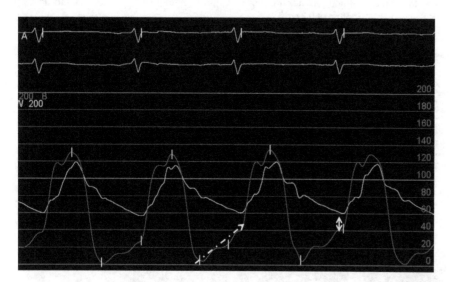

Figure 7.6 Hemodynamic tracing of acute aortic insufficiency. Relatively normal pulse pressure, but a marked increase and rapid rise of diastolic pressure and narrow end diastolic left ventricular–aortic pressures.

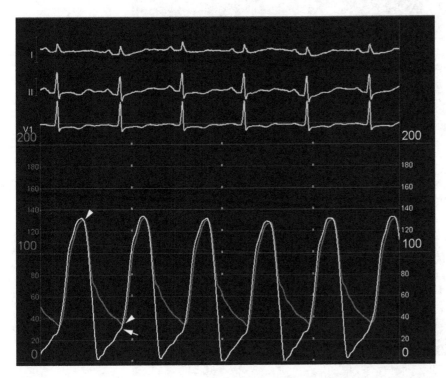

Figure 7.7 Hemodynamic tracing showing elevated left ventricular (LV) end-diastolic pressure (arrow), widened aortic pulse pressure (arrowheads), and near equalization of LV and aortic end-diastolic pressures. *Source:* Ren 2012 [8]. Reproduced with permission of Wolters Kluwer Health, Inc.

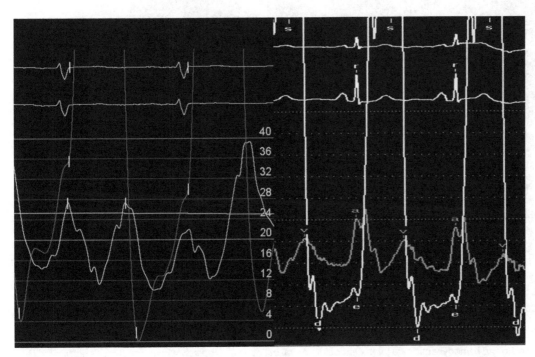

Figure 8.2 Hemodynamic tracings of (left) normal left atrial (LA, blue) and left ventricular (LV, red) pressures compared to those of mitral stenosis hemodynamics with LA in orange and LV in yellow (right). Note diastolic gradient and large "a" wave in mitral stenosis. Scale 0–50 mm Hg.

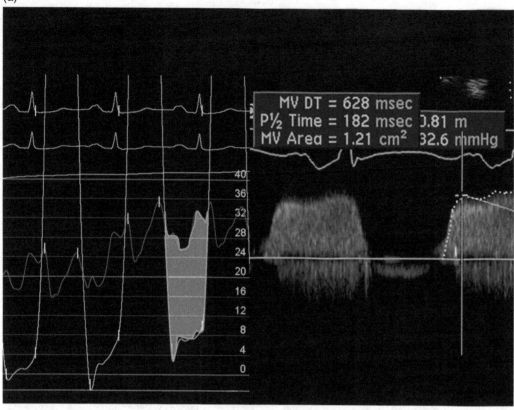

(a)

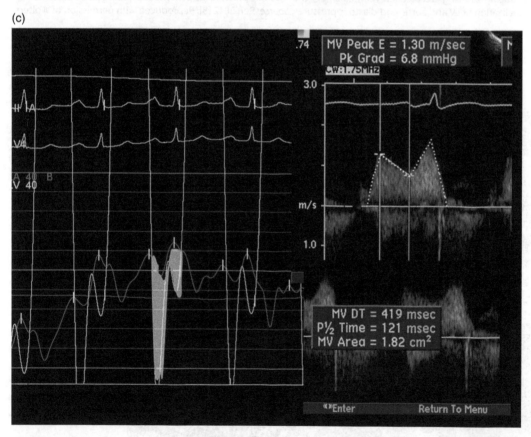

(c)

Figure 8.3 (a) Combined echo and hemodynamic data for patient before mitral balloon valvuloplasty with mitral stenosis (left), hemodynamic tracings with simultaneous left atrial (LA, red) and left ventricular (LV, blue) pressures, with diastolic gradient shaded in yellow. (Right) Doppler flow across mitral valve showing pattern of flat E–A slope and delayed chamber emptying. There is a significant mitral gradient. (c) Combined echo and hemodynamic data for the patient after mitral balloon valvuloplasty with mitral stenosis. (Left) Hemodynamic tracings with simultaneous LA (red) and LV (blue) pressures, with markedly reduced diastolic gradient shaded in yellow. (Right) Doppler flow across mitral valve showing normalized pattern of LA flow consistent with marked reduction in LA–LV. These comparisons indicated mitral gradient.

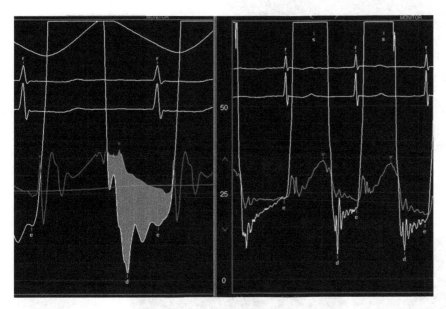

Figure 8.14 Pulmonary capillary wedge (PCW, red) and left ventricular (LV, yellow) tracings (left) compared to left atrial (LA, orange) and LV (yellow) tracings (right) in patient with mitral stenosis. Note the underdamped PCW tracing and large PCW–LV gradient compared to LA–LV gradient. The LA waveform is correctly damped without an "a" wave but a clear "c" notch and "v" wave. There is a much smaller mitral gradient, with end-diastolic pressure matching. Heart control is indicated over valvuloplasty from these data.

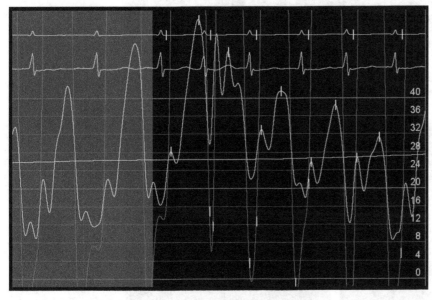

Figure 8.20 Left atrial (LA, blue) and left ventricular (LV, red) tracings show large "v" waves of mitral regurgitation. 0–40 mm Hg scale.

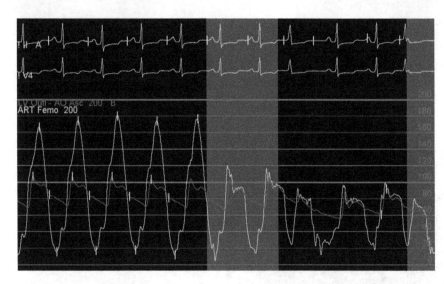

Figure 11.2 Hemodynamic left ventricular (LV, blue) and aortic (Ao, red) pressure tracings in a patient with hypertrophic cardiomyopathy. The LV catheter is pulled back from the distal LV (left side) to subaortic position (right side). Note the reduction in LV–Ao pressure gradient while still recording LV pressure. In addition, one can appreciate the configuration of the aortic pressure with a typical "spike and dome" appearance.

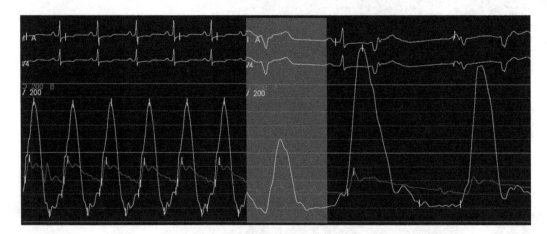

Figure 11.3 Hemodynamics in a patient with hypertrophic obstructive cardiomyopathy (HOCM). Left ventricular (blue) and aortic (red) pressure tracings demonstrate the vertical upstroke of aortic pressure, with a rapid early ejection and mid-systolic delay (spike and dome pattern). Following a PVC (shaded bar), the post-PVC reduction of the aortic pulse pressure is evident (called the Brockenbrough–Braunwald–Morrow sign), with a marked increase in the LVOT pressure gradient.

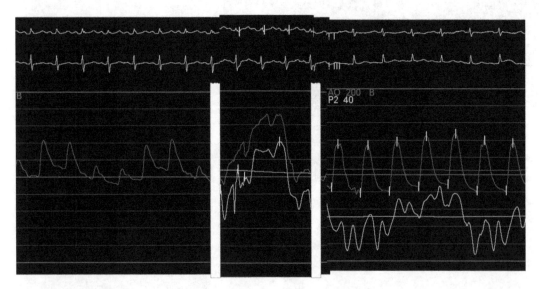

Figure 12.4 Hemodynamic findings in cardiac tamponade. (Left) Aortic pressure (0–200 mm Hg scale) before pericardiocentesis in patient with clinical and echocardiographic findings of tamponade. (Middle) Right atrial and pericardial pressures (0–40 mm Hg scale) before pericardiocentesis. (Right) Aortic pressure (0–200 mm Hg scale) and pericardial pressure (0–40 mm Hg scale) after pericardiocentesis. Note restoration of arterial pulse with loss of marked respiratory variance (pulsus paradoxus) and reduction of pericardial pressure from 22 to 12 mm Hg.

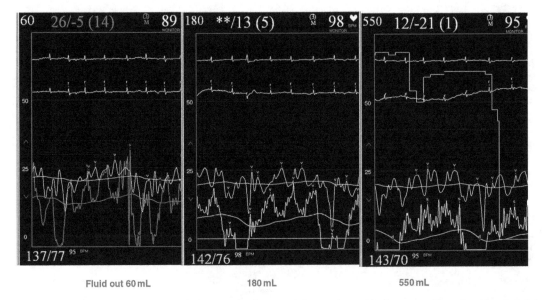

Figure 12.5 Hemodynamic tracings during pericardiocentesis in a patient with shortness of breath and pericardial effusion. The presumed cause of dyspnea was tamponade. (Left) Baseline hemodynamics. Right atrial (RA) pressure is yellow tracing. (Middle) RA and pericardial pressure after 180 mL removed. (Right) Pressures after 550 mL fluid removed from pericardium. However, the relief of pericardial pressure by pericardiocentesis demonstrated no change in RA pressure. No cardiac tamponade is present. The diagnosis is effusive constrictive pericardial disease with left ventricular dysfunction.

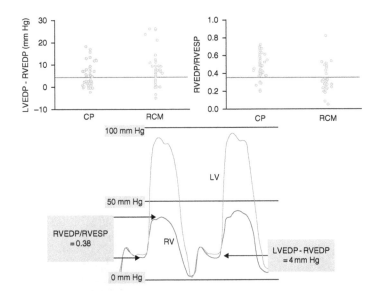

Figure 13.7 Differentiation of constriction and restriction by traditional hemodynamics. There have been a number of criteria proposed comparing left ventricular (LV) and right ventricular (RV) pressures at the time of cardiac catheterization in order to differentiate constrictive pericarditis (CP) from restrictive cardiomyopathy (RCM). These include the difference of left ventricular end-diastolic pressure (LVEDP) and right ventricular end-diastolic pressure (RVEDP); and the ratio of RVEDP to right ventricular end-systolic pressure (RVESP). Although there is a statistical difference when comparing the means of these criteria in a number of patients, the degree of overlap makes application to an individual case difficult. *Source:* Geske 2016 [10]. Reproduced with permission of Elsevier.

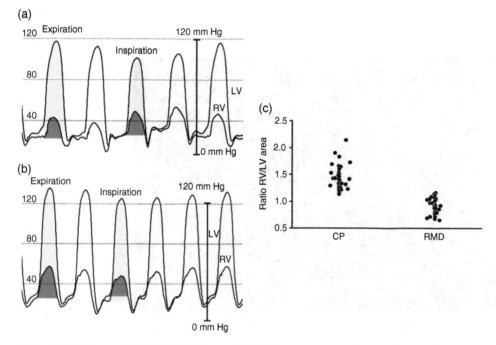

Figure 13.8 Left ventricular (LV) and right ventricular (RV) pressure traces in two patients with constriction (a) vs restriction (b) during respiration. Note that both patients have early rapid filling and elevation and end-equalization of the LV and RV pressures at end expiration. (a) Patient with surgically documented constrictive pericarditis (CP). During inspiration there is an increase in the area of the RV pressure curve (orange shaded area) compared with expiration. The area of the LV pressure curve (yellow shaded area) decreases during inspiration as compared with expiration. (b) Patient with restrictive cardiomyopathy (RMD) documented by endomyocardial biopsy. During inspiration there is a decrease in the area of the RV pressure curve (orange shaded area) as compared with expiration. The area of the LV pressure curve (yellow shaded area) is unchanged during inspiration as compared with expiration. (c) Scatter plot of the ratio of RV to LV areas comparing expiration and inspiration shows that patients with CP have consistently greater RV/LV systolic areas, indicative of ventricular interdependence. *Source:* Talreja 2008 [9]. Reproduced with permission of Elsevier.

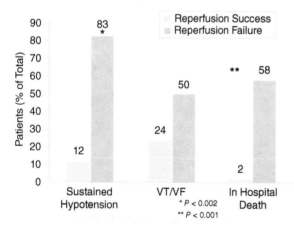

Figure 14.10 Reperfusion benefits in clinical outcomes in patients with acute right ventricular infarction. Reperfusion success including restoration of flow to the major right ventricular branches was associated with markedly lower prevalence of hypotension, arrhythmias, and superior survival compared to reperfusion failure. VF = ventricular fibrillation; VT = ventricular tachycardia. *Source:* Bowers 1998 [7]. Reproduced with permission of The New England Journal of Medicine.

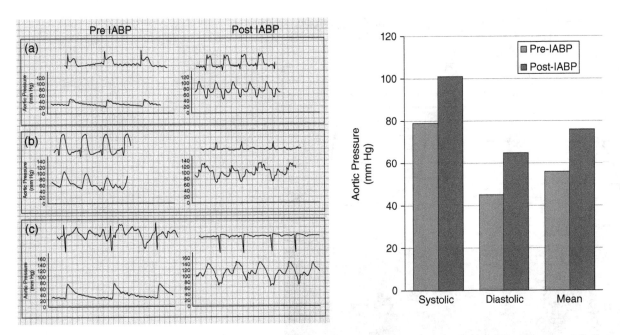

Figure 14.11 Patients with acute right ventricular infarction (RVI) and intractable hypotension may benefit from intra-aortic balloon pump (IABP) support to restore aortic perfusion pressure. In three patients with acute RVI and refractory shock, IABP support promptly improves aortic systolic, diastolic, and mean pressures. *Source:* McNamara 2014 [20]. Reproduced with permission of Wolters Kluwer Health, Inc.

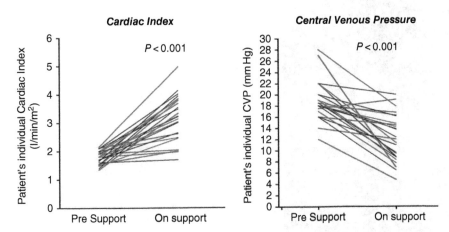

Figure 14.12 Mechanical support with Impella right percutaneous (RP) right ventricular (RV) assist device in patients with acute RV shock from right ventricular infarction, post-thoracotomy, or post-left ventricular assist device (LVAD) implantation. Immediately after initiation of Impella RP support, central venous pressure decreased and cardiac index increased. *Source:* Anderson 2015 [21]. Reproduced with permission of Elsevier.

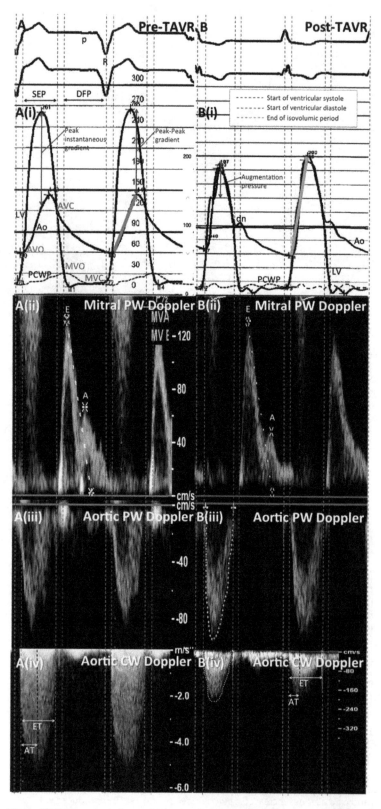

Figure 15.20 Transcatheter and Doppler waveforms in aortic stenosis before (a) and after (b) transaortic valve replacement (TAVR). SEP (systolic ejection period) in panel a(i) corresponds to the ET (ejection time) in panel a(iv). AVC = aortic valve closure; AVO = aortic valve opening; dn: dicrotic notch (onset corresponds to AVC); MVC: mitral valve closure; MVO = mitral valve opening; PW = pulsed-wave. *Source:* Courtesy of Dr. Raj Makkar.

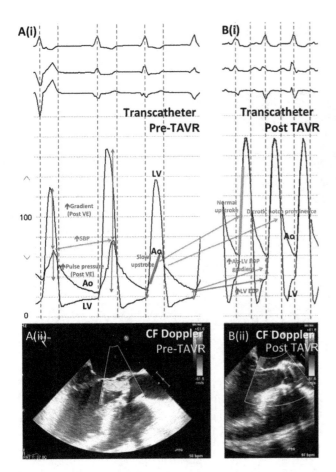

Figure 15.21 Mixed aortic stenosis and regurgitation. Assessment by catheter (top) and color-flow (CF) Doppler (bottom) before transaortic valve replacement (TAVR, A(i, ii), and after TAVR (B (i, ii)), with optimal bioprosthetic function. Ao = aorta; EDP = end-diastolic pressure; LV = left ventricle; SBP = systolic blood pressure; VE = ventricular ectopic. *Source:* Courtesy of Dr. Raj Makkar.

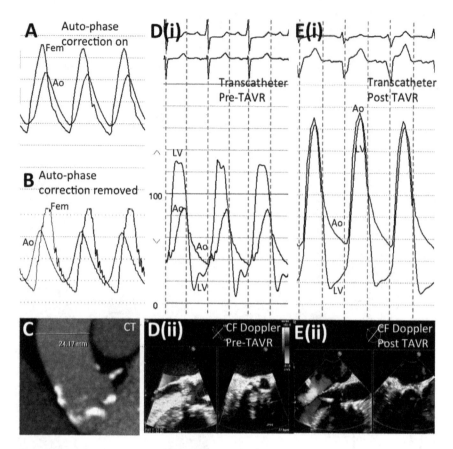

Figure 15.22 Demonstrates the phenomenon of pressure recovery in severe aortic stenosis (panels A (auto-phase correction 'on') and B (auto-phase correction 'off'))—simultaneous femoral artery (Fem) waveforms are higher than aortic (Ao) waveforms recorded just distal to the stenosed aortic valve. Pressure recovery is more common in patients with small aortas, as demonstrated on cardiac CT scan (panel C). Panels D (pre-TAVR) and E (postTAVR) show transcatheter waveforms (panel (i)) and color-flow Doppler TEE images (panel (ii)) of the aortic valve in long and short axes. There is severe mixed aortic stenosis and regurgitation, which is ameliorated following TAVR (panel E). A 'reverse' LV-femoral arterial gradient in panel E is attributable to pressure recovery.

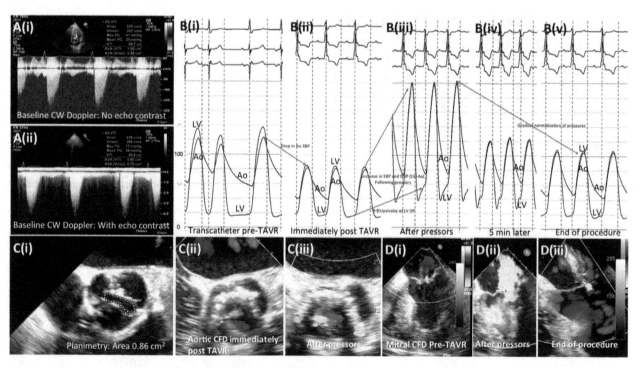

Figure 15.23 Mitral regurgitation after transaortic valve replacement (TAVR) by left ventricular (LV) dilatation. CW Doppler waveforms with (panel A(i)) and without (panel A(ii)) echocardiographic contrast agent use, and a shortaxis TEE (panel C(i)) confirming severe aortic stenosis. There is a precipitous drop in blood pressure immediately after valve implantation (likely due to rapid pacing during valve deployment) (panel B(ii)) that responds appropriately to vasopressor administration (panel B(iii))—note the change in the upstroke of LV end-diastolic pressure tracing. Ao = aorta; CFD = color-flow Doppler; CW = continuous-wave. *Source:* Courtesy of Dr. Raj Makkar.

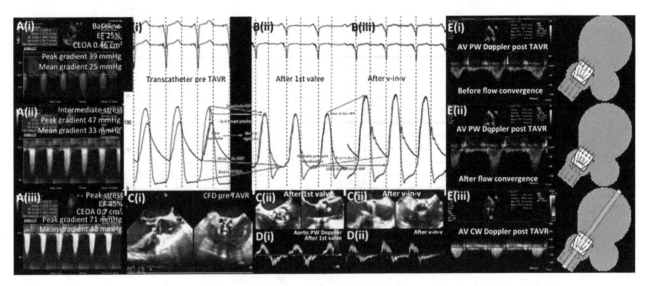

Figure 15.24 Low-flow, low-gradient aortic stenosis (AS) followed by severe aortic regurgitation (AR) post transaortic valve replacement (TAVR). AV = aorta; CEOA = continuous echo orifice area; CFD = color-flow Doppler; EF = ejection fraction; PW = pulsed-wave; v-in-v = valve-in-valve. A, B, C, D, E represent Doppler, 2D echo, C mitral valve echo, D pulmonary vein flow, E PW flow. i, ii, iii denote pre, immediately after and after final implant. *Source:* Courtesy of Dr. Raj Makkar.

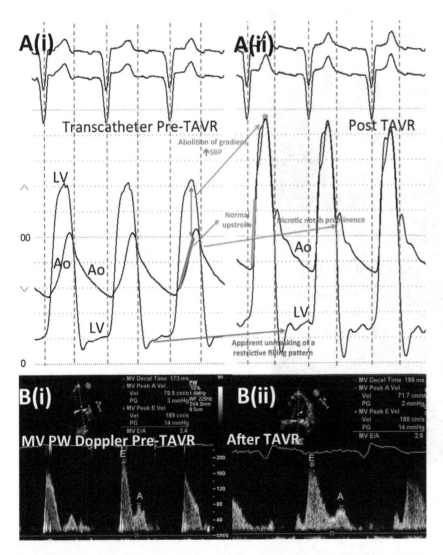

Figure 15.25 Diastolic dysfunction after transaortic valve replacement (TAVR). Ao = aorta; LV = left ventricle; MV = mitral valve; PW = pulsed-wave; SBP = systolic blood pressure. A and B represent hemodynamic and Doppler data, i, ii is pre and post TAVR periods. *Source:* Courtesy of Dr. Raj Makkar.

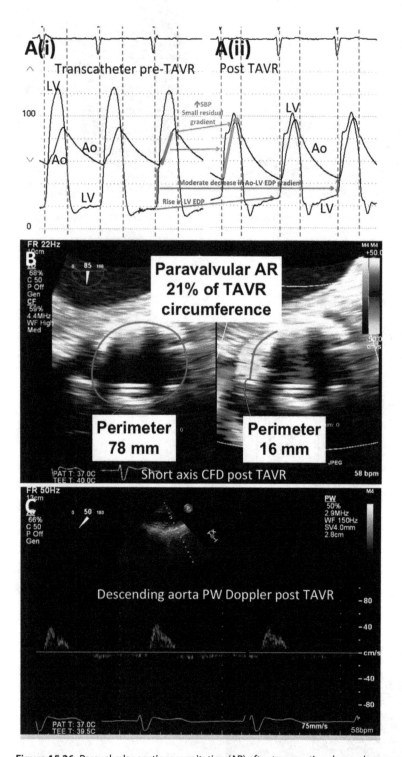

Figure 15.26 Paravalvular aortic regurgitation (AR) after transaortic valve replacement (TAVR). Ao = aorta; CFD = color-flow Doppler; LV = left ventricle; PW = pulsed-wave. A and B represent hemodynamic and Doppler data, i, ii is pre and post TAVR periods. C is descending aortic PW flow. *Source:* Courtesy of Dr. Raj Makkar.

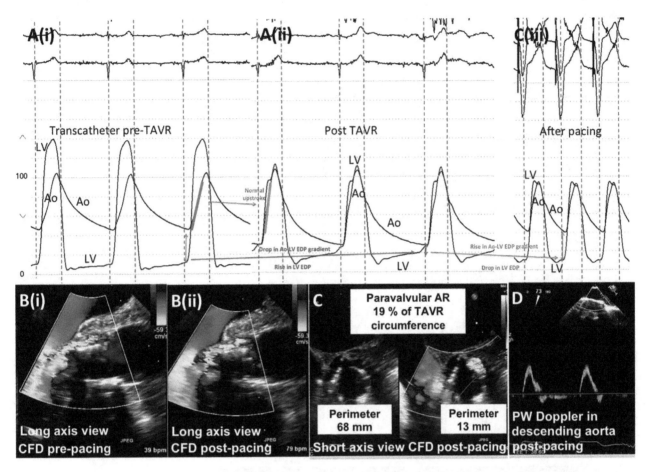

Figure 15.27 Aortic regurgitation (AR) with pacing. Ao = aorta; CFD = color-flow Doppler; LV = left ventricle; PW = pulsed-wave; TAVR = transaortic valve replacement. A and B represent hemodynamic and Doppler data, C is 2D echo and D is PW of aortic flow. i, ii is pre and post TAVR periods. *Source:* Courtesy of Dr. Raj Makkar.

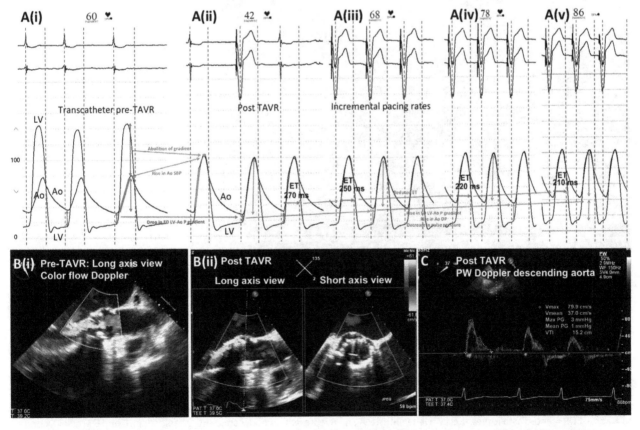

Figure 15.28 Diastolic dysfunction and aortic regurgitation (AR) after pacing. Ao = aorta; ET = ejection time; LV = left ventricle; PW = pulsed-wave; TAVR = transaortic valve replacement. A and B represent hemodynamic and Doppler data, i, ii, iii, iv, v is pre and post TAVR, pacing stablization, and final result. C is PW doppler of aortic flow. *Source:* Courtesy of Dr. Raj Makkar.

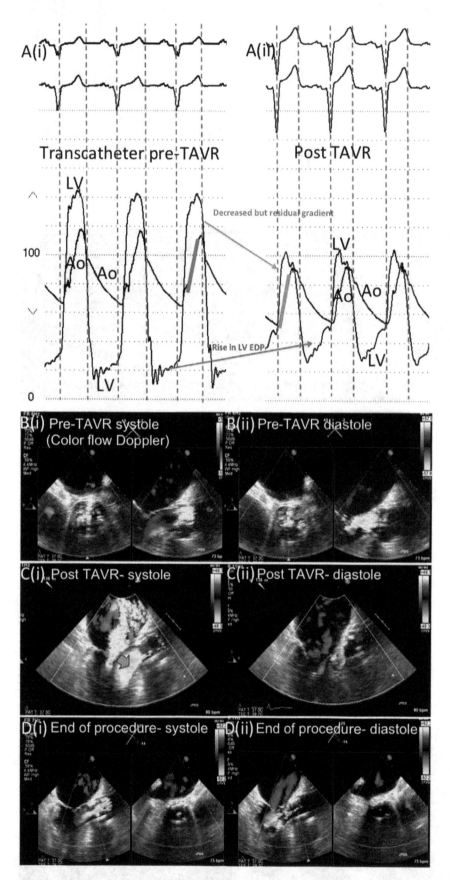

Figure 15.29 Mitral regurgitation after transaortic valve replacement (TAVR) by systolic anterior motion of the anterior leaflet (AMVL). Ao = aorta; EDP = end-diastolic pressure; LV = left ventricle. A and B represent hemodynamic and Doppler data, C and D is color Doppler signals. i, ii is pre and post TAVR periods. *Source:* Courtesy of Dr. Raj Makkar.

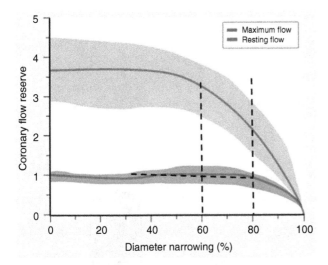

Figure 18.2 Coronary flow reserve expressed as the ratio of maximum to resting flow, plotted as a function of percentage diameter narrowing. With progressive narrowing, resting flow does not change (magenta line), whereas maximum potential increase in flow (blue line) and coronary flow reserve begin to be impaired at approximately 50% diameter narrowing. The shaded area represents the limits of variability of data about the mean. *Source*: Gould 1974 [4]. Reproduced with permission of Elsevier.

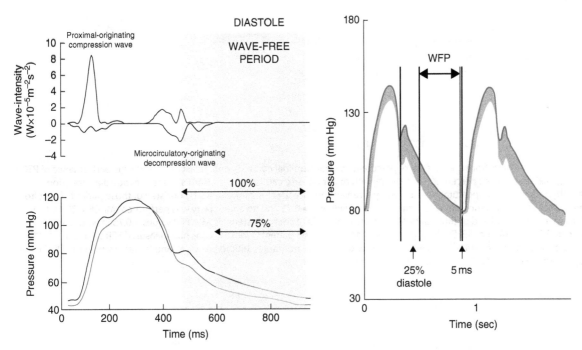

Figure 18.5 The instantaneous wave-free pressure ratio (iFR) is derived from a period of diastole in which equilibration or balance between pressure waves from the aorta and distal microcirculatory reflection is a "wave-free period" (WFP) with a low and fixed resistance. During this period the resistance may be sufficiently low—compared with adenosine hyperemia—to assess translesional hemodynamic significance. Modified from Sen S et al and Davies J et al (see references).

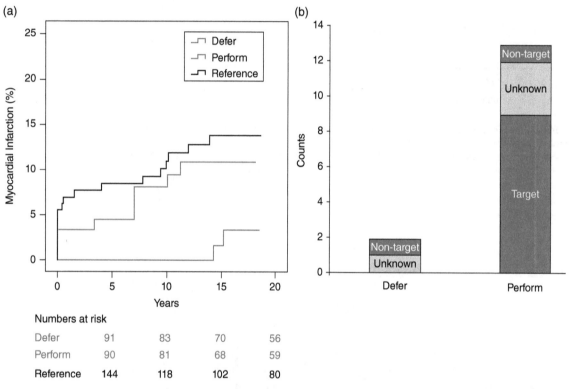

Figure 18.8 (a) Five-year results from the Deferral of percutaneous transluminal coronary angioplasty (PTCA) versus performance of PTCA (DEFER) trial. The y axis depicts the percentage of patients with major adverse cardiac events (MACEs): death, myocardial infarction, coronary artery bypass surgery, or percutaneous coronary intervention. The "DEFER" group (*n* = 91) consisted of those patients found to have an intermediate coronary stenosis in whom the measured FFR was > 0.75 and no angioplasty was performed (MACE = 20%). The "PERFORM" group (*n* = 90) consisted of those patients with an intermediate coronary stenosis with FFR values > 0.75 in whom angioplasty was performed (MACE = 28%). The "REFERENCE" group (*n* = 144) comprised patients whose lesions had measured FFR values of < 0.75 in whom angioplasty was performed (MACE = 37%). (b) Number of events in nontarget, unknown target, and target artery in the DEFER and treated groups. *Source:* Pijls 2007 [25]. Reproduced with permission of Elsevier.

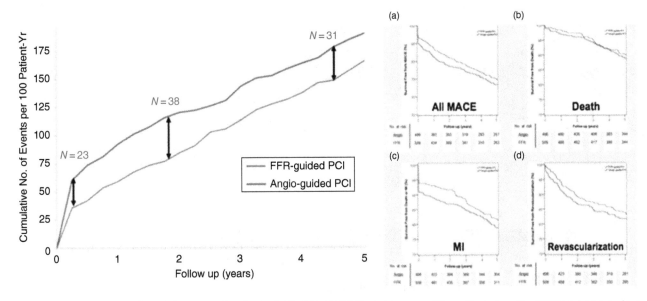

Figure 18.9 Two-year Kaplan–Meier curves showing individual and combined outcomes of the patients from the FAME trial. (a) Freedom from major adverse cardiac events (MACE); (b) Overall survival; (c) Freedom from death or myocardial infarction (MI); (d) Freedom from revascularization by percutaneous coronary intervention (PCI) or coronary artery bypass grafting (CABG). *Source:* Adapted from the New England Journal of Medicine, Tonino 2009 [29].

Primary End Point

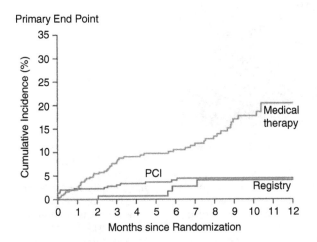

Figure 18.10 FAME II examined patients receiving optimal medical therapy (OMT) compared to percutaneous coronary intervention (PCI) + OMT for patients with abnormal FFR (i.e., ischemia). Kaplan–Meier curves for FAME II patients. Medical therapy had a more than tenfold incidence of major adverse cardiac events compared to the PCI group, which was similar to the nonischemic registry group. *Source:* De Bruyne 2012 [30]. Reproduced with permission of The New England Journal of Medicine.

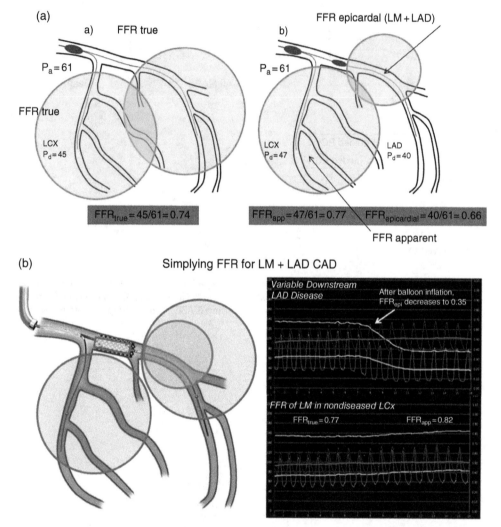

Figure 18.12 (a) Schematic example of physiologic measurements on animal model of left main with or without left anterior descending stenosis. (Left) True fractional flow reserve (FFR$_{true}$) of the left main coronary artery obtained during left main balloon inflation and no stenosis in the left anterior descending (LAD) artery (FFR$_{true}$ = distal pressure [P$_d$]) in the left circumflex (LCX) artery divided by proximal arterial pressure (P$_a$). (Right) FFR$_{app}$ obtained during balloon inflation in the LAD (FFR$_{app}$ = LCX P$_d$/P$_a$ during downstream balloon inflation). FFR$_{epicardial}$ represents FFR of left main plus LAD (FFR$_{epicardial}$ = LAD P$_d$/P$_a$ during LAD balloon inflation). *Source*: Modified from Yong 2013 [32]. (b) Experimental layout to test relationship between left main (LM) and left anterior descending (LAD) lesions of increasing severity. There is a deflated ("winged") balloon in the LM coronary artery with a variably inflated balloon within the newly placed LAD stent, and pressure wires down the LAD and the left circumflex (LCx) coronary artery. The circles represent smaller myocardial bed size, changing bed size when the LAD balloon is inflated. Only when the LAD lesion is very severe does the fractional flow reserve (FFR) become apparent in the LCx rise. CAD = coronary artery disease. *Source:* Fearon 2015 [33].

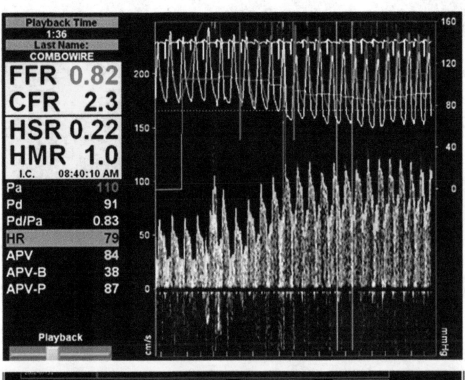

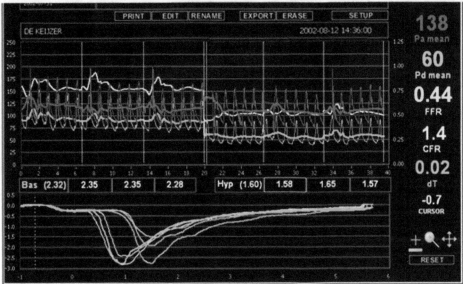

Figure 18.31 (Top) Combination of pressure signals and flow velocity tracings used to compute fractional flow reserve (FFR), coronary flow reserve (CFR) and hyperemic stenosis resistance (HSR). (Bottom) Thermodilution signals from the St. Jude pressure wire used to compute flow velocity by thermodilution curves. *Source:* Wilson 1986 [66]. Reproduced with permission of Wolters Kluwer Health, Inc.

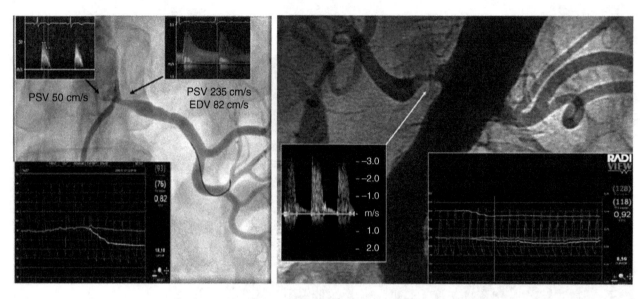

Figure 19.2 Renal artery stenosis, translesional flow velocity, and hemodynamics. (Left) Peak aortic systolic velocity (PSV) 50 cm/sec, with post-stenotic PSV of 235 cm/sec. Corresponding aortic (P_a) and distal renal artery pressure (P_d) ratio = 0.82. (Right) PSV is 300 cm/sec with P_d/P_a 0.90. EDV = end-diastolic volume. *Source:* Drieghe 2008 [3]. Reproduced with permission of Oxford University Press.

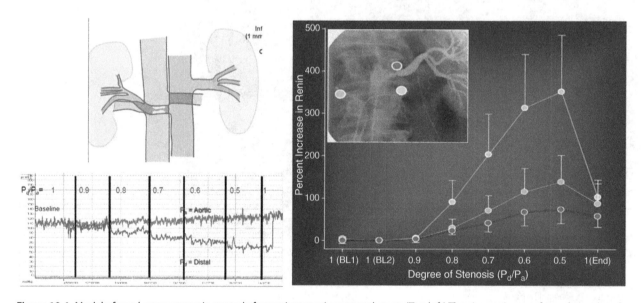

Figure 19.4 Model of renal artery stenosis created after patient receives a renal stent. (Top left) The cineangiogram frame has colored dots corresponding to the sampling locations for renal vein and artery renin. (Lower left) Pressure ratios (P_d/P_a) during partial artery occlusion created by balloon inflation. (Lower right) Renal vein begins to increase when P_d/P_a is less than 0.90. P_a = aortic pressure; P_d = distal pressure. *Source:* De Bruyne 2006 [1]. Reproduced with permission of Elsevier.

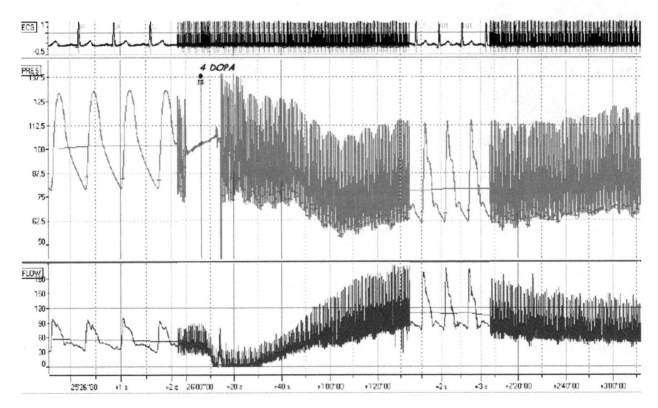

Figure 19.6 Effect of vasodilators on renal artery flow velocity. Example of simultaneous pressure and velocity pressure tracings before, during, and after intrarenal administration of a bolus of 50 μg·kg − 1 of dopamine (DOPA); immediately after administration of the bolus, a marked decrease in renal artery average peak velocity is observed, followed by an almost twofold increase in flow velocities, without changes in blood pressure nor in heart rate. *Source:* Manoharan 2006 [4]. Reproduced with permission of Elsevier.

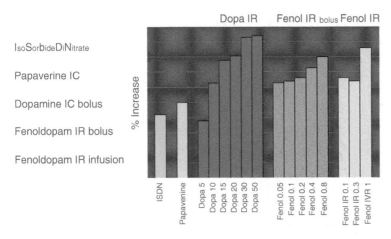

Figure 19.7 Effect of vasodilators on renal artery flow velocity. IC = intracoronary; IR = intrarenal. *Source:* Manoharan 2006 [4]. Reproduced with permission of Elsevier.

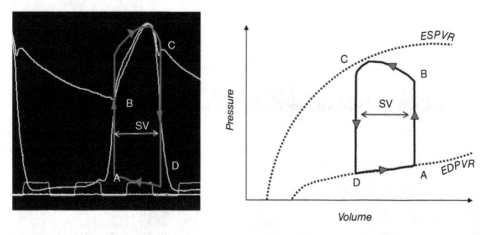

Figure 21.24 (Left) Left ventricular and aortic pressures obtained during cardiac catheterization. (Right) A pressure–volume loop is constructing moving from the initiation of systole, point A. Pressure in the left ventricle (LV) closes the mitral valve and isovolumetric contraction increases pressure, eventually exceeding aortic pressure, point B, when the aortic valve opens. LV ejection continues across systole until repolarization signals the onset of diastole and the LV ceases to eject. LV pressure falls and when below aortic pressure the aortic valve closes, point C. Isovolumetric relaxation occurs, with LV pressure falling to that below the left atrium, point D, at which time the mitral valve opens. The pressure–volume loop is bounded by the end-systolic and end-diastolic pressure–volume relationships, ESPVR and EDPVR. The pressure–volume area (PVA) is defined as the area between the ESPVR and EDPVR bounded by LV ejection (line A–B–C) and is a measure of oxygen consumption per beat. PVA is the sum of stroke work (stroke volume by heart rate, SV*HR) and potential energy (PE). Unloading occurs by reducing the PVA. Modified from Naidu S et al (refs).

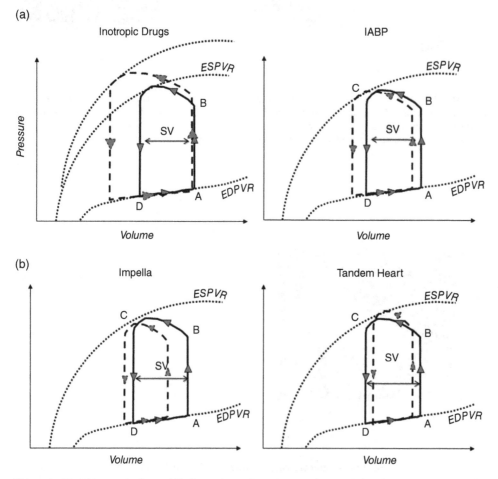

Figure 21.25 (a) Inotropic drugs shift the end-systolic pressure–volume relationship (ESPVR) upward and enlarge the stroke volume (SV) and pressure–volume area (PVA), increasing oxygen demand. The intra-aortic balloon pump (IABP) only minimally shifts the PV loop leftward by reducing afterload, resulting in a modest reduction in PVA and oxygen consumption. (b) Impella shifts the PV loop leftward, decreasing preload, PVA, and oxygen consumption. Tandem Heart decreases preload while also increasing afterload, resulting in modest changes (+/−) in the PVA. EDPVR = end-diastolic pressure–volume relationship. Modified from Naidu S et al (refs).

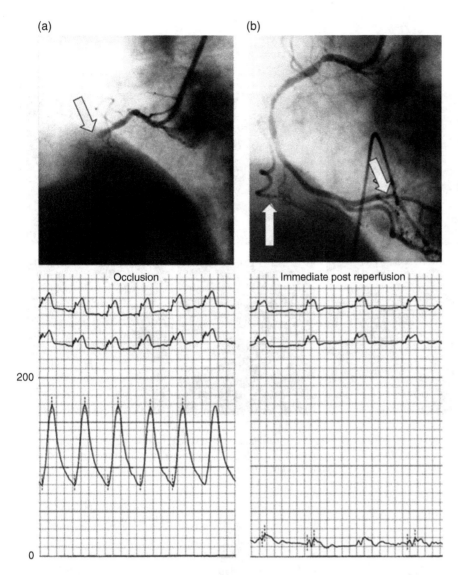

(a)

(b)

Occlusion

Immediate post reperfusion

200

0

Figure 14.7 Patient with acute inferior myocardial infarction with right ventricular infarction attributable to proximal right coronary artery occlusion, with normal sinus rhythm and excellent aortic blood pressure during occlusion. Immediately following successful reperfusion, the patient paradoxically developed profound hypotension and reflex-induced profound sinus bradycardia with a slow sub-junctional escape rhythm. ED = end-diastole; ES = end-systole. (a) during acute inferior STEMI, (b) after recanalization of the right coronary artery. *Source:* Goldstein 2005 [14]. Reproduced with permission of Wolters Kluwer Health, Inc.

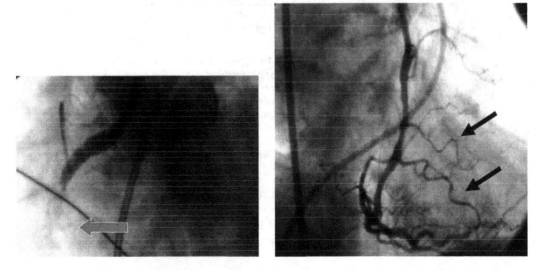

Figure 14.8 Proximal right coronary artery (RCA) occlusion which after successful stenting resulted in complete restoration of flow to the entire RCA, including the major right ventricular (RV) branches.

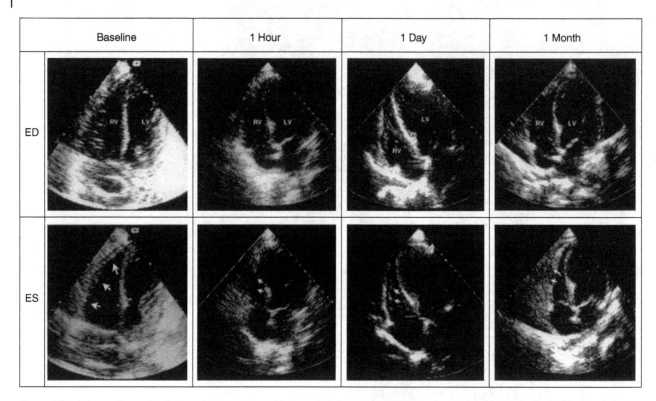

	Baseline	1 Hour	1 Day	1 Month
ED				
ES				

Figure 14.9 Echocardiographic images from a patient with acute inferior myocardial infarction and right ventricular (RV) ischemia in whom angioplasty was successful. The dilated dysfunctional RV improved rapidly and dramatically following successful reperfusion. *Source:* Bowers 1998 [7]. Reproduced with permission of The New England Journal of Medicine.

contractile function. These observations may have clinical implications for biventricular mechanical support in such cases.

Mechanical Support for Acute Right Ventricular Infarction

Given that ischemic RV failure is typically reversible, application of short-term percutaneous mechanical hemodynamic support may provide a "bridge to recovery" for refractory RV shock [5, 6]. First principles dictate that in the setting of acute MI, restoration of blood pressure sufficient to maintain organ and particularly coronary perfusion is essential. Recent findings in patients with acute inferior myocardial infarction complicated by predominant RV shock demonstrate the hemodynamic benefits of intra-aortic balloon pump (IABP) support [20], which promptly improves aortic pressure (Figure 14.11). It is hypothesized that balloon assist likely does not directly improve RV performance, but rather exerts salutary effects indirectly by improving coronary perfusion, which may augment left coronary flow and thereby benefit LV function, which imparts benefits to the failing RV via enhanced LV–septal contractile contributions.

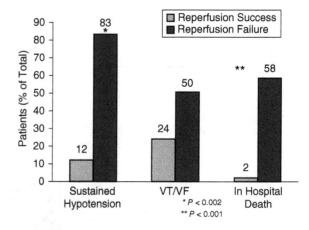

Figure 14.10 Reperfusion benefits in clinical outcomes in patients with acute right ventricular infarction. Reperfusion success including restoration of flow to the major right ventricular branches was associated with markedly lower prevalence of hypotension, arrhythmias, and superior survival compared to reperfusion failure. VF = ventricular fibrillation; VT = ventricular tachycardia. *Source:* Bowers 1998 [7]. Reproduced with permission of The New England Journal of Medicine. (*See insert for color representation of the figure.*)

Recent reports suggest temporary mechanical support with a novel percutaneous RV assist device (Impella RP, Abiomed Inc., Danvers, MA, USA) promptly improves hemodynamics in patients with severe RV failure

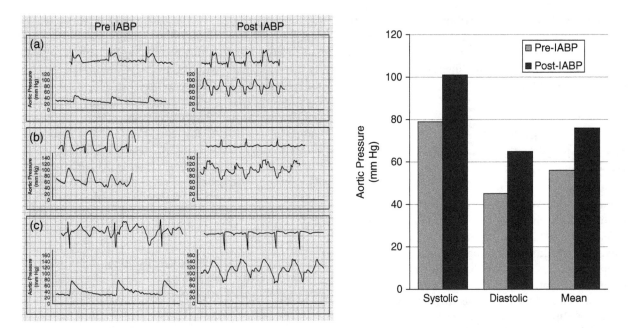

Figure 14.11 Patients with acute right ventricular infarction (RVI) and intractable hypotension may benefit from intra-aortic balloon pump (IABP) support to restore aortic perfusion pressure. In three patients with acute RVI and refractory shock, IABP support promptly improves aortic systolic, diastolic, and mean pressures. *Source:* McNamara 2014 [20]. Reproduced with permission of Wolters Kluwer Health, Inc. *(See insert for color representation of the figure.)*

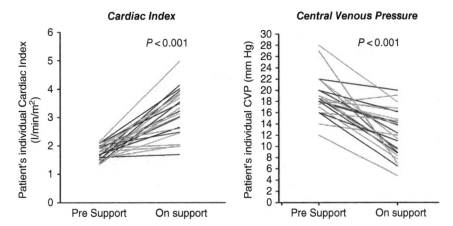

Figure 14.12 Mechanical support with Impella right percutaneous (RP) right ventricular (RV) assist device in patients with acute RV shock from right ventricular infarction, post-thoracotomy, or post-left ventricular assist device (LVAD) implantation. Immediately after initiation of Impella RP support, central venous pressure decreased and cardiac index increased. *Source:* Anderson 2015 [21]. Reproduced with permission of Elsevier. *(See insert for color representation of the figure.)*

complicated by refractory life-threatening low output, thereby providing a bridge to recovery. The pivotal study demonstrating clinical efficacy leading to FDA approval of this device has recently been published [21]. This prospective study included two populations: cohort A, patients who developed RV failure post–left ventricular assist device implantation; and cohort B, patients who developed RV failure post-cardiotomy cardiogenic shock or post-myocardial infarction. Hemodynamics improved immediately after initiation of Impella RP support, with an increase in cardiac index and a decrease in central venous pressure (Figure 14.12). The secondary effectiveness endpoint showed a significant decrease in need for inotropes and vasopressors after institution of Impella RP. Patients were supported on average for 3 days and the overall survival at 30 days or discharge and at 180 days was 73.3%. These data support the probable benefit of the percutaneous Impella RP RV assist device in this gravely ill patient population. It is important to emphasize the importance of delineating the extent to which both RV and LV dysfunction contribute to severe hemodynamic compromise in a given patient. In those with refractory hemodynamic compromise with concomitant LV dysfunction, biventricular mechanical support devices may be needed.

Differential Diagnosis of Hemodynamically Severe Right Ventricular Infarction

In its most severe form, the clinical syndrome of predominant RVI is characterized by right-heart failure with clear lung fields and hypotension, together with hemodynamic findings of elevated equalized diastolic filling pressures. It is important to consider the differential diagnosis of patients who present with low-output hypotension, clear lungs, and disproportionate right-heart failure. Important clinical entities to consider include cardiac tamponade, constrictive pericarditis or restrictive cardiomyopathy, acute severe tricuspid regurgitation, acute pulmonary embolism, severe pulmonary hypertension, and right-heart mass obstruction (Table 14.2). However, careful evaluation of the clinical presentation and hemodynamics together with echocardiographic imaging of the right heart help differentiate these conditions. First, RVI is usually easily distinguished by its absolute association with acute transmural ST-elevation inferior myocardial infarction, confirmed by ECG. Cardiac tamponade may appear identical to RVI and in fact may develop in the setting of acute MI and complicate RVI. The clinical and hemodynamic picture may be indistinguishable, but echocardiography is diagnostic

Table 14.2 Conditions with hypotension, clear lungs, and elevated jugular venous pressure.

Tamponade	Pulsus paradoxus Effusion on echo
Right ventricular infarction	Acute chest pain STEMI by ECG Large RV no fluid on echo
Acute pulmonary embolism	Shortness of breath/chest pain RV strain by ECG Large RV no fluid on echo
Pulmonary hypertension with RV failure	Chronic right-heart failure Large RV no fluid on echo
Constriction/restriction	Chronic biventricular congestive heart failure Small RV/LV on echo
Right-heart mass obstruction	Chronic right-heart failure RA/RV mass on echo

ECG = echocardiogram; LV = left ventricle; RA = right atrium; RV = right ventricle; STEMI = ST-elevation myocardial infarction.

with respect to both RV ischemic dysfunction and evidence of effusion resulting in tamponade physiology. Constrictive pericarditis presents typically with chronic right-heart failure without acute MI; although sharing some hemodynamic features similar to RVI, constriction is noteworthy for rapid unimpeded filling of the right ventricle in the first third of diastole, reflected in the RA waveform as a brisk Y descent, whereas RVI manifests a blunted Y. Restrictive cardiomyopathy mimics constriction and is a chronic condition lacking evidence of acute inferior MI. The general clinical presentation of chest pain with acute inferior MI, together with echocardiographic documentation of RV dilatation and dysfunction, effectively excludes tamponade, constriction, and restriction. Primary acute tricuspid regurgitation is confirmed by echocardiography, including delineation of primary valvular abnormalities such as vegetations. Severe pulmonary hypertension with RV decompensation may mimic severe RVI, but delineation of markedly elevated RV and PA systolic pressures by Doppler or invasive hemodynamic monitoring excludes RVI, in which RV pressure generation is depressed. Acute massive pulmonary embolism may also mimic severe RVI; and since the unprepared right ventricle cannot acutely generate elevated RV systolic pressures (>50–55 mm Hg), severe pulmonary hypertension may be absent. In such cases, although the clinical scenario and absence of inferior LV myocardial infarction by ECG and ultrasound point to embolism, further noninvasive studies (spiral CT) and ultimately angiography (pulmonary and coronary) may be necessary.

Case: Occlusion of the Mid-Right Coronary Artery—Right Ventricular Ischemic Dysfunction with Augmented Right Atrial Function

A 65-year-old man presented with an acute inferior myocardial infarction complicated by second-degree atrioventricular block, elevated jugular venous pressure, and hypotension. Echocardiography revealed marked RV dilatation, severe RVFW dysfunction, and an inferior LV wall motion abnormality, but overall normal LV ejection fraction. Coronary angiography demonstrated RCA occlusion proximal to the RV branches but distal to the RA branches.

Hemodynamic evaluation with a fluid-filled, balloon-tipped catheter (Figure 14.2) demonstrated a broadened, depressed RV systolic waveform with a diminished upstroke, decreased and bifid peak pressure, and delayed relaxation. These changes reflect depressed RV contractility and the compensatory effects of systolic ventricular interactions. RV filling pressure was elevated early in diastole, with a rapid rise to a plateau indicative of progressive pan-diastolic impedance to RV filling. Though mean RA pressure was elevated, the upstroke and peak amplitude of the "a" wave were increased ("W" pattern), indicating augmented RA contraction. A steep X descent was evident, reflecting enhanced RA relaxation, whereas the Y descent was blunted, representing pan-diastolic resistance to RV filling. Simultaneous superimposed RA and pulmonary capillary wedge pressures (not shown) revealed equalization of diastolic pressures, attributable to the effects of pericardial restraint.

Case: Proximal Right Coronary Artery Occlusion—Right Ventricular and Right Atrial Ischemic Dysfunction

A 72-year-old man presented with an acute inferior myocardial infarction complicated by severe hypotension with predominant right-heart failure. Echocardiography revealed severe RVFW dysfunction, RV dilatation, and an inferior LV wall motion abnormality, with overall normal LV ejection fraction. Coronary angiography demonstrated RCA occlusion proximal to the RA branches, with no evidence of collateral flow.

Hemodynamic evaluation (Figure 14.3) demonstrated RV waveform alterations similar to those in the previous case and characteristic of RV systolic dysfunction. The RV upstroke was depressed, with its peak pressure diminished, and a broad systolic wave with delayed relaxation was evident. RV diastolic pressure was elevated, with a dip and plateau pattern. As in the prior case, mean RA pressure was markedly elevated and the Y descent blunted, reflecting the effects of impedance to RV filling. In contrast, the upstroke and peak amplitude of the A wave were markedly depressed and the X descent diminished ("M" pattern), consistent with ischemic depression of RA contraction and relaxation (Figure 14.3). Gross RA dilatation and akinesis were observed at thoracotomy for emergency revascularization in this patient, indicating the presence of RA ischemia/infarction.

Summary

Acute RCA occlusion proximal to the RV branches results in RVFW dysfunction. The ischemic, dyskinetic RVFW exerts mechanically disadvantageous effects on biventricular performance. Depressed RV systolic function leads to a decrease in transpulmonary delivery of LV preload, resulting in diminished cardiac output. The ischemic right ventricle is stiff, dilated, and volume dependent, resulting in pan-diastolic RV dysfunction and septally mediated alterations in LV compliance, which are exacerbated by elevated intrapericardial pressure. Under these conditions, RV pressure generation and output are dependent on LV–septal contractile contributions, governed by both primary septal contraction and paradoxical septal motion. When the culprit coronary lesion is distal to the RA branches, augmented RA contractility enhances RV performance and optimizes cardiac output. Conversely, more proximal occlusions result in ischemic depression of RA contractility, which impairs RV filling, thereby resulting in further depression of RV performance and more severe hemodynamic compromise. Bradyarrhythmias limit the output generated by the rate-dependent noncompliant ventricles. Patients with RVI and hemodynamic compromise often respond to volume resuscitation and restoration of a physiologic rhythm. Vasodilators and diuretics should generally be avoided. In some, parenteral inotropic stimulation may be required. The right ventricle appears to be relatively resistant to infarction and has a remarkable ability to recover even after prolonged occlusion. Therefore, the term RV "infarction" appears to be somewhat of a misnomer, because in most patients a substantial proportion of acute RV dysfunction represents ischemic but viable myocardium. Although RV performance improves spontaneously even in the absence of reperfusion, recovery of function may be slow and associated with high in-hospital mortality. Reperfusion enhances the recovery of RV performance and improves the clinical course and survival of patients with ischemic RV dysfunction.

Hemodynamic Manifestations of Ischemic Right Heart Dysfunction (Morton J. Kern)

Patients with right ventricular infarction often present with striking abnormalities of right-heart hemodynamics. The extent and detail of these hemodynamic alterations have been eloquently elucidated by Dr. Goldstein in this chapter. The changes observed in right atrial pressure during different degrees of ischemic right ventricular dysfunction are discussed as new observations and interpretations of the traditional A, C, and V waveforms. Further striking changes can be observed with the addition of right atrial ischemia superimposed on right ventricular ischemia. These findings are unique and rarely described in earlier studies. The elegant investigational work of this author confirms commonly observed changes in right-heart hemodynamics, and accurately reflects and further clarifies the underlying physiologic mechanisms.

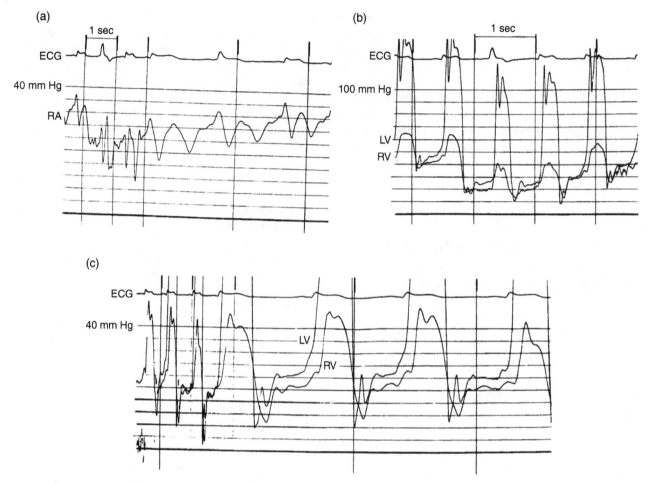

Figure 14.13 (a) Right atrial (RA) pressure in a patient with acute inferior myocardial infarction (0–40 mm Hg scale). (b) Simultaneous right ventricular (RV) and left ventricular (LV) pressures (0–100 mm Hg scale). (c) Simultaneous RV and LV pressures (0–40 mm Hg scale).

This chapter illustrates the changes in right atrial and ventricular pressures during the progressive ischemia of right coronary occlusion which may be commonly observed in patients. Simultaneous right and left ventricular hemodynamic patterns often demonstrate constrictive/restrictive physiology during acute right ventricular infarction. I have taken the liberty of adding the following clinical example to complete the common findings.

Right atrial and simultaneous right and left ventricular pressures (Figure 14.13) were measured in a 43-year-old woman with acute inferior myocardial infarction, persistent chest pain, and ventricular arrhythmias after receiving intravenous streptokinase. Coronary artery bypass grafting was performed in 1987, with saphenous vein grafts to the left anterior descending and diagonal branch. The right coronary artery had not been bypassed. The systolic pressure was 90 mm Hg. The electrocardiogram showed ST elevation in the inferior leads, and reciprocal ST depression in leads V_1–V_6. A right-sided electrocardiogram showed ST elevation in lead V_4. Periods of Mobitz's type I AV block were noted. Coronary arteriography revealed total occlusion of the proximal right coronary artery with patent vein grafts to the left system. The initial right atrial pressure (Figure 14.13) demonstrated a mean right atrial pressure of approximately 28 mm Hg, with nearly equal A and V waves and the "M"-shaped configuration as described by Dr. Goldstein. Right ventricular pressure was also elevated (approximately 50/128 mm Hg). Prior to coronary angioplasty, the configurations of the right and left ventricular diastolic pressure waveforms were nearly matched, with an early diastolic dip and a relatively flat period of diastasis prior to atrial systole (Figure 14.13b and 14.13c). Following coronary angioplasty, with resolution of chest pain and restoration of a consistent sinus rhythm, left and right ventricular end-diastolic pressure declined, with persistence of the matching of the diastolic waveforms similar to that of constrictive physiology. These tracings further illustrate the role of pericardial constraint in the patient with significant right ventricular ischemic dysfunction.

Review of the waveforms in this chapter should bring new insight into the hemodynamic mechanisms and consequences of right ventricular ischemia for the clinician.

Key Points

1) The RCA is the culprit vessel in nearly all cases with RV ischemic dysfunction.
2) RCA occlusion proximal to the RA branches results in RA ischemia/infarction and depressed RA function manifest by a depressed a wave and x-descent ("M"pattern).
3) During acute RVFW dysfunction, RV performance is dependent on LV-septal contractile activity with pressure generation mediated by the septum and identified by both paradoxical septal motion and primary septal thickening.
4) Additional mechanical complications of acute RVI infarction compounding hemodynamic compromise is ventricular septal rupture, a particularly disastrous complication, adding substantial overload stress to the ischemically dysfunctional right ventricle.
5) Reperfusion enhances the recovery of RV performance and improves the clinical course and survival of patients with ischemic RV dysfunction.

References

1 Cresci SG, Goldstein JA. Hemodynamic manifestations of ischemic right heart dysfunction. *Cathet Cardiovasc Diagn* 27(1):28–33, 1992.

2 Kern MJ, Lim MJ, Goldstein JA (eds). *Hemodynamic Rounds: Interpretation of Cardiac Pathophysiology from Pressure Waveform Analysis*, 3rd ed. Hoboken, NJ: John Wiley & Sons, Inc., 2009.

3 Cohn JN, Guiha NH, Broder MI, Limas CJ. Right ventricular infarction: Clinical and hemodynamic features. *Am J Cardiol* 33:209–214, 1974.

4 Lorell B, Leinbach RC, Pohost GM, Gold HK, Dinsmore RE, Hutter AM Jr, Pastore JO, Desanctis RW. Right ventricular infarction: Clinical diagnosis and differentiation from cardiac tamponade and pericardial constriction. *Am J Cardiol* 43:465–471, 1979.

5 Goldstein JA, Barzilai B, Rosamond TL, Eisenberg PR, Jaffe AS. Determinants of hemodynamic compromise with severe right ventricular infarction. *Circulation* 82:359–368, 1990.

6 Goldstein JA. State of the art review: Pathophysiology and management of right heart ischemia. *J Am Coll Cardiol* 40:841–885, 2002.

7 Bowers TR, O'Neill WW, Grines C, Pica MC, Safian RD, Goldstein JA. Effect of reperfusion on biventricular function and survival after right ventricular infarction. *N Engl J Med* 338:933–940, 1998.

8 Bowers TR, O'Neill WW, Pica M, Goldstein JA. Patterns of coronary compromise resulting in acute right ventricular ischemic dysfunction. *Circulation* 106(9):1104–1109, 2002.

9 Goldstein JA, Vlahakes GJ, Verrier ED, Schiller NB, Tyberg JV, Ports TA, Parmley WW, Chatterjee K. The role of right ventricular systolic dysfunction and elevated intrapericardial pressure in the genesis of low output in experimental right ventricular infarction. *Circulation* 65:513–522, 1982.

10 Goldstein JA, Vlahakes GJ, Verrier ED, Schiller NB, Botvinick E, Tyberg JV, Parmley WW, Chatterjee K. Volume loading improves low cardiac output in experimental right ventricular infarction. *J Am Coll Cardiol* 2:270–278, 1983.

11 Goldstein JA, Tweddell JS, Barzilai B, Yagi Y, Jaffe AS, Cox JL. Right atrial ischemia exacerbates hemodynamic compromise associated with experimental right ventricular dysfunction. *J Am Coll Cardiol* 18:1564–1572, 1991.

12 Goldstein JA, Tweddell JS, Barzilai B, Yagi Y, Cox JL. Importance of left ventricular function and systolic ventricular interaction to right ventricular performance during acute right heart ischemia. *J Am Coll Cardiol* 19:704–711; 1992.

13 Wei JY, Markis JE, Malagold M, Braunwald E. Cardiovascular reflexes stimulated by reperfusion of ischemic myocardium in acute myocardial infarction. *Circulation* 67:796–801, 1983.

14 Goldstein JA, Lee DT, Pica MC, Dixon SR, O'Neill WW. Patterns of coronary compromise leading to bradyarrhythmias and hypotension in inferior myocardial infarction. *Coron Artery Dis* 16:265–274, 2005.

15 Laster SB, Shelton TJ, Barzilai B, Goldstein JA. Determinants of the recovery of right ventricular performance following experimental chronic right coronary artery occlusion. *Circulation* 88:696–708, 1993.

16 Laster SB, Ohnishi Y, Saffitz JE, Goldstein JA. Effects of reperfusion on ischemic right ventricular dysfunction: Disparate mechanisms of benefit related to duration of ischemia. *Circulation* 90:1398–1409, 1994.

17 Kinn JW, Ajluni SC, Samyn JG, Bates ER, Grines CL, O'Neill W. Rapid hemodynamic improvement after reperfusion during right ventricular infarction. *J Am Coll Cardiol* 26:1230–1234, 1995.

18 Moore CA, Nygaard TW, Kaiser DL, Cooper AA, Gibson RS. Post infarction ventricular septal rupture: The importance of location of infarction and right ventricular function in determining survival. *Circulation* 74(1):45–55, 1986.

19 Goldstein JA, Kommuri N, Dixon SR. LV systolic dysfunction is associated with adverse outcomes in acute right ventricular infarction. *Coron Artery Dis* 27:277–286, 2016.

20 McNamara M, Dixon SD, Goldstein JA. Impact of intra-aortic balloon pumping on hypotension and outcomes in acute right ventricular infarction. *Coron Artery Dis* 25:602, 2014.

21 Anderson M, Goldstein JA, Morris L, Milano C, Kormos R, Bhama J, Kapur N, Bansal A, Garcia J, Sivestry S, Holman W, Douglas P, O'Neill WW. Benefits of a novel percutaneous ventricular assist device for right heart failure: The prospective RECOVER RIGHT Study of the Impella RP device. *J Heart Lung Transplant* 34:1549–1560, 2015.

Part Four

Hemodynamics of Structural Heart Disease

15

Percutaneous Balloon Aortic Valvuloplasty and Transaortic Valve Replacement

Williams M. Suh, Morton J. Kern, and Zoltan Turi

Although percutaneous balloon aortic valvuloplasty (PBAV) has distinctly inferior results compared to surgical aortic valve replacement (AVR) [1, 2], with a few useful but limited Class II indications [3], PBAV is now a required part of transaortic valve replacement (TAVR) and as such it provides an interesting study in partial relief of aortic stenosis prior to the TAVR. A full understanding of TAVR hemodynamics also becomes important in assessing the intraprocedural results.

In contrast to PBAV, percutaneous balloon mitral valvuloplasty (PBMV) has been shown to be superior to surgery in patients with appropriate anatomic features and is still the procedure of choice for patients with mitral valve stenosis [4]. PBMV requires an iterative process of balloon inflations and hemodynamic assessments during the procedure. Its success is highly dependent on interpreting the hemodynamics accurately, so that the operator knows when to stop or when to continue with the inflation of larger balloons.

Finally, balloon valvuloplasty is associated with a variety of complications, from life-threatening tamponade to severe regurgitation, all of which require early awareness by the operator of the hemodynamic features associated with these phenomena.

This chapter will present examples that demonstrate the subtleties referred to above in the context of pre-procedure evaluation and intra- and post-procedure assessment, along with some examples of important complications.

Percutaneous Balloon Aortic Valvuloplasty

Unfortunately, PBAV did not live up to its promise as an alternative to surgery for adult patients with severe aortic valve stenosis [5]. The mechanism of action of balloon dilatation in these patients is the fracturing of calcifications, resulting in multiple, frequently microscopic fracture lines that in turn result in improved compliance of the valve leaflets. Stretching of the commissures is a temporary result, resolving within hours, and the improvement in compliance lasts at best weeks to months as the fracture lines heal. A combination of mediocre early results and a very high recurrence rate have relegated this procedure to a pair of Class IIb indications. It is reserved for patients who are deemed too unstable to undergo aortic valve replacement or for whom PBAV is part of pre-AVR stabilization as part of a TAVR. PBAV once was considered as a palliative measure but is now superseded by TAVR [6], which provides dramatically better overall hemodynamic results than balloon dilatation (Figure 15.1).

Balloon valvuloplasty for young patients with congenital aortic stenosis is quite effective and is the procedure of choice in the absence of significant aortic insufficiency; a variety of Class I and Class II indications are predicated on a peak-to-peak gradient of at least 50 mm Hg systolic, the patient's lifestyle, symptoms, or the presence of electrocardiographic or other signs of left ventricular strain. The hemodynamics of severe aortic stenosis in young patients tend to be dramatic, with some of the highest gradients recorded; an example is seen in Figure 15.2.

Hemodynamic Screening for Aortic Stenosis

The classic features of aortic stenosis are shown in Figure 15.3a. In this patient, there is a gradient of 100 mm Hg across the aortic valve. Because the gradient is dependent on total flow across the valve and thus can be very high in patients with mild to moderate aortic stenosis in a high output state, or low in patients with depressed cardiac output, the gradient alone is not adequate to determine the severity of the obstruction. Thus, it is important to consider several other elements that are considered the sine qua non of severe aortic stenosis: the aortic upstroke and the pulse pressure. The tracing in

Hemodynamic Rounds: Interpretation of Cardiac Pathophysiology from Pressure Waveform Analysis, Fourth Edition.
Edited by Morton J. Kern, Michael J. Lim, and James A. Goldstein.
© 2018 John Wiley & Sons Ltd. Published 2018 by John Wiley & Sons Ltd.

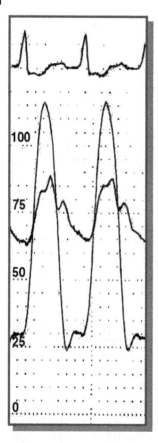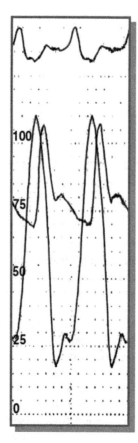

Figure 15.1 Aortic valve gradient before and after percutaneous aortic valve placement. The hemodynamics are similar to those seen after conventional aortic valve replacement, including a peak-to-peak gradient of only approximately 10 mm Hg, normal pulse pressure, and systemic pressure upstroke similar to left ventricular pressure rise. Compare to Figure 15.3, showing the result of balloon dilatation. *Source:* Cribier 2006 [6]. Reproduced with permission of Elsevier.

Figure 15.3a demonstrates not only a severe gradient, but also a markedly blunted upstroke of the systemic pressure (dP/dt, or the rate of rise of pressure over time) and a diminished pulse volume. Compare this to the tracing in Figure 15.4a. Here there is a nearly 50 mm Hg gradient, and the tracing could be considered suggestive of severe aortic stenosis. In fact, this patient had no aortic stenosis at all. As seen in Figure 15.4b, the gradient completely resolves with rebalancing of transducers. The sophisticated hemodynamicist would appreciate the lack of blunting of the systemic pressure, with identical dP/dt slopes for both systemic and left ventricular pressures, and the absence of any blunting of the pulse pressure.

Another important error in assessing the severity of aortic stenosis is caused by comparison of left ventricular pressure to systemic pressure, with the latter recorded at the level of the femoral artery instead of at the level of the central aorta [7]. Because of harmonic reflection of waveforms, the femoral arterial pressure, especially in the older patients typically found in the severe calcific aortic stenosis population, tends to have higher systolic and lower diastolic pressures as the distance from the pressure source (the heart) increases. Thus, compare the pressures seen in Figure 15.5a and 15.5b. With pressure recorded through the femoral sheath side arm, both the peak and mean gradients are substantially underestimated, and the systemic dP/dt and pulse pressure are both overestimated, suggesting much less severe aortic stenosis than is the actual case. Use of catheters capable of obtaining simultaneous left ventricular and central aortic pressures on either side of the aortic valve addresses this problem.

Finally, laboratories use either peak-to-peak or mean gradients, even though the ACC/AHA guidelines are based on mean gradients (except for congenital aortic stenosis in young adults). The accuracy of peak-to-peak gradients on catheter pullback across the aortic valve

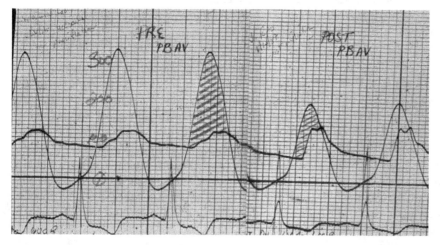

Figure 15.2 Tracing from a 17-year-old with bicuspid aortic valve stenosis, 400 mm Hg scale. The panel at left demonstrates a 200 mm Hg gradient, with marked blunting of the systemic pressure upslope and a pulse pressure of only approximately 40 mm Hg. After balloon dilatation (right), the gradient decreased to approximately 50 mm Hg, the upslope normalized, and the pulse pressure increased to 85 mm Hg. PBAV = percutaneous balloon aortic valvuloplasty.

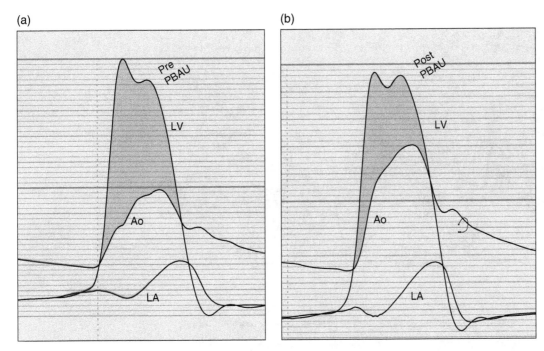

Figure 15.3 (a) Baseline left ventricular (LV), ascending aortic (Ao), and left atrial (LA) pressures. Note the gradient of approximately 100 mm Hg and markedly blunted upstroke of the ascending aortic pressure tracing. (b) Hemodynamics after balloon dilatation. The gradient has been reduced by approximately 50%, the upstroke has risen to nearly the equivalent of the LV pressure rise, and the pulse pressure has risen 50% (from 60 mm Hg to 90 mm Hg). A rise in pulse pressure should always raise the possibility of associated aortic insufficiency; in this case it was the result only of improved stroke volume. PBAV = percutaneous balloon aortic valvuloplasty.

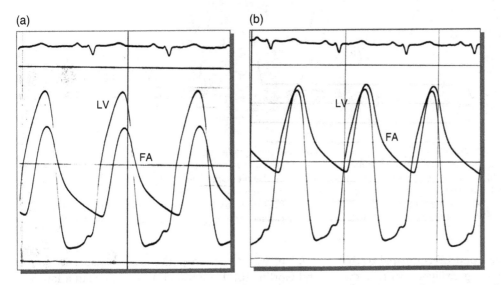

Figure 15.4 (a) Apparent aortic stenosis, with LV (left ventricular) and FA (femoral arterial) pressure recorded on a 200 mm Hg scale. The gradient of 50 mm Hg across the aortic valve, suggested by this tracing, should be recognized as false, given the wide pulse pressure and the identical upslope of left ventricular and systemic pressure. In fact, this was induced by a transducer balancing error, with no gradient seen in the same patient after rebalancing (b).

suffers from substantial beat-to-beat variability, compounded by respiratory changes, and does not take into account the effect of differences in the upslope of the left ventricular and central aortic pressures, which can underestimate the total gradient over time. The pullback

peak-to-peak gradient measurement is generally the least accurate technique. With mean gradients as well, there is considerable variability because there are three methods for assessing mean aortic valve gradient: left ventricle (LV) compared to central aorta, LV compared

(a)

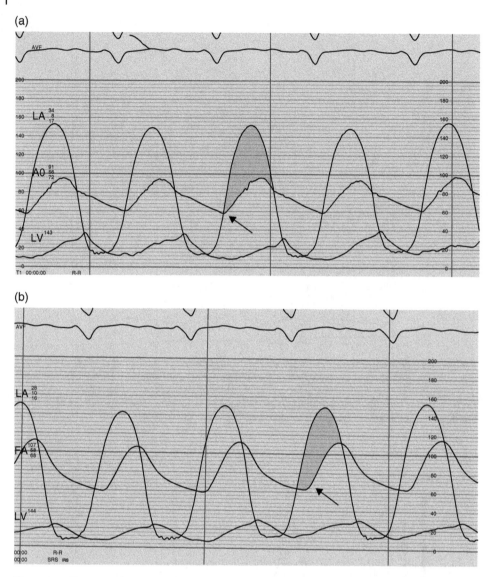

(b)

Figure 15.5 Two sets of aortic valve gradients on 200 mm Hg scale. (a) A peak-to-peak gradient of approximately 60 mm Hg, a pulse pressure of only approximately 35 mm Hg, and a markedly blunted upstroke of pressure vs. time (dP/dt) for systemic pressure compared to left ventricular (LV) pressure. (b) A peak-to-peak gradient of only 40 mm Hg, a pulse pressure of nearly 60 mm Hg, and a much less blunted pressure upstroke. In fact, the two tracings are from the same patient a few moments apart, with ascending aortic (AO) pressure recorded in a and femoral arterial (FA) pressure in b. These panels demonstrate the extent to which severity of aortic stenosis can be underestimated by the LV versus FA pressure technique used in the majority of cardiac catheterization laboratories. LA = left atrium.

to femoral artery as recorded, and LV compared to the femoral arterial pressure tracing realigned so that the upstroke of the systemic pressure coincides with the left ventricular upstroke. The effect of these different modalities is substantial, as shown in Figure 15.6. Given the additional errors in valve area calculations that are dependent on measured or estimated cardiac output, the assessment of the severity of aortic stenosis in the cardiac catheterization laboratory is a delicate art [8].

In addition to measurement techniques, the patient's physiological state needs to be considered. The nonlinear relationship between flow across the valve and

gradient was described in the original paper by Gorlin and Gorlin [10]. Diminished flow, such as in a low output, will result in marked diminution of the gradient. High flow, such as is seen with the increased blood volume and cardiac output of pregnancy, will tend to exaggerate the gradient. In a setting where low gradient is associated with depressed left ventricular function, it is essential to differentiate between (i) severe aortic stenosis with secondary depression of left ventricular ejection and (ii) moderate aortic stenosis with primary depressed LV function secondary to a cardiomyopathy. The administration of drugs to increase flow across the valve, such

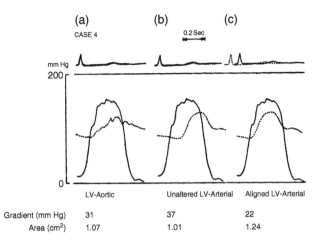

| Gradient (mm Hg) | 31 | 37 | 22 |
| Area (cm²) | 1.07 | 1.01 | 1.24 |

Figure 15.6 Simultaneous tracings showing the left ventricular (LV) pressure with the aortic (Ao, a) and femoral arterial (FA, b) pressures. The gradient is seen to be greater in the LV to FA comparison when contrasted to that of the LV to Ao comparison, resulting in a smaller calculated valve area. Tracing c depicts the "phase-shifted" femoral arterial pressure tracing from b, resulting in a decrease in gradient when compared to tracing a and a resultant larger valve area. *Source:* Folland 1984 [9]. Reproduced with permission of Elsevier.

as dobutamine, can differentiate the two physiologic subsets. If the gradient rises dramatically, the depressed LV function is typically secondary to the stenosis, and intervention for aortic stenosis is appropriate. An example of this maneuver is shown in the subsequent section on PBMV.

Balloon Dilatation

The typical results of PBAV are an approximately 50% acute reduction in aortic valve gradient and a rise in aortic valve area in the range of 0.2–0.3 cm². In contrast, in congenital aortic stenosis in young patients, the valve

area is reduced by 75% or greater and the valve area may double (Figure 15.2b). An excellent response is noted in an adult in Figure 15.3. Note that there is still a residual gradient sufficient to label the patient as having severe aortic stenosis. Nevertheless, the hallmarks of improvement are all present: the pulse pressure has widened from 60 mm Hg to 90 mm Hg, the dP/dt has improved dramatically, and left ventricular pressure has decreased by 10 mm Hg while systemic pressure has risen by 40 mm Hg. The improvement in pressure upslope can be seen and measured as in Figure 15.7. The extent of improvement may be related to the size of the balloon used; an example is seen in Figure 15.8. Here the gradient has decreased from a peak to peak of nearly 100 mm Hg to approximately 60 mm Hg after a 15 mm diameter balloon inflation, and it has decreased to approximately 40 mm Hg after an 18 mm diameter balloon inflation. Typical inflations in adults utilize 20 mm or larger balloons.

Hemodynamics during balloon inflation can be dramatic and quite variable, depending on the contractile reserve of the left ventricle, extent of occlusion of the aortic valve by the balloon, status of the conduction system, presence of any coronary artery disease, and overall hemodynamic status of the patient. Thus, left ventricular pressure may rise initially as contraction takes place against a balloon-obstructed aortic valve; and it can fall precipitously, along with systemic pressure, in patients with a compromised hemodynamic state. In patients in cardiogenic shock or a low-output state prior to inflation, the infinite relative afterload may result in a "spiraling down" where the left ventricle never recovers; this is the setting in which much early mortality associated with PBAV occurs. Hemodynamics during inflation were reported by Bittl *et al.* [12], who demonstrated a direct correlation between peak left ventricular systolic pressure after balloon inflation and left ventricular function,

Figure 15.7 Effect of balloon valvuloplasty on pressure rise (dP/dt) over time using micromanometer catheters. (a) Systemic pressure is 87 mm Hg, rising to 110 mm Hg after balloon dilatation in an 82-year-old woman presenting in pulmonary edema and shock. (b) The dP/dt has nearly doubled to 200 mm Hg/sec. Ao = aorta; LV = left ventricle.

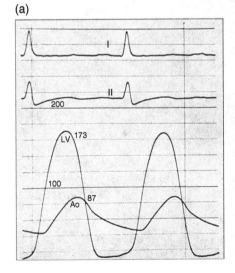

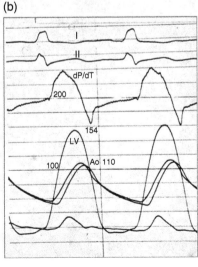

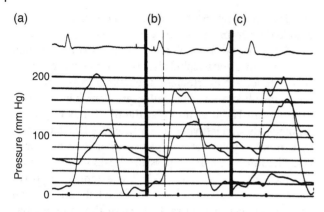

Figure 15.8 Hemodynamic tracings of aortic and left ventricular pressures during balloon valvuloplasty. (a) The control. (b) After 15 mm balloon inflation. (c) After 18 mm balloon inflation. See text for details. *Source:* Vandormael 1988 [11]. Reproduced with permission of John Wiley & Sons.

and an inverse correlation with end-systolic wall stress. Figure 15.9 demonstrates the decline in systemic pressure seen almost invariably during balloon inflation, along with an initial rise in left ventricular pressure characteristic of patients with relatively preserved left ventricular function. Most patients recover from the transient hypotension, although hemodynamic collapse, occasionally accompanied by seizures and complete heart block, is seen, particularly in the elderly.

Post-Dilatation Hemodynamics

A gradient reduction of 50%, such as is seen in Figure 15.3b, is traditionally viewed as an acceptable result. On occasion, there is a more dramatic decrease in gradient, which may reflect a superior result or loss of integrity of the aortic valve. Severe aortic regurgitation

as a complication of PBAV is uncommon (approximately 1–2%) [13, 14], particularly in patients with severe homogeneous calcification of the aortic valve, where tearing or avulsion of leaflets is unlikely. In contrast, younger patients and those with more heterogeneous fibrosis or calcification are more prone to this complication. An example is shown in Figure 15.10. Note the substantial decrease in gradient from more than 80 mm Hg to approximately 20 mm Hg, decrease in LV systolic pressure to 150 mm Hg from 230 mm Hg, and increase in pulse pressure from 70 mm Hg to 80 mm Hg. However, several factors here suggest an unfavorable outcome and point to the diagnosis. First, systemic pressure has fallen from 140 mm Hg to 130 mm Hg rather than risen; and left ventricular end-diastolic pressure, previously in the range of 22 mm Hg, has risen to 40 mm Hg. Also striking is the diastasis between aortic and left ventricular pressure seen during the last third of diastole, a hallmark of severe aortic insufficiency. These features suggest equilibration of central aortic and left ventricular pressures, with the rise in the latter reflecting the augmented volume entering the LV retrograde during diastole.

The decrease in aortic valve gradient in this setting reflects both (i) disruption of the aortic valve with consequent decrease in obstruction to forward flow and (ii) decreased cardiac output in the setting of decreased stroke volume, characteristic of severe acute aortic insufficiency. The latter is particularly poorly tolerated in the setting of severe aortic stenosis because these patients typically have significant LV hypertrophy and are already operating on the steep portion of their pressure–volume curve. These ventricles are relatively noncompliant and cannot dilate adequately to absorb the marked regurgitant LV volume. The forward stroke volume (antegrade minus regurgitant flow) is subsequently too low to maintain cardiac output.

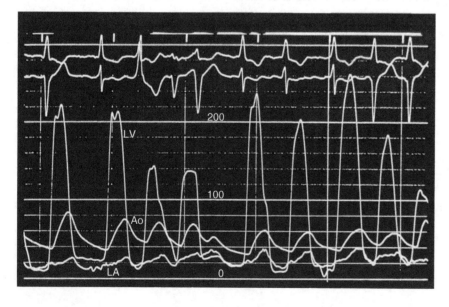

Figure 15.9 Hemodynamics during balloon inflation. Note the gradient at left of nearly 140 mm Hg. Aortic (Ao) pressure declines to approximately 60 mm Hg, while left ventricular (LV) systolic pressure rises to higher than baseline on the non-extra-systolic beats. LA = left atrium.

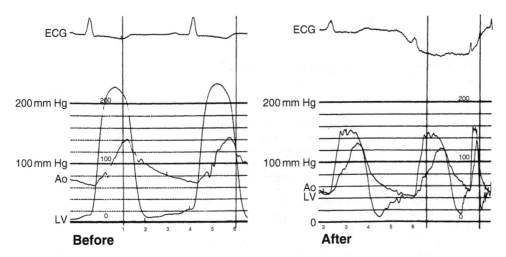

Figure 15.10 Aortic (Ao) and left ventricular (LV) pressure tracings during balloon valvuloplasty. The lower panel represents hemodynamic findings at the conclusion of the procedure. A new murmur was identified.

The situation is further compromised in this setting by the equilibration of diastolic LV and ascending aortic pressures. Because the gradient between these two drives blood flow to the subendocardium, coronary flow diminishes. This alone can cause severe ischemia, exacerbated by the characteristic increased wall mass in patients with aortic stenosis, which raises myocardial oxygen demand; if there is co-existent coronary artery disease, acute disruption of the aortic valve can be catastrophic. At the same time, myocardial oxygen demand is also increased by greater afterload and wall stress; this combination can lead to cardiogenic shock and death. The early closure of the mitral valve, a result of rapid rise of LV diastolic pressure and equilibration with left atrial pressure, can be protective of the pulmonary circulation.

In Figure 15.11, an 86-year-old woman undergoing a repeat PBAV had initial tracings (Figure 15.11a) consistent with a large transvalvular gradient. However, note a wide pulse pressure (100 mm Hg) and relatively low diastolic gradient between the LV and aorta. The calculated aortic valve area was 0.5 cm². The right side of Figure 15.11a demonstrates the results of the first balloon inflation. The gradient is nearly resolved, but the LV pressures are nearly identical in both systole and diastole with a wide pulse pressure, suggesting possible catastrophic disruption of the aortic valve or, in this case, possible contribution to tenting open of the valve by a stiff guidewire. With repositioning, the prior gradient is reestablished (Figure 15.11b), and the operators persisted with redilatation. The subsequent hemodynamics (right side of Figure 15.11b; Figure 15.11c) demonstrate shock, equilibration of LV, aortic, and pulmonary artery pressures, and a massive pulmonary wedge V wave to near systemic pressures. These hemodynamics, generally not compatible with survival without prompt surgical intervention,

suggest disruption of both the aortic valve and mitral or submitral apparatus. Catecholamine infusion improved systemic pressures (Figure 15.11d) and demonstrates complete equilibration of LV and aortic pressures, in keeping with the torn aortic valve leaflet found at surgery; echocardiography confirmed severe mitral insufficiency.

Case: Aortic Valvuloplasty in a Very Elderly Woman

Dr. Ted Feldman contributes this case of a 92-year-old woman in good health who was admitted to the hospital in 2007 with progressive fatigue and dyspnea. She had had a known heart murmur for many years. Her activity was limited only by arthritis. Over the last year, she had noted episodes of dyspnea on exertion, which had been intermittent and relatively infrequent; however, two weeks prior to admission, dyspnea became markedly worse, limiting her activity and even making it difficult to walk to the bathroom from her bedroom. She was admitted with congestive heart failure and found to have critical aortic stenosis with normal left ventricular function.

Cardiac catheterization revealed mild coronary artery disease with a heavily calcified porcelain aorta. She was evaluated by surgery, but risk of mortality and morbidity for AVR at her age was felt to be unacceptable. Since her activity is still limited by dyspnea on exertion, aortic balloon valvuloplasty was thought likely to improve her activities of daily life, at least in the short run. A cardiac catheterization procedure for aortic valvuloplasty was performed as follows. A 14 F sheath was inserted in the right femoral vein with pre-closure placement of a 6 F Perclose device. Left femoral artery with a 6 F and left

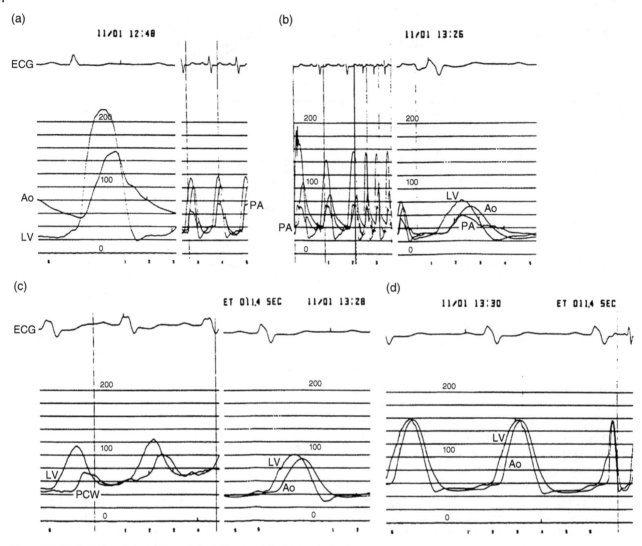

Figure 15.11 Serial hemodynamic tracings during aortic balloon valvuloplasty in an 86-year-old woman undergoing a repeat procedure. The patient required emergency surgery. See text for details. Ao = aorta; LV = left ventricle; PA = pulmonary artery; PCW = pulmonary capillary wedge. *Source:* Kern 1990 [15]. Reproduced with permission of American Heart Journal.

femoral vein with 8 F access was obtained. A 7 F balloon-tipped catheter was advanced to the right heart and pulmonary arteries for cardiac output determination, and left femoral vein access was used for left-sided hemodynamic measurements. Transseptal puncture via the right femoral vein was accomplished using a Mullins sheath and transseptal needle. A 7 F single-lumen balloon catheter was passed through the Mullins sheath into the left atrium and into the left ventricle. Anti-coagulation was then administered. A transaortic valve pressure gradient was measured (Figure 15.12). The balloon catheter was then passed antegrade across the stenotic aortic valve and into the aortic arch and descending aorta. A 260 cm long #0.032 guidewire was passed through the balloon-tipped catheter and into the descending aorta, where it was anchored by a 10 mm gooseneck snare

introduced retrograde via the 6 F arterial sheath. The Mullins sheath was removed and a 14 F rigid dilator passed across the atrial septum. An Inoue 26 mm diameter balloon catheter was then passed via the left atrium, positioned in the aortic valve for valvuloplasty. The balloon was inflated to 25 mm diameter and hemodynamic assessments of transvalvular gradients were repeated (Figures 15.13, 15.14, and 15.15). The balloon catheter was then removed. The right femoral venous sheath was removed using the existing suture over guidewire. Hemostasis was secured and the guidewire was removed. The left femoral arterial sheath was removed using suture closure and left femoral venous sheath was controlled with manual compression. There were no complications during the procedure. The findings of the procedure are shown in Table 15.1.

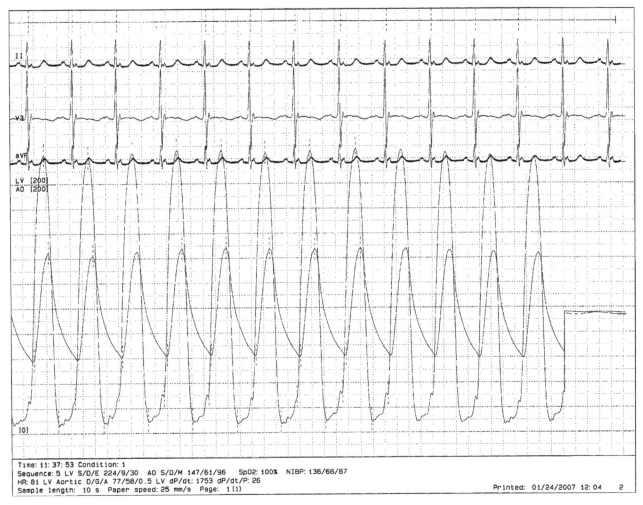

II

v3

aVF

LV [200]
AO [200]

[0]

Time: 11:37:53 Condition: 1
Sequence: 5 LV S/D/E 224/9/30 AO S/D/M 147/61/96 SpO2: 100% NIBP: 136/68/87
HR: 81 LV Aortic D/G/A 77/58/0.5 LV dP/dt: 1753 dP/dt/P: 26
Sample length: 10 s Paper speed: 25 mm/s Page: 1(1)
Printed: 01/24/2007 12:04 2

Figure 15.12 Aortic (AO) and left ventricular (LV) pressures, demonstrating aortic stenosis mean gradient of 57 mm Hg and peak gradient of 80 mm Hg.

The severe aortic stenosis was treated successfully with single antegrade balloon valvuloplasty, with improvement in valve area from 0.49 to 0.95 cm^2. The patient had symptomatic relief and returned to a functional status.

Case: Reduction of Mitral Regurgitation after Aortic Valvuloplasty

Dr. Ted Feldman contributed this case of an 80-year-old woman with symptomatic severe aortic stenosis who was referred for aortic balloon valvuloplasty. She had a history of coronary artery bypass graft surgery in 2001, complicated by acute renal failure following preoperative coronary angiography. At that time, she did not have a significant aortic stenosis. Coronary bypass vessels included saphenous vein graft to the posterior descending branch of the right coronary

artery and marginal branch of the circumflex. The left anterior descending artery was bypassed with a sequential Y graft as well. The internal mammary artery was used to bypass the distal left anterior descending coronary artery. At presentation, she complained of progressive exertional dyspnea in New York Heart Association Class III with dyspnea on showering and walking short distances. A recent echocardiogram showed atrial enlargement, severely reduced left ventricular function, moderate mitral regurgitation, and no significant aortic regurgitation. The calcified aortic stenosis was estimated at a valve area of 0.6–0.7 cm^2.

Using local anesthesia, a 14 F sheath was inserted into the right femoral vein after pre-closure with the 6 F Perclose device. Left femoral arterial access was obtained with a 6 F sheath and left femoral venous access with an 8 F sheath. A 5 F pacing wire was inserted to the right ventricle via the left femoral vein access. A 7 F

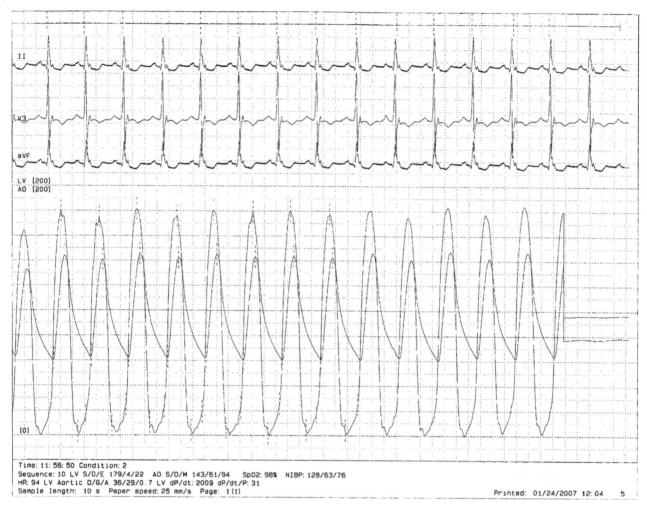

Time: 11: 56: 50 Condition: 2
Sequence: 10 LV S/D/E 179/4/22 AO S/D/M 143/61/94 SpO2: 98% NIBP: 128/63/76
HR: 94 LV Aortic D/G/A 36/29/0.7 LV dP/dt: 2009 dP/dt/P: 31
Sample length: 10 s Paper speed: 25 mm/s Page: 1 (1)
Printed: 01/24/2007 12: 04 5

Figure 15.13 Post-valvuloplasty arterial (AO) and left ventricular (LV) pressures showing post-valvuloplasty gradient of approximately 30 mm Hg.

balloon-tipped catheter was used for right-heart pressure measurements and cardiac output determination. A transseptal puncture was performed via the right femoral vein with standard technique using a Mullins sheath and a transseptal needle. A 7 F single-lumen balloon catheter was passed through the Mullins sheath into the left atrium and into the left ventricle. Anti-coagulant heparin was administered. The transaortic valve pressure gradient was measured (Figure 15.16). The balloon catheter was then passed antegrade across the stenotic aortic valve and into the aortic arch and descending aorta. A 0.032 inch guidewire was passed through the balloon-tipped catheter and a snare from the left femoral artery was used to fix the 0.032 guidewire in the descending aorta. The Mullins sheath was removed and a 14 F rigid dilator passed across the intra-atrial septum. An Inoue 26 mm diameter balloon catheter was passed via the left atrium and positioned in the aortic valve. The balloon was inflated twice to 25 mm to accomplish aortic dilatation. Hemodynamic assessments were repeated (Figure 15.17).

Left atrial and left ventricular pressures demonstrated significant V waves prior to aortic balloon valvuloplasty (Figure 15.18) and significant reduction of the atrial V wave following the valvuloplasty (Figure 15.19).

Catheters were removed and the right femoral vein sheath removed using the existing suture over a guidewire. When hemostasis was secure, the guidewire was removed. The left femoral arterial sheath was removed using suture closure, and the left femoral vein sheath was removed with manual compression. There were no complications of the procedure. Table 15.2 summarizes the hemodynamic data.

In summary, the severe aortic stenosis was successfully treated with balloon aortic valvuloplasty, resulting in improvement of the aortic valve area from 0.7 to 1.1 cm^2 and a reduction in left atrial pressure from 29 to 17 mm Hg. The relief of aortic stenosis resulted in afterload reduction with improved mitral regurgitation. The diminished left atrial V wave is the result.

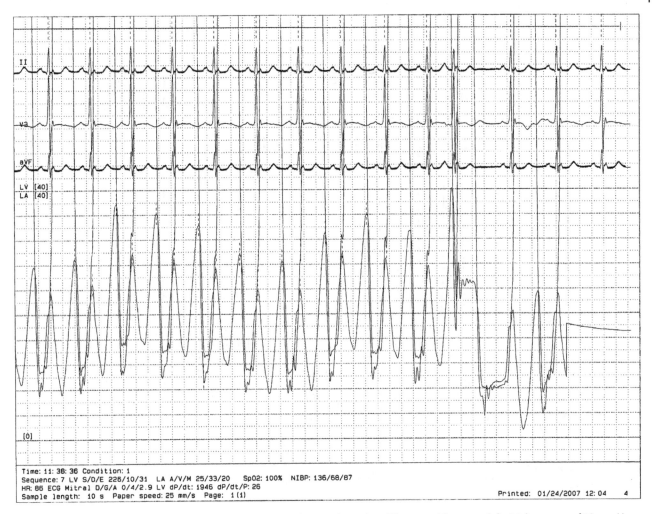

II

v3

aVF

LV [40]
LA [40]

[0]

Time: 11: 38: 36 Condition: 1
Sequence: 7 LV S/D/E 226/10/31 LA A/V/M 25/33/20 SpO2: 100% NIBP: 136/68/87
HR: 86 ECG Mitral D/G/A 0/4/2.9 LV dP/dt: 1946 dP/dt/P: 26
Sample length: 10 s Paper speed: 25 mm/s Page: 1 (1)

Printed: 01/24/2007 12: 04 4

Figure 15.14 Left atrial (LA) and left ventricular (LV) pressure showing large A and V waves with a mean left atrial pressure of 18 mm Hg.

Transcatheter and Doppler Waveforms before and after Transaortic Valve Replacement

Dr. Raj Makkar, pre-eminent interventional cardiologist at Cedar Sinai Medical Center in Los Angeles, CA, graciously provided us with examples of hemodynamics obtained before, during, and after the performance of TAVR.

Hemodynamics used to guide TAVR are obtained from both noninvasive and invasive modalities. The operator can use these techniques with confidence when understanding the limitations of each method. Figure 15.20 shows the similarities between observed intra-procedural transcatheter waveforms in panel a(i), top) with nonsimultaneous pulmonary capillary wedge pressure (PCWP) superimposed. The classic LV–aortic gradient with slow aortic upslope (red line) and loss of dichrotic notch are well demonstrated. The right side of this figure shows post TAVR the Edwards Sapien bioprosthesis (b(i)) result, with elimination of the aortic valve gradient, restoration of the anachrotic shoulder, and dichrotic notch. The PCW "v" wave was reduced after TAVR suggested reduced LV outflow resistance. The panels below the echocardiographic Doppler waveforms show (a(ii)) transcatheter hemodynamic tracings with left ventricular and aortic waveforms; (a(iii)) pulsed-wave (PW) Doppler at the tip of the mitral leaflets; (a(iv)) PW Doppler in the LVOT; and (a(iv)) CW Doppler across the aortic valve.

The duration of upstroke of the aortic arterial waveform as the solid red and solid green lines in panel b(i) corresponds to the AT (acceleration time) in panel b(iv). The DFP (diastolic filling period) in panel b(i) corresponds to the duration of the period between the start of the E wave (early passive LV filling) and the end of the A (atrial contraction) wave of the mitral inflow seen during diastole in panel b(ii). The "p" wave of the electrocardiogram corresponds to the A wave in panel b(ii), while the

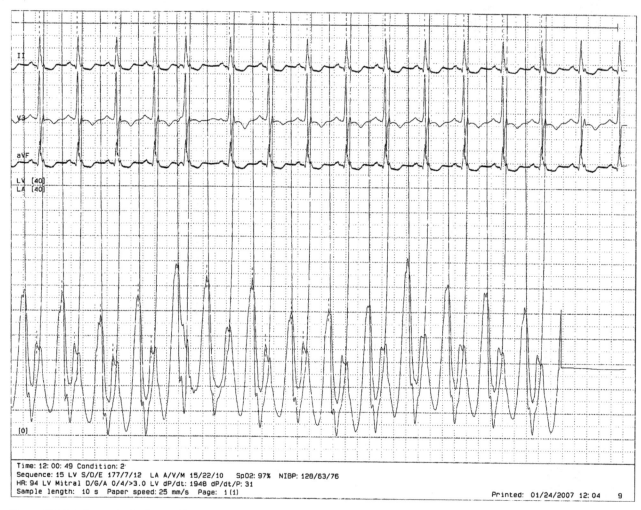

```
Time: 12: 00: 49 Condition: 2
Sequence: 15 LV S/D/E 177/7/12  LA A/V/M 15/22/10   SpO2: 97%  NIBP: 128/63/76
HR: 94 LV Mitral D/G/A 0/4/>3.0 LV dP/dt: 1948 dP/dt/P: 31
Sample length: 10 s  Paper speed: 25 mm/s  Page: 1 (1)
                                                          Printed: 01/24/2007 12: 04    9
```

Figure 15.15 Left ventricular (LV) and left atrial (LA) pressure measurements following valvuloplasty showing a mean left atrial pressure of 14 mm Hg.

Table 15.1 Hemodynamic data.

Site	Pressures at Rest (a/v/mean), (s/d/mean)	Pressures Following Valvuloplasty
Right atrial pressure	8/4/3	
Pulmonary artery pressure	43/6/27	43/17/29
Left atrial pressure	25/33/23	15/22/10
Left ventricular pressure	226/10/31	177/7/12
Aortic pressure	146/61/95	139/57/90
Cardiac output (L/min)	6.7	
SVR (W units)	114	
PAR (unit)	250	
Mean aortic valve gradient (mm Hg)	57	32
Aortic valve area (cm²)	0.49	0.94
Heart rate (beats/min)	80	91

PAR = pulmonary vascular resistance; SVR = systemic vascular resistance.

R wave corresponds to the onset of ventricular systole which occurs on mitral valve closure (blue dashed line).

Figure 15.21 shows the assessment by catheter (a) and color-flow Doppler (b) before TAVR (i), and after TAVR (ii), with optimal bioprosthetic function in a patient with mixed aortic stenosis (AS) and regurgitation. The increased pulse pressure following a ventricular ectopic (VE) in severe AS is shown (blue arrows). The amelioration of AS is shown by reduced gradients on transcatheter assessment and the increased angle of the arterial upstroke and the return of the dichrotic notch post TAVR. Using catheter hemodynamics, severe AR is suggested by the low aortic diastolic pressure, wide pulse pressure, and low left ventricular end-diastolic pressure (LVEDP) gradient, and is confirmed on transesophageal echocardiography (TEE, lower panel) with a wide regurgitant jet. The rise in the aortic diastolic pressure and the Ao–LV end-diastolic pressure gradient and the return of a dichrotic notch are also consistent with an amelioration in aortic regurgitation (AR), which can be clearly seen on TEE. Despite no significant AR post

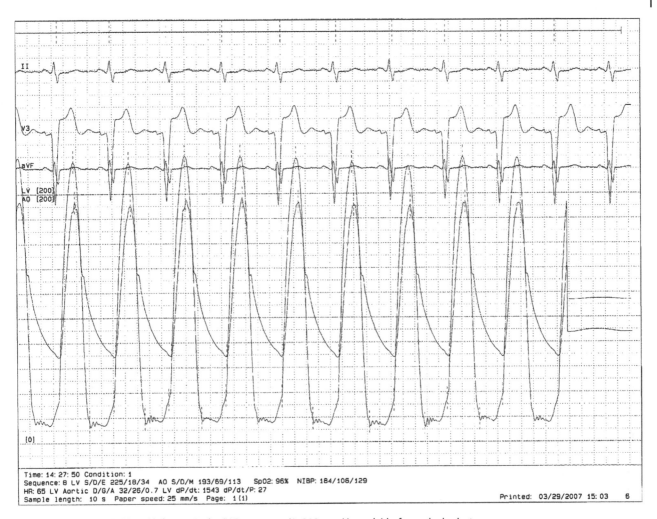

Time: 14: 27: 50 Condition: 1
Sequence: 8 LV S/D/E 225/18/34   AO S/D/M 193/69/113   SpO2: 96%   NIBP: 184/106/129
HR: 65 LV Aortic D/G/A 32/26/0.7 LV dP/dt: 1543 dP/dt/P: 27
Sample length: 10 s   Paper speed: 25 mm/s   Page: 1 (1)   Printed: 03/29/2007 15: 03   6

Figure 15.16 Aortic (AO) and left ventricular (LV) pressures (0–200 mm Hg scale) before valvuloplasty.

TAVR, there is a persistent wide pulse pressure. A rise in LVEDP is noted, but with an increase in LV pressures overall as well, again suggesting a degree of AR.

The pressure recovery of mixed aortic stenosis and regurgitation is illustrated in Figure 15.22. Auto-phase correction on (a) and removed (b) shows the simultaneous femoral artery waveform (Fem) higher than the aortic waveform (Ao) just distal to the valve. Pressure recovery is more common in small aortas (see CT, panel c). Transcatheter pressure waveforms (panel d) and color-flow Doppler (e), before TAVR (i, consistent with severe AS and AR) and after TAVR (ii), show trivial paravalvular AR and a reversed LV–femoral arterial gradient, attributable to pressure recovery.

Mitral regurgitation is often reduced to some degree after TAVR by the associated reduction of left ventricular pressure (and dilatation). Figure 15.23 shows continuous-wave (CW) Doppler without (a(i)) and with (a(ii)) echo contrast, confirming severe AS. Transcatheter (b) and accompanying short-axis color-flow Doppler (c) assessment, pre TAVR (i) and immediately post (ii), show

trivial AR, and after pressor administration (iii) show moderate AR. Mitral valve color-flow Doppler (d) is shown pre TAVR (i), after TAVR with hypotension and pressor administration (ii), and at the end of the procedure (iii). There is a progressive reduction in LV pressures (panels b(iv–v)), with an amelioration in mitral regurgitation (d(iii)).

One of the most difficult management problems for the TAVR operators is the decision to proceed in patients with low-flow, low-gradient AS. Figure 15.24 shows a patient with low-flow, low-gradient AS followed by severe AR after TAVR requiring a second valve implant (valve-in-valve). Panels a(i–iii) show dobutamine stress echocardiogram confirming severe AS and ejection fraction (EF) 25%, and peak gradient 39 mm Hg with mean gradient 25 mm Hg. Intermediate and peak stress increased peak and mean gradients from 47 to 71 mm Hg, and 33 to 40 mm Hg, respectively, with EF increasing to 45%. Transcatheter (b) and color-flow Doppler assessment (c) before TAVR (i) confirms resting peak-to-peak gradient of 25 mm Hg. Immediately post TAVR (ii), Doppler shows

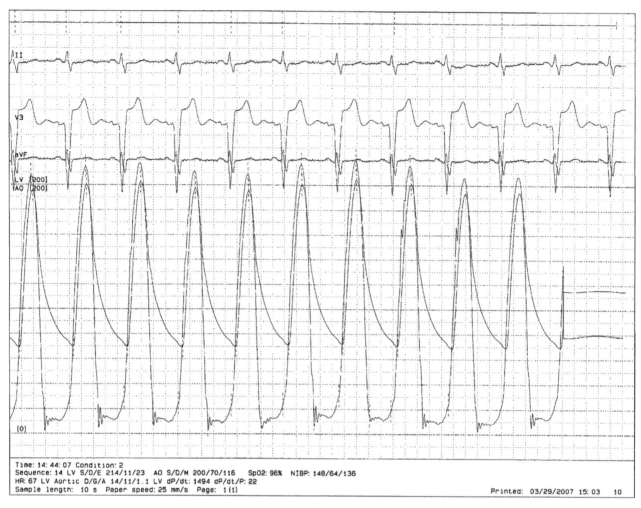

Time: 14: 44: 07 Condition: 2
Sequence: 14 LV S/D/E 214/11/23   AO S/D/M 200/70/116   SpO2: 96%   NIBP: 148/64/136
HR: 67 LV Aortic D/G/A 14/11/1.1 LV dP/dt: 1494 dP/dt/P: 22
Sample length: 10 s Paper speed: 25 mm/s Page: 1 (1)   Printed: 03/29/2007 15: 03   10

Figure 15.17 Aortic (AO) and left ventricular (LV) pressures (0–200 mm Hg scale) after valvuloplasty.

severe central aortic regurgitation at the time when aortic and LV pressures are superimposable, indicative of wide-open aortic regurgitation. This problem is remedied after valve-in-valve (iii) with only trivial central AR and optimal hemodynamic function and low gradients on color-wave Doppler (e(iii)). There is some evidence of native left coronary leaflet overhang, seen posteriorly (c(ii)), asterisk, right panel, on the long-axis view, although the AR appears to originate from failure of closure of the bioprosthetic anterior leaflet, left panel, short-axis view. In support of the evidence from the transcatheter hemodynamics (b(ii)), severe aortic regurgitation immediately post TAVR is suggested by significant diastolic flow reversal using color-wave Doppler of the descending aorta (d(i)), which ameliorates after valve-in-valve (d(ii)). Correct assessment of post TAVR CEOA includes pulsed-wave Doppler sampling (yellow squares in far right panels) in the left ventriculasr outflow tract (LVOT) before (e(i)) rather than after (e(ii)) flow convergence and color-

wave Doppler sampling (e(iii)) perpendicular to flow (yellow rectangle in far right panel).

TAVR reveals some remarkable changes in diastolic function once the aortic stenosis is resolved. Figure 15.25 is a good example of revealing mild diastolic dysfunction after TAVR. Transcatheter (a) and transmitral Doppler (b) assessment of diastology before (a(i)) and after (a(ii)) TAVR show the obvious improvement in the LV pressure ejection parameters. However, there appears to be a new restrictive filling pattern by transcatheter assessment (a(ii)) and evident on further scrutiny of the transmitral Doppler, pre (i) and post (ii) TAVR, is that this finding has not changed from baseline, with a high E/A ratio at both time points.

Paravalvular aortic regurgitation after TAVR presents with subtle changes in the LV diastolic pressure waveforms. Figure 15.26 shows (a) transcatheter hemodynamics before (i) and after (ii) TAVR. The increased slowing of the diastolic filling pressure with elevated

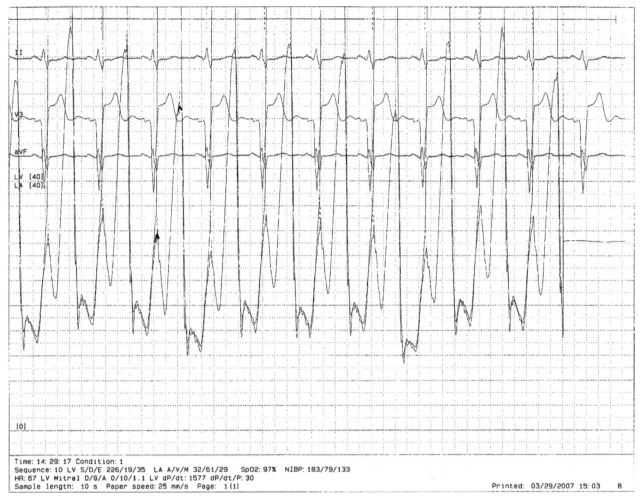

II

V3

aVF

LV [40]
LA [40]

[0]

Time: 14: 29: 17 Condition: 1
Sequence: 10 LV S/D/E 226/19/35 LA A/V/M 32/61/29 SpO2: 97% NIBP: 183/79/133
HR: 67 LV Mitral D/G/A 0/10/1.1 LV dP/dt: 1577 dP/dt/P: 30
Sample length: 10 s Paper speed: 25 mm/s Page: 1(1)   Printed: 03/29/2007 15: 03   B

Figure 15.18 Left ventricular (LV) and left atrial (LA) pressures (0–40 mm Hg scale) before aortic balloon and valvuloplasty. Note the large V waves and matching of the atrial and ventricular pressures.

LVEDP and wider pulse pressure (30 to 60 mm Hg) despite reduction of the LV–Ao gradient is highly suggestive of moderate AR. From the hemodynamics alone it is not possible to determine the origin of the AR. Use of color-flow Doppler in short-axis view after TAVR (b) nicely demonstrates paraprosthetic AR, with the circumferential extent greater than 20%, suggestive of severe AR by ASE/VARC criteria. Panel c shows color-wave Doppler in the descending aorta post TAVR with little diastolic flow reversal, suggestive of mild AR.

The acute management of TAVR-induced aortic regurgitation with rapid pacing is shown in Figure 15.27. Panel a shows transcatheter hemodynamics before (i) and after (ii) TAVR in a patient who developed heart block–related bradycardia, demonstrating widening pulse pressure with aortic and LV end-diastolic pressure equilibration at 45 mm Hg. The LV diastolic waveform increases across diastole with the increasing regurgitant volume. After right ventricular (RV) pacing post TAVR (iii), the short-

ened diastolic period produces resolution of most of the regurgitation, and reduced LV pressure rise during diastasis, increased aortic diastolic pressure and end-diastolic LV–Ao gradient, and drop in LVEDP point to no significant AR. Color-flow Doppler post TAVR (b) in the long-axis view before (i) and after (ii) post-TAVR RV pacing shows that a paravalvular color-flow jet is the cause of mild to moderate AR and does not appear to change after pacing. Color-flow Doppler post TAVR in the short-axis view (c) after post-TAVR RV pacing demonstrating a 19% circumferential extent is suggestive of moderate AR by ASE/VARC criteria. Color-wave Doppler in the descending aorta after post-TAVR RV pacing (d) shows minimal flow reversal and is suggestive of mild AR.

Diastolic dysfunction and aortic regurgitation after pacing following TAVR are shown in Figure 15.28. Panel a shows transcatheter hemodynamics and color-flow Doppler in long-axis view (b) before TAVR (i) and after

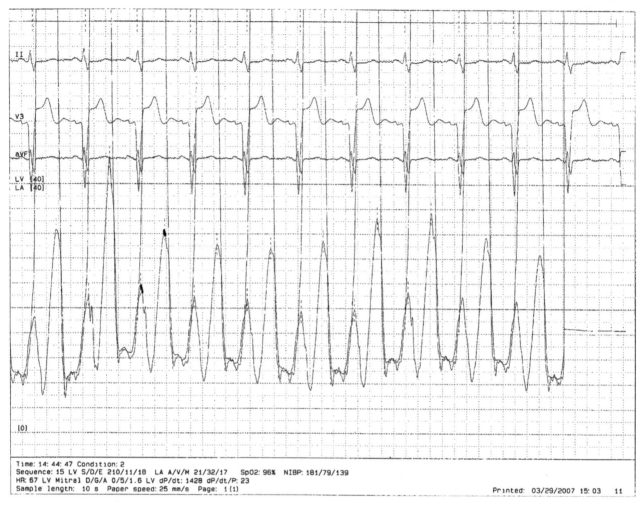

II

V3

aVF

LV [40]
LA [40]

[0]

Time: 14: 44: 47 Condition: 2
Sequence: 15 LV S/D/E 210/11/18 LA A/V/M 21/32/17   SpO2: 96% NIBP: 181/79/139
HR: 67 LV Mitral D/G/A 0/5/1.6 LV dP/dt: 1428 dP/dt/P: 23
Sample length: 10 s Paper speed: 25 mm/s Page: 1 (1)   Printed: 03/29/2007 15: 03   11

Figure 15.19 Left ventricular (LV) and left atrial (LA) pressures (0–40 mm Hg scale) after aortic balloon and valvuloplasty. Note the change in the V waves.

Table 15.2 Hemodynamic data for patient with mitral stenosis.

	Pre	Post
CO (L/min)	3.57	3.57
MV gradient (mm Hg)	26	11
MVA (cm^2)	0.69	1.12

CO = cardiac output; MV = mitral valve; MVA = mitral valve gradient.

TAVR (ii). Transcatheter and Doppler echocardiography pre TAVR are both suggestive of moderate to severe AR. Despite mild AR post TAVR seen on color-flow Doppler (b(ii)) and confirmed by the absence of significant flow reversal (c), the transcatheter findings post TAVR (a(ii)) are of a low diastolic pressure and end-diastolic LV–Ao gradient, although no rise in EDP is seen. Incremental RV pacing rate (a(iii–v)) shortens the ejection time (ET) and increases the aortic diastolic pressure without changing the LVEDP.

Mitral regurgitation after TAVR by systolic anterior motion of the anterior leaflet (AMVL) can be seen in Figure 15.29. Panel a shows transcatheter hemodynamic findings pre TAVR (i) and immediately after (ii). Color-flow Doppler findings are given at baseline (b), post TAVR (c), and at the end of the procedure, in systole (i) and diastole (ii). In the presence of a bulky intraventricular septum, relief of aortic valve stenosis increases contractility of an underfilled LV, resulting in systolic anterior motion of the AMVL (c(i), green arrow) and severe mitral regurgitation (MR). Fluid loading relieved the MR (d(i)).

Figure 15.20 Transcatheter and Doppler waveforms in aortic stenosis before (a) and after (b) transaortic valve replacement (TAVR). SEP (systolic ejection period) in panel a(i) corresponds to the ET (ejection time) in panel a(iv). AVC = aortic valve closure; AVO = aortic valve opening; dn: dicrotic notch (onset corresponds to AVC); MVC: mitral valve closure; MVO = mitral valve opening; PW = pulsed-wave. *Source:* Courtesy of Dr. Raj Makkar. (*See insert for color representation of the figure.*)

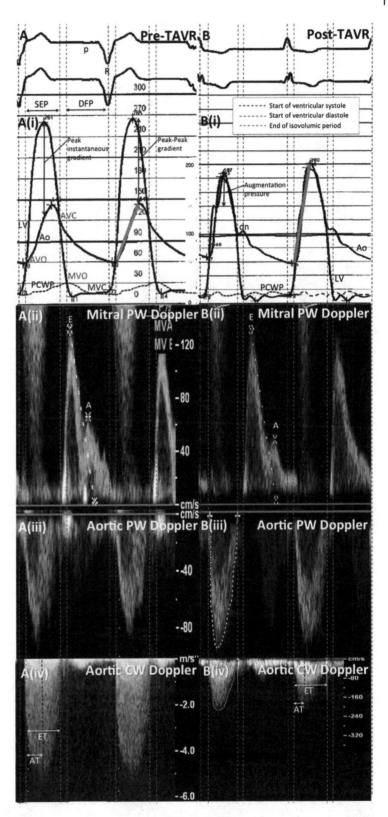

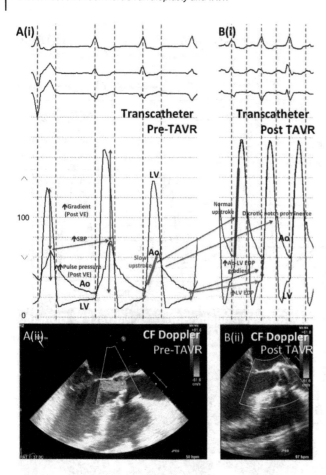

Figure 15.21 Mixed aortic stenosis and regurgitation. Assessment by catheter (top) and color-flow (CF) Doppler (bottom) before transaortic valve replacement (TAVR, A(i, ii), and after TAVR (B (i, ii)), with optimal bioprosthetic function. Ao = aorta; EDP = end-diastolic pressure; LV = left ventricle; SBP = systolic blood pressure; VE = ventricular ectopic. *Source:* Courtesy of Dr. Raj Makkar. (*See insert for color representation of the figure.*)

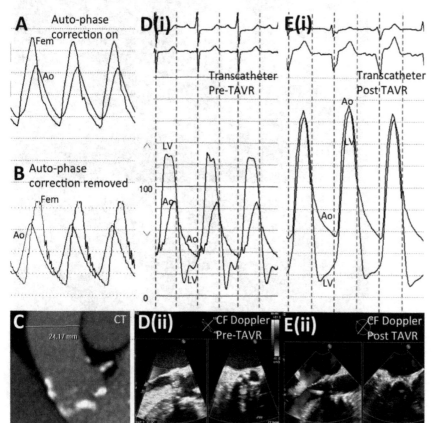

Figure 15.22 Demonstrates the phenomenon of pressure recovery in severe aortic stenosis (panels A (auto-phase correction 'on') and B (auto-phase correction 'off'))—simultaneous femoral artery (Fem) waveforms are higher than aortic (Ao) waveforms recorded just distal to the stenosed aortic valve. Pressure recovery is more common in patients with small aortas, as demonstrated on cardiac CT scan (panel C). Panels D (pre-TAVR) and E (postTAVR) show transcatheter waveforms (panel (i)) and color-flow Doppler TEE images (panel (ii)) of the aortic valve in long and short axes. There is severe mixed aortic stenosis and regurgitation, which is ameliorated following TAVR (panel E). A 'reverse' LV-femoral arterial gradient in panel E is attributable to pressure recovery. (*See insert for color representation of the figure.*)

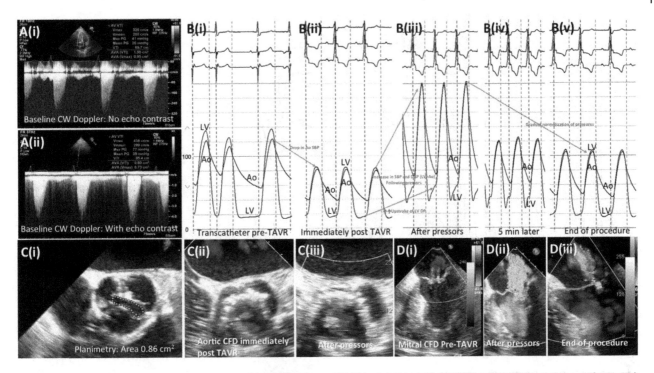

Figure 15.23 Mitral regurgitation after transaortic valve replacement (TAVR) by left ventricular (LV) dilatation. CW Doppler waveforms with (panel A(i)) and without (panel A(ii)) echocardiographic contrast agent use, and a shortaxis TEE (panel C(i)) confirming severe aortic stenosis. There is a precipitous drop in blood pressure immediately after valve implantation (likely due to rapid pacing during valve deployment) (panel B(ii)) that responds appropriately to vasopressor administration (panel B(iii))—note the change in the upstroke of LV end-diastolic pressure tracing. Ao = aorta; CFD = color-flow Doppler; CW = continuous-wave. *Source:* Courtesy of Dr. Raj Makkar. (*See insert for color representation of the figure.*)

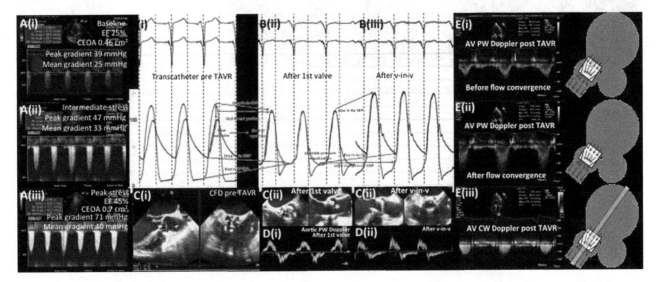

Figure 15.24 Low-flow, low-gradient aortic stenosis (AS) followed by severe aortic regurgitation (AR) post transaortic valve replacement (TAVR). AV = aorta; CEOA = continuous echo orifice area; CFD = color-flow Doppler; EF = ejection fraction; PW = pulsed-wave; v-in-v = valve-in-valve. A, B, C, D, E represent Doppler, 2D echo, C mitral valve echo, D pulmonary vein flow, E PW flow. i, ii, iii denote pre, immediately after and after final implant. *Source:* Courtesy of Dr. Raj Makkar. (*See insert for color representation of the figure.*)

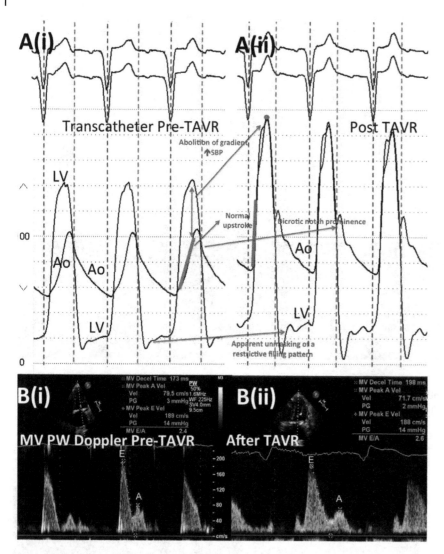

Figure 15.25 Diastolic dysfunction after transaortic valve replacement (TAVR). Ao = aorta; LV = left ventricle; MV = mitral valve; PW = pulsed-wave; SBP = systolic blood pressure. A and B represent hemodynamic and Doppler data, i, ii is pre and post TAVR periods. *Source:* Courtesy of Dr. Raj Makkar. (*See insert for color representation of the figure.*)

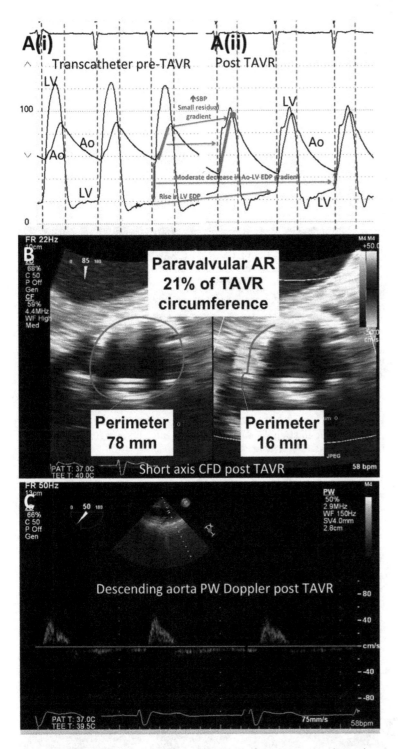

Figure 15.26 Paravalvular aortic regurgitation (AR) after transaortic valve replacement (TAVR). Ao = aorta; CFD = color-flow Doppler; LV = left ventricle; PW = pulsed-wave. A and B represent hemodynamic and Doppler data, i, ii is pre and post TAVR periods. C is descending aortic PW flow. *Source:* Courtesy of Dr. Raj Makkar. (*See insert for color representation of the figure.*)

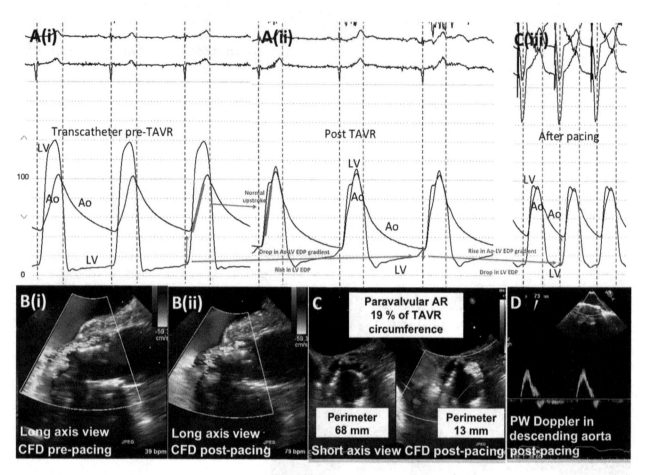

Figure 15.27 Aortic regurgitation (AR) with pacing. Ao = aorta; CFD = color-flow Doppler; LV = left ventricle; PW = pulsed-wave; TAVR = transaortic valve replacement. A and B represent hemodynamic and Doppler data, C is 2D echo and D is PW of aortic flow. i, ii is pre and post TAVR periods. *Source:* Courtesy of Dr. Raj Makkar. (*See insert for color representation of the figure.*)

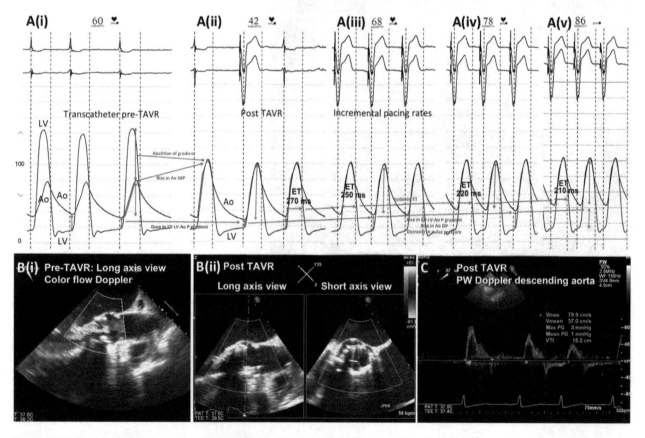

Figure 15.28 Diastolic dysfunction and aortic regurgitation (AR) after pacing. Ao = aorta; ET = ejection time; LV = left ventricle; PW = pulsed-wave; TAVR = transaortic valve replacement. A and B represent hemodynamic and Doppler data, i, ii, iii, iv, v is pre and post TAVR, pacing stablization, and final result. C is PW doppler of aortic flow. *Source:* Courtesy of Dr. Raj Makkar. (*See insert for color representation of the figure.*)

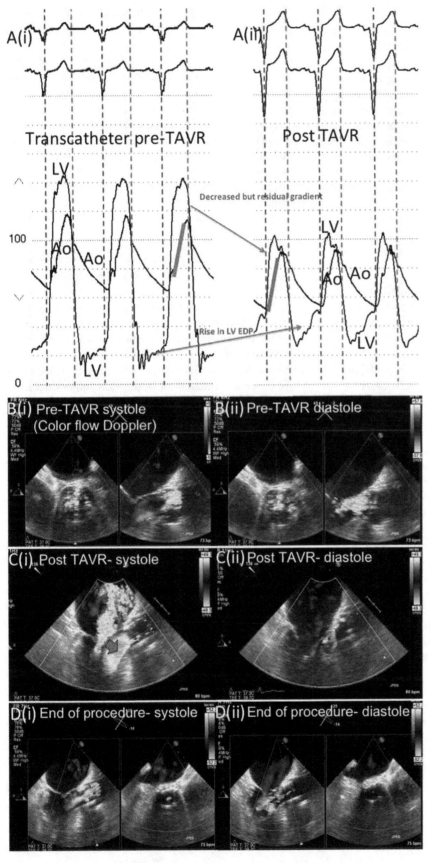

Figure 15.29 Mitral regurgitation after transaortic valve replacement (TAVR) by systolic anterior motion of the anterior leaflet (AMVL). Ao = aorta; EDP = end-diastolic pressure; LV = left ventricle. A and B represent hemodynamic and Doppler data, C and D is color Doppler signals. i, ii is pre and post TAVR periods. *Source:* Courtesy of Dr. Raj Makkar. (*See insert for color representation of the figure.*)

Key Points

1) In contrast to percutaneous balloon aortic valvuloplasty, percutaneous balloon mitral valvuloplasty has been shown to be superior to surgery in patients with appropriate anatomic features and is still the procedure of choice for patients with mitral valve stenosis.
2) For most accurate hemodynamic data collection in aortic stenosis, use a dual = lumen catheter or two catheters (or pressure wire) above and below the aortic valve.
3) The relief of aortic stenosis reduces left ventricular afterload and can improve mitral regurgitation in some patients.
4) One of the most difficult decisions for the transaortic valve replacement operators is the decision proceed in patients with low-flow, low-gradient aortic stenosis. Additional testing is usually required.
5) Paravalvular aortic regurgitation after transaortic valve replacement presents with subtle changes in the left ventricular diastolic pressure waveforms.

References

1 Kern MJ. Pulmonary valvuloplasty. In MJ Kern (ed.), *Hemodynamic Rounds*, 2nd ed. New York: Wiley-Liss, 1993, pp. 129–136.
2 Lieberman EB, Bashore TM, Hermiller JB, Wilson JS, Pieper KS, Keeler GP, *et al.* Balloon aortic valvuloplasty in adults: Failure of procedure to improve long-term survival. *J Am Coll Cardiol* 26:1522–1528, 1995.
3 Bonow RO, Carabello BA, Chatterjee K, de Leon AC Jr, Faxon DP, Freed MD, *et al.* ACC/AHA 2006 guidelines for the management of patients with valvular heart disease: A report of the American College of Cardiology/American Heart Association Task Force on Practice Guidelines (Writing Committee to Revise the 1998 guidelines for the management of patients with valvular heart disease) developed in collaboration with the Society of Cardiovascular Anesthesiologists endorsed by the Society for Cardiovascular Angiography and Interventions and the Society of Thoracic Surgeons. *J Am Coll Cardiol* 48:e1–e148, 2006.
4 Reyes VP, Raju BS, Wynne J, Stephenson LW, Raju R, Fromm BS, *et al.* Percutaneous balloon valvuloplasty compared with open surgical commissurotomy for mitral stenosis. *N Engl J Med* 331:961–967, 1994.
5 Roberts WC, Ko JM. Frequency by decades of unicuspid, bicuspid, and tricuspid aortic valves in adults having isolated aortic valve replacement for aortic stenosis, with or without associated aortic regurgitation. *Circulation* 111:920–925, 2005.
6 Cribier A, Eltchaninoff H, Tron C, Bauer F, Agatiello C, Nercolini D, *et al.* Treatment of calcific aortic stenosis with the percutaneous heart valve: Mid-term follow-up from the initial feasibility studies: The French experience. *J Am Coll Cardiol* 47:1214–1223, 2006.
7 Carabello BA. Advances in the hemodynamic assessment of stenotic cardiac valves. *J Am Coll Cardiol* 10:912–919, 1987.
8 Turi ZG. Whom do you trust? Misguided faith in the catheter- or Doppler-derived aortic valve gradient. *Catheter Cardiovasc Intervent* 65:180–182, 2005.
9 Folland ED, Parisi AF, Carbone C. Is peripheral arterial pressure a satisfactory substitute for ascending aortic pressure when measuring aortic valve gradients? *J Am Coll Cardiol* 4:1207–1212, 1984.
10 Gorlin R, Gorlin SG. Hydraulic formula for calculation of the area of the stenotic mitral valve, other cardiac valves, and central circulatory shunts. *Am Heart J* 41:1–29, 1951.
11 Vandormael M, Deligonul U, Gabliani G, Chaitman B, Kern MJ. Percutaneous balloon valvuloplasty and coronary angioplasty for the treatment of calcific aortic stenosis and obstructive coronary artery disease in an elderly patient. *Cathet Cardiovasc Diagn* 14:49–52, 1988.
12 Bittl JA, Bhatia SJ, Plappert T, Ganz P, St John Sutton MG, Selwyn AP. Peak left ventricular pressure during percutaneous aortic balloon valvuloplasty: Clinical and echocardiographic correlations. *J Am Coll Cardiol* 14:135–142, 1989.
13 Isner JM. Acute catastrophic complications of balloon aortic valvuloplasty. The Mansfield Scientific Aortic Valvuloplasty Registry Investigators. *J Am Coll Cardiol* 17:1436–1444, 1991.
14 McKay RG. The Mansfield Scientific Aortic Valvuloplasty Registry: Overview of acute hemodynamic results and procedural complications. *J Am Coll Cardiol* 17:485–491, 1991.
15 Kern MJ, Deligonul U, Serota H, Gudipati C, Ring M, Aguirre F. Acute combined aortic and mitral regurgitation during balloon catheter valvuloplasty for a third recurrence of critical aortic stenosis. *Am Heart J* 120:1007–1011, 1990.

16

Percutaneous Balloon Mitral Valvuloplasty

Morton J. Kern, Paul Sorajja, and Zoltan Turi

In contrast to aortic valve dilatation, the percutaneous approach to mitral stenosis is the preferred treatment if subvalvular disease, calcification, thickening, and mobility of the valve leaflets are moderate or less, mitral valve regurgitation is no greater than mild, and thrombus is not present in the left atrium. The results of percutaneous balloon mitral valvuloplasty (PBMV) are equal to [1] or superior to surgical commissurotomy [2, 3]. There is a steep learning curve for this procedure, and the rate of success and complications correlate strongly with experience; both success and avoidance of complications are predicated in part on appreciating the subtleties of hemodynamics during the screening and intra-procedure phases of management.

Hemodynamic Screening for Mitral Stenosis

Several factors may confound the baseline hemodynamic evaluation of mitral valve stenosis. As with aortic stenosis, the gradient is dependent on flow across the valve; because of the lower overall pressures in the atria, changes in volume, such as those caused by fasting prior to catheterization, can have a significant impact on gradient. In addition, the compliance of the left atrium can be quite variable. Figure 16.1a demonstrates the effect of 100 mL of intravenous saline on the gradient across the mitral valve in a patient catheterized in the late afternoon after having fasted for nearly 18 hours. Note the near doubling of the gradient. Similarly, exercise can demonstrate a striking increase in gradient; in the same patient (Figure 16.1b), the gradient nearly tripled with arm exercise. Exercise at least has two effects that increase the gradient: (i) it increases heart rate, which disproportionately decreases the diastolic filling period; and (ii) it increases contractility, which increases flow across the valve. Finally, in both mitral and aortic

stenosis patients with depressed left ventricular (LV) function, the infusion of an inotrope, which also increases contractility and transvalvular flow, can have a dramatic effect on the gradient, as seen in Figure 16.1c.

As with aortic valve stenosis, there are distinct pitfalls in the assessment of the mitral valve gradient. Figure 16.2 demonstrates the gradient seen in a 58-year-old woman with known mitral stenosis referred to us for PBMV. Her valve area was reported to be $1.5 \, cm^2$ by echocardiography, and she was appropriately symptomatic. The initial LV versus pulmonary wedge tracing is seen in Figure 16.2a. The gradient appears to be substantial; by failing to appreciate the hemodynamic significance of the rest of the findings on this tracing, such patients are unfortunately subjected to balloon dilatation. In fact, attention should be paid to two factors. First, there is a V wave to more than 40 mm Hg, always a concern for possible mitral regurgitation. Second, there is diastasis in late cycle, which is not characteristic of mitral stenosis (see subsequent examples in Figures 16.3 and 16.4). Occasionally, on very long cycles, because the diastolic filling period is enhanced with bradycardia, diastasis can be seen even with moderate mitral stenosis (Figure 16.5), but in Figure 16.2a the heart rate was in the 70s. Transseptal puncture and direct left atrial pressure recording solved the mystery: the wedge tracing was characteristic of mixed mitral stenosis and insufficiency, with predominantly the latter. A rapid falloff of the left atrial pressure can be seen in Figure 16.2b, with minimal gradient during most of diastole. Figure 16.2c highlights the limitation of relying on the wedge pressure for determining the mitral valve gradient: the reflection of left atrial pressure across the pulmonary capillary bed results in damping and phase delay and consequent gross overestimation of the gradient [4]. Thus there is a substantial incremental gradient between the pulmonary wedge and left atrial pressures, clearly seen in the right panel.

Hemodynamic Rounds: Interpretation of Cardiac Pathophysiology from Pressure Waveform Analysis, Fourth Edition.
Edited by Morton J. Kern, Michael J. Lim, and James A. Goldstein.
© 2018 John Wiley & Sons Ltd. Published 2018 by John Wiley & Sons Ltd.

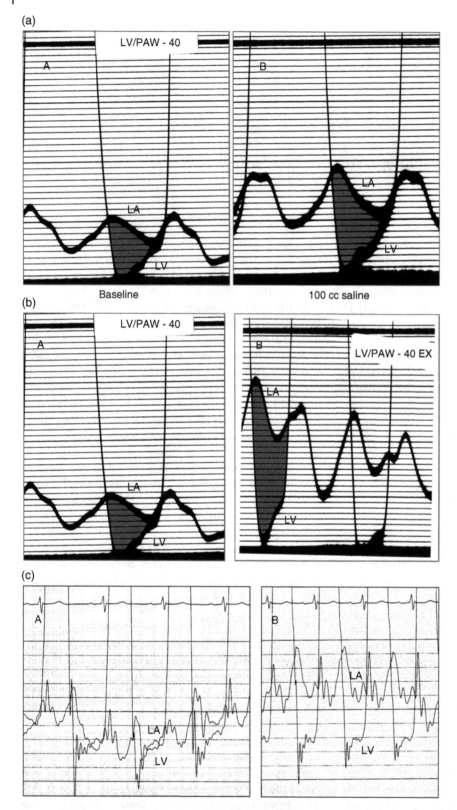

Figure 16.1 Three manipulations that affect mitral valve gradient, all 40 mm Hg scale. (a) Before and after 100 mL of volume infusion. (b) Before and after exercise (note the threefold increase in gradient with increased heart rate). (c) After dobutamine infusion, 10 µg/kg. In the latter case, the gradient was virtually absent in a sedated and somewhat volume-depleted patient. LA = left atrium; LV = left ventricle; PAW = pulmonary artery wedge.

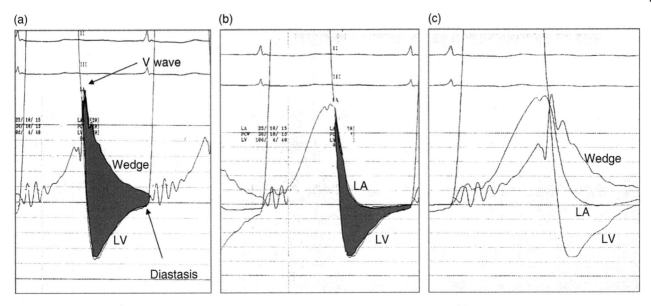

Figure 16.2 Pulmonary wedge, transseptal left atrial (LA), and left ventricular (LV) pressures, all on a 40 mm Hg scale. The pressures were recorded within one minute of each other. (a) Pulmonary capillary Wedge pressure, Wedge with LV, (b) LA with LV pressure, (c) both Wedge and LA with LV pressures. The gray shade illustrates the valve gradient measured with each technique. See text for discussion.

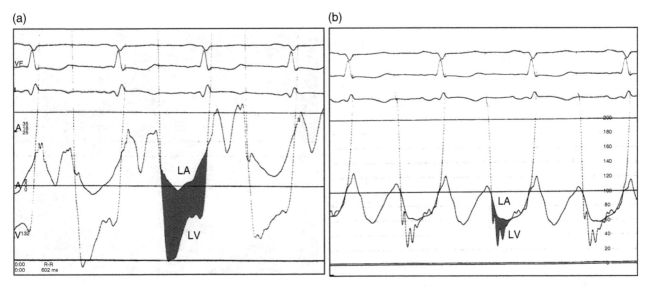

Figure 16.3 Left atrial (LA) and left ventricular (LV) pressures on 40 mm Hg scale. Note the gradient pre-dilatation (a) of approximately 12 mm Hg reduced to essentially 0 mm Hg with diastasis early during diastole (b). A single balloon inflation resulted in an abolition of the gradient that should not be the goal; the absence of a gradient after percutaneous balloon mitral valvuloplasty more commonly correlates with severe mitral insufficiency. In this case, the left atrial mean pressure has fallen from 24 to 14 mm Hg and the V wave has fallen from 34 to 21 mm Hg, while left ventricular end-diastolic pressure has risen from 12 to 15 mm Hg. The latter does not suggest significant mitral regurgitation: increasing forward flow from the left atrium to the left ventricle typically causes a mild increase in LV end-diastolic pressure due to the displacement along the LV pressure–volume curve.

Balloon Dilatation

PBMV results in a gradient decrease of 50% or more and a valve area increase to 1.5 cm^2, the definition of success in most of the literature. In ideal valve anatomy the mitral valve area will typically increase to 1.8 cm^2 or more.

Figure 16.3 demonstrates the results of PBMV in an ideal patient, a 27-year-old Caribbean native with complete resolution of the gradient after a single balloon inflation. Although occasionally seen, this result should not be sought out: in many cases with an absent gradient after balloon dilatation, there is severe mitral insufficiency.

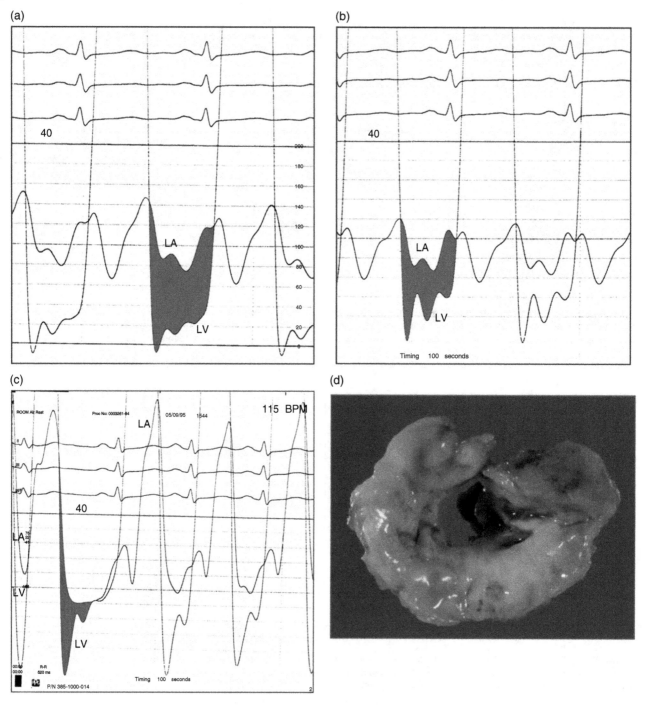

Figure 16.4 Hemodynamics (a) at baseline, (b) post first inflation, and (c) after second inflation. (d) Appearance of the mitral valve at surgery. See text for discussion. LA = left atrium; LV = left ventricle.

However, the hemodynamics suggest a competent valve; in fact, no mitral regurgitation was detected by echo except for the characteristic minimal peri-commissural leak seen with successful PBMV.

The typical stepwise Inoue balloon technique for PBMV involves assessing a maximal balloon size using the patient's height; inflations usually begin with a bal-

loon size several millimeters smaller. After each inflation the patient is assessed for reduction of gradient and induction of any new mitral regurgitation. This is done by a combination of echocardiography (transesophageal or intracardiac echo and occasionally by transthoracic echo, though the latter has technical limitations in a recumbent patient) and hemodynamics, and in many

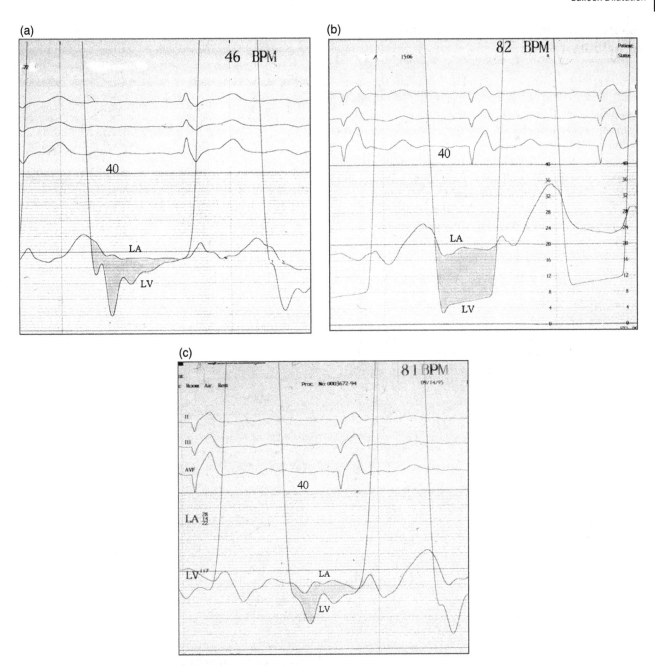

Figure 16.5 (a) Left atrial (LA) and left ventricular (LV) pressures before balloon dilatation in a patient with severe mitral stenosis at baseline; note heart rate of 46 beats/min. (b) After institution of pacing, the gradient has risen dramatically. (c) After balloon dilatation, the final gradient is again minimal despite pacing to a heart rate of 81 beats/min.

developing countries it is done by careful physical examination between inflations. A decrease in gradient of at least 50% and particularly an increase in mitral insufficiency by one grade will usually be indications to discontinue further inflations; otherwise the balloon is increased in size by 1 mm and repeat inflation is performed. Figure 16.4 shows this stepwise dilatation technique with an unfortunate result. The initial tracing (Figure 16.4a) is consistent with severe mitral stenosis in a 38-year-old severely symptomatic woman. After initial inflation the gradient is significantly lowered (Figure 16.4b), but the improvement was judged to be moderate only, with substantial residual gradient and no diastasis at late cycle. The subsequent inflation with a 1 mm larger balloon resulted in abolition of the gradient, but a rise in the V wave to 70 mm Hg (Figure 16.4c), consistent with wide open mitral insufficiency. A picture of the patient's valve taken at surgery (Figure 16.4d) shows a catastrophic tear of the valve leaflet. She did well after emergency mitral valve replacement.

Cases: Percutaneous Balloon Mitral Valvuloplasty

A 44-year-old woman with mitral stenosis had dyspnea (New York Heart Association Class III symptoms). Before the valvuloplasty (Figure 16.6, upper panel), the mean mitral valve gradient (shaded area) was 16 mm Hg and the mitral valve area was 1.0 cm². A double balloon technique (two 18 mm × 4 cm balloons) was used. Immediately after BMV (Figure 16.6, lower panel), the mean gradient decreased to 5 mm Hg and the mitral valve area increased to 2.1 cm². Note the reduction of the V wave. These tracings depict a fairly typical result.

As in the case shown in Figure 16.3, in some patients it is possible to achieve completely normal-appearing diastolic left atrial and left ventricular pressure tracings. The patient was a 75-year-old man with increasing exertional dyspnea (New York Heart Association Class III symptoms) and hemophilia B. The hemodynamics before BMV (Figure 16.7, upper panel) showed a significant mean mitral gradient with prominent V waves. After BMV (Figure 16.7, lower panel), there was a marked decrease in mitral gradient with normal appearance of

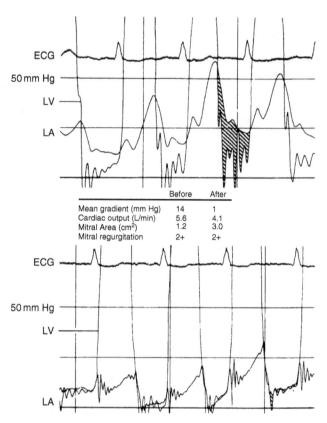

	Before	After
Mean gradient (mm Hg)	14	1
Cardiac output (L/min)	5.6	4.1
Mitral Area (cm²)	1.2	3.0
Mitral regurgitation	2+	2+

Figure 16.7 Hemodynamic tracings obtained before and after mitral valvuloplasty. LA = left atrium; LV = left ventricle. See text for details. *Source:* Kern 2015 [5]. Reproduced with permission of Elsevier.

left atrial pressure tracing. Mitral valve area increased from 1.2 cm² to 3.0 cm².

With a successful BMV the pulmonary vascular resistance decreases significantly as a result of decreased pulmonary wedge pressure and increased cardiac output. The pulmonary artery pressure may continue to decrease gradually after PBMV.

Mitral Regurgitation and Percutaneous Balloon Mitral Valvuloplasty

Although a mild increase in pre-existent mitral regurgitation or the new appearance of mild mitral regurgitation after BMV may occur in up to 55% of patients, severe mitral regurgitation requiring valve replacement is uncommon [6]. Figure 16.8 depicts a somewhat less dramatic hemodynamic response to severe mitral regurgitation after balloon inflation than that seen in Figure 16.4. Before BMV (Figure 16.8, upper panel), the A wave was greater than the V wave. There was no angiographic mitral regurgitation, and the V wave morphology, likewise, did not suggest

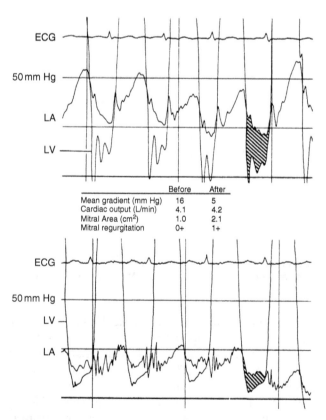

	Before	After
Mean gradient (mm Hg)	16	5
Cardiac output (L/min)	4.1	4.2
Mitral Area (cm²)	1.0	2.1
Mitral regurgitation	0+	1+

Figure 16.6 Hemodynamic tracings obtained before and after mitral valvuloplasty. LA = left atrium; LV = left ventricle. See text for details. *Source:* Kern 2015 [5]. Reproduced with permission of Elsevier.

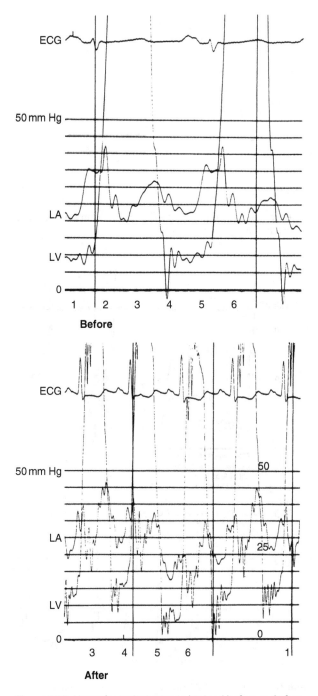

Figure 16.8 Hemodynamic tracings obtained before and after balloon valvuloplasty in a patient who developed an increased systolic murmur. See text for details. LA = left atrium; LV = left ventricle.

significant hemodynamic mitral regurgitation. After BMV (Figure 16.8, lower panel), the V wave is somewhat larger and more peaked, but there is no "giant" V wave as would be expected in acute severe mitral regurgitation. The enlarged and compliant left atrium (due to longstanding mitral stenosis) and left atrial decompression via the new

"atrial septal defect" created to facilitate atrial septal balloon passage are potential mechanisms influencing the V wave morphology, despite severe angiographic mitral regurgitation.

The mitral regurgitation may improve or occasionally may worsen during follow-up [7]. We have observed a patient with severe mitral stenosis and mild aortic regurgitation who had no mitral regurgitation after BMV, but returned eight months later with severe mitral regurgitation and congestive heart failure [8]. Simultaneous left atrial and left ventricular pressure tracings before, immediately after, and eight months after BMV for this patient are shown in Figure 16.9. On the later hemodynamic study (Figure 16.9c), the development of a large V wave in the left atrial tracing and elevated left ventricular end-diastolic pressure with no significant gradient at end-diastole was a striking new finding. During mitral valve surgery, no mitral leaflet tears or perforations were found. Only one elongated and thin chord attaching to the posterior leaflet was noted to be ruptured. In this patient, worsening aortic regurgitation after relief of mitral stenosis may also have played a role in cardiac decompensation.

Mitral Stenosis and Valvuloplasty

Case #1

Examine the hemodynamic data obtained in a 52-year-old woman with mitral stenosis and Class III symptoms (Figure 16.10, upper panel). The tracings show atrial fibrillation with well-demarcated left atrial C waves and large V waves (up to 55 mm Hg). The mitral gradient was 16 mm Hg before valvuloplasty with a cardiac output of 4.1 L/min, yielding a calculated mitral valve area of 1.0 cm^2. There was no angiographic mitral regurgitation, also confirmed by transesophageal echocardiography, which is now performed in all our patients to document the absence of left atrial thrombus prior to mitral valvuloplasty. Balloon mitral valvuloplasty using a standard two-balloon technique [1, 9] produced a marked reduction in the left atrial pressure and mitral valve gradient (Figure 16.10, lower panel). After valvuloplasty, the mean gradient was 5 mm Hg, cardiac output was unchanged (4.2 L/min), and the calculated mitral valve area increased to 2.1 cm^2 with new but mild (1+) mitral regurgitation. Note the differences in the left atrial pressure waveform after valvuloplasty. Sinus rhythm with first-degree AV block produced an A wave. Both the C and V waves are markedly reduced. The atrial pressure waveform after balloon mitral valve commissurotomy is the result of multiple factors relating to improved flow and mostly likely a concomitant

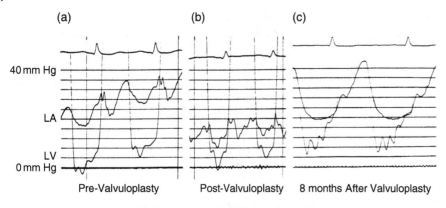

Figure 16.9 Hemodynamic tracings in a patient before (a), immediately after (b), and eight months after valvuloplasty (c) in a patient who developed progressive increase in shortness of breath. See text for details. LA = left atrium; LV = left ventricle.

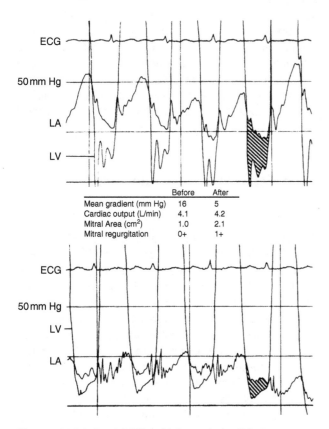

	Before	After
Mean gradient (mm Hg)	16	5
Cardiac output (L/min)	4.1	4.2
Mitral Area (cm²)	1.0	2.1
Mitral regurgitation	0+	1+

Figure 16.10 Left atrial (LA) and left ventricular (LV) pressures before (top) and after (bottom) balloon catheter mitral commissurotomy. Reproduced with permission [32].

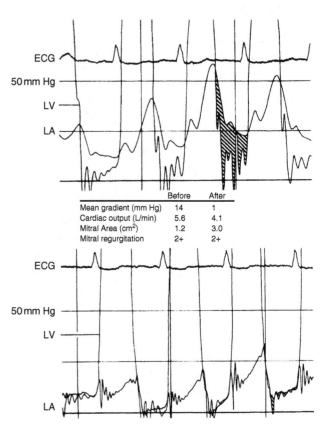

	Before	After
Mean gradient (mm Hg)	14	1
Cardiac output (L/min)	5.6	4.1
Mitral Area (cm²)	1.2	3.0
Mitral regurgitation	2+	2+

Figure 16.11 Left atrial (LA) and left ventricular (LV) pressures before (top) and after (bottom) balloon catheter mitral commissurotomy. Reproduced with permission [33].

shift in the left atrial compliance [10, 11]. The hemodynamic factors influencing the atrial pressure are strongly dependent on chamber compliance and peak transmitral pressure gradient, two variables that change dramatically with valvuloplasty, rendering the pressure half-time method unreliable in the setting of rapidly changing mitral valve function after balloon valvular dilatation and commissurotomy [10, 12].

Case #2

Mitral valve gradients may be completely eliminated in some patients with balloon valvuloplasty. Compare the hemodynamics of the mitral valve in a 29-year-old woman with mitral stenosis and regurgitation (Figure 16.11) to the previous patient. Before valvuloplasty (Figure 16.11, upper panel), large left atrial V waves (to 50 mm Hg) and 2+ mitral regurgitation on ventriculography were present.

The left atrial pressure wave is damped (compared to Figure 16.10), with slightly delayed and rounded C and V wave peaks. The left ventricular pressure was underdamped with a "ringing" artifact. The mean mitral gradient was 14 mm Hg. Atrial fibrillation produced marked differences among valve gradients, evident when comparing beats #1 and 3 (the shaded beat). Cardiac output was 5.6 L/min, yielding a calculated mitral valve area of 1.2 cm^2. After mitral valvuloplasty (Figure 16.11, lower panel), left atrial and ventricular catheters (and pressure manifolds) were flushed. The left atrial pressure corresponds closely to left ventricular pressure throughout diastole. There is virtually no mitral valve gradient. The cardiac output, although decreased to 4.1 L/min, yields a mitral valve area of 3.0 cm^2. There was no change in the angiographic degree of mitral regurgitation. The diminution of left atrial V waves again indicates improved left atrial chamber compliance without a change in valvular regurgitation.

Mitral Regurgitation after Balloon Valvuloplasty

Inherent to balloon mitral valvuloplasty or surgical commissurotomy is excessive valvular dilatation or leaflet tearing, resulting in malcoaptation of the leaflets with valvular regurgitation. Fortunately, mitral regurgitation is an infrequent complication [1, 9, 13, 14]. Of 40 patients undergoing mitral commissurotomy randomized to the balloon catheter or surgical approach, only two had severe mitral regurgitation at the completion of either procedure [9].

Consider the hemodynamic tracings obtained in a 56-year-old woman with severe mitral stenosis undergoing balloon catheter mitral valvuloplasty (Figure 16.12, upper panel). Before valvuloplasty, the left atrial pressure mean was 23 mm Hg with V waves to 45 mm Hg and an evident absence of atrial activity (atrial fibrillation). The downslope of the V wave was moderately delayed, consistent with severe mitral stenosis. Angiographic mitral regurgitation was minimal. The corresponding left ventricular end-diastolic pressure was approximately 20 mm Hg. The mitral valve gradient of 12 mm Hg yielded a valve area of calculation of 0.95 cm^2.

After valvuloplasty (Figure 16.12, lower panel), large V waves (twice the mean pressure) to 70 mm Hg are seen and are associated with the new severe angiographic mitral regurgitation. The V waves now have a steep downslope (Y descent) with only a modest reduction in the mean left atrial–ventricular gradient (approximately 8 mm Hg with an increased heart rate). The left atrial–left ventricular end-diastolic gradient is still evident. Although valve area was enlarged (1.6 cm^2), severe

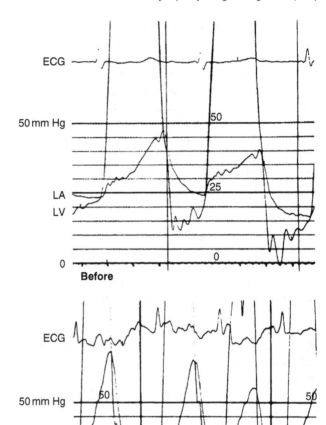

Figure 16.12 Left atrial (LA) and left ventricular (LV) pressures in a patient with mitral stenosis before (top) and after (bottom) balloon catheter mitral valvuloplasty. Note the larger V waves after the procedure.

mitral regurgitation produced congestive heart failure, requiring mitral valve replacement two days after the procedure.

Use of the Pulmonary Capillary Wedge during Valvuloplasty

Mitral valve area calculations using pulmonary capillary wedge pressure tracings can be misleading [15], an especially critical issue when using the pulmonary capillary wedge pressure for monitoring the progress of valve dilation during valvuloplasty. A 31-year-old woman with rheumatic mitral stenosis had Class III congestive heart failure four months postpartum. Fatigue and shortness of breath occurred with minimal activity during the course of routine newborn child care. Noninvasive evaluation confirmed mitral stenosis. Balloon catheter mitral valve commissurotomy was requested. Left ventricular and pulmonary capillary wedge pressures were measured simultaneously using fluid-filled systems (Figure 16.13a). Despite attention to manifold and catheter flushing and to catheter positioning, the pulmonary capillary wedge tracing shown was the best that could be obtained with the balloon-tipped thermodilution catheter. Are the pressure tracings satisfactory for mitral valve area assessment? Based on the pressures, is the patient in sinus rhythm?

The pulmonary capillary wedge tracing is of poor quality. A poor waveform may be due to improper positioning (over-wedging); damping due to a bubble, catheter, or pressure line kink; or inadequate flushing of the fluid path. The placement of a balloon-tipped catheter in this patient was difficult. Repositioning of the catheter and flushing did not produce a much better tracing. Left atrial pressure was then obtained with the transseptal technique (Figure 16.13b). One can appreciate the distinct A and V waves and elevated left atrial–left ventricular end-diastolic pressure, with a mean gradient of 14 mm Hg. The more precise atrial pressure wave with a distinct "a" wave emphasizes the limitation of using the pulmonary capillary wedge in this case and easily confirms sinus rhythm.

The pulmonary capillary wedge pressure can be improved by checking four steps: (i) repositioning the catheter; (ii) flushing the entire fluid to transducer path; (iii) checking for catheter kinks; and (iv) using a stiffer end-hold catheter. Confirm pulmonary capillary wedge pressure by pulmonary capillary wedge saturation (>95%).

Before mitral valvuloplasty, the matching of left atrial and pulmonary capillary wedge pressures permits the operator to use (or exclude) a pulmonary capillary wedge pressure during intraprocedural monitoring periods when left atrial pressure is unobtainable. Compare the left atrial and pulmonary capillary wedge pressures in this patient (Figure 16.13c). Although the two pressure means track together, phasic responses are not well matched.

During and after balloon valvuloplasty, the hemodynamic result was initially assessed by pulmonary capillary wedge and left ventricular pressures (Figure 16.13d; a 5 F pigtail catheter is positioned in the left ventricle for the duration of the procedure). A lower but persistent mitral gradient can be appreciated. Is the valve dilation satisfactory? Because the pulmonary capillary wedge tracing was suboptimal, the success of the procedure must be confirmed by direct measurement of the simultaneous left atrial and left ventricular pressures. Figure 16.13e shows that there is no residual mitral valve gradient with matching of left ventricular–left atrial diastolic pressures. One interesting feature of the left atrial pressure wave is the sharp C wave (Figure 16.13e, last beat from right) produced by catheter migration into the left ventricular cavity in early systole. Repositioning of the left atrial catheter eliminated this waveform artifact.

Mitral Valve Gradient with Dobutamine Stress Testing

Dr. Ted Feldman provides a case of a 36-year-old female who was first diagnosed with murmur at age 16 and has been followed for many years for rheumatic mitral stenosis. She now presents with dyspnea. Despite being asymptomatic, her initial evaluation in 2001 demonstrated a valve area of 1.4 cm^2 with a mean gradient of 10 mm Hg. Pulmonary artery pressure was 15 mm Hg, increasing to 23 mm Hg on exercise. In 2007, the patient reported mild external dyspnea and palpitations. Although she plays tennis and notes that singles tennis is difficult due to dyspnea, she can play doubles for several hours. She walks five flights of stairs several times a day to her office without stopping to rest. She denies paroxysmal nocturnal dyspnea (PND), orthopnea, or lower-extremity edema. Three episodes of rapid heart rate and profound dizziness occurred recently, which required her to lie down and elevate her legs. One episode lasted for 20 minutes. Home arrhythmia monitoring demonstrated only atrial tachycardia. On repeat echocardiography, the resting mean transmitral gradient of 8 mm Hg, mitral valve area of 1.2 cm^2, and pulmonary artery pressure of 36 mm Hg were identified. On exercise, the mean gradient increased to 25 mm Hg while pulmonary artery systolic pressure increased to 80 mm Hg. On exercise, she complained primarily of leg fatigue and moderate dyspnea and noted some atypical chest pain. Cardiac catheterization was performed with a view to performing percutaneous transluminal mitral commissurotomy (PTMC).

Cardiac catheterization was performed using bilateral femoral access. A 14 F venous sheath was placed in the right femoral vein followed by a Perclose pre-closure suture system with a 6 F Perclose device. An 8 F left femoral venous sheath and a 6 F left femoral arterial sheath were also placed. A 7 F balloon-tipped catheter was used to measure hemodynamics and cardiac output values. A pigtail catheter was placed in the pulmonary artery for levophase of the left atrial and left ventricular angiography. An 8 F long sheath and transseptal needle were advanced through the right femoral venous system, and access to the left atrium was obtained. Anti-coagulation using heparin was then given. Hemodynamic parameters were measured before and again after the dobutamine

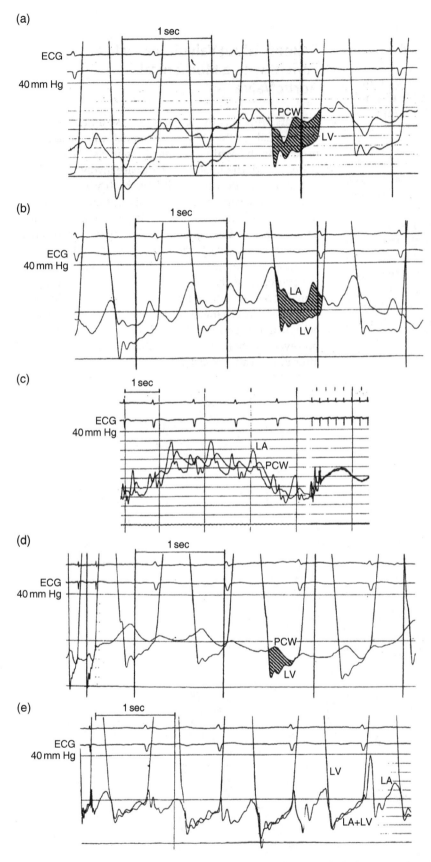

Figure 16.13 (a) Pulmonary capillary wedge (PCW) and left ventricular (LV) pressures in a patient with mitral stenosis before valvuloplasty. From the pressure tracings, what is the rhythm? Should this tracing be used to compute mitral valve area? (b) Left atrial (LA) and left ventricular pressures in the patient in tracing a. From this pressure tracing, what is the rhythm? Should this tracing be used to compute mitral valve area? (c) Simultaneous pulmonary capillary wedge (PCW) and left atrial pressures in a patient with mitral stenosis. Is pulmonary capillary wedge satisfactory for gradient determination in this case? (d) Pulmonary capillary wedge and left ventricular pressures after mitral valvuloplasty. Is this a successful procedure? (e) Left atrial and left ventricular pressures after mitral valvuloplasty obtained at the same time as the pressures in tracing d. Explain the large C wave on the last beat.

stress testing of 20 μg/kg/min, increasing cardiac output, gradient, and pulmonary artery pressure.

The mitral gradient before dobutamine was 5 mm Hg (Figure 16.14), pulmonary artery pressure 28/17 mm Hg (Figure 16.15), and cardiac output 5.57 L/min (see Table 16.1). With dobutamine infusion, mitral valve gradient increased to approximately 12 mm Hg (Figure 16.16), pulmonary artery pressure 46/20 mm Hg (Figure 16.17), with cardiac output 9.88 L/min and valve area changing from 2.32 to 2.15 cm² (see Table 16.2). Mitral valvuloplasty was deferred.

In conclusion, following dobutamine stress hemodynamics, increasing cardiac output increased the transmitral gradient and pulmonary artery pressure, but the mitral valve gradient did not rise to a sufficient level to warrant PTMC. Hence PTMC was not performed; the right femoral vein was closed with Perclose, and left femoral vein and femoral artery access was then controlled with manual pressure. There were no complications during the procedure, and the patient has done well.

Balloon Mitral Valvuloplasty in a Patient with a Mechanical Aortic Valve

Patients with rheumatic heart disease and a history of mechanical aortic valve replacement will occasionally present with significant mitral stenosis. While most patients with rheumatic heart disease involving both the mitral and aortic valves will have both valves replaced, those with severe aortic valve disease and progressive mitral stenosis may be referred for percutaneous mitral valvuloplasty subsequently. Traditional retrograde transaortic left-heart catheterization is not available, because catheter access to the left ventricle is limited by the presence of the prosthetic valve in the aortic position. Retrograde catheterization of the left ventricle with a bileaflet mechanical prosthetic valve can lead to complications and may be fatal [16–18]. It is important, however, to obtain left ventricular pressure prior to and after mitral valvuloplasty.

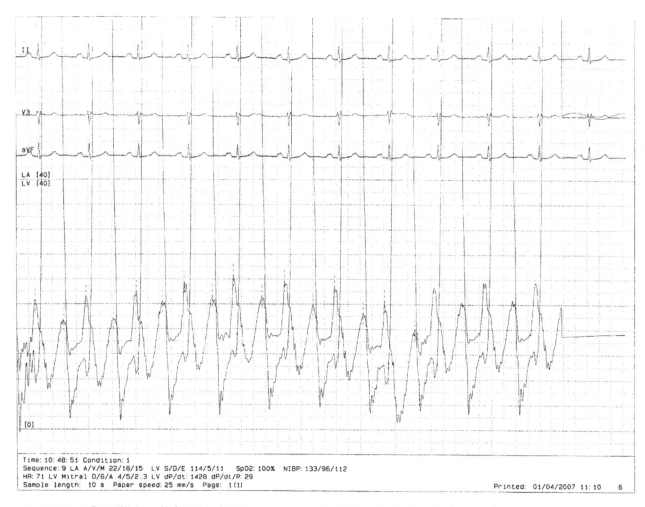

Figure 16.14 Left atrial (LA) and left ventricular (LV) pressures on a 0–40 scale at rest before dobutamine.

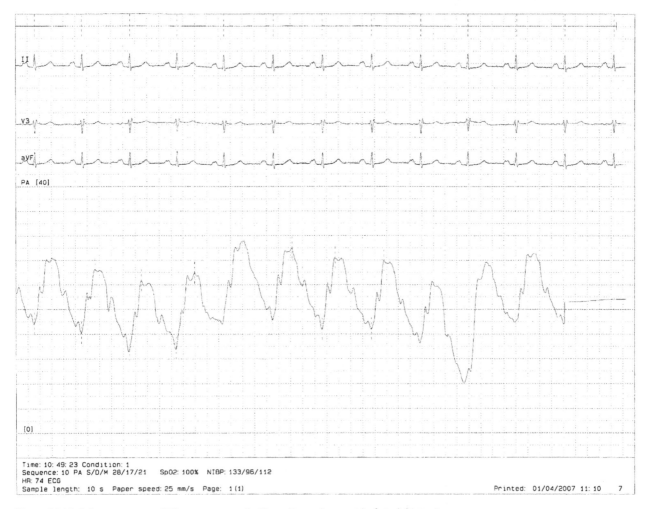

Figure 16.15 Pulmonary artery (PA) pressure on a 0–40 mm Hg scale at rest before dobutamine.

Table 16.1 Before dobutamine.

Site	Pressures (mm Hg)	Heart Rate (beats/min)
Right atrial pressure	6/4/3	71
Right ventricular pressure	24/3/5	71
Pulmonary artery pressure	28/17/21	74
Left atrial pressure	22/18/15	71
Left ventricular pressure	114/5/11	71
Aortic pressure	128/74/97	74

Cardiac output: 5.57 L/min TD
Mean valve gradient: 5 mm Hg
Valve area 2.32 cm^2
TD = thermodilution.

Transseptal left atrial access to the left ventricle is one option, with either a single or double interatrial puncture to allow performance of the Inoue balloon mitral valvuloplasty and to obtain pressures simultaneously in the left ventricle and left atrium. A second option is direct percutaneous left ventricular puncture along with a single transseptal puncture for left atrial pressure. Another option is placing a 0.014 inch diameter pressure sensor guidewire across the bileaflet aortic mechanical valve. There are two case reports of this being performed safely and providing accurate hemodynamics [19, 20]. We present another technique utilizing (i) a single transseptal, pre- and post-procedure direct hemodynamic assessment; and (ii) echocardiography. The infrequency of this presentation, in addition to multiple available techniques for left ventricular access, makes review of this topic worthwhile.

This discussion concerns a patient with rheumatic valvular disease and a history of mechanical aortic valve replacement, who presented with heart failure symptoms

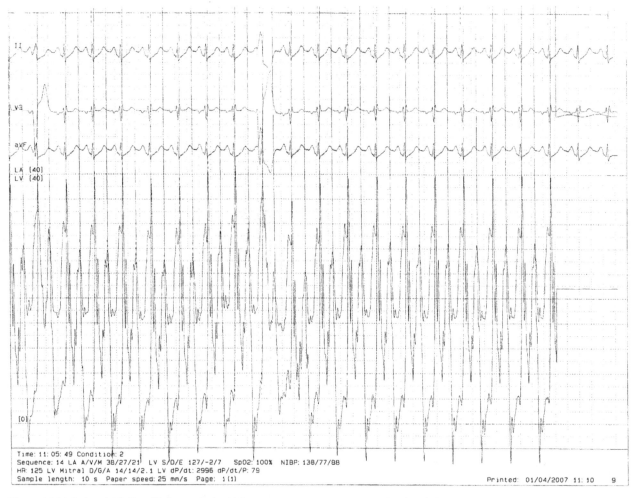

Figure 16.16 Left atrial (LA) and left ventricular (LV) pressures on a 0–40 mm Hg scale after dobutamine.

attributed to worsening rheumatic mitral valvular stenosis. We describe a modified technique of Inoue balloon mitral valvuloplasty involving only femoral venous access in the setting of a mechanical aortic valve.

Case History

A 38-year-old Hispanic female was referred to our institution for consideration of percutaneous balloon mitral valvuloplasty after being followed in a general cardiology clinic for moderate mitral stenosis [21]. She has a history of rheumatic heart disease and had undergone aortic valve replacement eight years ago (19 mm St. Jude Medical, Minneapolis, MN) for rheumatic aortic stenosis. Recently, she developed Class III heart failure manifested by less than one flight of stairs dyspnea and two-pillow orthopnea. She also described episodic palpitations that were evaluated with an event monitor. She was found to have short runs of 2:1 atrial flutter at a rate of 150 beats/min lasting up to 15 sec. She had no orthostatic symptoms or syncope. She continued to work full time making cabinets in a factory. She is a nonsmoker

and does not drink alcohol or use illicit drugs. Her medications included digoxin and Coumadin. On physical examination her blood pressure was 106/64 mm Hg with a regular pulse of 66 beats/min. Cardiovascular examination was remarkable for a crisp mechanical A2. S1 was slightly accentuated. There was an II/VI early diastolic rumble at the apex without an opening snap. An S3 or S4 was not detected. The point of maximal impulse was normal, and there was no parasternal heave. She had no peripheral edema. Transesophageal echocardiogram demonstrated typical rheumatic deformities of the mitral valve, with a mitral valve area of 1.5 cm² and a mean gradient of 10 mm Hg. There was trivial mitral regurgitation present, with no calcification or fibrosis of the subvalvular apparatus. The mechanical aortic valve was normal. Because she had New York Heart Association Class III heart failure symptoms, moderate mitral stenosis, and acceptable valve morphology, we decided to proceed with valvuloplasty after a discussion with the patient and her family.

The patient was brought to the catheterization laboratory and a 7 F venous access was achieved in the left

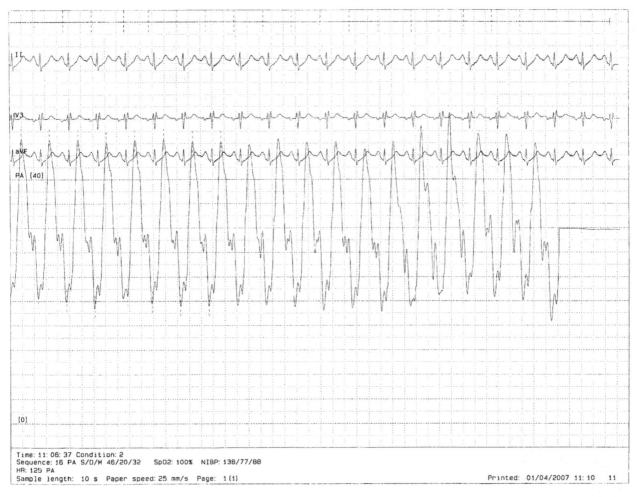

Time: 11: 06: 37 Condition: 2
Sequence: 16 PA S/D/M 46/20/32   SpO2: 100% NIBP: 138/77/88
HR: 125 PA
Sample length: 10 s Paper speed: 25 mm/s Page: 1 (1)   Printed: 01/04/2007 11: 10   11

Figure 16.17 Pulmonary artery (PA) pressure on a 0–40 mm Hg scale after dobutamine.

Table 16.2 After dobutamine.

Site	Pressures (mm Hg)	Heart Rate (beats/min)
Pulmonary artery pressure	46/20/32	133
Left atrial pressure	38/27/21	125
Left ventricular pressure	129/1/7	125
Aortic pressure	131/63/88	107

Cardiac output: 9.88 L/min TD
Mean valve gradient: 12 mm Hg
Valve area: 2.15 cm^2
Ejection fraction: 65%
TD = thermodilution.

femoral vein, through which the Swan Ganz catheter was placed in the pulmonary artery. An 8 F venous sheath was placed in the right femoral vein. A transthoracic echocardiogram was obtained, demonstrating trace mitral regurgitation and moderate mitral stenosis, with a mean gradient of 10 mm Hg and an area of 1.5 cm^2.

Right-heart catheterization demonstrated mild postcapillary pulmonary hypertension and an elevated pulmonary capillary wedge pressure (Table 16.3). A 7 F Berman catheter was used to do a right atrial angiogram, which demonstrated normal right ventricular (RV) and left ventricular (LV) function with a moderately enlarged left atrium. A 0.032″ J-wire was advanced into the superior vena cava (SVC) from the right femoral vein (RFV), and the 8 F sheath was exchanged for an 8 F Mullins sheath. The Brockenbrough needle was advanced to the tip of the Mullins sheath. Using the landmarks from the right atrial angiogram, transseptal catheterization by the standard Brockenbrough technique was performed, placing the Mullins sheath into the left atrium. After heparinization, a 5 F pigtail catheter was advanced into the LV through the 8 F Mullins sheath over a J wire to obtain simultaneous LV and left atrial (LA) pressures (Figure 16.18). Simultaneous LV and LA pressures were obtained, demonstrating a mean gradient of 10 mm Hg and a MVA of 1.4 cm^2 (Figure 16.19).

The pigtail catheter was removed, the Inoue coiled wire was inserted into the left atrium, and the Mullins

Table 16.3 Hemodynamics before and after Mitral Valvuloplasty.

Parameter	Before Valvuloplasty	After Valvuloplasty
Heart rate, beats/min	74 sinus rhythm	92 sinus rhythm
Right atrial pressure (a,v,m), mm Hg	16/14/12	14/13/12
Right ventricular pressure (s,d), mm Hg	45/12	39/9
Pulmonary artery pressure (s,d,m), mm Hg	45/18 (29)	39/20 (28)
Pulmonary capillary wedge pressure (a,v,m), mm Hg	26/23/21	24/22/21
Left atrial pressure (a,v,m), mm Hg	32/17/23	18/16/13
Left ventricular pressure (s,ed,ld), mm Hg	116/6/14	84/10/15
Cardiac output, L/min		
Fick	4.5	4.7
Thermodilution	4.0	4.4
Cardiac index, L/min/m^2		
Fick	2.5	2.6
Thermodilution	2.2	2.4
Pulmonary vascular resistance, Wood units	2.0	1.0
Mitral valve mean gradient, mm Hg	9.6	6.4
Mitral valve area, cm^2	1.4	2.1

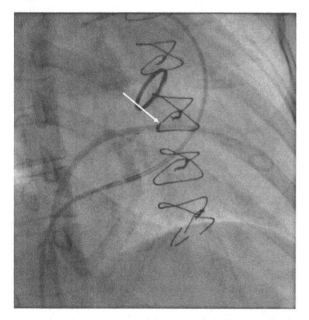

Figure 16.18 Cineangiographic frame of the 8 F Mullins sheath in the left atrium with the 5 F pigtail catheter through the Mullins sheath into the left ventricle. The arrow identifies the tip of the Mullins sheath. The mechanical aortic valve and pulmonary artery catheter are also seen in this right anterior oblique projection.

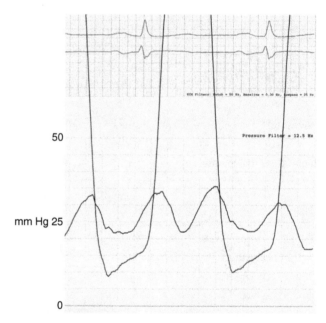

Figure 16.19 Simultaneous pressure recording of left atrial and ventricular pressure (50 mm Hg scale at 100 mm/sec paper speed), showing severe mitral stenosis.

sheath was removed. The 14 F dilator was advanced across the septum. The prepped, slenderized 26 mm Inoue balloon was advanced into the left atrium and the wire was removed. The stretching tube was removed and the preshaped J stylet was introduced into the Inoue balloon to advance it across the mitral valve. Initial inflation to 24.5 mm showed no improvement in mitral valve gradient by echo and no change in trace mitral regurgitation. LA pressure was monitored between balloon inflations by removing the stylet and obtaining pressure through the Inoue balloon. The Inoue balloon was inflated to 26 mm twice, with no improvement in the gradient by echo. The 26 mm Inoue balloon was exchanged for a 28 mm Inoue balloon, and this was inflated to 27 mm and then finally 28 mm (Figure 16.20). After the 28 mm inflation, the mitral mean gradient had improved to 5 mm Hg and there was continued trace mitral regurgitation by echocardiography. The Inoue coiled wire was inserted into the left atrium and the Inoue balloon was exchanged for the Mullins sheath. The 5 F pigtail was again inserted through Mullins sheath into the left ventricle over a J wire. Simultaneous LV and LA pressures were obtained.

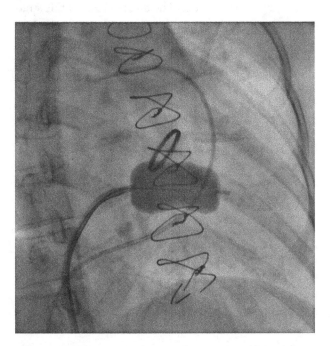

Figure 16.20 The Inoue balloon is inflated in the mitral orifice.

The patient had some venous bleeding around the femoral venous sheath, so direct pressure was applied around the sheath. The initial simultaneous LV and LA pressures showed complete resolution of the mitral valve gradient (Figure 16.21). However, it was recognized that the patient had become bradycardic and hypotensive. She was treated for a vagal response with atropine and intravenous (IV) fluids, with improvement of the hemodynamics over 5 minutes. The simultaneous LA and LV pressures then demonstrated improvement of gradient to 6 mm Hg and mitral valve area of 2.1 cm^2 (Figure 16.22).

The patient was followed up in clinic four weeks after the procedure and was doing very well. She had significant improvement in her heart failure symptoms from New York Heart Association Class III to Class I.

Discussion

Patients with rheumatic heart disease and a mechanical aortic valve will occasionally be referred for percutaneous balloon mitral valvuloplasty. Repeat thoracotomy in such patients would carry significant perioperative morbidity and mortality. Traditional left-heart catheterization via the retrograde transaortic route is not possible, because the mechanical aortic valve cannot be safely crossed with a pigtail catheter due to the risk of entrapment. Left ventricular pressure is generally performed to confirm the echocardiographic hemodynamics and to assess the procedural outcome.

There are several other options available to obtain the gradient across the mitral valve. Direct transthoracic puncture is one option. However, it has been mostly abandoned except in cases of mitral and aortic mechanical

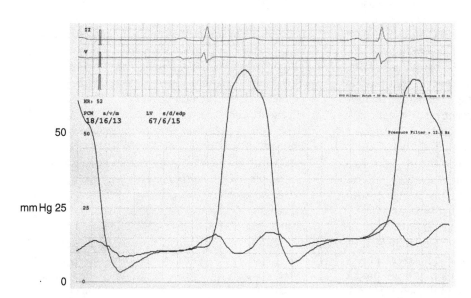

Figure 16.21 Simultaneous left ventricular (LV) and left atrial (LA) pressures during a vasovagal reaction after mitral valvuloplasty. During this low cardiac output state with decreased preload and systemic hypotension, there is near resolution of the mitral valve gradient (50 mm Hg scale at 100 mm/sec paper speed).

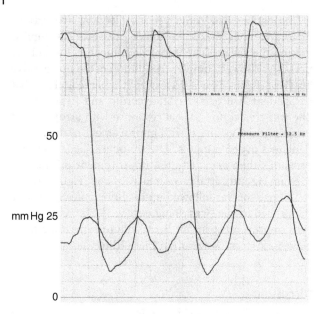

Figure 16.22 Final left ventricular (LV) and left atrial (LA) pressures following 28 mm Inoue balloon inflation, after treatment of the vasovagal reaction (at 50 mm Hg scale at 100 mm/sec paper speed). The patient is left with mild residual mitral stenosis.

valves, because it is hazardous and most interventional cardiologists have not performed this technique. A second option is the double transseptal puncture. This is being performed frequently now by electrophysiologists conducting pulmonary vein isolation procedures. Interventional cardiologists are not performing double transseptal punctures frequently, and they are not as facile with this procedure. Small case series indicate that it can be safely performed by appropriately trained individuals [22]. A modified version of the double transseptal has been described where a second guidewire is passed through a double-lumen catheter, thereby avoiding a second interatrial puncture [23]. Most iatrogenic atrial septal defects seal off by 12 months post-balloon mitral valvuloplasty, when a single Inoue balloon is placed across the septum [24–26]. However, there is concern that placing two catheters across a single transseptal puncture, thereby creating a larger defect, will significantly increase the risk of a residual iatrogenic atrial septal defect [27]. Another technique reported by Doorey [20] and Parham [21] is using a 0.014 in. pressure sensor guidewire placed retrograde across the bileaflet aortic valve. In the four patients reported and in ex vivo demonstrations, the guidewire was easily advanced across the bileaflet valve and subsequently withdrawn. Wire entrapment appeared to be unlikely, and has only been reported in these few patients.

A safe alternative to the other described techniques is proposed. This technique involves placing a 5 F pigtail catheter through the Mullins sheath to the left ventricle, for simultaneous left atrial and ventricular pressure assessment. The advantage of our technique is that there is no

increased risk of placing two catheters across the interatrial septum, either by single or double transseptal puncture. In 1998, Gupta *et al.* [28] described venous-only access for PBMV using transthoracic echocardiography for guidance. They only obtained invasive hemodynamics of the gradient and valve area if there was an unsatisfactory result. More recently, Chiang *et al.* [29] described performing balloon mitral valvuloplasty under transesophageal echocardiography guidance. The advantage of our technique is that prior to performing the valvuloplasty, we can correlate the invasive hemodynamics with the echocardiographic assessment. The disadvantage of this strategy is that it relies on echocardiography and left atrial pressure alone for determining the success of the balloon inflations. Another disadvantage of relying of echocardiography is the possibility of inaccuracy of mitral pressure half-time after percutaneous mitral valvotomy [10]. However, the ability to correlate the echocardiogram with the invasive assessment provides a good assessment of the area and gradient, with the ability to monitor for worsening mitral regurgitation by echocardiogram.

This case also demonstrates nicely the effect of heart rate and preload on mitral stenosis, as demonstrated by Figure 16.21. The patient had a vasovagal reaction after femoral venous compression, with a significant decrease in left atrial and left ventricular pressure and almost complete resolution of the mitral valve gradient. After being treated for the vagal reaction with atropine and IV fluids, the final LA and LV pressures likely demonstrated a gradient that she will reach with normal daily activities and with her occupation (Figure 16.22).

Key Points

1) Balloon mitral commissurotomy in many patients will be as satisfactory as closed surgical commissurotomy.
2) The pulmonary capillary wedge pressure may not be satisfactory to assess the success of gradient reduction after mitral valvuloplasty.
3) In patients with a mechanical aortic valve, left-heart catheterization is possible via a transseptal puncture, via direct left ventricular puncture, or using a 0.014 inch pressure guidewire from the retrograde transaortic approach.
4) In patients with a mechanical aortic valve undergoing mitral valvuloplasty, simultaneous left ventricular and left atrial pressure measurements for the mitral valve gradient are possible through a single transseptal puncture.
5) The mitral valve gradient changes significantly with changes in cardiac output. To assess changes in the mitral valve area, it is essential to simultaneously assess cardiac output. For example, during a vagal reaction, both the cardiac output and mitral valve gradient will decrease significantly.

References

1 Turi ZG, Reyes VP, Raju BS, Raju AR, Kumar DN, Rajagopal P, *et al*. Percutaneous balloon versus surgical closed commissurotomy for mitral stenosis: A prospective, randomized trial. *Circulation* 83:1179–1185, 1991.

2 Reyes VP, Raju BS, Wynne J, Stephenson LW, Raju R, Fromm BS, *et al*. Percutaneous balloon valvuloplasty compared with open surgical commissurotomy for mitral stenosis. *N Engl J Med* 331:961–967, 1994.

3 Ben Farhat M, Ayari M, Maatouk F, Betbout F, Gamra H, Jarra M, *et al*. Percutaneous balloon versus surgical closed and open mitral commissurotomy: Seven-year follow-up results of a randomized trial. *Circulation* 97:245–250, 1998.

4 Schoenfeld MH, Palacios IF, Hutter AM Jr, Jacoby SS, Block PC. Underestimation of prosthetic mitral valve areas: Role of transseptal catheterization in avoiding unnecessary repeat mitral valve surgery. *J Am Coll Cardiol* 5:1387–1392, 1985.

5 Kern MJ. Hemodynamic Waveforms, in *The Cardiac Catheterization Handbook*, Mosby–Year Book, 2015, pp. 173–199.

6 Kern MJ, Lim MJ, Goldstein JA (eds). *Hemodynamic Rounds: Interpretation of Cardiac Pathophysiology from Pressure Waveform Analysis*, 3rd ed. Hoboken, NJ: John Wiley & Sons, Inc, 2009.

7 Abascal VM, Wilkins GT, Choong CY, Thomas JD, Palacios IF, Block PC, Weyman AE. Echocardiographic evaluation of mitral valve structure and function in patients followed for at least 6 months after percutaneous balloon mitral valvuloplasty. *J Am Coll Cardiol* 12:606–615, 1988.

8 Tatineni S, Deligonul U, Kaiser G, Kern MJ. Delayed onset of severe mitral regurgitation after successful percutaneous mitral balloon valvuloplasty. *Am Heart J* 122:235–238, 1991.

9 Palacios IF, Block PC, Wilkins GT, Weyman AE. Follow-up of patients undergoing percutaneous mitral balloon valvotomy. *Circulation* 79:573–579, 1989.

10 Thomas JD, Wilkins GT, Choong CYP, Abascal VM, Palacios IF, Block PC, Weyman AE. Inaccuracy of mitral pressure half-time immediately after percutaneous mitral valvotomy: Dependence on transmitral gradient and left atrial and ventricular compliance. *Circulation* 78:980–993, 1988.

11 Kern MJ. Hemodynamic rounds: Interpretation of cardiac pathophysiology from pressure waveform analysis: The left-sided V wave. *Cathet Cardiovasc Diagn* 23(3):211–218, 1991.

12 Hatle L, Angelsen B, Tromsdal A. Noninvasive assessment of atrioventricular pressure half-time by Doppler ultrasound. *Circulation* 60:1096–1104, 1979.

13 Deligonul U, Kern MJ. Hemodynamic rounds: Interpretation of cardiac pathophysiology from pressure waveform analysis: Percutaneous balloon valvuloplasty. *Cathet Cardiovasc Diagn* 24(2):111–120, 1991.

14 McKay CR, Kawanishi DT, Kotlewski A, Parise K, Odom-Maryon T, Gonzales A, *et al*. Improvement in exercise capacity and exercise hemodynamics 3 months after double-balloon catheter balloon valvuloplasty treatment of patients with symptomatic mitral stenosis. *Circulation* 77:1013–1021, 1988.

15 Lange RA, Moore DM, Cigarroa RG, Hillis LD. Use of pulmonary capillary wedge pressure to assess severity of mitral stenosis: Is true left atrial pressure needed in this condition? *J Am Coll Cardiol* 13:825–829, 1989.

16 Horstkotte D, Jehle J, Loogen F. Death due to transprosthetic catheterization of a Bjork–Shiley prosthesis in the aortic position. *Am J Cardiol* 58(6):566–567, 1986.

17 Horstkotte D. Retrograde catheterization of left ventricle through mechanical aortic prostheses. *Eur Heart J* 9(2):194–195, 1988.

18 Rigaud M, Dubourg O, Luwaert R, Rocha P, Hamoir V, Bardet J, Bourdarias JP. Retrograde catheterization of left ventricle through mechanical aortic prostheses. *Eur Heart J* 8(7):689–696, 1987.

19 Doorey AJ, Gakhal M, Pasquale MJ. Utilization of a pressure sensor guidewire to measure bileaflet mechanical valve gradients: Hemodynamic and echocardiographic sequelae. *Cathet Cardiovasc Intervent* 67(4):535–540, 2006.

20 Parham W, El Shafei A, Rajjoub H, Ziaee A, Kern MJ. Retrograde left ventricular hemodynamic assessment across bileaflet prosthetic aortic valves: The use of a high-fidelity pressure sensor angioplasty guidewire. *Cathet Cardiovasc Intervent* 59(4):509–513, 2003.

21 Kosmicki DL, Michaels AD. Hemodynamic rounds series: Left heart catheterization and mitral balloon valvuloplasty in a patient with a mechanical aortic valve. *Cathet Cardiovasc Intervent* 71:429–433, 2008.

22 Hildick-Smith DJ, Shapiro LM. Balloon mitral valvuloplasty employing double transseptal puncture. *Cathet Cardiovasc Diagn* 45(1):33–36, 1998.

23 Yamada T, McElderry HT, Epstein AE, Plumb VJ, Kay GN. One-puncture, double-transseptal catheterization manoeuvre in the catheter ablation of atrial fibrillation. *Europace* 9(7):487–489, 2007.

24 Casale P, Block PC, O'Shea JP, Palacios IF. Atrial septal defect after percutaneous mitral balloon valvuloplasty: Immediate results and follow-up. *J Am Coll Cardiol* 15(6):1300–1304, 1990.

25 Cequier A, Bonan R, Serra A, Dyrda I, Crepeau J, Dethy M, Waters D. Left-to-right atrial shunting after percutaneous mitral valvuloplasty: Incidence and long-term hemodynamic follow-up. *Circulation* 81(4):1190–1197, 1990.

26 Ishikura F, Nagata S, Yasuda S, Yamashita N, Miyatake K. Residual atrial septal perforation after percutaneous transvenous mitral commissurotomy with Inoue balloon catheter. *Am Heart J* 120(4):873–878, 1990.

27 Hammerstingl C, Lickfett L, Jeong KM, Troatz C, Wedekind JA, Tiemann K, *et al*. Persistence of iatrogenic atrial septal defect after pulmonary vein isolation: An underestimated risk? *Am Heart J* 152(2):362 e1–5, 2006.

28 Gupta S, Schiele F, Xu C, Meneveau N, Seronde MF, Breton V, *et al*. Simplified percutaneous mitral valvuloplasty with the Inoue balloon. *Eur Heart J* 19(4):610–616, 1998.

29 Chiang CW, Hsu LA, Chu PH, Ho WJ, Lo HS, Chang CC. Feasibility of simplifying balloon mitral valvuloplasty by obviating left-sided cardiac catheterization using online guidance with transesophageal echocardiography. *Chest* 123(6): 1957–1963, 2003.

17

The Pulmonary Valve and Valvuloplasty

Morton J. Kern

Abnormalities of the pulmonary valve occur most frequently in children, with rare individuals having clinically significant pulmonary valve disease in adulthood. The hemodynamics of pulmonary valve disease most often reflect that of a congenitally narrowed, domed valve of pulmonic stenosis [1, 2]. A minority of individuals may have a thickened or dysplastic valve. Infundibular hypertrophy may present as pulmonic stenosis with normal valve structures. Occasionally, ventricular septal defects will also accompany the deformed valve. The diagnosis of pulmonary valvular (and sub- and supra-) lesions is made from echocardiography, right-heart pressure recordings, and right ventricular angiography [3–6]. Although such abnormalities are uncommon, it is important to recognize the different waveforms associated with pulmonary stenosis and regurgitation and conditions that may mimic or be confused with pulmonary stenosis in the absence of true valvular abnormalities. This hemodynamic round will deal with right-heart pressure tracings reflecting abnormalities of the pulmonary valve.

Pulmonary Stenosis: Valvular or Nonvalvular?

A 23-year-old woman with a history of congenital disease developed progressive exertional shortness of breath with atypical chest pain. At 8 months of age the patient had repair of an atrial septal defect with pulmonary artery banding. The ventricular septal defect was not repaired. At age 14 years the patient had debanding of the pulmonary artery and ventricular septal patch repair. Despite a small residual ventricular septal defect, right ventricular volume overload and increased right ventricular pressures were identified by echocardiography.

Because of increasing dyspnea on exertion with normal exercise tolerance, repeat echocardiography on the current examination revealed normal left ventricular systolic function, right ventricular enlargement with right ventricular overload, biatrial enlargement, and a small muscular persistent ventricular septal defect. Echocardiography suggested an increased pulmonary flow velocity and a pressure gradient across the pulmonary artery. Systemic blood pressure was 120/80 mm Hg. Pulse was 60 beats/min. There was no jugular vein distension. Heart examination revealed normal S_1 and S_2 without gallops. A III/VI systolic murmur was heard across the precordium with radiation to the back. Lungs were clear. Electrocardiogram showed normal sinus rhythm and pseudoinferior infarction pattern.

Right- and left-heart catheterization was performed. The mean pulmonary capillary wedge pressure was 14 mm Hg. There was no systolic gradient across the aortic valve. There was no clinically detectable shunt by oxygen saturation measurements through the right heart. Left ventriculography revealed a left ventricular ejection fraction of 53% without mitral regurgitation. Right ventriculography revealed a trace of right to left ventricular contrast flow.

To assess the right-heart pressures, two catheters were placed in the pulmonary artery and pressures zeroed, matched, and recorded. Examine the pressure waveforms in Figure 17.1. The pressure tracings are superimposed from two fluid-filled catheters. On pullback of the first catheter into the right ventricular cavity, a pressure gradient is easily identified, with right ventricular pressure equal to 95/10 mm Hg and pulmonary artery pressure equal to 30/12 mm Hg. This finding is consistent with pulmonary stenosis. Does this patient have pulmonary stenosis? Examine the pressure tracings in Figure 17.2 from the same patient. A large gradient between the higher pressure (PP) and the pulmonary artery pressure is obvious. From examining this tracing, localize where the gradient is produced. This patient does not have valvular but instead supravalvular stenosis. In Figure 17.2, the tracing labeled PP is a proximal pulmonary artery pressure obtained above the pulmonary

Hemodynamic Rounds: Interpretation of Cardiac Pathophysiology from Pressure Waveform Analysis, Fourth Edition.
Edited by Morton J. Kern, Michael J. Lim, and James A. Goldstein.
© 2018 John Wiley & Sons Ltd. Published 2018 by John Wiley & Sons Ltd.

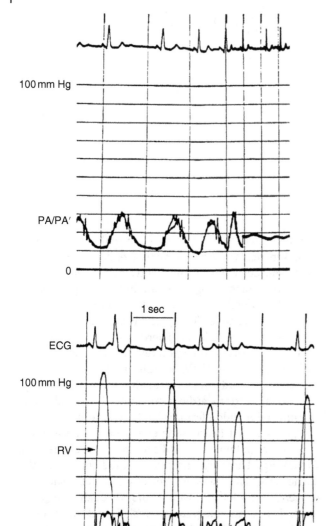

Figure 17.1 (Top) Two simultaneously matched pressures measuring pulmonary artery pressure beyond the pulmonary valve (0–100 mm Hg scale). The mean pressures also matched. Peak pulmonary artery pressure was 30 mm Hg. (Bottom) Right ventricular pressure and simultaneous pulmonary artery pressure. Note the prominent systolic gradient. PA = pulmonary artery; RV = right ventricle. See text for details.

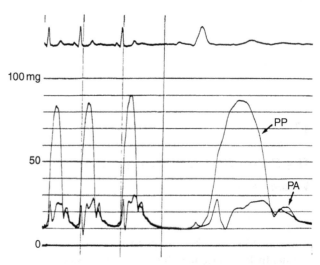

Figure 17.2 Simultaneous pressures from patient example in Figure 17.1 measured as in Figure 17.1. Note the decline in peak systolic pressure. Is this pulmonic valve stenosis? PA = pulmonary artery; PP = proximal pulmonary.

The diastolic pressures of both tracings are superimposable. The finding of valvular pulmonary artery disease is excluded by this tracing. In all patients with suspected pulmonary valvular stenosis, a careful pullback of pressures measured from the distal pulmonary artery to the left main and to the pulmonary valve, and then careful matching of the pressure to the right ventricle, is essential. Compare this tracing to that of the next patient.

Pulmonic Stenosis and ECG Abnormalities

Examine the right-heart hemodynamics (Figure 17.3) of a 77-year-old woman who had a myocardial infarction in April 1984. Because of new-onset chest pain in July 1990, the patient returned to the cardiac catheterization laboratory. This pain was similar to that of the previous myocardial infarction. Because of signs of dyspnea and a systolic murmur heard in the left parasternal area, simultaneous right- and left-heart catheterization was performed prior to coronary arteriography. On passage of the balloon-tipped pulmonary artery catheter, a right ventricular systolic pressure of 40 mm Hg was recognized; and on passage into the pulmonary artery beyond the pulmonic valve, the pulmonary artery pressure was 20/10 mm Hg. Simultaneous pressures were then obtained using a second right-heart catheter to identify the pulmonary artery–right ventricular gradient. Cardiac output was 4.9 L/min and the planimetered mean pulmonary artery gradient was 20 mm Hg. Compare the right ventricular and pulmonary artery pressures obtained in Figure 17.3 with the tracings in Figures 17.1 and 17.2. Note that the pulmonary artery pressure

valve, but below the area of narrowing (the site of the prior pulmonary banding) just proximal to the bifurcation of the left and right pulmonary arteries. The pressure in the distal pulmonary artery was 34/12 mm Hg at the proximal site of the narrowing which was the previous location of the pulmonary artery band (85/12 mm Hg) and right ventricular pressure was 95/10 mm Hg. Clues to the fact that this proximal pulmonary artery pressure was not the right ventricular pressure were evident by the reduction in peak systolic pressure and the matching of the diastolic to the pulmonary artery diastolic pressure.

Figure 17.3 (Top) Hemodynamics in a patient with a systolic pulmonic murmur. Right ventricular (RV) pressure is 42 mm Hg, pulmonary artery (PA) systolic pressure is 20 mm Hg. On continuous pullback from the pulmonary artery into the right ventricle, the two pressures match. There is no subpulmonic gradient identified. (Bottom) Right ventricular and pulmonary artery pressures (100 mm Hg paper speed). Note that the end-diastolic pressures for both pulmonary artery and right ventricular tracings are separated by 4 mm Hg. Also evident is the "a" wave on right ventricular tracing due to first-degree A–V block (arrow).

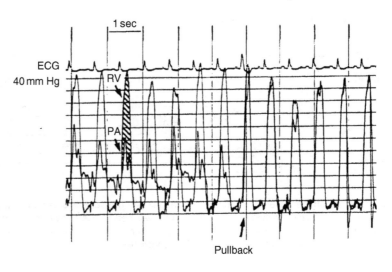

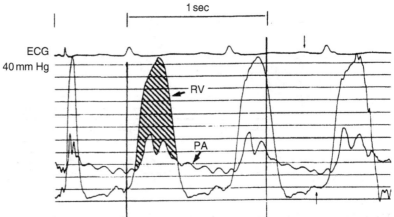

upstroke is slightly delayed and that the right ventricular pressure on pullback across the right ventricular infundibular area into the right ventricle (Figure 17.3, top) shows no supra- or subpulmonic gradient. The demonstration of the matching right ventricular pressures on pullback across the pulmonary artery valve is needed to identify unsuspected infundibular narrowing as a cause of the murmur.

An aside of special interest is the effect of pulmonary stenosis with right ventricular hypertrophy and bundle branch block on the right ventricular and left ventricular pressure patterns. The normal timing of the right ventricular pressure rise relative to left ventricular pressure (shown in Figure 17.4) can be delayed by abnormal impulse conduction to the right (or left) ventricle. Simultaneous right and left ventricular pressure measurements were made in patient #2 with pulmonary stenosis and myocardial ischemia (Figure 17.5). Note the early onset of the right ventricular pressure relative to the left ventricular pressure, and the leftward shift of right ventricular pressure beneath the left ventricular pressure curve. This timing shift may reflect the intraventricular conduction abnormality. However, with bundle branch block, a delay in right ventricular pressure

would be expected. The earlier right ventricular pressure seems to indicate an earlier excitation pathway. Alternatively, one might also attribute this earlier pressure rise to a different mechanism. The widened QRS is a nonspecific conduction defect.

The possible left ventricular hypertrophy with QRS widening may cause a delay in the onset of the left ventricular upstroke, delaying the timing of left ventricular relative to right ventricular pressure. Compared to the normal simultaneous right and left ventricular pressures in Figure 17.4, the left ventricular pressure upstroke in Figure 17.5 occurs later after the R wave, suggesting delay of left ventricular pressure rather than earlier activation of right ventricular pressure. The clinical significance of these findings is unknown.

Combined Pulmonary Stenosis and Insufficiency

A 36-year-old woman had progressive shortness of breath, systolic heart murmur, and combined diastolic murmur. Echocardiography revealed high-velocity jets across the pulmonary valve in systole and diastole.

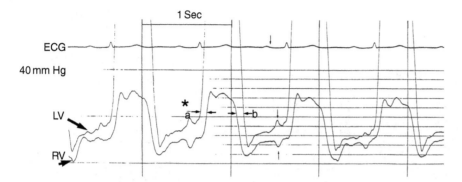

Figure 17.4 Simultaneous left (LV) and right ventricular (RV) pressures in a patient with ischemic heart disease without intraventricular conduction delay on electrocardiogram. The time intervals between left and right ventricular pressures (a and b) are normal and nearly identical. Because of first-degree heart block, note the prominent A wave on both left ventricular and right ventricular diastolic pressures (arrows) and the unusual configuration of the right ventricular A wave.

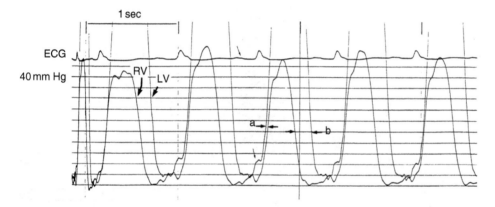

Figure 17.5 Simultaneous right ventricular (RV) and left ventricular (LV) pressures in the patient in Figure 17.3. Note the early onset of right ventricular pressure upstroke as indicated by the distance between arrows at a on beat #3. During ventricular relaxation, the right ventricular pressure declines earlier and more rapidly than the left ventricular pressure. The time interval between decline in right and left ventricular pressures is indicated by the distance between arrows at b and is markedly prolonged. See text for discussion.

Simultaneous hemodynamics measuring the pulmonary artery, right ventricular, and right atrial pressures (0–50 mm Hg scale) are shown in Figure 17.6. These pressure waves show a modest gradient between right ventricular and pulmonary artery systolic pressures, with matching of low pulmonary artery and right ventricular end-diastolic pressures. There is a normal decline in pulmonary artery pressure across the diastolic period. Compare this tracing to Figure 17.3 (bottom) in which the pulmonary artery pressure declines across the diastolic period, but is maintained and elevated above right ventricular end-diastolic pressure, analogous to the hemodynamics of aortic stenosis without insufficiency, in which aortic diastolic pressure is maintained at levels well above left ventricular end-diastolic pressure, in distinction to the reduced aortic diastolic pressure seen in chronic aortic insufficiency. The wide pulmonary pulse pressure of Figure 17.6 was associated with echocardiographically demonstrated pulmonic insufficiency. From these tracings (Figure 17.6), we can also deduce that

there is no tricuspid stenosis or regurgitation. The pulmonary stenosis (and less so insufficiency) can be well characterized by the combined techniques. These findings correlated angiographically with an insufficient pulmonic valve, as well as with a mild doming and deformation of the pulmonary valve leaflets.

A Diastolic Murmur and Elevated Right Ventricular End-Diastolic Pressure

In a 45-year-old woman, elevated and matching pulmonary artery systolic pressures (Figure 17.7) were observed with continuous diastolic murmur across the right upper sternal border. There was no right ventricular–pulmonary artery systolic gradient. The end-diastolic right ventricular pressure is elevated (25 mm Hg) and matches the pulmonary artery diastolic pressure at the onset of right

Figure 17.6 Simultaneous right ventricular (RV), pulmonary artery (PA), and right atrial (RA) pressures (0–50 mm Hg scale) in a patient with systolic and diastolic murmurs. See text for details.

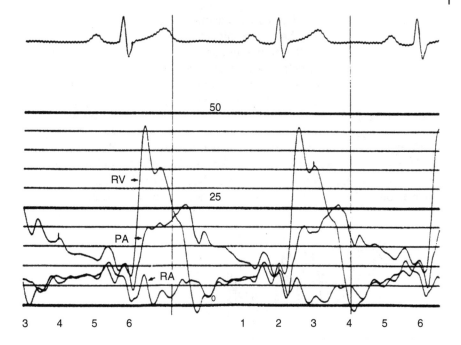

Figure 17.7 Simultaneous right ventricular (RV) and pulmonary artery (PA) pressures in a patient with continuous diastolic murmur (0–100 mm Hg scale). See text for details.

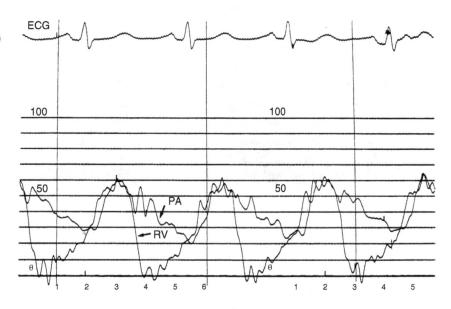

ventricular contraction. Compare the waveforms of Figure 17.7 to Figures 17.3 and 17.6. The elevated pulmonary artery diastolic pressure does not normally indicate pulmonary insufficiency, but the marked distortion of the diastolic right ventricular pressure, especially at end-diastole, suggests continued filling of the right ventricle or a very noncompliant chamber. Coupled with clinical and echocardiographic findings, the diagnosis is clear. Less obvious would be hemodynamic pulmonic insufficiency of Figure 17.6 without the striking right ventricular pressure increase during diastole. These tracings (Figure 17.7) might well correspond to those seen for acute aortic insufficiency, where end-diastolic left ventricular pressure increases to nearly equal aortic diastolic pressure.

Pulmonary Balloon Valvuloplasty

Pulmonary balloon valvuloplasty (PBV) is now the routine treatment for significant congenital pulmonic stenosis. A significant, longlasting decrease in the pulmonary-right ventricular gradient can be achieved with relatively low morbidity and mortality [7]. PBV is also an effective treatment for adult patients with pulmonic stenosis [8]. An unusual hemodynamic phenomenon sometimes seen after PBV is the development of a subvalvular gradient despite effective opening of the stenotic valve [9, 10]. Review the pressure tracings obtained from an 18-year-old man with pulmonary stenosis during PBV (Figure 17.8). The baseline right ventricular systolic pressure is markedly increased (150 mm Hg; Figure 17.8, upper left panel) and is higher than the systemic arterial pressure (not shown). On catheter pullback from the pulmonary artery to the right ventricle before PBV, no significant subvalvular gradient was noted (Figure 17.8, upper right panel). After PBV, catheter pullback reveals development of significant subvalvular gradient at the right ventricular outflow tract (Figure 17.8, lower panel). Because of the outflow obstruction, the net right ventricular to pulmonary artery gradient did not change significantly. A similar situation may be seen after surgical valvotomy, probably related to hypertrophy and hyperdynamic contraction of the outflow portion of the right ventricle. However, the subvalvular obstruction has been shown to decrease gradually after PBV. In a group of 22 patients aged 16–45 years, Fawzy *et al.* [11] showed that the peak pulmonary

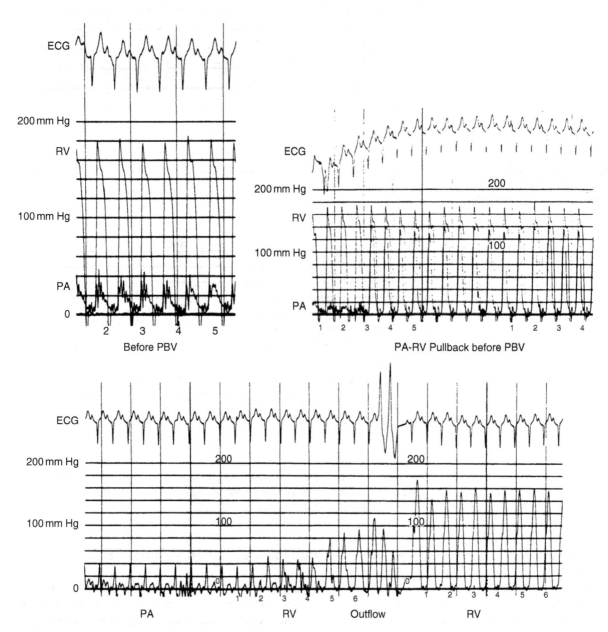

Figure 17.8 Right ventricular (RV) and pulmonary artery (PA) hemodynamic tracings before and after pulmonic balloon valvuloplasty (PBV). Note the pressure in the right ventricular outflow tract. See text for details.

gradient decreased from an average 38 mm Hg immediately after PBV to 18 mm Hg after an average 35 months follow-up. The outflow gradient was also reduced from an average 35 mm Hg to 15 mm Hg, with a significant increase in measured right ventricular outflow tract diameter.

Case Studies

Case #1: Pulmonary Valvuloplasty in Adults

A 39-year-old woman complained of progressive dyspnea on exertion [12]. She had relatively normal childhood growth and development, but was noted to have had a murmur during a high school medical evaluation. No therapy was sought and the patient had been well until recently. She had had several successful deliveries without hemodynamic compromise. The patient had no risk factors for coronary artery disease and was being treated for mild systemic hypertension.

On physical examination, there was a systolic murmur over the left and right sternal borders, a single S_2, and a hyperdynamic right ventricular contraction without a diastolic murmur. There was no peripheral edema or hepatomegaly. The electrocardiogram demonstrated right ventricular hypertrophy. Two-dimensional echocardiography documented pulmonic stenosis, a large right ventricle, and minimal tricuspid regurgitation. The peak valvular gradient was estimated to be greater than 60 mm Hg by Doppler.

At cardiac catheterization, coronary arteriography and left ventriculography were normal. There was a significant pulmonic valvular gradient (Figure 17.9). The pulmonary artery pressure was 22/12 mm Hg, with a right ventricular pressure of 135/12 mm Hg. The aortic pressure was 195/90 mm Hg, and the left ventricular pressure was 195/12 mm Hg with a restrictive diastolic filling pattern. Cardiac output was 3.8 L/min. Oximetry was normal.

To identify infundibular or subvalvular narrowing of the right ventricular outflow tract, a second catheter was placed across the pulmonic valve. While continuously recording both pressures, the catheter was then withdrawn (Figure 17.10). Right ventricular pressures beneath the pulmonic valve in the outflow tract were compared to the right ventricular pressures in the right ventricular apex (Figure 17.10, top). The right ventricular pressure pullback demonstrated a small infundibular gradient of approximately 35 mm Hg (right ventricular outflow, 100/22 mm Hg; right ventricular body, 135/22 mm Hg), appreciated at both low and high recording speeds (Figure 17.10, bottom).

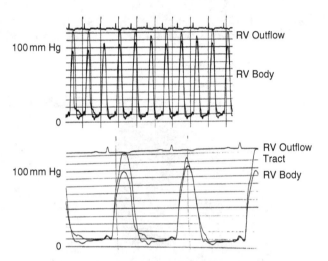

Figure 17.10 In evaluation of the subvalvular contribution to the pulmonic gradient, catheter pullback from the pulmonary artery to the right ventricle was performed. The subpulmonic gradient was 20 mm Hg. The two right ventricular (RV) pressures are shown during pullback maneuver on a 0–100 mm Hg scale. The RV pullback shows the small infundibular tract outflow gradient between the RV infundibulum and outflow and the RV body. The pressures are recorded at 25 mm/sec paper speed on a 0–100 mm Hg scale (top) and at 100 mm/sec paper speed (bottom).

Figure 17.9 Hemodynamic tracings obtained before pulmonary valvuloplasty, demonstrating aortic (Ao), right ventricular (RV), and pulmonary artery (PA) pressures on a 0–200 mm Hg scale. The systolic gradient across the pulmonic valve is 110 mm Hg.

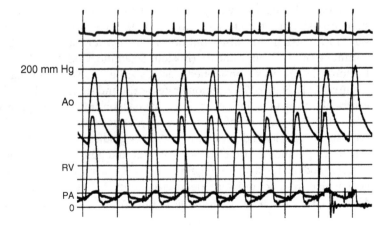

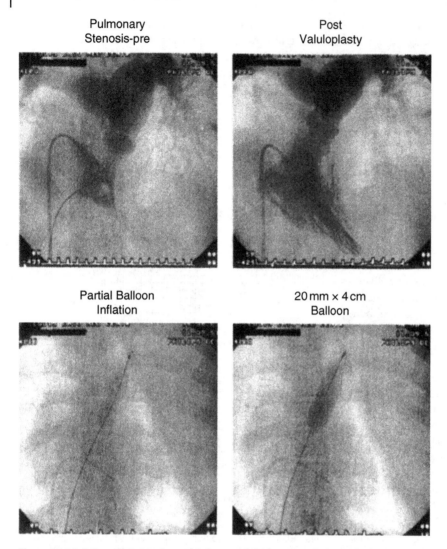

Pulmonary
Stenosis-pre

Post
Valuloplasty

Partial Balloon
Inflation

20 mm × 4 cm
Balloon

Figure 17.11 Selected cineangiographic frames of right ventriculography before pulmonary valvuloplasty. The valve and infundibulum are viewed from the AP cranial projection at end systole before valvuloplasty (top left) and after valvuloplasty (right top). (Below left) A single 20 mm × 4 cm balloon catheter (Mansfield Inc., Boston, MA) was used to dilate the pulmonary stenosis. The waist of the balloon can be seen during partial balloon inflation. (Below right) At completion of balloon inflation, valvular narrowing is eliminated.

Balloon valvuloplasty was performed with a single standard balloon catheter. A 300 cm exchange guidewire was positioned in the distal pulmonary artery, and a 20 mm × 4 cm balloon catheter (Boston Scientific Co., Boston, MA) was positioned across the valve (Figure 17.11). Figure 17.12 demonstrates aortic and right ventricular pressures during a pulmonary balloon inflation. After two balloon inflations, hemodynamics demonstrated a significant decrease in pulmonary gradient.

Following removal of the balloon catheter and guidewire, hemodynamic data were again measured. The right ventricular systolic pressure decreased from 135 to 45 mm Hg, with a corresponding reduction of the pulmonary gradient from 110 to 25 mm Hg. The pulmonary artery pressure was minimally affected (20–24 mm Hg; Figure 17.13).

The residual subvalvular obstruction was measured during pulmonary artery catheter pullback (Figure 17.14). The pulmonary artery systolic pressure was 22 mm Hg (Figure 17.14, left) and as the catheter entered the right ventricle, two new observations were evident. First, the systolic pressure increased to 26–28 mm Hg; also, the diastolic pressure waveform matched the right ventricular pressure. This region is the subvalvular right ventricular outflow tract, from which the residual gradient is formed.

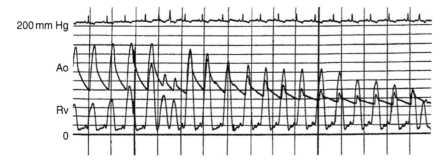

Figure 17.12 Hemodynamic alterations during pulmonary valvuloplasty (0–200 mm Hg scale). The right ventricular (RV) pressure after the second balloon inflation is recorded at initiation of balloon inflation. Aortic (Ao) pressure and cardiac output fall during pulmonary artery balloon obstruction. Ventricular premature contractions can be seen. Right ventricular pressure increases to equal systemic pressure for the first three beats, and then both systemic pressure and right ventricular pressure fall during balloon inflation and deflation.

Figure 17.13 Hemodynamic data before and after pulmonary valvuloplasty, demonstrating reduction in the right ventricular (RV) to pulmonary artery (PA) systolic pressure gradient from 110 mm Hg to approximately 25 mm Hg. The residual outflow tract gradient represents that of the infundibulum, which was not affected by the balloon inflation. Ao = aortic pressure.

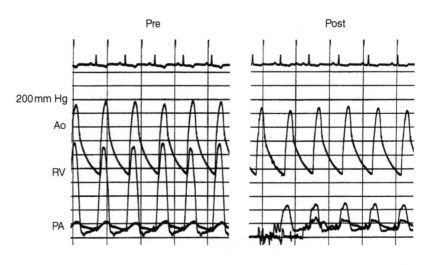

Figure 17.14 Demonstration of right ventricular (RV) outflow tract gradient. Catheter pullback to just beneath the pulmonary valve shows an increase in pulmonary artery (PA) systolic pressure simultaneous with RV diastolic pressure (0–40 mm Hg scale). As the catheter is pulled farther back, two RV pressures become superimposed (not shown).

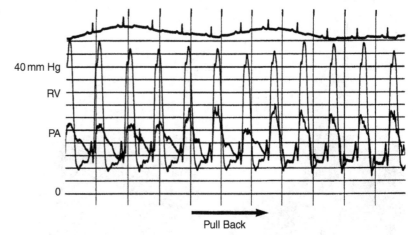

Case #2: Pulmonary Valvuloplasty in Adult Patient with Repaired Congenital Heart Disease

A 29-year-old man had Tetralogy of Fallot with a large ventricular septal defect, infundibular obstruction, and valvular pulmonic stenosis detected at birth. At age 7 years, he underwent surgical closure of the ventricular septal defect using a Dacron patch, resection of infundibular muscle, and incision of the pulmonic valve commissures, with excellent results. He was asymptomatic until several months before admission, when he noted progressive dyspnea on mild exertion, easy fatigability, and intermittent pedal edema. His examination was notable for clear lungs, a diminished second heart sound, and a loud, harsh III/VI systolic crescendo–decrescendo murmur at the upper left sternal border. There was no peripheral edema. The electrocardiogram demonstrated right ventricular hypertrophy.

Cardiac catheterization demonstrated normal left ventricular wall motion and normal coronary arteries. A peak systolic transvalvular pulmonic gradient of 60 mm Hg was produced by a right ventricular pressure of 85/15 mm Hg and a pulmonary artery pressure of

25/15 mm Hg (Figure 17.15, top left). There was no infundibular gradient. Right ventriculography in a lateral projection showed limited motion and doming of the pulmonic valve leaflets (Figure 17.16, left). Pulmonary artery angiography showed mild pulmonic insufficiency. There was poststenotic dilatation of the main pulmonary artery. Cardiac output was 4.5 L/min, and oximetry showed no evidence of intracardiac shunt.

Balloon valvuloplasty was performed. From right ventricular angiography in the left lateral projection, the pulmonic annulus was measured at 22–23 mm. After 5000

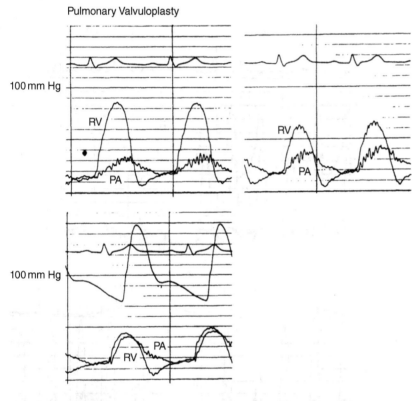

Pulmonary Valvuloplasty

Figure 17.15 Hemodynamic data for pulmonary valvuloplasty, before (top left) and after (top right) initial balloon inflations, and after (bottom) Inoue balloon inflations. RV = right ventricular pressure; PA = pulmonary artery pressure.

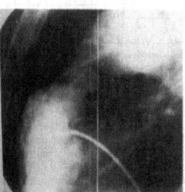
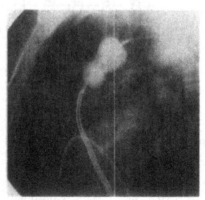
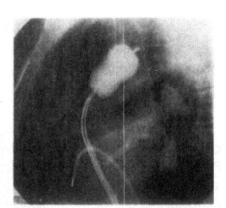

Figure 17.16 Cine frames during pulmonary valvuloplasty. (Left) Lateral view right ventriculogram demonstrating doming stenotic pulmonary valve. (Middle) Inoue balloon partially inflated. (Right) Inoue balloon fully inflated. Pulmonic valvuloplasty with the Inoue balloon is an off-label usage.

Table 17.1 Hemodynamic data for two cases of pulmonary stenosis.

	Right Ventricular Pressure (mm Hg)	Pulmonary Artery Pressure (mm Hg)	Pressure Gradient (mm Hg)	Cardiac Output (L/min)	Left Ventricular Pressure (mm Hg)	Aortic Pressure (mm Hg)
Case #1						
Before pulmonary valvuloplasty	135/12	22/12	115	3.8	195/12	195/90
After pulmonary valvuloplasty	45/12	24/12	25			190/90
Case 2						
Before pulmonary valvuloplasty	85/20	32/18	53			
After pulmonary valvuloplasty	45/18	42/15	3			

units of intravenous heparin had been administered, a stiff 0.038 inch Amplatz guidewire was placed into a distal pulmonary artery segment via a balloon-tipped wedge catheter. Multiple dilatations with a 23 mm × 4 cm balloon catheter (Boston Scientific Co.) were performed across the pulmonic valve. The balloon was noted, at times, to slip backward or forward at full inflation. These dilatations resulted in improvement, but there remained a residual 30–40 mm Hg transvalvular gradient (Figure 17.15, top right). Therefore, a 0.018 inch guidewire was exchanged for a 0.025 inch Amplatz wire and a 28 mm Inoue balloon (Toray, Inc., Tokyo, Japan) situated across the pulmonic valve. Careful torquing of the Inoue catheter through the right atrium and across the tricuspid valve was required. Taking advantage of the Inoue balloon characteristics, the tip was partially inflated in the main pulmonary artery and the balloon was pulled into the appropriate position at valve level (Figure 17.16, middle and right). Sequential stepwise dilatations from 24 to 28 mm by increasing balloon volume resulted in marked reduction in the transvalvular gradient to 6–8 mm Hg, with a reduction in right ventricular systolic pressure to 45 mm Hg (Figure 17.15, bottom). Pulmonary angiography showed moderate pulmonic insufficiency. Following the procedure, the patient noted resolution of his symptoms, which has been sustained for over 9 months. Follow-up echocardiography at 6 months post valvuloplasty showed no valvular restenosis and mild pulmonic insufficiency. A summary of the hemodynamics is shown in Table 17.1.

Clinical Outcomes of Pulmonary Valvuloplasty

Chen *et al.* [13] described their experience in 53 adolescent or adult patients (age 13–55 years) with follow-up studies at a mean of 7 ± 3 years after the procedure. After

pulmonic balloon valvuloplasty, the systolic pressure gradient across the pulmonic valve decreased from 91 ± 46 to 38 ± 32 mm Hg, and the pressure gradient of the pulmonic valve orifice increased from 9 ± 4 to 17 ± 5 mm Hg. At follow-up, hemodynamic data indicated that the systolic gradient continued to decrease from 107 ± 48 before to 50 ± 9 mm Hg after valvuloplasty, and a follow-up remained at 30 ± 16 mm Hg. Pulmonary valve incompetence was noted in 7 of 53 patients (13%) after balloon valvuloplasty, but was absent in the follow-up examination in all patients. Investigators concluded that late adolescent or adult patients with congenital pulmonic stenosis can be treated with balloon valvuloplasty successfully, with excellent short- and long-term results similar to those in children.

Residual Transpulmonic Gradients

A persistent systolic gradient suggests that subvalvular stenosis of the right ventricular outflow tract may occur after successful balloon valvuloplasty. The reduction in systolic gradient at follow-up examination of the patients undergoing pulmonary valvuloplasty suggests that a delayed reduction of the gradient produces results similar to those of surgical pulmonic valvulotomy, and that the systolic gradient measured immediately after balloon valvuloplasty underestimates the long-term results of the procedure. As noted in the case associated with Figure 17.9 through 17.14, infundibular hypertrophy caused by longstanding pulmonary stenosis may result in residual outflow tract obstruction, which can regress over time. The regression of infundibular hypertrophy is more notable in the younger population as compared to adults [14]. The systolic gradient, measured across both the valve and the infundibulum at follow-up, although markedly reduced after valvuloplasty, suggests that there is some degree of regression of the hypertrophic infundibulum and that surgical resection for adults may not be required. This finding also supports the idea that stenosis of the infundibulum is not an absolute contraindication to percutaneous balloon pulmonic valvuloplasty.

Although the mechanism of infundibular tract systolic gradients is incompletely understood, the subvalvular muscular hypertrophy and activity of contraction in the unrestrained phase immediately on relief of valvular resistance probably produce a hyperkinetic effect. Beta blockers have been recommended, although in most adult series these medications have not been necessary.

Complications of Pulmonic Valvuloplasty

Pulmonic insufficiency after valvuloplasty occurred in 13% of patients in the study by Chen *et al.* [13], none of which was of major hemodynamic consequence. Similar data have been reported by others [15, 16] and appear to be due to the more precise sizing of the pulmonic valve by a variable balloon catheter method. Unique to pulmonic stenosis is the situation of the dysplastic valve associated with complex intracardiac defects. David *et al.* [17] reported on the results of percutaneous balloon dilatation for pulmonic stenosis in 38 patients ranging from 9 months to 63 years in age. Thirty-four patients had typical pulmonary stenosis, with five having complex congenital cardiac anomalies. Thirteen patients also had a patent foramen ovale.

For the group, there was significant reduction in the immediate postvalvuloplasty transpulmonic gradient from 97 to 26 mm Hg. There was one death in the postvalvuloplasty period of a patient with Class IV congestive heart failure due to right ventricular decompensation. There were no other cardiovascular complications encountered, with a mean hospital stay of 3 days. At 8-month follow-up, the transpulmonic gradient in 12 patients was 27 mm Hg, compared to the prevalvuloplasty value of 84 mm Hg. Two patients had restenosed, one required open-heart surgical valvotomy, and one had successful repeat balloon valvuloplasty.

Key Points

1) Although it is an uncommon lesion, when pulmonary stenosis is considered, pulmonary artery and right ventricular pressures should be assessed simultaneously on two-catheter pullback to appreciate the precise location of pulmonary–right ventricular pressure gradients.
2) Peripheral pulmonic stenosis can mimic pulmonary valve stenosis, and pulmonary artery insufficiency may be difficult to delineate on pressure alone (as is often the case with the hemodynamics of aortic insufficiency).
3) Conduction defects or ventricular hypertrophy can affect the right ventricular pressure tracing and either delay or increase the timing of pressure rise and decline, depending on the conduction disturbance and abnormality of myocardial contraction.

References

1 Kern MJ. Hemodynamic rounds: Interpretation of cardiac pathophysiology from pressure waveform analysis: The pulmonary valve. *Cathet Cardiovasc Diagn* 24:209–213, 1991.
2 Kern MJ, Lim MJ, Goldstein JA (eds). *Hemodynamic Rounds: Interpretation of Cardiac Pathophysiology from Pressure Waveform Analysis*, 3rd ed. Hoboken, NJ: John Wiley & Sons, Inc., 2009.
3 Grossman W. Profiles in valvular heart disease. In W Grossman (ed.), *Cardiac Catheterization and Angiography*. Boston, MA: Lea and Febiger, 1986, pp. 359–381.
4 Freed MD, Keane JR. Profiles in congenital heart disease. In W Grossman (ed.), *Cardiac Catheterization and Angiography*. Boston, MA: Lea and Febiger, 1986, pp. 446–469.
5 Hirshfeld JW. Valve function: Stenosis and insufficiency. In CJ Pepine (ed.), *Diagnostic and Therapeutic Cardiac Catheterization*. Baltimore, MD: Williams & Wilkins, 1989, pp. 390–410.
6 Conti CR. Cardiac catheterization and the patient with congenital heart disease. In CJ Pepine (ed.), *Diagnostic and Therapeutic Cardiac Catheterization*. Baltimore, MD: Williams & Wilkins, 1989, pp. 508–522.
7 Beekman RH, Rocchini AP. Pulmonary valvuloplasty. In EJ Topol (ed.), *Textbook of Interventional Cardiology*. Philadelphia, PA: WB Saunders, 1990, pp. 900–911.
8 Fawzy ME, Mercer EN, Dunn B. Late results of pulmonary balloon valvuloplasty in adults using double balloon technique. *J Intervent Cardiol* 1:35–32, 1988.
9 Ben-Shachar G, Cohen MH, Sivakoff MC, Portman MA, Riemenschneider TA, Van Heeckeren DW. Development of infundibular obstruction after percutaneous pulmonary balloon valvuloplasty. *J Am Coll Cardiol* 5:754–756, 1985.

10 Griffith BP, Hardesty RL, Siewers RD, Lerberg DB, Ferson PF, Bahnson HT. Pulmonary valvulotomy alone for pulmonary stenosis: Results in children with and without muscular infundibular hypertrophy. *J Thorac Surg* 83:577–583, 1982.

11 Fawzy ME, Galal O, Dunn B, Shaikh A, Sriram R, Duran CMG. Regression of infundibular pulmonary stenosis after successful balloon pulmonary valvuloplasty in adults. *Cathet Cardiovasc Diagn* 21:77–81, 1990.

12 Kern MJ. Pulmonary valvuloplasty. In MJ Kern (ed.), *Hemodynamic Rounds*, 2nd ed. New York: Wiley-Liss, 1999, pp. 129–136.

13 Chen C, Cheng T, Huang T, Zhou Y, Chen J, Huang Y, Li H. Percutaneous balloon valvuloplasty for pulmonic stenosis in adolescents and adults. *N Engl J Med* 335:21–25, 1996.

14 Ben-Shachar G, Cohen MH, Sivakoff MC, Portman MA, Riemenschneider TA, Van Heeckeren DW. Development of infundibular obstruction after percutaneous pulmonary balloon valvuloplasty. *J Am Coll Cardiol* 5:754–756, 1985.

15 Gutgesell HP. Pulmonary valve insufficiency: Malignant or benign? *J Am Coll Cardiol* 20:174–175, 1992.

16 O'Connor BK, Beekman RH, Lindauer A, Rocchini A. Intermediate-term outcome after pulmonary balloon valvuloplasty: Comparison with a matched surgical control group. *J Am Coll Cardiol* 20: 169–173, 1992.

17 David SW, Goussous YM, Harbi N, Doghmi F, Hiari A, Krayyem M, Ferlinz J. Management of typical and dysplastic pulmonic stenosis, uncomplicated or associated with complex intracardiac defects in juveniles and adults: Use of percutaneous balloon pulmonary valvuloplasty with eight-month hemodynamic follow-up. *Cathet Cardiovasc Diagn* 29:105–112, 1993.

Part Five

Coronary, Renal, Congenital, and Left Ventricular Support Hemodynamics

18

Coronary Hemodynamics: The Basics of Pressure and Flow Measurements, Coronary Vasodilatory Reserve, and Fractional Flow Reserve

Morton J. Kern and Crystal Medina

In the last decade, studies have demonstrated favorable outcomes for revascularization decisions based on determination of lesion-specific ischemia by in-laboratory coronary physiologic measurements. Coronary physiologic lesion assessment in the catheterization laboratory is required to overcome the inability of anatomy (either angiographic or intravascular ultrasound imaging) to accurately predict the ischemic potential of a coronary luminal narrowing. Measurements of coronary pressure and flow in the catheterization laboratory are now used in daily clinical practice.

Coronary Blood Flow and Resistance

Coronary arterial resistance (R, pressure/flow) is the summed resistances of the epicardial coronary conductance (R1), precapillary arteriolar (R2), and intramyocardial capillary (R3) resistance circuits (Figure 18.1). Normal epicardial coronary arteries in humans typically taper gradually from the base of the heart to the apex. The epicardial vessels (R1) do not offer significant resistance to blood flow in their normal nondiseased state. Coronary epicardial resistance would be manifest as a pressure drop along the length of human epicardial arteries [1]. Epicardial vessel resistance (R1) is trivial until atherosclerotic obstructions develop.

Precapillary arterioles (R2) are small (100–500 microns in size), resistive vessels connecting epicardial arteries to myocardial capillaries, and are the main controllers of coronary blood flow [1]. Precapillary arterioles autoregulate the perfusion pressure at their origin within a finite pressure range.

The microcirculatory resistance (R3) consists of a dense network of capillaries perfusing each myocyte adjacent to a capillary. Several conditions, such as left ventricular (LV) hypertrophy, myocardial ischemia, or diabetes, can impair the microcirculatory resistance (R3) and blunt the normal increases in coronary flow in response to demand or pharmacologic agents. Increased R3 resistance may increase resting blood flow, resulting in reduced coronary flow reserve (i.e., the hyperemic/basal flow ratio).

Coronary vasodilator flow reserve (CFR), the ratio of maximal hyperemic to resting coronary flow or flow velocity, is the ability of the coronary vascular bed to increase flow from a basal level to a maximal (or near maximal) hyperemic level in response to a mechanical or pharmacologic stimuli. Normal CFR ranges from 2 to 5x resting flow in humans [2].

Gould [3] showed that increasing coronary stenosis severity was associated with a predictable decline in coronary flow reserve. CFR begins to decline at about a 60% artery diameter narrowing, and hence it was thought that such stenoses carried physiologic importance; a truth in the animal but not the human experimental models. At diameter stenoses greater than 80–90%, all available coronary reserve has been exhausted and resting flow begins to decline (Figure 18.2).

Pressure Loss across a Stenosis

As blood traverses a diseased arterial segment, turbulence, friction, and separation of laminar flow cause energy loss, resulting in a pressure gradient (ΔP) across the stenosis. Morphologic features of the stenosis are also responsible for resistance to flow changing exponentially with lumen cross-sectional area (the most commonly used measure of severity) and linearly with lesion length [5] (Figure 18.3). Additional factors contributing to stenosis resistance include the shape of the entrance and exit orifices. Using a simplified Bernoulli formula for fluid dynamics, pressure loss across a stenosis can be estimated from blood flow as follows:

$$\Delta P = fQ + sQ^2$$

Hemodynamic Rounds: Interpretation of Cardiac Pathophysiology from Pressure Waveform Analysis, Fourth Edition.
Edited by Morton J. Kern, Michael J. Lim, and James A. Goldstein.

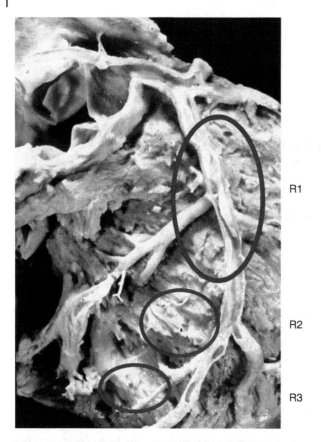

Figure 18.1 Pathological specimen demonstrating sources of myocardial perfusion. (R1) Epicardial arteries; (R2) Precapillary arterioles; (R3) Microcirculation. Fractional flow reserve is specific for epicardial coronary stenosis (R1 resistance), whereas coronary flow reserve measures the sum of both the epicardial (R1) and microvascular (R2, R3) resistances.

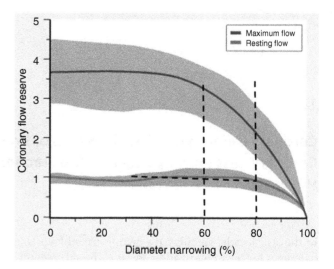

Figure 18.2 Coronary flow reserve expressed as the ratio of maximum to resting flow, plotted as a function of percentage diameter narrowing. With progressive narrowing, resting flow does not change (magenta line), whereas maximum potential increase in flow (blue line) and coronary flow reserve begin to be impaired at approximately 50% diameter narrowing. The shaded area represents the limits of variability of data about the mean. *Source:* Gould 1974 [4]. Reproduced with permission of Elsevier. (*See insert for color representation of the figure.*)

Intracoronary Pressure and Fractional Flow Reserve

Significant atherosclerotic stenosis produces epicardial conduit resistance. In response to the loss of perfusion pressure and flow to the distal (poststenotic) vascular bed, the small resistance vessels dilate to maintain satisfactory basal flow appropriate for myocardial oxygen demand. Viscous friction, flow separation forces, and flow turbulence at the site of the stenosis produce energy loss at the stenosis (Figure 18.3). Energy (heat) is extracted, reducing pressure distal to the stenosis and thereby producing a pressure gradient between proximal and distal artery regions. The pressure loss or gradient increases with increasing coronary flow.

Fractional Flow Reserve and Method of Guidewire Pressure Measurements

The measurement of coronary pressure is similar to performing an angioplasty, in that a sensor guidewire is passed through an angioplasty Y-connector attached to a guiding catheter. Anti-coagulation (intravenous [IV] heparin 70 U/kg) and often intracoronary (IC) nitroglycerin (100–200 mg) are given before the guidewire is advanced into the artery.

Before inserting the guidewire into the patient, the sensor wire and guide catheter pressure signals are calibrated and zeroed. The sensor wire is then introduced and positioned at the tip of the guiding catheter, where

where ΔP is the pressure drop across the stenosis (mm Hg) and Q is the flow across the stenosis (mL/sec). The components of these two terms are shown below:

$$f = \frac{1}{A_s^2} \times L \times Q \quad s = \frac{1}{A_s^2} \times \frac{1}{A_n^2} \times Q^2$$

The first term (f) accounts for energy losses owing to viscous friction of laminar flow, and the second term (s) reflects energy loss when normal arterial flow accelerates to high-velocity flow in the stenosis and then back to slower turbulent nonlaminar distal flow on exiting the stenosis. A_s is stenotic segment cross-sectional area, p = blood density, μ = blood viscosity, L = stenosis length, A_n = normal artery cross-sectional area.

Because of the second term, the increases in coronary blood flow increase the associated pressure gradient in a quadratic manner. As an additional consequence, for a given stenosis with potentially variable area and size of reference normal vessel, there may be a family of pressure–flow relationships reflecting altered stenosis diameter and variable distending pressure.

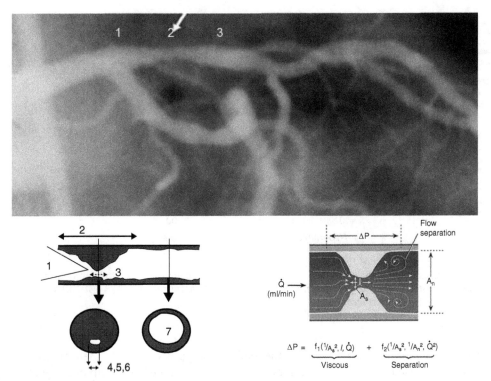

Figure 18.3 Morphologic features of the stenosis are also responsible for resistance to flow changing exponentially with lumen cross-sectional area (the most commonly used measure of severity) and linearly with lesion length. 1 = entrance angle, 2 = lesion narrowing, 3 = exit angle. Arrow indicates lesion. (Bottom left) Diagram of coronary stenosis showing seven factors producing resistance to flow: 1 = entrance angle, 2 = disease segment length, 3 = stenosis length, 4, 5, 6 = shape factors of lumen area, 7 = size of reference vessel. (Bottom right) Total pressure loss across a stenosis is derived from two sources: frictional losses along the leading edge of the stenosis; and inertial losses stemming from the sudden expansion, which causes flow separation and eddies (exit losses). Frictional losses are linearly related to flow by the law of Poiseuille, and exit losses increase with the square of the flow (law of Bernoulli). The total change in pressure gradient (ΔP) is the sum of the two. The loss coefficients, f_1 and f_2, are functions of stenosis geometry and rheologic properties of blood (viscosity and density). The graphic representation of this equation results in a quadratic relationship, in which the curvilinear shape demonstrates the presence of nonlinear exit losses. If no stenosis is present, the second term is zero, and the curve becomes a straight line (with a positive slope that depends on the diameter of the vessel, based on the law of Poiseuille). An = area of the normal segment; As = area of the stenosis; L = length. *Source:* Kern 2000 [6]. Reproduced with permission of Wolters Kluwer Health, Inc.

the guiding catheter and wire pressures are equalized (assuming an accurate baseline before advancing down the artery). The wire is then advanced across the stenosis, or to the most distal part of the coronary artery for assessment of serial lesions or diffuse disease. The sensor should be at least 1 cm distal to the coronary stenosis being assessed.

Stenosis severity should always be assessed using measurements obtained during maximal hyperemia. A pharmacologic hyperemic stimulus is then administered through the guide catheter (intracoronary) or intravenously. The mean and phasic pressure signals are continuously recorded and at peak hyperemia (represented by the nadir or lowest distal pressure). Pijls *et al.* [7] derived an estimate of the percentage of normal coronary blood flow expected to go through a stenotic artery from the distal/aortic pressure ratio at maximal hyperemia, called the fractional flow reserve (FFR; Figure 18.4). FFR can be subdivided into three components describing the flow contributions by the coronary artery (FFR_{cor}), the myocardium (FFR_{myo}), and the collateral supply.

Fractional Flow Reserve of the Coronary Artery

The following equations are used to calculate the FFR of a coronary artery and its dependent myocardium:

$$FFR_{cor} = \left(P_d - P_w \right) / \left(P_a - P_w \right)$$
$$FFR_{myo} = \left(P_d - P_v \right) / \left(P_a - P_v \right)$$
$$FFR_{collateral} = FFR_{myo} - FFR_{cor}$$

where P_a, P_d, P_v, and P_w are pressures of the aorta, distal artery, venous (or right atrial), and coronary wedge (during balloon occlusion), respectively; because FFR_{cor} uses P_w, it can be calculated only during coronary angioplasty.

FFR_{myo}, generally referred to just as FFR, can be readily calculated during either diagnostic or interventional

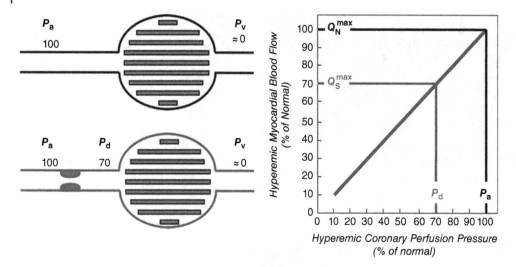

Figure 18.4 Fractional flow reserve (FFR) is an estimate of the percentage of normal coronary blood flow expected to go through a stenotic artery from the distal/aortic pressure ratio at maximal hyperemia. N = normal vessel; P_a = aortic pressure; P_d = distal arterial pressure; P_v = venous pressure; Qmax = maximal flow; S = stenotic vessel.

procedures. In most clinical circumstances P_v is negligible relative to aortic pressure and is omitted from the calculations. FFR reflects both antegrade and collateral perfusion. Because it is calculated only at peak hyperemia, it excludes the microcirculatory resistance from the computation. FFR is largely independent of basal flow, driving pressure, heart rate, systemic blood pressure, or status of the microcirculation [8].

FFR is strongly related to provocable myocardial ischemia, using different clinical stress testing modalities in patients with stable angina as the comparative standard. The nonischemic threshold value of FFR is > 0.80. Even in patients with an abnormal microcirculation, a normal FFR indicates that the epicardial conduit resistance (i.e., a stenosis) is not a major contributing factor to perfusion impairment, and that focal conduit enlargement (e.g., stenting) would not restore normal perfusion. Errors and pitfalls of measuring FFR have been described in detail elsewhere [9].

Pressure Guidewire Pullback Tracings

To study the distribution of abnormalities along a diseased coronary artery (with serial lesions or diffuse disease), the pressure wire can be pulled back slowly during intravenously induced hyperemia. Pressure loss due to diffuse atherosclerosis is differentiated from a focal stenosis, which is identified by an abrupt increase in pressure proximal to the lesion. By moving the sensor back and forth, the exact location of a pressure drop representing a focal obstruction to flow can be determined.

After pressures are measured, the sensor wire coupler is disconnected. The pressure wire is then used as a routine wire and the angioplasty procedure performed as per normal.

At the end of the procedure, the sensor wire is withdrawn and then positioned at the tip of the guiding catheter to verify equal guiding catheter and guidewire pressures if present. Pressure signal drift can be seen. A more complete description of the application and pitfalls of coronary pressure measurements can be found elsewhere [9].

Nonhyperemic Indices of Lesion Severity

The assessment of stenosis severity by FFR requires that coronary resistance is stable and minimal, usually achieved by the administration of adenosine. Utilization of an adenosine-free or adenosine-independent pressure-derived index of coronary stenosis severity may facilitate the incorporation of physiology into the catheterization laboratory. Using wave intensity analysis, Sen *et al.* (10) identified a period of diastole in which equilibration or balance between pressure waves from the aorta and distal microcirculatory reflection was a "wave-free period" with a low and fixed resistance. During this period the resistance may be sufficiently low—compared with adenosine hyperemia—to assess translesional hemodynamic significance (Figure 18.5). The ratio of P_d/P_a during the wave-free period was called the instantaneous wave-free pressure ratio (iFR). In the ADVISE study, 157 stenoses were assessed with pressure and flow distal to the lesion, and another 118 stenoses were assessed using pressure alone. The intracoronary resistance at rest during the wave-free period was similar in variability and magnitude to that during FFR, and the iFR correlated closely with FFR, r = 0.90 (Figure 18.6). However, there were limitations to this analysis despite having high

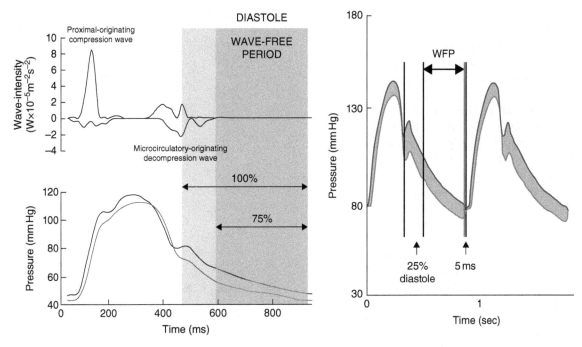

Figure 18.5 The instantaneous wave-free pressure ratio (**iFR**) is derived from a period of diastole in which equilibration or balance between pressure waves from the aorta and distal microcirculatory reflection is a "wave-free period" (WFP) with a low and fixed resistance. During this period the resistance may be sufficiently low—compared with adenosine hyperemia—to assess translesional hemodynamic significance. (*See insert for color representation of the figure.*)

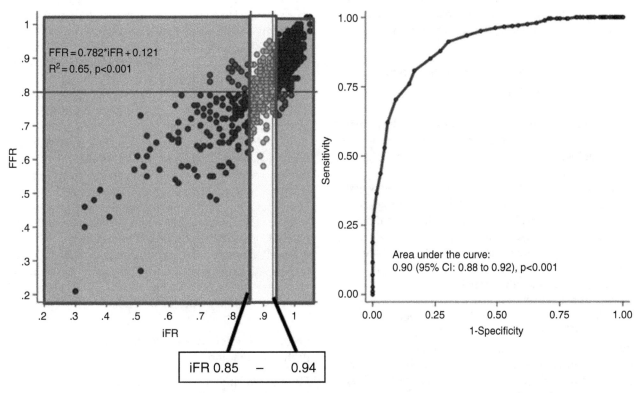

Figure 18.6 The intracoronary resistance at rest during the wave-free period was similar in variability and magnitude to that during fractional flow reserve (FFR), and the instantaneous wave-free pressure ratio (iFR) correlated closely with FFR, r = 0.90.

sensitivity, specificity, and negative and positive predictive values for iFR versus FFR. In particular, there is concern that the iFR at rest was different than the iFR during hyperemia, suggesting that the wave-free period does not have as low a resistance as a hyperemic period would.

Subsequently, Petraco *et al.* [11] demonstrated that at iFR cutoff points of > 0.93 or < 0.86, there was a strong correlation with normal and abnormal FFR values (using 0.80 as an FFR cutoff point). Thus, potentially 57% of the patients with intermediate stenosis could be assessed without the need for hyperemic stimulus.

The RESOLVE study [12] compared the diagnostic accuracy of iFR and resting pressure ratio P_d/P_a to FFR in a core laboratory. The iFR, P_d/P_a, and FFR were measured in 1,768 patients from 15 clinical sites. Core lab technicians were used to analyze the data. Thresholds corresponding to 90% accuracy in predicting ischemic versus nonischemic FFR were then identified. In 1,974 lesions, the optimal iFR to predict an FFR < 0.8 was 0.90 with accuracy of 80%. For the resting P_d/P_a ratio, the cutoff point was 0.92 with an overall accuracy of 80%, with no significant differences between iFR and P_d/P_a. Both measures have 90% accuracy to predict positive or negative FFR in 65% and 48% of lesions, respectively. These data suggest that the overall accuracy of iFR with FFR was about 80%, which can be improved to 90% in a subset of lesions. The benefit of a nonhyperemic index of lesion severity may simplify the technique of lesion assessment and improve decision-making. Studies of the value and accuracy of such indices are in progress.

Clinical Application of Intracoronary Pressure Measurements

The usefulness of any index is the validity of the ischemic thresholds established for that measurement. A summary of physiologic thresholds values for common clinical applications is provided in Table 18.1.

In order to define the threshold of FFR_{myo} below which inducible ischemia is present, Pijls and colleagues [14] compared FFR_{myo} with the unique ischemic standard of common noninvasive testing modalities in 45 patients with moderate coronary stenoses and chest pain syndromes. When the FFR_{myo} was lower than 0.75 (21 patients), reversible myocardial ischemia was demonstrated unequivocally on at least one noninvasive test (bicycle exercise testing, thallium scintigraphy, stress echocardiography with dobutamine), and all these positive test results were reversed after percutaneous transluminal coronary angioplasty (PTCA) or coronary artery bypass graft surgery. In 21 of 24 patients with an FFR_{myo} greater than 0.75, all the tests showed no demonstration of ischemia, and no revascularization procedure was

Table 18.1 Fractional flow reserve (FFR) and other FFR-like indices.

Index	Normal Value	Ischemic Threshold	Comments
FFR	1.0	≤ 0.80	—
cFFR	1.0	≈ 0.83	Avoids adenosine by using contrast media; may correlate with FFR better than iFR and P_d/P_a
iFR	1.0	≈ 0.89	Avoids need for hyperemia; 80% accurate when compared with FFR
Rest P_d/P_a	1.0	≈ 0.91	Avoids need for hyperemia; 80% accurate when compared with FFR

cFFR = contrast FFR; FFR = fractional flow reserve; iFR = instantaneous wave-free pressure ratio; P_d/P_a = distal coronary pressure/proximal coronary pressure.
Source: Fearon [13].

performed. Importantly, no revascularization was required after 14 months of follow-up. The sensitivity of FFR_{myo} in the identification of reversible ischemia was 88%, the specificity 100%, the positive predictive value 100%, the negative predicted value 88%, and the accuracy 93%.

FFR values less than 0.75 are associated with ischemic stress testing in numerous comparative studies with high sensitivity (88%), specificity (100%), positive predicted value (100%), and overall accuracy (93%). FFR values greater than 0.80 are associated with negative ischemic results with a predictive accuracy of 95%. Single stress testing comparisons with variations in testing methods and patient cohorts have produced a zone of FFR with overlapping positive and negative results (0.75–0.80). The use of FFR in this zone requires clinical judgment. A meta-analysis of 31 studies [15] found that quantitative coronary angiography (QCA) had a random effects sensitivity of 78% and specificity of 51% against FFR (<0.75 cutoff) and that, compared with noninvasive imaging (21 studies, 1,249 lesions), FFR versus perfusion scintigraphy (976 lesions) had sensitivity 75%, specificity 77%, and versus dobutamine stress echocardiography (273 lesions) had sensitivity 82%, specificity 74%. From the ischemia validation studies over the last 15 years, FFR can be used as a vessel-specific index of ischemia.

Coronary Physiology and Myocardial Perfusion Imaging

Strong correlations exist between myocardial stress testing and FFR_{myo} or CFR. An FFR_{myo} less than 0.75 identifies physiologically significant stenoses associated with

Table 18.2 Ischemic stress testing and coronary physiologic measurements.

FFR Study	N	Ischemic Test	Threshold	Physiologic Sensitivity	Specificity	PV+	PV-	Accuracy
Pijls *et al.* [14]	45	Four-test standard*	<0.75	88	100	100	88	93
de Bruyne *et al.* [15]	60	Ex ECG	<0.72	100	87	—	—	—
Bartunek *et al.* [16]	37	Dobu/Ex echo	<0.68	95	90	—	—	—
Chamuleau *et al.* [17]	127	Dipy MIBI	<0.75	—	—	—	—	75
Caymaz *et al.* [20]	30	Ex thallium	<0.75	—	—	91	100	—
Fearon *et al.* [21]	10	Ex thallium	<0.75	90	100	—	—	93

*Four tests were used: electrocardiogram, echocardiogram, pacing, and nuclear stress tests.
Adeno/Dipy MIBI = adenosine or dipyridamole sestamibi scan; CFR = coronary flow reserve; Dobu = dobutamine; ECG = electrocardiogram; Echo = echocardiagram; Ex = exercise; Pharm = pharmacologic; PV+/PV– = predictive value positive/negative; rCFR = relative coronary flow reserve.

inducible myocardial ischemia, with high sensitivity (88%), specificity (100%), positive predicted value (100%), and overall accuracy (93%). Although no longer used for stenosis assessment, an abnormal CFR (<2.0) corresponds to reversible myocardial perfusion imaging defects with high sensitivity (86–92%), specificity (89–100%), predictive accuracy (89–96%), and positive and negative predictive values (84–100% and 77–95%, respectively) [16]. A summary of ischemic stress testing and coronary physiologic measurements is provided in Table 18.2.

Fractional Flow Reserve and Intravascular Imaging Measurements

As another method of assessing a coronary artery beyond coronary angiography, intravascular ultrasound (IVUS) offers a high degree of anatomic detail that can aid the operator in making clinical decisions. A study comparing IVUS, QCA, and FFR in 42 patients with 51 stenoses also demonstrated that QCA alone was not accurate in determining physiologic lesion significance assessed by either IVUS or FFR [22]. There was, however, a strong correlation of minimum lumen area (MLA) IVUS less than $3.0 \, mm^2$ and cross-sectional area (CSA) IVUS stenosis greater than 60% with a measured FFR less than 0.75 (IVUS sensitivity 83%, specificity 92%).

Briguori and colleagues [23] related anatomy and physiology in 53 lesions. The percent area stenosis and lesion length had a significant inverse correlation with FFR ($r = -0.58$, $P < 0.001$ and $r = -0.41$, $P < 0.004$, respectively). Minimum lumen diameter (MLD) and MLA showed significant positive correlation with FFR. By receiver operating characteristic (ROC) curves, a percent

area stenosis > 70%, MLD < 1.8 mm, MLA < $4.0 \, mm^2$, and lesion length > 10 mm were the best cutoff values to fit FFR < 0.75. Optical coherence tomography and intravascular ultrasound cross-sectional areas have similar weak relationships to FFR (Figure 18.7).

Hemodynamic Assessment of an Intermediately Severe Angiographic Stenosis

The clinical outcomes of deferring coronary intervention for intermediate stenoses with normal physiology are remarkably consistent, with clinical event rates of less than 10% over a two-year follow-up period. No study has deferred treatment in symptomatic patients with abnormal translesional physiology. Pijls and colleagues have recently reported the results of a large, randomized study (Deferral of PTCA versus performance of PTCA [DEFER]) of 325 patients for whom PTCA was planned and who did not have documented ischemia [25]. FFR of the stenosis was measured and, when it was more than 0.75, patients were randomly assigned to deferral (deferral group; $n = 91$) or performance (performance group; $n = 90$) of PTCA. If FFR was less than 0.75, PTCA was performed as planned (reference group; $n = 144$). Clinical follow-up was obtained at 1, 3, 6, 12, and 24 months. Event-free survival was similar between the deferral and performance groups (92% vs. 89% at 12 months and 89% vs. 83% at 24 months), but was significantly lower in the reference group (80% at 12 months and 78% at 24 months; Figure 18.8). In addition, the percentage of patients free from angina was similar between the deferral and performance groups (49% vs. 50% at 12 months and 70% vs. 51% at 24 months), but was significantly higher in the reference group (67% at 12 months and 80% at 24 months). It could

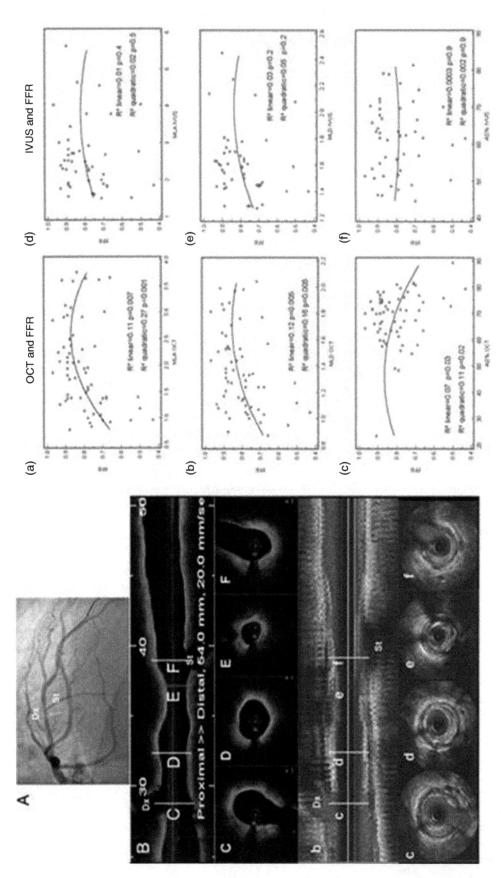

Figure 18.7 Matching of optical coherence tomography (OCT) and intravascular ultrasound (IVUS) pullbacks. (A) Angiographic view showing an intermediate stenosis in the mid left anterior descending coronary artery (yellow arrow). Distal to the lesion there is a septal branch (St) and proximal there is a diagonal branch (Dx). (B, b) Longitudinal optical coherence tomography and intravascular ultrasound reconstructions showing the two side branches (St and Dx) and the stenosis. (C, c; D, d; E, e; F, f) Corresponding cross-sectional optical coherence tomography and intravascular ultrasound images. (C, c) Diagonal branch. (D, d) Reference cross-section. (E, e) Minimum lumen area. (F, f) Septal branch. FFR = fractional flow reserve. *Source:* Gonzalo 2012 [24]. Reproduced with permission of Elsevier.

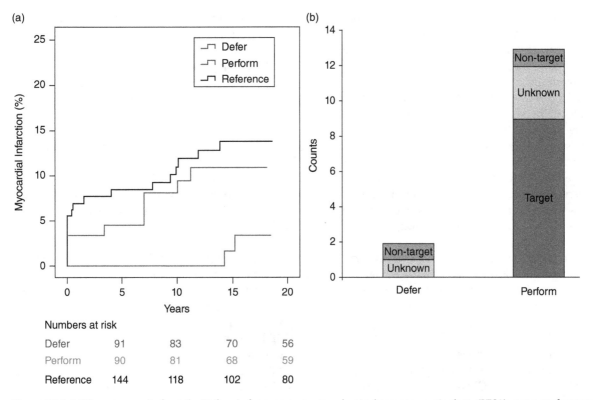

Figure 18.8 (a) Five-year results from the Deferral of percutaneous transluminal coronary angioplasty (PTCA) versus performance of PTCA (DEFER) trial. The y axis depicts the percentage of patients with major adverse cardiac events (MACEs): death, myocardial infarction, coronary artery bypass surgery, or percutaneous coronary intervention. The "DEFER" group (*n* = 91) consisted of those patients found to have an intermediate coronary stenosis in whom the measured FFR was > 0.75 and no angioplasty was performed (MACE = 20%). The "PERFORM" group (*n* = 90) consisted of those patients with an intermediate coronary stenosis with FFR values > 0.75 in whom angioplasty was performed (MACE = 28%). The "REFERENCE" group (*n* = 144) comprised patients whose lesions had measured FFR values of < 0.75 in whom angioplasty was performed (MACE = 37%). (b) Number of events in nontarget, unknown target, and target artery in the DEFER and treated groups. *Source:* Pijls 2007 [25]. Reproduced with permission of Elsevier. (*See insert for color representation of the figure.*)

be concluded that in patients with a coronary stenosis without evidence of ischemia, coronary pressure–derived FFR identifies those who will benefit from PTCA.

Safety of Intracoronary Lesion Assessment

Despite excellent safety, some patients with deferred procedures may still have recurrent angina, requiring continued medical therapy. Nonetheless, when they are physiologically normal, the functional and clinical impact of angiographically intermediate stenoses is associated with an excellent clinical outcome. Like other tests at a single point in time, in-laboratory translesional hemodynamics may not reflect the episodic ischemia-producing conditions of daily life, particularly those related to vasomotor changes during exercise or emotional stress. Fortunately, most dynamic conditions are often highly responsive to medical therapy. Physiologic thresholds validated by ischemic stress testing and clinical outcomes support decisions to defer intervention while continuing medical therapy for endothelial dysfunction, hypertension, hyperlipidemia, and episodic coronary vasoconstriction.

Fractional Flow Reserve in Multivessel Disease

With the increasing use of coronary stents in an ever more complex patient population, a frequent application of physiologic assessment involves lesion selection in patients with multivessel disease. Accurate lesion selection is important, because noninvasive studies have demonstrated that MIBI-SPECT (single-photon emission computed tomography) fails to correctly indicate all ischemic areas in 90% of patients [26]. In 35% of such patients, no perfusion defect was present, possibly due to balanced ischemia. Often, one ischemic area was masked by another more severely under-perfused area. Furthermore, when several stenoses or diffuse disease are present within one coronary artery, an abnormal MIBI-SPECT hypoperfusion image cannot discriminate among the different stenoses along the length of that vessel. For clinical practice, coronary pressure measurements are particularly useful to localize regions of suspected ischemia.

In patients with multivessel disease referred for bypass surgery, patients who underwent selective percutaneous coronary intervention (PCI) of hemodynamically significant stenoses with medical therapy for all other nonsignificant lesions had a similar prognosis to patients who had coronary artery bypass surgery of all angiographic diseased vessels [27]. In a similar study, 150 patients with multivessel disease referred for bypass surgery had FFR performed [28]. If three vessels were significant (FFR < 0.75) or two vessels were significant (with one being the proximal left anterior descending [LAD]), bypass surgery was performed. Otherwise, significant lesions were treated with stenting. After a two-year follow-up, there was no difference in event-free survival, including repeat revascularization, showing that a tailored approach to patients with multivessel disease can be accomplished by determining the hemodynamic significance of each lesion.

In a larger prospective randomized, multicenter trial, Tonino *et al.* [29] for the FAME (FFR versus Angiography for Multivessel Evaluation study) investigators tested outcomes for two PCI strategies: a physiologically guided PCI approach (FFR-PCI) compared to a conventional angiographic guided PCI (Angio-PCI) in patients with multivessel coronary artery disease (CAD). After identifying which of the multiple lesions required treatment, 1,005 patients undergoing PCI with drug-eluting stents were randomly assigned one of the two strategies. For the FFR-PCI group, all lesions had FFR measurements and were only stented if the FFR was less than 0.80. The primary endpoints of death, myocardial infarction (MI), or repeat revascularization (coronary artery bypass grafting [CABG] or PCI) were obtained at one year. Of the 1,005 patients, 496 were assigned to Angio-PCI and 509 to FFR-PCI. Clinical characteristics and angiographic findings were similar in both groups. The

SYNTAX (Synergy between PCI with Taxus and Cardiac Surgery) scores for gauging risk in multivessel disease involvement were identical at 14.5, indicating low- to intermediate-risk patients.

Compared to the Angio-PCI group, the FFR-PCI group used fewer stents per patient (1.9 ± 1.3 vs. 2.7 ± 1.2, $P < 0.001$), less contrast, had lower procedure cost, and a shorter hospital stay. More importantly, at two-year follow-up, the FFR-PCI group had fewer major adverse cardiac events (MACE; 13.2% vs. 18.4%, $P = 0.02$), fewer combined deaths or MI (7.3% vs. 11%, $P = 0.04$), and a lower total number of MACE (76 vs. 113, $P = 0.02$) compared with the Angio-PCI group (Figure 18.9).

The FAME study also demonstrated that not all angiographic three-vessel (3v) CAD is physiologic 3v CAD. A functional SYNTAX score (SYNTAX grading excluding any vessel that has FFR > 0.80) adds the prognostic value of FFR to angiographic grading in patients with multivessel CAD. The economic impact of the FFR-guided strategy produces superior results at lower cost.

FAME II (Fractional Flow Reserve versus Angiography for Multivessel Evaluation 2) was a randomized trial of 888 stable angina patients testing whether optimal medical therapy (OMT) alone compared to OMT and coronary revascularization with stenting was better in patients with demonstrated ischemia in at least one vessel (i.e., FFR < 0.80). Patients with angiographically assessed one-, two, or three-vessel coronary artery disease that was amenable to PCI had FFR measured and were randomized to OMT or OMT + PCI if FFR was < 0.80, or if FFR > 0.80 assigned to a registry and followed. Enrollment in the study was terminated after 19 months due to a highly significant difference in MACE

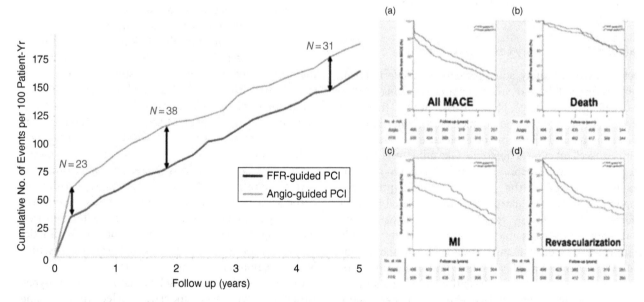

Figure 18.9 Two-year Kaplan–Meier curves showing individual and combined outcomes of the patients from the FAME trial. (a) Freedom from major adverse cardiac events (MACE); (b) Overall survival; (c) Freedom from death or myocardial infarction (MI); (d) Freedom from revascularization by percutaneous coronary intervention (PCI) or coronary artery bypass grafting (CABG). *Source:* Adapted from the New England Journal of Medicine, Tonino 2009 [29]. (*See insert for color representation of the figure.*)

Primary End Point

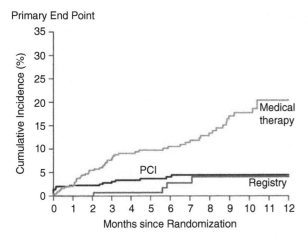

Figure 18.10 FAME II examined patients receiving optimal medical therapy (OMT) compared to percutaneous coronary intervention (PCI) + OMT for patients with abnormal FFR (i.e., ischemia). Kaplan–Meier curves for FAME II patients. Medical therapy had a more than tenfold incidence of major adverse cardiac events compared to the PCI group, which was similar to the nonischemic registry group. *Source:* De Bruyne 2012 [30]. Reproduced with permission of The New England Journal of Medicine. (*See insert for color representation of the figure.*)

between the groups: 12.7% of the patients with OMT compared to only 4.3% of the FFR-guided PCI group reached the primary endpoint [30]. This result was primarily driven by an eightfold increase in the need for urgent revascularization, which included unstable angina (52%), but also myocardial infarction or unstable angina with electrocardiographic changes in 48%. A registry group of participants with documented coronary disease, but no functionally significant stenosis by FFR, did not receive PCI and shared the low event rates seen in the PCI group (Figure 18.10). FFR-guided PCI dramatically reduced the need for urgent revascularization in ischemic patients treated with only medical therapy.

Fractional Flow Reserve and Left Main Coronary Artery Disease

FFR can be used to assess left main (LM) narrowings with specific technical considerations regarding guiding catheter seating and IV adenosine. Because of the potential of guiding catheter obstruction to blood flow across an ostial narrowing, FFR measurements should be performed with the guiding catheter disengaged from the coronary ostium and hyperemia induced with IV adenosine. Initially, the guiding catheter and wire pressures should be matched (equalized) before seating the guiding catheter. Then, the guiding catheter is seated and the pressure wire is advanced into the left anterior descending or left circumflex artery. The guiding catheter is then disengaged and IV adenosine infusion initiated. After 1–2 minutes, the FFR is calculated and thereafter the wire can be pulled back slowly, identifying the exact location of the pressure drop. In the case of a distal left main narrowing, this procedure may be performed twice, once

(a)

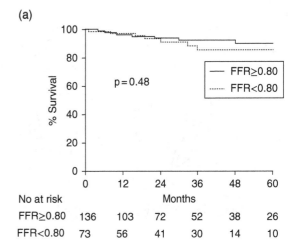

(b)

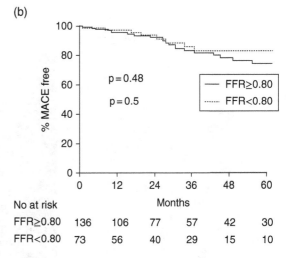

Figure 18.11 Kaplan–Meier mortality curves showing percent survival (a) and major adverse cardiac events (MACE; b) in the two study groups. There is no difference between the nonsurgical and surgical groups. *Source:* Hamilos 2009 [31]. Reproduced with permission of Wolters Kluwer Health, Inc. (*See insert for color representation of the figure.*)

with the pressure wire in the left anterior descending artery and then again in the circumflex artery.

Nonischemic FFR values (>0.80) in left main lesions are associated with excellent long-term outcomes. The largest and longest follow-up trial published to date, by Hamilos *et al.* [31], found a low incidence of MACE including cardiac death or MI between groups with FFR greater than 0.80 (treated medically) compared to those undergoing CABG when FFR was less than 0.80. Reporting their five-year outcomes with the use of FFR for LM stenoses treated with medical or surgical therapy based on FFR less than 0.80 (Figure 18.11), Hamilos *et al.* [31] found similar low MACE rates using FFR to assign suitable surgical revascularization or continued medical therapy.

The FFR of a LM stenosis with downstream CAD may be difficult to interpret, as the FFR reflects flow through both the LAD and circumflex (CFX). The LM FFR alone cannot be accurately measured when there are significant serial

(a)

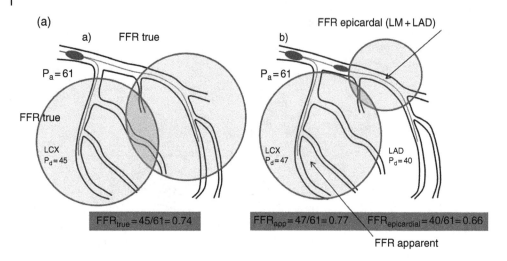

(b)   Simplying FFR for LM + LAD CAD

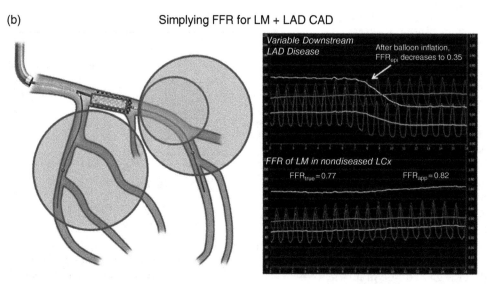

Figure 18.12 (a) Schematic example of physiologic measurements on animal model of left main with or without left anterior descending stenosis. (Left) True fractional flow reserve (FFR$_{true}$) of the left main coronary artery obtained during left main balloon inflation and no stenosis in the left anterior descending (LAD) artery (FFR$_{true}$ = distal pressure [P$_d$]) in the left circumflex (LCX) artery divided by proximal arterial pressure (P$_a$). (Right) FFR$_{app}$ obtained during balloon inflation in the LAD (FFR$_{app}$ = LCX P$_d$/P$_a$ during downstream balloon inflation). FFR$_{epicardial}$ represents FFR of left main plus LAD (FFR$_{epicardial}$ = LAD P$_d$/P$_a$ during LAD balloon inflation). *Source*: Modified from Yong 2013 [32]. (b) Experimental layout to test relationship between left main (LM) and left anterior descending (LAD) lesions of increasing severity. There is a deflated ("winged") balloon in the LM coronary artery with a variably inflated balloon within the newly placed LAD stent, and pressure wires down the LAD and the left circumflex (LCx) coronary artery. The circles represent smaller myocardial bed size, changing bed size when the LAD balloon is inflated. Only when the LAD lesion is very severe does the fractional flow reserve (FFR) become apparent in the LCx rise. CAD = coronary artery disease. *Source:* Fearon 2015 [33]. (*See insert for color representation of the figure.*)

lesions. If the LAD and CFX are hemodynamically insignificant, the LM FFR will be accurate [32, 33] (Figure 18.12).

Serial (Multiple) Lesions in a Single Vessel

An accurate FFR requires maximum translesional flow across the stenosis. This condition cannot be met in serial lesions wherein the blood flow through one stenosis will be submaximal because of the second stenosis. The FFR can assess the summed effect across any series of stenoses, but individual lesion FFR in the series will be more difficult to appreciate without special calculations [34].

The most practical technique to assess serial lesions involves passing the pressure wire distal to the last lesion and measuring the summed FFR across all lesions. If FFR = 0.84 then no lesion would need treatment. If the summed FFR is less than 0.80 then a wire pullback during IV adenosine hyperemia can identify the largest change in gradient (ΔP) between lesions. Stenting should

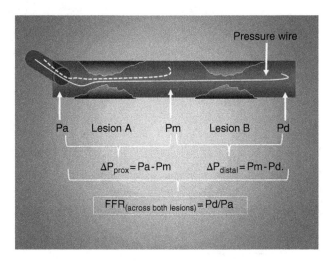

Figure 18.13 Serial lesion assessment. If multiple stenoses are present in the same vessel, the hyperemic flow and pressure gradient through the first stenosis will be attenuated by the presence of the second one, and vice versa. Each stenosis will mask the true effect of its serial counterpart by limiting the achievable maximum hyperemia. Although calculation of the exact fractional flow reserve (FFR) for each lesion separately is possible, it remains largely academic. In clinical practice, the use of the pressure pullback recording is particularly well suited to identify the several regions of a vessel with large pressure gradients that may benefit from treatment. The one stenosis with the largest gradient can be treated first, after which the FFR can be remeasured for the remaining stenoses to determine the need for further treatment. ΔP = pressure gradient; P_a arterial pressure; P_d distal coronary pressure; P_m pressure between stenoses.

then start with the lesion with the most significant gradient (largest ΔP). After treating this lesion, the remaining lesion(s) can be measured using the standard FFR technique (Figure 18.13).

The fluid dynamic interaction between two serial stenoses depends on the sequence, severity, and distance between the lesions as well as the flow rate. The gradient is the sum of the individual pressure losses at any given flow rate.

When addressing two stenoses in series, equations have been derived to predict the FFR (FFR_{pred}) of each stenosis separately (i.e., as if the other one were removed) using arterial pressure (P_a), pressure between the two stenoses (P_m), distal coronary pressure (P_d), and coronary occlusive pressure (P_w). FFR_{app} (ratio of the pressure just distal to that just proximal to each stenosis) and FFR_{true} (ratio of the pressures distal and proximal to each stenosis but after removal of the other one) have been compared in patients [35]. FFR_{true} was more overestimated by FFR_{app} than by FFR_{pred}. It was clearly demonstrated that the interaction between two stenoses is such that the FFR of each lesion separately cannot be calculated by the equation for isolated stenoses applied to each separately, but can be predicted by more complete equations taking into account P_a, P_m, P_d, and P_w.

Although calculation of the exact FFR of each lesion separately is possible, it remains academic. In clinical practice, the use of the pressure pullback recording is particularly well suited to identifying the several regions of a vessel with large pressure gradients which may benefit from treatment. The stenosis with the largest gradient can be treated first and the FFR can be remeasured for the remaining stenoses to determine the need for further treatment.

Diffuse Coronary Disease

A diffusely diseased atherosclerotic coronary artery has a gradually diminishing flow along the length of the narrowed conduit. Using FFR_{myo} during continuous pressure wire pullback from a distal to proximal location, the impact of a specific area of angiographic narrowing can be examined and the presence of diffuse atherosclerosis can be documented. De Bruyne and coworkers have demonstrated the influence of diffuse atherosclerosis [36]. FFR_{myo} measurements were obtained from 37 arteries in 10 individuals without atherosclerosis (group I) and from 106 nonstenotic arteries in 62 patients with angiographic stenoses in another coronary artery (group II). In group I, the pressure gradient between aorta and distal coronary artery was minimal at rest (1 ± 1 mm Hg) and during maximal hyperemia (3 ± 3 mm Hg). Corresponding values were significantly larger in group II (5 ± 4 mm Hg and 10 ± 8 mm Hg, respectively; both $P < 0.001$). The FFR_{myo} was near unity (0.97 ± 0.02; range 0.92 to 1) in group I, indicating no resistance to flow in truly normal coronary arteries, but it was significantly lower (0.89 ± 0.08; range 0.69 to 1) in group II, indicating a higher resistance to flow. Diffuse disease is associated with myocardial ischemia and has consequences for decision-making during PCI.

Fractional Flow Reserve for Ostial Lesions and "Jailed" Side Branches

Determining the physiologic significance of ostial lesions, particularly in side branch vessels, remains difficult with current angiographic techniques and equipment. This is particularly problematic after the side branch has been stented over or "jailed" by a stent in the parent vessel. Koo *et al.* [37] examined the physiologic assessment of jailed side branches using FFR.

In 94 lesions the mean FFR was 0.94+/-0.04 and 0.85+/-0.11 at the main branches and jailed side branches, respectively. There was a negative correlation between the percent stenosis and FFR ($r = 0.41$, $P < 0.001$). However, no lesion with less than 75% stenosis had FFR less than 0.75. Among 73 lesions with more than 75% stenosis, only 20 lesions were functionally significant.

Measurement of FFR in jailed side branch lesions is both safe and feasible. FFR across ostial lesions suggests that most of these lesions do not have functional significance and that intervention on these nonsignificant lesions may not be necessary. Similar findings have been reported for native ostial and branch lesions that have not been "jailed" during routine coronary angiography [38].

Coronary Physiology for Acute Coronary Syndromes

Acute myocardial injury produces transient microvascular dysfunction to various degrees and impairs maximal coronary hyperemia, thereby reducing flow across a stenosis. After the patient recuperates, myocardial recovery may increase coronary flow across the stenosis, and higher flow would lower the FFR, perhaps below the ischemic threshold, thus changing a treatment decision from that made during the acute event. As a result, the FFR of a vessel (i.e., a lesion different from the culprit lesion, but in the same vessel) that is involved in a ST-elevation myocardial infarction (STEMI) or large non-STEMI can result in a false-negative result. FFR has been demonstrated to be accurate after four to six days in most unstable angina patients and small non-STEMI patients. In the FAME study, FFR was accurate and equally beneficial in the 328 patients in the trial with positive troponin, but creatinine kinase (CK) levels were less than 1000 U/L, compared with the stable angina patients. These researchers posit that the degree of microvascular dysfunction for such small myocardial injury is minimal, and the benefit of FFR applies equally to such patients [39].

In an acute STEMI, FFR of most nonculprit lesions at a distance from the infarct-related artery has also been shown to be accurate. Therefore, in this setting, a low FFR indicates hemodynamic significance of the nonculprit lesion, but a normal FFR may not be definitive. Ntalianis *et al.* [39] measured the FFR of 112 nonculprit lesions during an acute MI (75 patients with STEMI, 26 patients with non-STEMI) and again 35 ± 24 days later. Only two lesions had a clinically meaningful change where FFR was greater than 0.80 during the acute episode and less than 0.75 at follow-up (Figure 18.14).

De Bruyne *et al.* [40] and Samady *et al.* [41] obtained FFR measurements of culprit vessels three or more days after acute MI and compared them to subsequent SPECT imaging to identify true positives and negatives. Both studies showed that an FFR less than 0.75 had high sensitivity, specificity, and overall accuracy for detecting reversible ischemia identified by SPECT imaging, and they both reached the same best cutoff value for FFR of 0.78. Trials that have evaluated the use of FFR in the

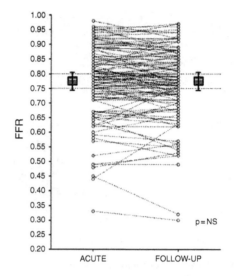

Figure 18.14 Plot of fractional flow reserve (FFR) values of nonculprit coronary artery stenoses during the acute phase and at follow-up. *Source:* Ntalianis 2010 [39].

setting of an acute coronary syndrome are summarized in Table 18.3.

In patients following an acute myocardial infarction, the predictive ability of FFR has some theoretic limitations, as the microvascular bed in the infarct zone does not necessarily have a uniform and constant resistance. However, DeBruyne *et al.* [40] demonstrated that a threshold of 0.75 was also valid in 57 patients who had sustained a MI more than six days earlier. Myocardial perfusion SPECT imaging and FFR_{myo} were obtained before and after angioplasty. The sensitivity and specificity of the 0.75 value of FFR_{myo} to detect flow maldistribution on SPECT imaging were 82% and 87%, respectively. The concordance between the FFR and SPECT imaging was 85% ($P < 0.001$). When only truly positive and truly negative SPECT imaging was considered, the corresponding values were 87%, 100%, and 94% ($P < 0.001$). Patients with positive SPECT imaging before angioplasty had a significantly lower FFR_{myo} than patients with negative SPECT imaging (0.52 ± 0.18 vs. 0.67 ± 0.16; $P = 0.0079$), but a significantly higher left ventricular ejection fraction (63% ± 10% vs. 52% ± 10%; $P = 0.0009$), despite a similar percent diameter stenosis (% DS; 67% ± 13% vs. 68% ± 16%; $P = NS$). A significant inverse correlation was found between left ventricular ejection fraction and FFR_{myo} ($R = 0.29$, $P = 0.049$). It appears that, for a similar degree of stenosis, the value of FFR_{myo} depends on the mass of viable myocardium. The possibility of analyzing truly positive and negative SPECT imaging confirmed the validity of the 0.75 threshold, which could not be derived from those studies based solely on angiographic parameters.

Table 18.3 Fractional flow reserve (FFR) and acute coronary syndrome (ACS) trials.

Setting	Culprit/Nonculprit	Validity	Author	N	Comments
Acute MI	Culprit vessel	Unreliable	Tamita 2002 [42]	33 STEMI	Mean FFR after successful PCI was higher (0.95 ± 0.04) than in reference group of stable angina patients (0.90 ± 0.04, $P = 0.002$) despite identical IVUS parameters, likely reflecting microvascular stunning and dysfunction.
Acute MI	Nonculprit vessel	Reliable	Ntalianis 2010 [39]	75 STEMI, 26 NSTEMI	112 nonculprit lesions measured acutely and 35 ± 24 days later. Only 2 lesions had clinically meaningful change: FFR > 0.80 during the acute episode and < 0.75 at follow-up.
Recent MI	Culprit vessel	Reliable	De Bruyne 2001 [40]	57 acute MI with viable myocardium on LVgram	FFR after acute MI (≥6 days, mean 20 days) compared to SPECT before and after PCI. FFR < 0.75 had high sensitivity (87%) and specificity (100%) for detecting ischemia on true positive/negative SPECT. BCV for FFR 0.78. Inverse correlation between FFR and LVEF: for a similar degree of stenosis, FFR depends on mass of viable myocardium.
Recent MI	Culprit vessel	Reliable	Samady 2006 [41]	36 STEMI, 12 NSTEMI	FFR after acute MI (STEMI ≥3 days, NSTEMI ≥2 days, mean 3.7 days) compared to SPECT at 11 weeks. FFR ≤ 0.75 had high sensitivity (88%), specificity (93%), and overall accuracy (91%) for detecting reversibility on true positive/negative SPECT. BCV for FFR 0.78.
Recent MI	Nonculprit vessel	FFR-guided PCI = good clinical outcomes	Potvin 2006 [43]	125 ACS, 60 SIHD, 16 atypical CP	201 consecutive pts (62% unstable angina, NSTEMI, or >24hrs after STEMI) with ~50% stenosis in which PCI was deferred based on FFR ≥ 0.75. No difference in clinical outcomes between ACS and stable angina patients.
Recent MI	Culprit vessel	FFR-guided PCI = good clinical outcomes	Fischer 2006 [44]	35 ACS	FFR-guided PCI of intermediate lesions (50–70%). Deferring PCI for FFR ≥ 0.75 in patients with recent ACS. Similar MACE rates at 12 months compared to patients without ACS.
UA/NSTEMI	Culprit vessel	FFR-guided PCI = good clinical outcomes	Leesar 2003 [45]	70 UA/NSTEMI	Recent NSTE-ACS with intermediate single-vessel lesion randomized to immediate FFR-guided PCI vs. post-angiography SPECT. FFR-guided treatment reduced hospital stay and cost, with no increase in procedure time, radiation exposure, or clinical event rates at 1 year.
UA/NSTEMI	Culprit + nonculprit vessel	FFR-guided PCI = good clinical outcomes	Sels 2011 [46]	326 UA/NSTEMI	FAME study. FFR-guided PCI vs. angiography-guided PCI for multivessel disease. In subset of patients with recent NSTE-ACS, significantly lower MACE rate with FFR-guided PCI.

BCV = best cutoff value; CP = chest pain; IVUS = intravascular ultrasound; LVgram = left ventricular angiogram; MACE = major adverse cardiac event; MI = myocardial infarction; NSTE-ACS = non-ST elevation acute coronary syndrome; NSTEMI = non-ST-elevation myocardial infarction; PCI = percutaneous coronary intervention; SIHD = stable ischemic heart disease; SPECT = single-photon emission computed tomography; STEMI = ST-elevation myocardial infarction;

Case: Coronary Physiology after Myocardial Infarction

A 44-year-old man presented with an anterior myocardial infarction and ventricular fibrillatory arrest at an outside hospital. Intravenous thrombolysis using reptelase was administered and the patient was transferred for further evaluation. He had been taking aspirin, capoten, lopressor, albuterol, and zocor and continued to smoke cigarettes.

In the catheterization laboratory, his blood pressure was 100/60 mm Hg, pulse 70 beats/min. There was no neck vein distention. He had a grade III/VI systolic murmur at the left sternal border radiating to the base of the heart. The remainder of the examination was normal. The electrocardiogram showed Q waves in leads V_j–V_3 of anterior myocardial infarction in evolution.

Left ventriculography demonstrated mild anterolateral hypokinesis with an ejection fraction of 72%. Coronary arteriography found a 50% mid left anterior descending eccentric lesion with TIMI grade 3 flow. There was a 30% mid right coronary artery stenosis. The left circumflex artery was normal.

In view of TIMI grade 3 flow and intermediately severe coronary stenoses, intervention was deferred and the patient was transferred to the coronary care unit for further medical therapy. Eleven days later, after undergoing a negative low-level risk stratification test, the patient complained of having anterior chest pain at home during various activities such as bending over. He denied exertional chest discomfort, but had not experienced high activity levels. He continued to smoke cigarettes during this recovery period.

The patient was readmitted to the cardiac catheterization laboratory for coronary artery lesion assessment and potential intervention. Coronary angiography again revealed a 50–60% mid left anterior descending stenosis (Figure 18.15, top). Anterior left ventricular wall motion (by ventriculography) was improved, with normal systolic contraction and a global ejection fraction of 65%.

Intracoronary flow velocity reserve measurements were made in the circumflex and left anterior descending coronary arteries in the standard fashion. The circumflex (reference artery) coronary flow reserve was 3.1 (Figure 18.15, bottom right). Coronary flow reserve in the (target) left anterior descending artery distal to the intermediate stenosis was 1.9 (Figure 18.15, bottom left). Relative coronary artery flow reserve (RCFR; CFRtarget/CFRreference) was 0.61.

Translesional pressure was obtained with a 2.2 F tracking catheter. The resting pressure gradient of 10 mm Hg increased during maximal hyperemia to 30 mm Hg (FIgure 18.16). The calculated fractional flow reserve of the myocardium (FFRmyo; pressure distal/pressure aortic at maximal hyperemia) was 58/80 = 0.73 (normal value 2:0.75; Figure 18.16, right). Because of the borderline flow and pressure values and suggestive ischemic symptoms, angioplasty and stent placement were performed. After balloon dilatation with 3.5 mm balloons, there was no change in the coronary hemodynamics or flow velocity data. A 3.5 x 15 mm J&J stent was positioned and dilated with a high-pressure inflation. The final percent diameter stenosis was less than 10%. It was noted during the procedure that severe, somewhat atypical chest pain persisted despite having an open artery

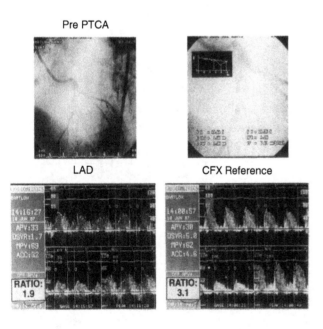

Pre PTCA

LAD   CFX Reference

RATIO: 1.9   RATIO: 3.1

Figure 18.15 (Top) Coronary cineangiograms before angioplasty demonstrating a 45% QCA diameter stenosis in the left anterior descending (LAD) artery. (Bottom left) Coronary flow reserve in the target LAD artery was 1.9. (Bottom right) Coronary flow reserve in the reference circumflex (CFX) artery was 3.1. The relative coronary vasodilatory reserve ratio was 0.61. The velocity panels are split into top and bottom, with lower panels divided into base (left) and hyperemic (right) flow. The spectral signals are shown on a 0–120 cm/sec scale. The electrocardiogram and aortic pressure are displayed above the velocity spectra. ACC = acceleration; APV = average peak velocity; DSVR = diastolic/systolic velocity ratio; MPV = maximal peak velocity; PTCA = percutaneous transluminal coronary angioplasty; ratio = coronary vasodilatory reserve.

Figure 18.16 Distal coronary and aortic pressures before angioplasty at baseline, during adenosine, and during catheter pullback, demonstrating a small diastolic pressure gradient (0–200 mm Hg scale). The fractional flow reserve of the myocardium (FFRmyo) computed from values measured at peak adenosine response was 58/80 = 0.71. PTCA = percutaneous transluminal coronary angioplasty.

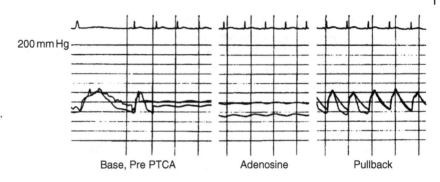

200 mm Hg

Base, Pre PTCA   Adenosine   Pullback

Figure 18.17 (Top left) Coronary angiogram after stent placement. (Right) Coronary flow velocity reserve after angioplasty was 1.4 and after stent placement increased to 2.1, improving (but not normalizing) relative coronary vasodilatory flow reserve to 0.67. The velocity panels are split into top and bottom, with lower panels divided into base (left) and hyperemic (right) flow. The spectral signals are shown on a scale of 0–120 cm/sec. The electrocardiogram and aortic pressure are displayed above the velocity spectra. (Bottom left) Intravascular ultrasound imaging in the reference and post stent region with a fully expanded stent. Acc = acceleration; APV = average peak velocity; DSVR = diastolic systolic velocity ratio; MPV = maximal peak velocity; PTCA = percutaneous transluminal coronary angioplasty; ratio = coronary vasodilatory reserve.

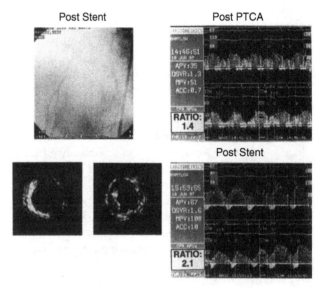

Post Stent   Post PTCA

Post Stent

with no electrocardiographic changes. Intravascular ultrasound revealed a well-expanded stent and large lumen (Figure 18.17, bottom left). Final flow velocity measurements demonstrated that coronary flow reserve in the target vessel increased to 2.1. RCFR increased to 0.68 (Figure 18.17, right). The FFRmyo also remained unchanged at 55/78 = 0.71 (Figure 18.18).

The patient was discharged home and recurrent atypical chest pain occurred. A low-level stress test was negative. Medical therapy was increased, but due to persistent complaints during the cardiac rehabilitation activities, the patient underwent a repeat cardiac catheterization one month after discharge. The left anterior descending stent site was widely patent. There was a stenotic diagonal branch (<0.5 mm diameter) adjacent to the stent. There were minimal diffuse luminal irregularities of the circumflex and right coronary artery. Ergonovine challenge was negative, without evidence of focal coronary vasospasm, angina, or electrocardiographic changes. The patient was discharged on analgesics and anti-ischemic therapy. He has been well for four months.

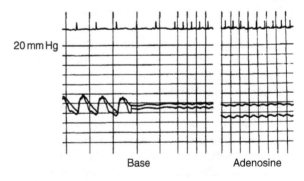

20 mm Hg

Base   Adenosine

Figure 18.18 Post-stent coronary hemodynamics are similar to the pre-angioplasty hemodynamics, with fractional flow reserve (FFR) of 55/78 mm Hg = 0.71.

Coronary blood flow assessment for ischemia in the post-infarct patient is important, but can be problematic. The finding of an intermediately severe coronary stenosis often prompts the cardiologist to proceed with intervention on the target vessel, despite having relatively little or no objective evidence of ischemia. The intermediate coronary stenosis in this patient was likely not solely responsible for the persistent chest pain syndrome. Coronary hemodynamics were at the borderline of normal and changed minimally after eliminating the target stenosis. The symptoms persisted even after complete elimination of the major coronary narrowing.

In such a case, the pressure–flow relationship may be influenced by factors other than the stenosis alone, such as basal myocardial oxygen demands and microcirculatory abnormalities. The limitations of using coronary lumenography (angiography or intravascular ultrasound imaging) to precisely gauge lesion severity have been acknowledged.

Doppler Coronary Flow Velocity

The measurement of coronary blood flow in patients has been of interest to cardiologists since the beginning of cardiac catheterization. Until 1980, blood flow methodologies had been cumbersome and technically difficult. Indicator dilution and washout techniques had time constants too slow to measure rapid, precise changes in blood flow responses. Electromagnetic flow probes were limited to anesthetized patients in the operating suite. Historically, the measurement of coronary venous efflux by the coronary sinus thermodilution technique, as described by Ganz *et al.* [47] and refined by Pepine *et al.* [48], was used to estimate the left ventricular myocardial flow indirectly. This method was replaced by direct measurement of intra-arterial blood flow velocity, initially using miniaturized Doppler crystals placed on small catheters [49, 50], followed by sensor-tipped Doppler angioplasty guidewires. With the use of the intracoronary Doppler wire, examination of coronary physiology under a variety of circumstances was easily and safely obtained, offering new insights into coronary circulation in awake, unanesthetized patients.

The use of intracoronary flow velocity is no longer considered important for lesion assessment in clinical decision-making. However, it is a valuable tool to study the coronary physiology, its phasic variations, and the effects of interventions.

Principles of Doppler Velocimetry

An observer moving toward a sound source will hear a tone with higher frequency than at rest; an observer moving away from the source will hear a tone of lower frequency. This change in frequency is called the Doppler effect, after Christian Johann Doppler (1803–1853), an Austrian physicist who was the first to describe this phenomenon. This principle is applied in interventional cardiology practice by mounting a piezoelectric crystal that emits and receives high-frequency sounds on the tip of an intravascular catheter. The blood flow velocity alters the return frequency, causing the Doppler shift. Electronic circuits performing spectral analysis of the received signal allow continuous determination of the Doppler shift, and of blood flow velocity, based on the following equation:

$$V = \frac{(F_1 - F_0) \times C}{2 \times F_0 \times \cos(\phi)}$$

where F_0 = transmitting (transducer) frequency; F_1 = returning frequency; C = constant, speed of sound in blood; and ϕ = angle of incidence.

Maximum velocity can be recorded, provided the transducer beam is nearly parallel to blood flow, cos (φ) ~1. With continuous-wave Doppler, the signal reflects all the flow velocities encountered by the exploring ultrasound beam. In contrast, a pulsed-wave Doppler permits determination of both magnitude and direction of the flow changes at a predetermined distance from the transducer.

The Doppler guidewire is a 0.014 inch diameter, 175 cm long, flexible and steerable guidewire with handling characteristics similar to traditional angioplasty guidewires. It has a 12 MHz piezoelectric ultrasound transducer integrated onto the tip. Its minimal CSA is only 0.1 mm^2. The CSA of the Doppler guidewire causes a 9% area reduction of a circular lumen of 1.2 mm diameter, whereas a 1 mm diameter catheter induces a 70% obstruction. The wire creates less disturbance of the flow profile distal to its tip when placed within a vessel, and can be passed into smaller coronary arteries without creating significant stenoses. The forward-directed ultrasound beam diverges at 35 degrees, so that the Doppler sample volume is approximately 0.65 mm thick by 3.1 mm in diameter when maintained 5.2 mm beyond the transducer, distal to the area of flow velocity profile distortion induced by the Doppler guidewire [51]. This broad ultrasound beam provides a relatively large area of insonification, sampling a large portion of the flow velocity profile. The signal transmitted from the piezoelectric transducer is processed from the quadrature Doppler audio signal by a real-time spectral analyzer using online fast Fourier transform, providing a scrolling gray-scale spectral display. The frequency response of this system calculates approximately 90 spectra per second. The spectral analysis of the signal and the Doppler audio signals are videorecorded for later review. Simultaneous electrocardiogram and blood pressure measurements are displayed with the spectral velocity. The quadrature signals can also be acquired with an independent personal computer–based analog-to-digital board for archiving and post-processing of the Doppler spectra [51]. The Doppler FlowWire has been validated during intravascular measurement of coronary arterial flow velocity.

Techniques of Intracoronary Blood Flow Velocity Measurements

In 1991, an angioplasty Doppler guidewire became available to measure intracoronary blood flow velocity, making earlier Doppler catheters obsolete. A Judkin's-type Doppler catheter was used to measure nonselective coronary velocity in the LM segment [52]. Two smaller Doppler angioplasty-style catheters were used to obtain subselective coronary artery flow velocity (Figure 18.19). Only the Doppler guidewire was able to cross a stenosis to accurately assess post-stenotic blood flow.

Employing the Doppler principle [47], accurate measurement of red cell velocity moving down the coronary artery could be made. The nonselective Judkin's Doppler catheter technique used a standard Judkin's catheter placement, interrogating only the LM flow. The subselective Doppler catheter methods were identical to placement of a coronary angioplasty balloon catheter, but the catheter did not cross the stenosis. The Doppler guidewire was used identically to that of a typical angioplasty guidewire with a standard guiding catheter, valved "y" connector, and IV heparin (40–70 U/kg).

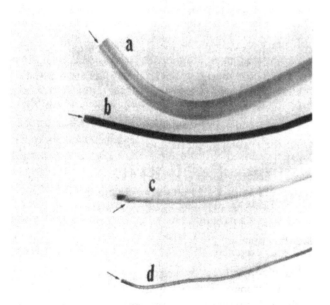

Figure 18.19 Coronary flow velocity catheters and guidewires. (a) Judkin's-style Doppler; (b) Millar (end-mounted crystal); (c) Numed Doppler (side-mounted crystal); (d) Cardiometrics 0.018 inch guidewire. Arrows indicate location and angle of Doppler beam.

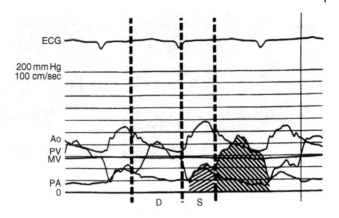

Figure 18.20 Coronary flow velocity tracing with aortic and pulmonary artery pressures in a patient with normal coronary arteries. Ao = aortic pressure; D = diastole; MV = mean velocity; PA = pulmonary artery pressure; PV = phasic velocity; S = systole.

The intracoronary Doppler guidewire can be placed in any arterial branch. Once the Doppler guidewire is positioned, the velocity signal is adjusted, moving wire tip orientation and range. The Doppler catheters used a zero-crossing method, while the guidewire Doppler employs spectral signal analysis.

Coronary velocity signals are processed by two methods. The more common and less expensive is the zero-cross method. The velocimeter detects the direction and rate at which the signal changes frequency (frequency shift) past a zero-velocity point. The frequency shift is proportional to the velocity. The signals are easily acquired and recorded on a standard physiologic catheterization laboratory recorder (Figure 18.20). The zero-cross technique was used with most 20 MHz subselective and nonselective Doppler catheters.

The second method of Doppler signal processing is spectral analysis. Time-averaged and instantaneous peak velocity values are processed by a computer using fast Fourier transformation techniques, displaying a gray-scale depiction of all velocities recorded in the sample volume at one point in time. As with standard transthoracic echocardiographic technique, the more homogenous the velocity, the more intense and uniform the velocity spectrum. Spectral analysis is applied to the 12 MHz signal obtained with the angioplasty Doppler flow wire (Figure 18.20 and 18.21).

Components of the Coronary Flow Velocity Signal

Although routinely studied in the physiology classes of medical school, the responses of the coronary circulation as observed in patients in the cardiac catheterization laboratory are not generally familiar to cardiologists commonly performing the procedures. The phasic

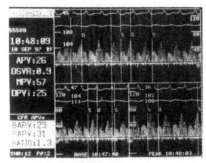
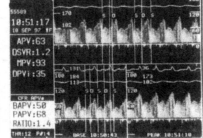

Pre PTCA   Post PTCA

Figure 18.21 Doppler spectral flow velocity signals in right coronary artery obtained with a 0.018 inch Doppler guidewire before (top) and after (bottom) coronary balloon angioplasty. Note that systolic/diastolic velocity integrals (areas) have normalized in the distal region after dilation (bottom flow signals). PTCA = percutaneous transluminal coronary angioplasty.

patterns of coronary blood flow velocity signals easily obtained with Doppler catheters or guidewires reflect typical coronary physiology during common respiratory maneuvers, hyperemic stimulation, and cardiac arrhythmias. Examples of these follow.

The coronary hemodynamic tracings obtained in the left anterior descending coronary artery in a 52-year-old woman with an atypical chest pain syndrome are shown in Figure 18.20. Coronary flow velocity was measured with a Doppler catheter to assess coronary vasodilatory reserve. The aortic pressure is used to demarcate the onset of diastolic and systolic flow periods. Figure 18.20 shows the simultaneously recorded aortic and pulmonary artery pressure, phasic and mean coronary flow velocity signals, along with the electrocardiogram. The typical waveform of coronary flow velocity has the predominant diastolic flow velocity wave, with a relatively rapid increase in diastolic flow velocity immediately following the aortic dichrotic notch and a rapid falling off of the flow velocity signal just after the onset of systole. There is usually a small systolic component, approximately 25% of the diastolic flow velocity at rest. The (electronic) mean velocity is computed from the integrated area of flow during both systole and diastole. The flow velocity signal is generally stable during respiratory maneuvers. If the ultrasound beam is directed into the arterial wall, the signal can be obscured, producing an artifactually low waveform. The waveform of flow velocity may be altered to various degrees by atherosclerosis within the artery. In this example, the patient had normal coronary arteries with a normal flow velocity pattern. Figure 18.22 demonstrates several features of the flow velocity wave that can be easily quantitated.

Coronary Blood Flow Velocity during Respiratory Maneuvers

A 60-year-old woman undergoing diagnostic coronary angiography has a 3 sec sinus arrest during contrast injection of the right coronary artery. The operator asks the patient to cough vigorously. What does coughing do to coronary blood flow? Although in the early years of angiography coughing was thought to clear contrast

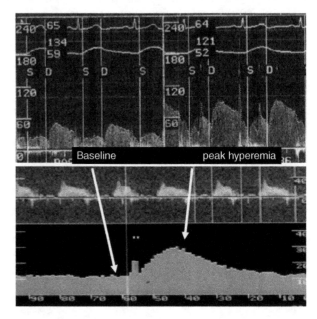

Figure 18.22 Coronary flow velocity tracing and measurements. (Top left) Baseline flow velocity with predominant diastolic flow and smaller systolic flow. ECG and arterial pressure waves are shown at the top of this tracing. Scale is 0–240 cm/sec. (Top right) Hyperemic peak flow velocity with larger phasic diastolic and systolic flow components. (Bottom) Continuous trend of average peak velocity. ** denotes injection of IC adenosine with peak hyperemic response about 15–20 sec. *Source:* Kern 1989 [53]. Reproduced with permission of Elsevier.

from the coronary arteries, we now know that its only mechanism is maintenance of arterial pressure until normal cardiac rhythm is restored. The effect of increased intrathoracic pressure on coronary blood flow velocity has been previously examined both echocardiographically [54] and by direct flow measurement [55], demonstrating that neither coughing nor Valsalva augments coronary blood flow velocity.

Examine the hemodynamic tracings in a patient with normal coronary arteries (Figure 18.23). Cough increases both aortic pressure (>240 mm Hg) and right atrial pressure (210 mm Hg), together producing a marked and parallel pressure increase. The pulse pressure (the difference between aortic diastolic and right atrial pressure, A)

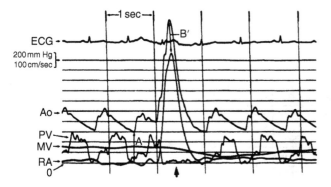

Figure 18.23 Coronary flow velocity signals during cough (arrow). A = diastolic aortic (Ao) pressure and right atrial (RA) pressure; B' = pulse pressure during cough. Arrow shows phasic flow velocity signal during diastolic period of cough. MV = mean velocity; PV = phasic velocity. *Source:* Kern 1990 [55]. Reproduced with permission of Elsevier.

remains the same or decreases during coughing (B'). The cough pulse pressure (B') is associated with a marked decrease in coronary flow velocity without any augmentation of either peak or mean flow on the subsequent beat(s). The limited and often reduced flow velocity is present whether single or multiple coughs are performed. With the sustained increase of intrathoracic pressure that occurs with continuous coughing (Figure 18.24), there is a prolonged and sustained decrease in coronary flow velocity.

The same physiology appears to apply for the coronary flow velocity changes occurring during the increased intrathoracic pressure of the Valsalva maneuver (Figure 18.25). Although intrathoracic pressure is markedly increased during phase III, coronary blood flow velocity does not increase and, for most studies, declines slightly or remains unchanged [56, 57].

Benign sinus arrhythmia and normal respiratory activity cause cyclical alterations in aortic pressure. Small changes in myocardial oxygen demand occur, consistent with the increasing and decreasing heart rate–pressure products. Examine the corresponding coronary flow velocity signal measured in a patient without coronary artery disease during sinus arrhythmia (Figure 18.26). The mean and peak phasic flow velocity signals demonstrate parallel changes in response to alteration in arterial pressure during respiration. Coronary flow velocity, as shown in this patient, accurately reflects the autoregulatory response of the normal coronary circulation. With the appreciation of autoregulation and its effect on coronary flow velocity, can one predict what the result of loss of atrial activity would do to coronary flow velocity? Examine the data record in a patient who had temporary ventricular pacing for transient heart block during coronary arteriography (Figure 18.27). Aortic pressure and mean and phasic coronary flow velocity were measured during a period of transition from sinus rhythm to paced rhythm and return to sinus rhythm. The

coronary flow velocity remained nearly constant, with a slight decline in the peak flow velocity during the period of ventricular pacing with loss of atrial activity. As the atrial contribution returns to the rhythm, flow velocity undergoes only an insignificant change. Although loss of atrial activity with decreased aortic pressure would likely reduce demand, the result on autoregulation in this patient was not reflected in a reduction in coronary flow velocity. Compare this response with the marked changes seen in the patient in Figure 18.26 during sinus arrhythmia.

Coronary Flow Velocity during Atrial Fibrillation

Atrial fibrillation is a common arrhythmia in which very rapid ventricular depolarizations may cause ineffective arterial pressure generation. Although a loss of coronary flow during the pulse deficit might be anticipated, coronary flow velocity has not been commonly observed in these patients. Consider the systemic and pulmonary artery pressures and coronary flow velocity measured in a patient with atrial fibrillation and periods of rapid ventricular response (Figure 18.28). During the cardiac cycles of different durations, coronary flow, as measured by the flow–velocity area (time x flow = integral), varied in proportion to the RR cycle length, with the mean flow remaining relatively constant. On beats #1 and 2, the flow–velocity area was reduced from 23.7 to 13.0 units, with reduced RR intervals of 933 to 667 msec. After beat #3 (Figure 18.28), the ventricular rhythm exceeds 150 beats/min (ventricular couplet). Coronary blood flow in beat #4 was abbreviated by the next early ventricular beat (flow integral = 5.8 units). Arterial pressure continued to decline and was not affected. The flow velocity was maintained during the subsequent rapid beats despite the loss of arterial pressure. A small arterial pressure wave, generated by beat #5, was associated with significant augmentation of the coronary blood flow integral (20.0 units), despite the minimal contribution to peripheral or coronary pressure.

Coronary Flow during Ventricular Tachycardia

Although rarely witnessed, as one might expect, coronary blood flow ceases during the disorganized rhythm of ventricular tachycardia. Ineffective ventricular systole limits pressure generation and the markedly shortened diastole fails to permit ventricular relaxation, curtailing coronary flow. Coronary flow velocity was measured in a patient undergoing diagnostic catheterization to determine coronary vasodilatory reserve. Intracoronary papaverine (10 mg) was used as the hyperemic stimulus to produce maximal coronary flow. Intracoronary papaverine has been associated with prolongation of the QT interval and rare episodes of

(a)

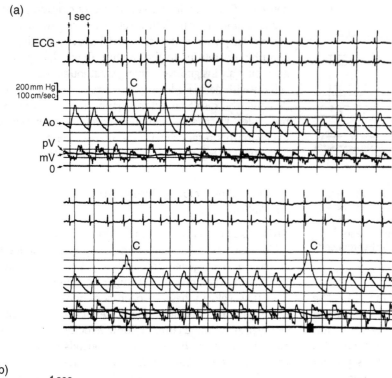

(b)

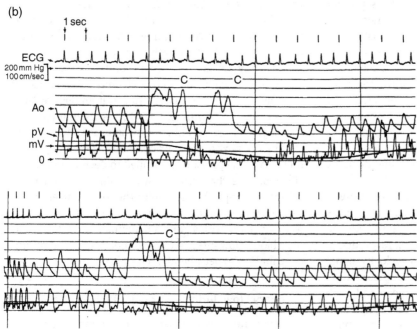

Figure 18.24 Aortic (Ao) and coronary flow velocity tracings during coughing. (a) Single and multiple coughs (C). (b) Sustained coughing reducing coronary flow velocity for a more prolonged period. These effects on coronary flow are present whether coronary flow velocity is measured proximally (top tracings of panels) or distally (bottom tracings of panels). mV = mean velocity; pV = phasic velocity. *Source:* Kern 1990 [55]. Reproduced with permission of Elsevier.

Torsade de Pointes and ventricular tachycardia [58]. Examine the hemodynamic and coronary blood flow velocity tracings in Figure 18.29. Premature ventricular contractions preceded ventricular tachycardia. During ventricular tachycardia, when aortic pressure was not produced, coronary blood flow velocity rapidly fell to zero. Immediate defibrillation restored both rhythm

and coronary flow, with no residual adverse effects. Unlike ventricular fibrillation and depending on the rate, slow ventricular tachycardia (as seen on the couplet after beat #3, Figure 18.28) could maintain some degree of coronary flow [58]. Regardless of the coronary flow patterns, restoration of a normal rhythm for these patients is of obvious importance.

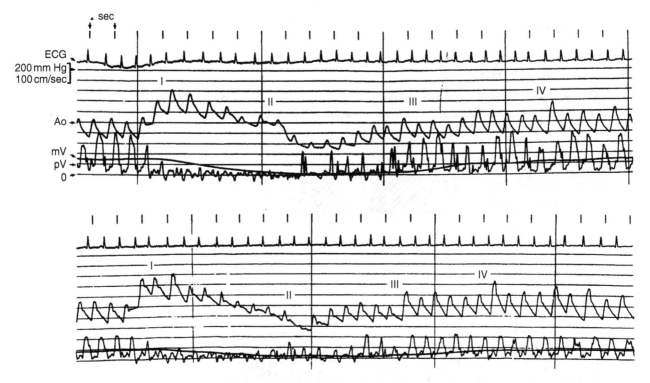

Figure 18.25 Coronary flow velocity during Valsalva maneuver. Ao = aortic pressure; mV = mean velocity; pV = phasic velocity. *Source:* Kern 1990 [55]. Reproduced with permission of Elsevier.

Figure 18.26 Coronary flow velocity during sinus arrhythmia and respiratory variation. Note the marked decline in arterial pressure (c, first arrow) with return on the next respiratory cycle (second arrow). AO = aortic pressure; mVEL = mean velocity; pVEL = phasic velocity.

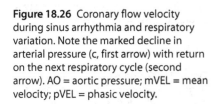

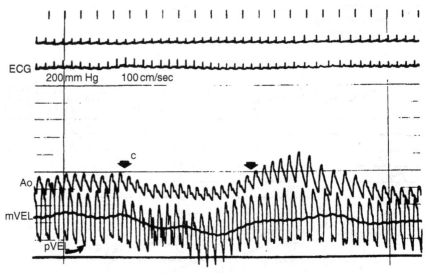

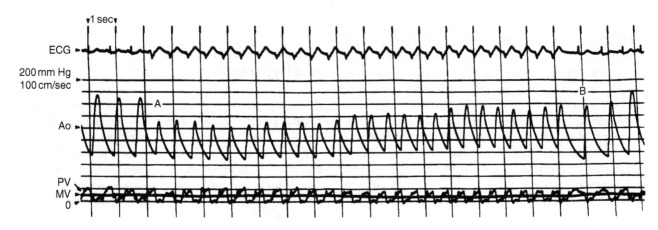

Figure 18.27 Arterial (Ao) pressure and coronary flow velocity during temporary pacing. Pacemaker rhythm begins at beat #4 (A) and terminates 14 sec later. MV = mean velocity; PV = phasic velocity.

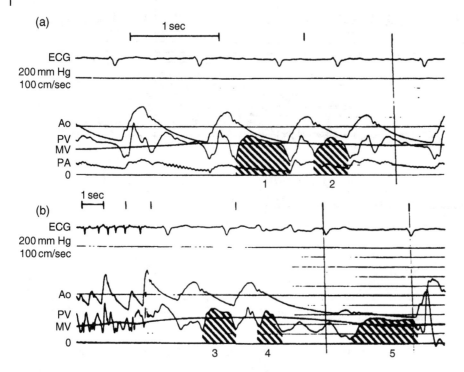

Figure 18.28 Coronary flow velocity during atrial fibrillation for long and short cardiac cycles. (a) Cycle length during beats #1 and 2 is 933 and 667 msec with flow velocity integrals (23.7 and 13.0 units, shaded areas), respectively. (b) During beat #5 coronary flow velocity is augmented over a long RR interval (1000 msec) with flow velocity integral (20.0 units). Ao = aortic pressure; MV = mean velocity; PV = phasic velocity.

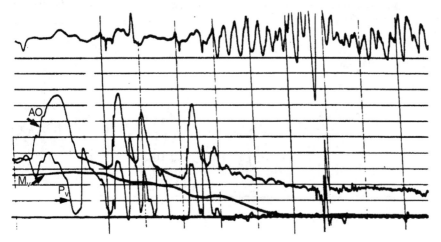

Figure 18.29 Coronary flow velocity during an episode of Torsade de Pointes and ventricular fibrillation. AO = aortic pressure; M_V = mean velocity; P_V = phasic velocity. *Source:* Kern 1990 [58]. Reproduced with permission of John Wiley & Sons.

These specialized tracings illustrate several important patterns of coronary blood flow velocity that may occur in patients during diagnostic cardiac catheterization. Recent advances in Doppler methodologies permit easy measurement of coronary blood flow during routine coronary angiography. At the current time, measurement of coronary blood flow velocity remains principally a research technique, but is of continuing interest in clinical syndromes of atypical angina, myocardial hypertrophy and infarction, early transplant rejection, or premature (subangiographic) atherosclerosis in some patients.

Coronary Flow Reserve and Hyperemia

Coronary flow reserve is the ratio of maximal to basal coronary blood and is a measure of the heart's ability to increase flow in response to increases in myocardial demand. Impaired CFR results from either obstructed epicardial arteries or abnormal microvascular circulation or both, and can be computed in several ways. First, coronary reserve can be calculated as the ratio of mean hyperemic to basal coronary flow velocity. Second, CFR can be normalized for mean arterial pressure as follows:

(hyperemic flow velocity/
mean arterial pressure at peak hyperemia)/
(basal velocity/mean arterial pressure at basal pressure)

A coronary resistance index may be computed as the ratio of mean arterial pressure and mean coronary flow velocity. Normal coronary vasodilatory reserve has been reported as a range depending on the clinical characteristics, but greater than 3.0 (a threefold increase of the basal value) is widely considered the lower limit of normal. Coronary hyperemic responses may be altered by metabolic, vascular, myocardial, and endothelial factors [59], and additional considerations beyond the scope of this discussion. Hemodynamic changes in the mean arterial pressure heart rate and left ventricular contraction markedly influence the reproducibility of measured CFR. From an interstudy assessment of variability, when measured serially over an 11-month interval, the major changes in CFR determinations appeared to be related to changes in heart rate more than other variables [60].

Coronary hyperemia is needed to measure CFR and FFR. Coronary hyperemia is defined as a transient or permanent increase in coronary flow above the basal level in response to exercise, pharmacologic stimulation, or relief of ischemia. Reactive hyperemia describes the coronary flow response occurring after relief of transient arterial occlusion, producing ischemia. Animal models used coronary ligature and release (Figure 18.30). In patients, reactive hyperemia can be produced following balloon deflation during coronary angioplasty. Pharmacologic hyperemia can be induced with a number of common drugs such as papaverine, adenosine, ATP, dipyridamole, nitroglycerin, nitroprusside, and radiographic contrast media. Coronary vasodilatory reserve, the ratio of basal to maximal hyperemic flow, is considered to be the maximal increase in flow that can be achieved by the stimulated coronary bed. CFR is thought to be the result of several complex, interrelating processes. Although measurements of coronary hyperemia and coronary reserve can be easily obtained in the cardiac catheterization laboratory with coronary Doppler techniques, the application of this technique currently remains principally for research.

There are two methods available for measuring coronary blood flow reserve in the catheterization laboratory: intracoronary Doppler flow velocity and coronary artery thermodilution.

Coronary Doppler Flow Velocity

Unlike the pressure wire, measuring flow velocity with the Doppler sensor wire requires no zeroing or central signal matching. Once sensor connections and the velocity settings on the screen display are set, the Doppler wire is passed beyond the stenosis with the Doppler guidewire tip positioned at least 5–10 artery-diameter lengths (>2 cm) beyond the target stenosis. Resting flow velocity is recorded, and then coronary hyperemia is induced by IC or IV adenosine (or another suitable agent), with continuous recording of the flow velocity signals. CFR is computed as the ratio of maximal hyperemic to basal average peak velocity. Because of the highly position-dependent signal, poor signal acquisition may occur in 10–15% of patients even within normal arteries. As with transthoracic echo Doppler studies, the operator must adjust the guidewire position (sample volume) to optimize the velocity signal. See above on Doppler coronary flow velocity.

Variations in Normal Coronary Vasodilatory Reserve

Variations of CFR (defined as the ratio of maximal coronary flow in hyperemia to baseline flow) in multiple arteries in large numbers of patients in the cardiac catheterization laboratory have led to controversy regarding normal values. This issue is especially pertinent for assessing the significance of coronary stenosis in patients

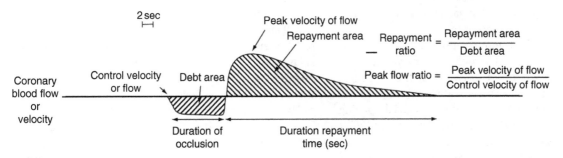

Figure 18.30 Diagram of coronary blood flow velocity tracing demonstrating the reactive hyperemic response of transient coronary occlusion. *Source:* Marcus 1981 [61]. Reproduced with permission of the American Heart Association.

with angiographically near-normal coronary arteries and early atherosclerotic disease, who may have concomitant impairment of the microcirculation. Absolute CFR measures the capacity of the two-component system of coronary artery and supplied vascular bed to achieve maximal blood flow in response to a given hyperemic stimulation. Studies with intravascular ultrasound (IVUS) of normal arteries in animals and in young patients demonstrated an absolute CFR of 3.5–5 [60]. However, the spectrum of CFR in 450 coronary arteries of patients undergoing cardiac catheterization was found to be lower [16]. Maximal hyperemia was stimulated with IC adenosine (12–18 mcg bolus) and CFR was computed as hyperemia/basal average peak (mean) velocity (BAPV). CFR in normal patients with chest pain syndromes was approximately 2.9 ± 0.6, similar to the angiographically normal artery in patients with coronary artery disease (2.5 ± 0.95), with both values higher than the post-stenotic diseased-vessel CFR (1.8 ± 0.6). Transplant arteries had the highest CFR (3.1 ± 0.9). Among different normal arteries, there was no difference in CFR for circumflex artery, right coronary artery (RCA), or left coronary artery (LCA). Regional differences were not present, suggesting that relative CFR should be 1.0 ± 0.2. The overall incidence of impaired coronary vasodilatory reserve less than 2.0 in these 220 patients undergoing angiographic evaluation for chest pain or cardiac transplantation follow-up was approximately 12%.

Influence of Hemodynamics on Coronary Flow Reserve

CFR is subject to variations in conditions that may alter resting flow and limit maximal hyperemic flow. Tachycardia increases basal flow; CFR is reduced by 10% for each 15 beats of heart rate [60]. Increasing mean arterial pressure reduces maximal vasodilation, reducing hyperemia with less alteration in basal flow. CFR may be reduced in patients with essential hypertension and normal coronary arteries, and in patients with aortic stenosis and normal coronary arteries [63]. De Bruyne and associates [8] have analyzed the short-term reproducibility of CFR measurements. CFR was measured twice at a 3-minute interval and under atrial pacing, nitroprusside administration, and then dobutamine administration. The coefficient of variation of CFR was 10.5% between the two baseline measurements. CFR did not change during infusion of nitroprusside, but decreased during atrial pacing and dobutamine infusion. Interpretation of CFR measurements should thus account for the variable hemodynamic conditions at which the flow velocity measurements are obtained.

Guidewire Thermodilution Blood Flow Technique

The coronary thermodilution technique uses thermistors on a pressure-sensor angioplasty guidewire and measures the arrival time of room-temperature saline bolus indicator injections through the guiding catheter into the coronary artery [64, 65]. The shaft of the angioplasty pressure-monitoring guidewire (St. Jude Medical Systems) has a temperature-dependent electrical resistance and acts as a proximal thermistor, which allows for the detection of the start of the indicator (saline) injection (Figure 18.31). Thermodilution CFR (CFR_{thermo}) is defined as the ratio of hyperemic flow divided by resting coronary flow (F):

$$CFR = \frac{\text{Fat hyperemia}}{\text{Fat rest}}$$

Simultaneous measurements of CFR and FFR are currently obtained for research studies on coronary and myocardial resistance. When combined with pressure measurements, coronary flow reserve measurements can provide a complete description of the pressure–flow relationship and the response of the microcirculation.

Pharmacologic Agents for Coronary Hyperemia

Stenosis severity should always be assessed using measurements obtained during maximal hyperemia. The most widely used maximal vasodilator agent for determination of coronary vasodilatory reserve is adenosine. The hyperosmolar ionic and low-osmolar nonionic contrast media do not produce maximal vasodilation. Nitrates increase volumetric flow, but, because these agents also dilate epicardial conductance vessels, the increase in coronary flow velocity is less than with adenosine or papaverine. Table 18.4 summarizes hyperemic agents used for FFR.

Adenosine

Both IC and IV adenosine have the advantage of short half-lives. The total duration of the hyperemic response to IC adenosine is only 25% that of papaverine or dipyridamole [67]. Adenosine is benign in the appropriate dosages (to 30–50 mcg in the RCA or 100–200 mcg in the LCA, or infused IV at 140 mcg/kg/minute), although many have reported safety at much higher dosages. Transient atrioventricular block and bradycardia may occur. Intravenous administration tends to have a higher incidence of flushing, chest tightness, and A-V block as compared with intracoronary dosing.

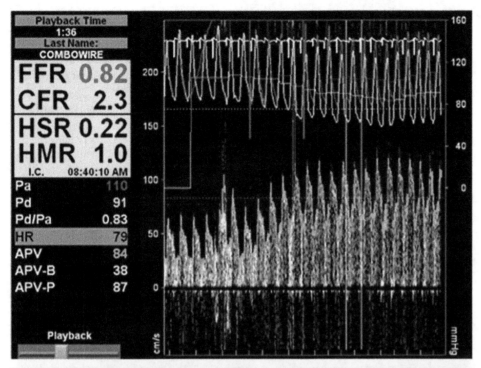

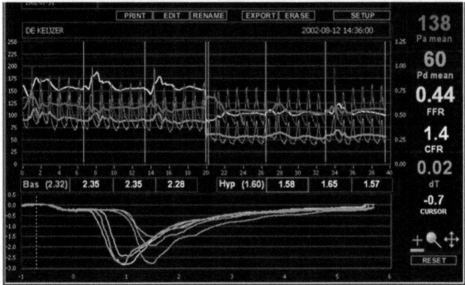

Figure 18.31 (Top) Combination of pressure signals and flow velocity tracings used to compute fractional flow reserve (FFR), coronary flow reserve (CFR) and hyperemic stenosis resistance (HSR). (Bottom) Thermodilution signals from the St. Jude pressure wire used to compute flow velocity by thermodilution curves. *Source:* Wilson 1986 [66]. Reproduced with permission of Wolters Kluwer Health, Inc. (*See insert for color representation of the figure.*)

Jeremias and colleagues [68] found that IC adenosine is equivalent to IV infusion for determination of FFR in the large majority of patients. However, in a small percentage of cases, coronary hyperemia was suspected to be suboptimal with IC adenosine, suggesting a repeated higher IC adenosine dose may be helpful in some patients [69].

Dipyridamole

IV dipyridamole, which acts by blocking uptake of adenosine, increases coronary blood flow velocity four to five times basal levels in normal subjects. Dipyridamole (0.56 mg/kg infused over 4 min) has been shown to increase flow velocity 4.8 ± 0.4 times basal flow velocity, a result that was significantly greater than contrast-induced

Table 18.4 Hyperemic agents used for coronary physiology assessment.

Agent	Route	Dose	Comments
Adenosine	IV infusion	140 mcg/kg/min	Reference standard. Side effects include dyspnea and chest pain. Prolonged hyperemia allows pressure wire pullback.
Adenosine	IC bolus	>100 mcg	Easy to use, inexpensive, and no significant side effects. Transient heart block at high doses. Hyperemia lasts only 10–15 sec.
Adenosine	IC infusion	240–360 mcg/min	Inconvenient set-up. Fewer side effects compared with IV infusion. Prolonged hyperemia allows pullback. Not well validated.
Regadenoson	IV bolus	400 mcg	Convenient, single IV bolus. Expensive. Side effects similar to IV adenosine. but less severe and briefer. Hyperemia lasts 20 sec to 10 min.
Papaverine	IC bolus	10–20 mg	Easy to use, inexpensive. Rare but significant side effects of polymorphic VT. Hyperemia lasts 30 sec, allowing pullback.
Nitroprusside	IC bolus	0.3–0.9 mcg/kg	Easy to use, inexpensive. Major side effect is hypotension. Hyperemia last 50 sec, allowing pullback. Not well validated.
Dobutamine	IV infusion	50 mcg/kg/min	Inconvenient, as it takes time for onset and offset. Side effects include palpitations and hypotension. Not well validated for FFR.
Nicorandil	IC bolus	2 mg	Not available in United States. Fewer side effects compared with IV adenosine. Hyperemia lasts 30 sec. Not well validated.

FFR = fractional flow reserve; IC = intracoronary; IV = intravenous; VT = ventricular tachycardia.
Source: Fearon [13].

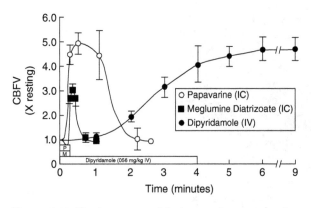

Figure 18.32 The time course of the hyperemic responses of papaverine, meglumine diatrizoate, and dipyridamole. CBFV = coronary blood flow velocity; IC = intracoronary; IV = intravenous. Reprinted with permission [57].

hyperemia (meglumine diatrizoate, 3.1 ± 0.2, $P < 0.01$) [70]. Dipyridamole has a longer time to onset (6–10 minutes, see Figure 18.32) than the other agents, with persistent effects for more than 20 min, making it unsuitable for repetitive studies. Patients receiving methylxanthines or similar drugs may have a markedly reduced effect from dipyridamole. Side effects from dipyridamole, including flushing, chest pain, and nausea, are rapidly reversed by theophylline administration.

Dobutamine

Bartunek and associates [71] examined FFR in response to IC adenosine and IV dobutamine (10–40 mcg/kg/min) in 22 patients with single-vessel coronary artery disease. Peak dobutamine infusion produced similar distal coronary pressure and pressure ratios (P_d/P_a 60 ± 18 and 59 ± 18 mm Hg, FFR 0.68 ± 0.18 and 0.68 ± 0.17, respectively; all $P = $ NS). An additional bolus of IC adenosine given at peak dobutamine in nine patients failed to change the FFR. By angiography, high-dose IV dobutamine did not modify the area of the epicardial stenosis and, much like adenosine, fully exhausted myocardial resistance regardless of inducible left ventricular dysfunction.

Nitroglycerin

IC nitroglycerin does not induce maximal hyperemia, but rather produces submaximal vasodilation between 1.5 and 2.5 times basal flow velocity (Figure 18.33). IC nitroglycerin in doses of 100–200 mcg produces vasodilation and doubles coronary venous efflux and arterial flow velocity [72]. Doses above 200 mcg are associated with significant decreases in mean arterial pressure and fall in coronary hyperemia. Nitroglycerin-induced hyperemic effects occur within 20 ± 5 sec, with a duration of up to 90–110 sec. Coronary hyperemia after balloon deflation during angioplasty-induced ischemia is not attenuated by intracoronary nitroglycerin.

Sodium Nitroprusside

IC nitroprusside may be an alternative to IC adenosine. Parham *et al.* [73] examined coronary blood flow velocity, heart rate, and blood pressure in unobstructed left anterior descending coronary arteries in 21 patients at rest, after IC adenosine (30–50 mcg boluses), and after

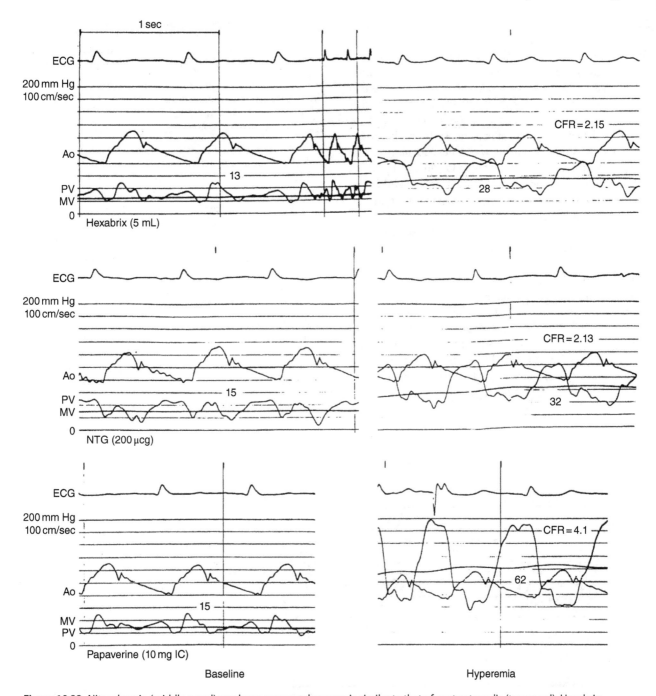

Figure 18.33 Nitroglycerin (middle panel) produces coronary hyperemia similar to that of contrast media (top panel). Hexabrix, nitroglycerin, and papaverine (bottom panel) demonstrate increases in mean coronary blood flow velocity of 28, 32, and 64 cm/sec, with coronary flow reserve (CFR) of 2.15, 2.13, and 4.1, respectively, in a 38-year-old woman 4 years after orthotopic cardiac transplantation. Ao = aortic pressure; MV = mean velocity; NTG = nitroglycerin; PV = phasic velocity.

three serial doses (0.3, 0.6, and 0.9 mcg/kg boluses) of IC nitroprusside. IC nitroprusside produced equivalent coronary hyperemia with a longer duration (about 25%) compared with IC adenosine. IC nitroprusside (0.9 mcg/kg) decreased systolic blood pressure by 20%, with minimal change in heart rate, whereas IC adenosine had no effect on these parameters. FFR measurements with IC nitroprusside were identical to those obtained with IC adenosine ($r = 0.97$). IC nitroprusside, in doses commonly used for the treatment of the no-reflow phenomenon, can produce sustained coronary hyperemia without detrimental systemic hemodynamics. Sodium nitroprusside also appears to be a suitable hyperemic stimulus for coronary physiological measurements.

Papaverine

IC papaverine 10 mg markedly increases coronary blood flow within 30 sec. Maximal hyperemia occurs 28 ± 15 sec after intracoronary injection and returns to baseline within 128 ± 15 sec [66]. Coronary flow velocity increases by an average of 3–5 times basal flow velocity in normal vessels (Figure 18.34). Although the short duration of action and lack of major effects on systemic hemodynamics suggested papaverine was a near-ideal agent for human studies, papaverine-induced QT interval prolongation and rare episodes of ventricular tachycardia have been reported. Since low doses of papaverine may not elicit maximal hyperemia, an initial dose of 8–10 mg is administered, with a second 12 mg dose to confirm a maximal vasodilatory response.

Regadenoson

Regadenoson is an α2A adenosine receptor agonist that induces coronary vasodilatation and increases myocardial blood flow in a manner reportedly equivalent to adenosine, with fewer adverse effects. Regadenoson has a half-life of 2–3 min in the initial phase, 30 min in the intermediate phase, and 2 hours in the terminal phase. It is administered as an IV bolus [74, 75].

Measurements of Microvascular Disease

The ratio of distal coronary pressure to the inverse of the mean transit time during maximal hyperemia defines an index of microvascular resistance (IMR; Figure 18.31). IMR is superior to CFR because it is not affected by resting hemodynamics, making it more reproducible, even after hemodynamic perturbations. It is also specific for the microvasculature, whereas CFR is affected by epicardial stenosis. IMR, when measured immediately after primary PCI for STEMI, predicts the amount of myocardial damage as well as left ventricular recovery better than other indices, such as CFR, ST-segment resolution, or TIMI myocardial perfusion grade. IMR can also be useful for identifying microvascular dysfunction in patients with chest pain and no epicardial artery disease.

For the determination of IMR, small bolus injections of 3 mL of saline in triplicate at maximal are given to the target artery, as described by Fearon *et al.* [76]. Mean transit time (T_{mn}) and P_d are measured simultaneously. IMR is calculated by multiplying the mean P_d by the hyperemic T_{mn}. IMR is taken as the average of the three consecutive measurements at hyperemia.

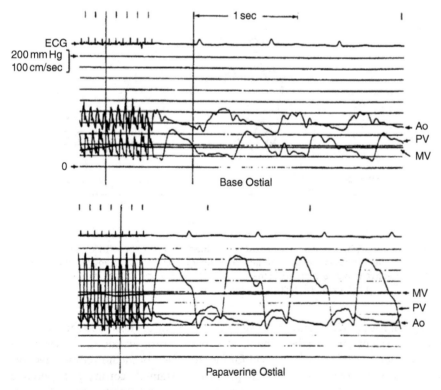

Figure 18.34 Since low doses of papaverine may not elicit maximal hyperemia, an initial dose of 8–10 mg is administered, with a second 12 mg dose to confirm a maximal vasodilatory response. Ao = aortic pressure; MV = mean velocity; PV = phasic velocity. *Source:* Wilson 1985 [49].

Coronary Hemodynamic Tracings in the Catheterization Laboratory: Catheter Tip Pressures

Observing the arterial pressure waveform from the tip of the catheter during coronary angiography is an important key to a safe procedure [77–79]. One of the earliest clues to the presence of left main coronary stenosis is a characteristically abnormal arterial pressure immediately upon catheter engagement of the coronary ostium. The pressure waves in these patients are often referred to as ventricularized or damped. Ventricularization or damping of coronary arterial pressure has a recognized association with left main coronary stenosis by experienced angiographers over several decades [80, 81]. Because of a potentially fatal complication, related to LM stenosis and occlusion, it is critical to identify and understand these coronary catheter pressure waveforms. All angiographers, especially those early in their training, should learn the importance of LM pressure damping to avoid the catastrophic outcome after diagnostic angiography that has been associated with some patients with LM coronary stenosis.

Cases: Pressure Ventricularization

A 60-year-old woman had a one-year history of exertional chest pain, with progressive pain over the past three months. In the past month, episodes of chest pain had occurred with minimal exertion and at rest. An exercise test performed one day prior to coronary angiography revealed a reduced exercise tolerance (3 min, 40 sec) with 2 mm ST segment flattening in leads V_2–V_5 II, III and A VF (at 2 min), which accompanied anginal chest pain. Exercise testing was stopped after 2 mm ST segment depression was identified. The ST segment depression persisted 8 min into recovery. The patient was admitted to the hospital and scheduled for cardiac catheterization the next day.

In the cardiac catheterization laboratory, coronary arteriography was performed from the routine (femoral) approach using a 6 F Judkin's diagnostic catheter. Catheter tip pressure from this patient during angiography is shown on Figure 18.35. On catheter tip engagement, arterial pressure dropped from 140 to 60 mm Hg (systolic), with diastolic pressures dropping from 80 to 35 mm Hg. A brief coronary injection was performed with immediate withdrawal of the catheter, as evidenced by the rapid return of arterial pressure to normal. Note the wide pulse pressure, rapid diastolic decline, and small positive deflection immediately before systolic upstroke. This pressure pattern, sometimes called ventricularized, can be commonly seen in patients with left main steno-

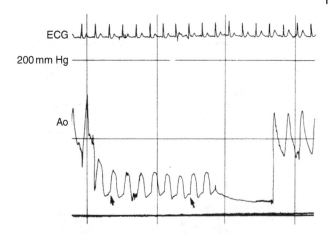

Figure 18.35 Coronary catheter pressure before and during engagement of the left main coronary artery and during pullback of catheter immediately following injection. Arrow indicates presystolic positive deflection. Ao = aortic pressure.

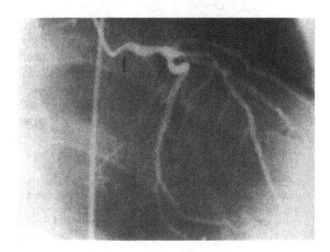

Figure 18.36 Coronary angiogram (shallow right anterior oblique projection) showing left coronary ostial stenosis (arrow). Note the absence of contrast reflux into the aorta.

sis. To limit the time of impaired perfusion with the catheter partially obstructing the coronary ostium, the operator performed a "hit-and-run" maneuver with brief contrast injection and rapid removal of the catheter. After catheter withdrawal, normal pressure and blood flow are restored. Figure 18.36 is a line angiogram frame in the shallow right anterior oblique (RAO) projection.

A similar hemodynamic tracing was obtained in a 65-year-old man with chest pain following coronary artery bypass graft surgery. The left main coronary was previously known to be narrowed by 50%. On engagement of the coronary catheter (Figure 18.37), the arterial pressure pattern showed characteristic changes of ventricularization. Coronary arteriography was performed with immediate withdrawal of the catheter tip ("hit-and-run" maneuver). In this patient, the arterial systolic pressure dropped from 140

(a)

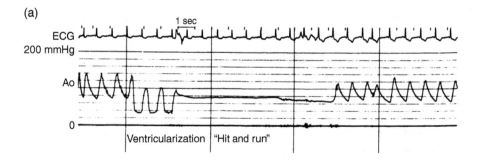

(b)

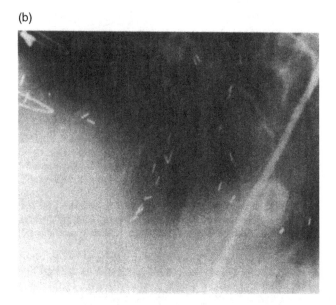

Figure 18.37 (a) Hemodynamic and electrocardiographic tracings during coronary angiography of a patient with left main coronary stenosis. On engagement of the left main coronary artery, ventricularization of the pressure waveform is noted. Contrast injection occurs during a brief "hit-and-run" period lasting approximately 5–7 sec after withdrawal of the catheter. Note the alterations of electrocardiogram immediately after contrast injection with marked T wave inversion. This contrast-induced ischemic pattern generally will revert to normal. (b) Left anterior oblique frame from cineangiogram demonstrating 80% left main coronary narrowing.

to 100 mm Hg and diastolic pressure dropped from 75 to 40 mm Hg (remember that left ventricular end-diastolic pressure is usually less than 25 mm Hg, especially if clinical congestion is absent). Note the electrocardiogram, which showed characteristic ST and T wave changes associated with contrast media injection. Should these "pseudo-ischemic" changes persist after angiography, myocardial ischemia should be suspected and immediate therapy be instituted to prevent the downward spiral of left ventricular ischemic decompensation with hypotension after contrast injection in the setting of LM stenosis.

Pressure Damping

Significant pressure changes occurring when a coronary catheter tip obstructs artery flow into a flattening of the pressure wave are called "damping." Damping can commonly occur during angiography of the right coronary artery. In general, right coronary waveform pressure alterations are more common, due, in part, to a smaller artery, subselective conus branch engagement, or catheter-induced coronary spasm. Ostial right coronary stenosis may give a ventricularized pattern. These changes carry less significant consequences unless left main or severe multivessel left coronary stenoses are also present.

The coronary pressure (Figure 18.38) was recorded during injection of a right coronary artery in a patient with angina and a positive exercise test. Thallium scintigraphic redistribution was present in the inferior and lateral regions. The coronary pressure damped on catheter tip engagement. Contrast was injected 15 sec after rapid positioning of the X-ray c-arm. The injector syringe pressure was recorded, demonstrating the time, duration, and intensity (pressure) of hand injection during the right coronary artery angiogram. The hit-and-run maneuver also shows the immediate return of normal arterial pressure upon completion of catheter withdrawal during contrast injection.

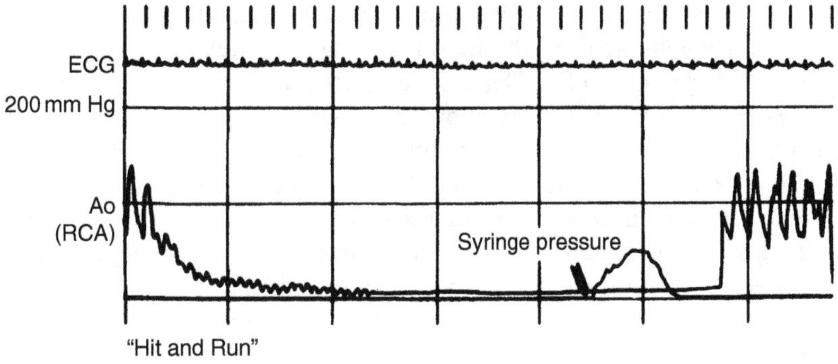

Figure 18.38 Right coronary pressure during contrast injection using a "hit-and-run" maneuver. Damping of pressure during right coronary artery (RCA) does not show the ventricularization pattern. The technique of contrast injection is demonstrated by the injection syringe pressure (arrow), which was measured during this study. On immediate pullback of the catheter, aortic (Ao) pressure is restored. There were no significant electrocardiographic abnormalities during this injection.

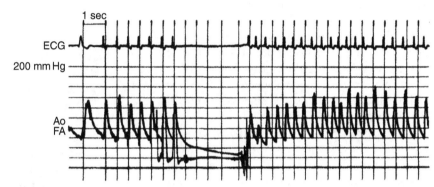

Figure 18.39 Simultaneous aortic (Ao) and femoral artery (FA) pressures measured prior to coronary angiography. Is this coronary ventricularization?

Ventricularization or Ventricular Pressure?

Simultaneous 8 F femoral artery sheath and 7 F Judkin's coronary catheter pressures were recorded prior to left coronary angiography (Figure 18.39). Pressure ventricularization was observed followed by transient asystole. The catheter was rapidly removed, with return of sinus rhythm. Examine these tracings closely. Is this ventricularization? Why is there immediate asystole? From examination of the two pressures, the coronary pressure was actually left ventricular pressure. The catheter had fallen into the left ventricle. Coronary pressure ventricularization (Figure 18.37) differs from true left ventricular pressure in several important respects. Left ventricular systolic pressure is equivalent to systolic aortic pressures and LV diastolic pressure is considerably lower (in this example 20 mm Hg). The characteristic waveform pattern of true ventricular pressure is evident. This catheter had slipped into the left ventricle and, prior to contrast injection, asystole occurred, probably by stimulation of the left bundle creating transient left bundle block in the setting of a preexisting right bundle branch block. On catheter removal, restoration of the left bundle conduction occurred and cardiac rhythm was restored with normal blood pressure. The morphology of ventricularized coronary pressure also has a distinct presystolic deflection, resembling an "a" wave. The upstroke is also slower than aortic pressure and the downstroke steeper than aortic pressure. The pressure tracing of Figure 18.39 demonstrates that not all ventricularization is due to coronary pressure damping, and that complications during coronary angiography may occur from causes other than catheters limiting coronary flow. The problem presented on Figure 18.39 is obvious during fluoroscopy and its identification immediately apparent. However, an inattentive operator may take several seconds to react promptly to limit asystole and hypotension.

Mechanisms of Ventricularization

The mechanisms of coronary pressure damping have been studied by Pacold *et al.* [80]. Variable degrees of intracoronary pressure changes upon cannulation of diseased left main coronary arteries were observed in 20 consecutive patients with ventricularization of coronary pressure. Confirmation of these pressure waveforms was obtained in an animal model by inserting a balloon-tipped catheter and producing partial degrees of occlusion of the left main coronary artery.

The ventricularized pressure wave is derived from aortic pressure, which is altered by its transmission across the narrowed left main coronary artery. Advancing a catheter into the ostium of a narrowed coronary artery reduces both systolic and diastolic pressures, as well as causing a steep decline of the pressure in diastole. A characteristic increase in pressure at end-diastole with a pre-systolic positive deflection was thought to be related to atrial contraction. This "a" waveform (seen on

Figure 18.35, arrow), although at times inconspicuous, is more likely generated by the motion of the ascending aorta during systole [80]. The degree of pressure drop between the ascending aorta and a stenosed left main coronary artery is variable, depending on the degree of stenosis. Pacold *et al.* [80] also note that ventricularization may be seen in conditions other than left main coronary artery stenosis, such as matching diameters of the coronary artery and catheter, or a deeply seated subselective position into a stenosed branch artery. Pressures from small right coronary arteries and stenosed proximal vein grafts may also demonstrate this phenomenon. The concept that ventricularization may occur by an unfavorable position of the catheter tip against an arterial wall without stenosis does not appear to be supported by the demonstration of Pacold *et al.* [80]. Ventricularization remains a critical observation related to left main coronary artery stenosis. Appropriate special techniques to obtain safe angiograms for this situation should be employed [81].

Appropriate precautions in patients with suspected left main disease involve performing a nonselective aortic cusp flush, or a brief hit-and-run injection in a shallow RAO or anteroposterior projection. Minimizing the number of contrast injections is important. Performance of ventriculography depends on a low-risk/high-benefit ratio. A low-volume, digital subtraction ventriculogram may be a helpful "one-test" study for immediate surgical consultation. In patients with critical left main stenosis, insertion of an intra-aortic balloon pump and rapid transfer for emergency cardiac surgery may be required.

Pressure Damping Due to Catheter Tip Abutment against the Arterial Wall

Pressure damping due to true left main stenosis must be differentiated from damping due to the tip of the catheter set flush against the vessel wall. With a JL4 catheter angled upward into the LM, pressure may appear identical to that of a stenotic obstruction. Catheter withdrawal, repositioning, reangulation, and cusp injection should be performed. Give nitroglycerin if coronary spasm is suspected. Pressure damping can also occur with subselective engagement in the ostium of the LAD. Despite these maneuvers, it may be difficult to confirm angiographically the significance of the LM narrowing. In this case, a pressure wire with FRR or an IVUS examination becomes diagnostic.

The coronary pressure waveforms described in this chapter are an integral part of the angiographer's approach to patients, especially those with suspected left main coronary stenosis. Patient management will differ according to the laboratory experience and training of the operators. Recognition and appreciation of abnormal coronary pressure waveforms may directly affect the life and death of these patients.

Key Points

1) Measurements of coronary pressure and flow in the catheterization laboratory are now used in daily clinical practice and associated with improved clinical outcomes for percutaneous coronary intervention decision-making.
2) The morphology of the stenosis from angiography or intravascular ultrasound (IVUS) does not account for the several factors contributing to resistance to flow, which include lumen cross-sectional area (the most commonly used measure of severity), lesion length, the shape of the entrance and exit orifices, and the size of the reference vessel.
3) Fractional flow reserve (FFR) is strongly related to provocable myocardial ischemia using different clinical stress testing modalities in patients with stable angina as the comparative standard.
4) Instantaneous wave-free pressure ratio (iFR) was found to be noninferior to FFR in two recent studies for major adverse cardiac events over the first year.
5) FFR and iFR can be used to assess the non-infarct-related artery in the acute coronary syndrome patient.
6) Left main (LM) FFR in the setting of severe downstream left anterior descending (LAD) artery disease (LAD FFR < 0.6) may require IVUS, since LM FFR will be artifactually higher when measured in the circumflex.

References

1 Chilian WM. Coronary microcirculation in health and disease: Summary of an NHLBI workshop. *Circulation* 95: 522–528, 1997.
2 Gould KL, Kirkeeide RL, Buchi M. Coronary flow reserve as a physiologic measure of stenosis severity. *J Am Coll Cardiol* 15:459–474, 1990.
3 Gould KL. Noninvasive assessment of coronary stenoses by myocardial perfusion imaging during pharmacologic coronary vasodilation: Physiologic basis and experimental validation. *Am J Cardiol* 41:267–272, 1978.
4 Gould KL, Lipscomb K, Hamilton GW. Physiologic basis for assessing critical coronary stenosis: Instantaneous

flow response and regional distribution during coronary hyperemia as measures of coronary flow reserve. *Am J Cardiol* 33:87–94, 1974.

5 Siebes M, Campbell CS, D'Argenio DZ. Fluid dynamics of a partially collapsible stenosis in a flow model of the coronary circulation. *J Biomech Eng* 118:489–497, 1996.

6 Kern MJ. Coronary physiology revisited: Practical insights from the cardiac catheterization laboratory. *Circulation* 101:1344–1351, 2000.

7 Pijls NHJ, Van Gelder B, Van der Voort P, Peels K, Bracke FA, Bonnier HJ, el Gamal MI. Fractional flow reserve: A useful index to evaluate the influence of an epicardial coronary stenosis on myocardial blood flow. *Circulation* 92:318–319, 1995.

8 De Bruyne B, Bartunek J, Sys SU, Pijls NH, Heyndrickx GR, Wijns W. Simultaneous coronary pressure and flow velocity measurements in humans: Feasibility, reproducibility and hemodynamic dependence of coronary flow velocity reserve, hyperemic flow versus pressure slope index and fractional flow reserve. *Circulation* 94:1842–1849, 1996.

9 Pijls NHJ, Kern MJ, Yock PG, De Bruyne B. Practice and potential pitfalls of coronary pressure measurement. *Cathet Cardiovasc Interv* 49:1–16, 2000.

10 Sen S, Asrress KN, Nijjer S, Petraco R, Malik IS, Foale RA, *et al.* Diagnostic classification of the instantaneous wave-free ratio is equivalent to fractional flow reserve and is not improved with adenosine administration. *J Am Coll Cardiol* 61(13):1409–1420, 2013.

11 Petraco R, Park JJ, Sen S, Nijjer SS, Malik IS, Echavarría-Pinto M, *et al.* Hybrid iFR-FFR decision-making strategy: Implications for enhancing universal adoption of physiology-guided coronary revascularisation. *EuroIntervention* 8(10):1157–1165, 2013.

12 Jeremias A, Maehara A, Genereux P, Asrress KN, Berry C, De Bruyne B, *et al.* Multicenter core laboratory comparison of the instantaneous wave-free ratio and resting Pd/Pa with fractional flow reserve: the RESOLVE study. *J Am Coll Cardiol* 63(13):1253–1261, 2014.

13 Fearon WF. Invasive coronary physiology for assessing intermediate lesions. *Circ Cardiovasc Interv* 8(2):e001942, 2015.

14 Pijls NH, De Bruyne B, Peels K, Van Der Voort PH, Bonnier HJ, Bartunek J, Koolen JJ. Measurement of fractional flow reserve to assess the functional severity of coronary-artery stenoses. *N Engl J Med* 334(26):1703–1708, 1996.

15 Christou MA, Siontis GC, Katritsis DG, Ioannidis JP. Meta-analysis of fractional flow reserve versus quantitative coronary angiography and noninvasive imaging for evaluation of myocardial ischemia. *Am J Cardiol* 99(4):450–456, 2007.

16 Kern MJ, Bach RG, Mechem CJ, Caracciolo EA, Aguirre FV, Miller LW, Donohue TJ. Variations in normal coronary vasodilatory reserve stratified by artery, gender, heart transplantation and coronary artery disease. *J Am Coll Cardiol* 28:54–1160, 1996.

17 De Bruyne B, Bartunek J, Sys SU, Heyndrickx GR. Relation between myocardial fractional flow reserve calculated from coronary pressure measurements and exercise-induced myocardial ischemia. *Circulation* 92:39–46, 1995.

18 Bartunek J, Van Schuerbeeck E, de Bruyne B. Comparison of exercise electrocardiography and dobutamine echocardiography with invasively assessed myocardial fractional flow reserve in evaluation of severity of coronary arterial narrowing. *Am J Cardiol* 79:478–481, 1997.

19 Chamuleau SA, Meuwissen M, van Eck-Smit BL, Koch KT, de Jong A, de Winter RJ, *et al.* Fractional flow reserve, absolute and relative coronary blood flow velocity reserve in relation to the results of technetium-99 m sestamibi single-photon emission computed tomography in patients with two-vessel coronary artery disease. *J Am Coll Cardiol* 37: 1316–1322, 2001.

20 Caymaz O, Fak AS, Tezcan H, Inanir SS, Toprak A, Tokay S, *et al.* Correlation of myocardial fractional flow reserve with thallium-201 SPECT imaging in intermediate-severity coronary artery lesions. *J Invasive Cardiol* 12:345–350, 2000.

21 Fearon WF, Takagi A, Jeremias A, Yeung AC, Joye JB, Cohen DJ, *et al.* Use of fractional myocardial flow reserve to asses the functional significance of intermediate coronary stenosis. *Am J Cardiol* 86:1013–1014, 2000.

22 Takagi A, Tsurumi Y, Ishii Y, Suzuki K, Kawana M, Kasanuki H. Clinical potential of intravascular ultrasound for physiological assessment of coronary stenosis: Relationship between quantitative ultrasound tomography and pressure-derived fractional flow reserve. *Circulation* 100:250–255, 1999.

23 Briguori C, Anzuini A, Airoldi F, Gimelli G, Nishida T, Adamian M, *et al.* Intravascular ultrasound criteria for the assessment of the functional significance of intermediate coronary artery stenoses and comparison with fractional flow reserve. *Am J Cardiol* 87:136–141, 2001.

24 Gonzalo N, Escaned J, Alfonso F, Nolte C, Rodriguez V, Jimenez-Quevedo P, *et al.* Morphometric assessment of coronary stenosis relevance with optical coherence tomography: A comparison with fractional flow reserve and intravascular ultrasound. *J Am Coll Cardiol* 59(12):1080–1089, 2012.

25 Pijls NHJ, Van Schaardenburgh P, Manoharan G, Boersma E, Bech JW, Van't Veer M, *et al.* Percutaneous

coronary intervention of functionally non-significant stenoses: 5 year follow-up of the Defer study. *J Am Coll Cardiol* 49:2105–2111, 2007.

26 Ragosta M, Bishop AH, Lipson LC, Watson DD, Gimple LW, Sarembock IJ, Powers ER. Comparison between angiography and fractional flow reserve versus single-photon emission computed tomographic myocardial perfusion imaging for determining lesion significance in patients with multivessel coronary disease. *Am J Cardiol* 99:896–902, 2007.

27 Chamuleau SAJ, Meuwissen M, Koch KT, van Eck-Smit BLF, Tio RA, Tijssen JGP, Piek JJ. Usefulness of fractional flow reserve for risk stratification of patients with multivessel coronary artery disease and an intermediate stenosis. *Am J Cardiol* 89:377–380, 2002.

28 Berger A, Botman KJ, MacCarthy PA, Wijns W, Bartunek J, Heyndrickx GR, *et al.* Long-term clinical outcome after fractional flow reserve-guided percutaneous coronary intervention in patients with multivessel disease. *J Am Coll Cardiol* 46:438–442, 2005.

29 Tonino PAL, DeBruyne B, Pijls NHJ, Siebert U, Ikeno F, van' t Veer M, *et al.* Fractional flow reserve versus angiography for guiding percutaneous coronary intervention. *N Engl J Med* 360(3):213–224, 2009.

30 De Bruyne B, Pijls NH, Kalesan B, Barbato E, Tonino PA, Piroth Z, *et al.* Fractional flow reserve–guided PCI versus medical therapy in stable coronary disease. *N Engl J Med* 367:991–1001, 2012.

31 Hamilos M, Muller O, Cuisset T, Ntalianis A, Chlouverakis G, Sarno G, *et al.* Long-term clinical outcome after fractional flow reserve-guided treatment in patients with angiographically equivocal left main coronary artery stenosis. *Circulation* 120:1505–1512, 2009.

32 Yong AS, Daniels D, De Bruyne B, Kim HS, Ikeno F, Lyons J, *et al.* Fractional flow reserve assessment of left main stenosis in the presence of downstream coronary stenoses. *Circ Cardiovasc Interv* 6:161–165, 2013.

33 Fearon WF, Yong AS, Lenders G, Toth GG, Dao C, Daniels DV, *et al.* The impact of downstream coronary stenosis on fractional flow reserve assessment of intermediate left main coronary artery disease: Human validation. *JACC Cardiovasv Interv* 8(3):398–403, 2015.

34 Pijls NHJ, de Bruyne B, G. Bech GJ, Liistro F, Heyndrickx GR, Bonnier HJ, Koolen JJ. Coronary pressure measurement to assess the hemodynamic significance of serial stenoses within one coronary artery validation in humans. *Circulation* 102:2371–2377, 2000.

35 De Bruyne B, Pijls NH, Heyndrickx GR, Hodeige D, Kirkeeide R, Gould KL. Pressure-derived fractional flow reserve to assess serial epicardial stenoses: Theoretical basis and animal validation. *Circulation* 101:1840–1847, 2000.

36 De Bruyne B, Hersbach F, Pijls NH, Bartunek J, Bech J-W, Heyndrickx GR, *et al.* Abnormal epicardial coronary resistance in patients with diffuse atherosclerosis but "normal" coronary angiography. *Circulation* 104:2401–2406, 2001.

37 Koo BK, Kang HJ, Youn TJ, Chae IH, Choi DJ, Kim HS, *et al.* Physiologic assessment of jailed side branch lesions using fractional flow reserve. *J Am Coll Cardiol* 46; 633–637, 2005.

38 Ziaee A, Parham WA, Herrmann SC, Stewart RE, Lim MJ, Kern MJ. Lack of relationship between imaging and physiology in ostial coronary artery narrowings. *Am J Cardiol* 93:1404–1407, 2004.

39 Ntalianis A, Sels JW, Davidavicius G, Tanaka N, Muller O, Trana C, *et al.* Fractional flow reserve for the assessment of nonculprit coronary artery stenoses in patients with acute myocardial infarction. *JACC Cardiovasc Interv* 3(12):1274–1281, 2010.

40 De Bruyne B, Pijls NH, Bartunek J, Kulecki K, Bech JW, De Winter H, *et al.* Fractional flow reserve in patients with prior myocardial infarction. *Circulation* 104:157–162, 2001.

41 Samady H, Lepper W, Powers ER, Wei K, Ragosta M, Bishop GG, *et al.* Fractional flow reserve of infarct-related arteries identifies reversible defects on noninvasive myocardial perfusion imaging early after myocardial infarction. *J Am Coll Cardiol* 47:2187–2193, 2006.

42 Tamita K, Akasaka A, Takagi T, Yamamuro A, Yamabe K, Katayama K, *et al.* Effects of microvascular dysfunction on myocardial fractional flow reserve after percutaneous coronary intervention in patients with acute myocardial infarction. *Cath Cardiovasc Interv* 57:452–459, 2002.

43 Potvin JM, Rodés-Cabau J, Bertrand OF, Gleeton O, Nguyen CN, Barbeau G, *et al.* Usefulness of fractional flow reserve measurements to defer revascularization in patients with stable or unstable angina pectoris, non-ST-elevation and ST-elevation acute myocardial infarction, or atypical chest pain. *Am J Cardiol* 98:289–297, 2006.

44 Fischer JJ, Wang XQ, Samady H, Sarembock IJ, Powers ER, Gimple LW, Ragosta M. Outcome of patients with acute coronary syndromes and moderate lesions undergoing deferral of revascularization based on fractional flow reserve assessment. *Cath Cardiovasc Interv* 68:544–548, 2006.

45 Leesar MA, Abdul-Baki T, Akkus NI, Sharma A, Kannan T, Bolli R. Use of fractional flow reserve versus stress perfusion scintigraphy after unstable angina: Effect on duration of hospitalization, cost, procedural characteristics, and clinical outcome. *J Am Coll Cardiol* 41:1115–1121, 2003.

46 Sels JW, Tonino PA, Siebert U, Fearon WF, Van't Veer M, De Bruyne B, Pijls NH. Fractional flow reserve in unstable angina and non-ST-segment elevation myocardial infarction experience from the FAME (Fractional flow reserve versus Angiography for Multivessel Evaluation) study. *JACC Cardiovasc Interv* 4(11):1183–1189, 2011.

47 Ganz W, Tamura K, Marcus HS, Donoso R, Yoshida S, Swan HJC. Measurement of coronary sinus blood flow by continuous thermodilution in man. *Circulation* 44:181–195, 1971.

48 Pepine CJ, Mehta J, Webster WW, Nichols WW. In vivo validation of a thermodilution method to determine regional left ventricular blood flow in patients with coronary disease. *Circulation* 58(5):795–802, 1978.

49 Wilson RF, Laughlin DE, Ackell PH, Chilian WM, Holida MD, Hartley CI, *et al.* Transluminal, subselective measurement of coronary artery blood flow velocity and vasodilator reserve in man. *Circulation* 72:82, 1985.

50 Kern MJ. Intracoronary Doppler blood flow velocity catheters. In CJ White, SR Ramee (eds.), *Interventional Cardiology: Clinical Application of New Technologies.* New York: Raven Press, 1991, pp. 55–100.

51 Doucette JW, Corl PD, Payne HM, Flynn AE, Goto M, Nassi M, Segal J. Validation of a Doppler guidewire for assessment of coronary arterial flow. *Circulation* 82:621, 1990.

52 Kern MJ, Courtois M, Ludbrook P. A simplified method to measure coronary blood flow velocity in patients: Validation and application of a Judkin's-style Doppler-tipped angiographic catheter. *Am Heart J* 120:1202–1212, 1990.

53 Kern MJ, Diligently U, Vendome M, Lavovitz A, Gudipati R, Gabliani G, *et al.* Impaired coronary vasodilatory reserve in the immediate post-coronary angioplasty period: Analysis of coronary arterial velocity flow indices and regional cardiac venous efflux. *J Am Coll Cardiol* 13:868–872, 1989.

54 Cohen A, Gottdiener J, Wish M, Fletcher R. Limitations of cough in maintaining blood flow during asystole: Assessment by two dimensional and Doppler echocardiography. *Am Heart J* 118:474, 1989.

55 Kern MJ, Gudipati C, Tatineni S, Aguirre F, Serota H, Deligonul D. Effect of abruptly increased intrathoracic pressure on coronary blood flow velocity in patients. *Am Heart J* 119:863–870, 1990.

56 Benchimol A, Wang TF, Desser KB, Gartlan JL Jr. The Valsalva maneuver and coronary arterial blood flow velocity. *Ann Intern Med* 77:357, 1972.

57 Wilson RF, Marcus ML, White CW. Pulmonary inflation reflex: Its lack of physiological significance in coronary circulation of humans. *Am J Physiol* 255(*Heart Circ Physiol* 24):H866, 1988.

58 Kern MJ, Deligonul U, Serota H, Gudipati C, Buckingham T. Ventricular arrhythmia due to intracoronary papaverine: Analysis of clinical and hemodynamic data with coronary vasodilatory reserve. *Cathet Cardiovasc Diagn* 19:229–236, 1990.

59 Olsson RA. Myocardial reactive hyperemia. *Circ Res* 37:263–270, 1975.

60 McGinn AL, White CW, Wilson RF. Interstudy variability of coronary flow reserve: Influence of heart rate, arterial pressure and ventricular preload. *Circulation* 81:1319–1330, 1990.

61 Marcus Ml, Wright C, Doty D, Eastham CL, Laughlin DE, Krumm P, *et al.* Measurement of coronary velocity and reactive hyperemia in the coronary circulation of humans. *Circ Res* 49:871–871, 1981.

62 Strauer B. The significance of coronary reserve in clinical heart disease. *J Am Coll Cardiol* 5:775–783, 1990.

63 Marcus ML, Doty DB, Hiratzka LF, Wright CB, Eastham CL. Decreased coronary reserve: A mechanism for angina pectoris in patients with aortic stenosis and normal coronary arteries. *N Engl J Med* 307:1362–1366, 1982.

64 Pijls NH, De Bruyne B, Smith L, Aarnoudse W, Barbato E, Bartunek J, *et al.* Coronary thermodilution to assess flow reserve: Validation in humans. *Circulation* 105: 2482–2486, 2002.

65 De Bruyne B, Pijls NHJ, Smith L, Wievegg M, Heyndrickx GR. Coronary thermodilution to assess flow reserve: Experimental validation. *Circulation* 104:2003, 2001.

66 Wilson RF, White CW. Intracoronary papaverine: An ideal coronary vasodilator for studies of the coronary circulation in conscious humans. *Circulation* 73:444–451, 1986.

67 Wilson RF, Wyche K, Christensen BV, Zimmer S, Laxson DD. Effects of adenosine on human coronary arterial circulation. *Circulation* 82:1595–1606, 1990.

68 Jeremias A, Whitbourn RJ, Filardo SD, Fitzgerald PJ, Cohen DJ, Tuzcu EM, *et al.* Adequacy of intracoronary versus intravenous adenosine-induced maximal coronary hyperemia for fractional flow reserve measurements. *Am Heart J* 140:651–657, 2000.

69 De Luca, G., L. Venegoni, S. Iorio, Giuliani L, Marino P. Effects of increasing doses of intracoronary adenosine on the assessment of fractional flow reserve. *JACC Cardiovasc Interv* 4(10):1079–1084, 2011.

70 Marchant E, Pichard A, Rodriguez JA, Casanegra P. Acute effect of systemic versus intracoronary dipyridamole on coronary circulation. *Am J Cardiol* 57:1401, 1986.

71 Bartunek J, Wijns W, Heyndrickx GR, de Bruyne B. Effects of dobutamine on coronary stenosis physiology and morphology: Comparison with intracoronary adenosine. *Circulation* 100:243–249, 1999.

72 Kern MJ, Vandormael M, Deligonul U, Labovitz A, Harper M, Gibson P, *et al.* Intracoronary nitroglycerin and regional coronary blood flow responses during coronary angioplasty in patients. *J Interv Cardiol* 1:49–57, 1988.

73 Parham WA, Bouhasin A, Ciaramita JP, Khoukaz S, Herrmann S, Kern MJ. Coronary hyperemic dose responses to intracoronary sodium nitroprusside. *Circulation* 109:1236–1243, 2004.

74 Nair PK, Marroquin OC, Mulukutla, Khandhar S, Gulati V, Schindler JT, Lee JS. Clinical utility of regadenoson for assessing fractional flow reserve. *JACC Cardiovasc Interv* 4(10):1085–1092, 2011.

75 Hodgson JMcB, Dib N, Kern MJ, Bach RG, Barrett RJ. Coronary circulation responses to binodenoson, a selective adenosine A2a receptor agonist. *Am J Cardiol* 99:1507–1512, 2007.

76 Fearon WF, Shah M, Ng M, Brinton T, Wilson A, Tremmel JA, *et al.* Predictive value of the index of microcirculatory resistance in patients with ST-segment elevation myocardial infarction. *J Am Coll Cardiol* 51:560–565, 2008.

77 Kern MJ. Hemodynamic rounds: Interpretation of cardiac pathophysiology from pressure waveform analysis. Coronary hemodynamics part II: Patterns of coronary flow velocity. *Cathet Cardiovasc Diagn* 25:154–160, 1992.

78 Kern MJ, Aguirre F, Donohue T, Bach R. Hemodynamic rounds: Interpretation of cardiac pathophysiology from pressure waveform analysis. Coronary hemodynamics part III: Coronary hyperemia. *Cathet Cardiovasc Diagn* 26:204–211, 1992.

79 Kern MJ, Puri S, Craig WR, Bach RG, Donohue TJ. Coronary hemodynamics for angioplasty and stenting after myocardial infarction: Use of absolute, relative coronary velocity and fractional flow reserve. *Cathet Cardiovasc Diagn* 45:174–182, 1998.

80 Pacold I, Hwang MH, Piao ZE, Scanlon PJ, Loeb HS. The mechanism and significance of ventricularization of intracoronary pressure during coronary angiography. *Am Heart J* 118:1160–1166, 1989.

81 Kern MJ. Hemodynamic rounds: Interpretation of cardiac pathophysiology from pressure waveform analysis. Coronary hemodynamics: I. Coronary catheter pressures. *Cathet Cardiovasc Diagn* 25:57–60, 1992.

19

Renal Artery Stenosis

Morton J. Kern

Renal autoregulation seeks to maintain a constant glomerular filtration rate by maintenance of renal artery pressure despite having loss of pressure across the stenosis. The afferent arteriole leads into the glomerular circulation, with an efferent arteriole providing tubuloglomerular feedback. The proximal afferent arteriole is subject to myogenic reflex and the changes in pressure control the resisters at each of the afferent and efferent arteriole circulations. For example, in a patient with a 30 mm Hg gradient across the renal artery, the myogenic reflex dilates the afferent arteriole, producing renin which increases the systemic pressure, thus raising the translesional perfusion pressure to 90 mm Hg from its starting 60 mm Hg for this gradient. Thus, the renin produces increased perfusion pressure to the glomeruli, and the constricted tone of the afferent arteriole is then reduced on sensation of this increased perfusion pressure (Figure 19.1).

The incidental finding of the renal artery stenosis can be detected angiographically and assessed by measurement of translesional pressure, using the guide catheter and pressure guidewire as shown in Figure 19.2. On the left, a 45-year-old woman with asymptomatic hypertension on three antihypertensive medications has a significant pressure gradient across the ostial stenosis of the left renal artery, with distal pressure of 66 mm Hg and proximal pressure of 107 mm Hg. Compare this to the images of the patient on the right, a 62-year-old woman again with asymptomatic hypertension who had renal artery stenting 12 months earlier and now has a near-zero pressure gradient across this stenosis. Thus angiograms are important, but not entirely revealing as to the significance. The prediction of whether a stenosis is associated with hemodynamic significant impairment can be seen in Figure 19.3, in which a 2010 study by Mangiacapra *et al.* [1] demonstrates a poor correlation between percent diameter and baseline gradient, or percent diameter and dobutamine-induced gradient in this series. The eccentric nature of the stenosis, similar

to that of coronary artery disease, is responsible for exactly that problem.

Renal Artery Stenosis Pressure Gradient and Ratio

De Bruyne *et al.* [2] addressed what constitutes a significant renal artery pressure gradient. These investigators created an artificial stenosis with a balloon catheter after stenting of the renal artery (Figure 19.4). The results demonstrate that as the renal artery stenosis increases (i.e., P_d/P_a [distal pressure/aortic pressure] falls), renal vein renin increases in the renal vein. On the contralateral control side, no increase in renal vein renin was noted.

Drieghe *et al.* [3] assessed renal artery stenosis (RAS) in a side-by-side comparison of angiography-ultrasound standard (Figure 19.5). A percent diameter stenosis greater than 50% was associated with P_d/P_a less than 0.90, whereas the minimal lumen diameter did not correlate well with P_d/P_a ratios less than 0.8. Of note is that there was a curvilinear relationship between P_d/P_a for both peak systolic and mean gradient (Figure 19.5).

Renal hyperemia in the kidney is reproduced through different pharmacologic stimulation than hyperemic in the heart. In a small study by Manoharan *et al.* in 2006 [4], patients were challenged with isosorbide dinitrate, papaverine, dobutamine, and felodipine in several doses, and dopamine in 3, 5, 10, 20, and 30 µg/kg infusions. Figure 19.6 shows an example of aortic pressure and renal flow velocity signals in response to dopamine infusion. The results of hyperemia demonstrated that dopamine intrarenal produced the highest hyperemic response in renal flow velocity and this occurred in a dose– response fashion (Figure 19.7). Felodipine, both intrarenal and infusion, produced near-optimal hyperemia relative to nitrates and papaverine. Based on the available data, renal doses of dobutamine increase renal blood flow in

Hemodynamic Rounds: Interpretation of Cardiac Pathophysiology from Pressure Waveform Analysis, Fourth Edition.
Edited by Morton J. Kern, Michael J. Lim, and James A. Goldstein.
© 2018 John Wiley & Sons Ltd. Published 2018 by John Wiley & Sons Ltd.

normal patients, but not in patients with moderate renal dysfunction.

Based on the physiologic measurement of the translesional gradient, how does one know whether benefit will occur to the dilated area? Figure 19.8 shows a severe renal artery stenosis with a peak systolic gradient between aorta and left renal artery of about 50 mm Hg. The relief of the stenosis produced symptomatic change for preservation of renal function. The May 2014 SCAI expert consensus statement for the appropriate use of renal artery stenting by Parikh *et al.* [5] indicates that patients with intermediate

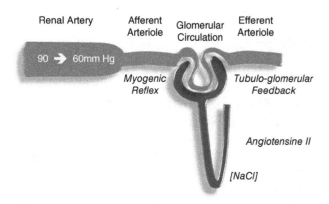

Figure 19.1 Renal artery and glomerular circulation. A renal artery stenosis may reduce perfusion pressure (90 to 60 mm Hg), setting in motion changes in afferent and efferent arteriolar resistance to preserve perfusion. NaCl = sodium chloride. *Source:* De Bruyne 2006 [2]. Reproduced with permission of Elsevier.

stenosis between 50 and 70% should undergo physiologic testing. A mean resting gradient greater than 10 mm Hg or systolic hyperemic pressure gradient greater than 20 mm Hg or renal P_d/P_a less than 0.8 are all consider hemodynamically significant. When these criteria are met, systolic blood pressure with the treatment of the physiologically important stenosis can reduce both systolic and diastolic blood pressure, according to Mitchell *et al.* [6]. However, the CORAL study by Murphy *et al.* [7] was disappointing, in that the results of stenting versus medical therapy failed to demonstrate a substantial benefit in almost any subgroup. Indications for renal stenting thus include hemodynamically significant renal artery stenosis with recurrent and unexplained congestive heart failure, or flash pulmonary edema, or unstable angina. Renal artery stenting may benefit those with resistant hypertension and those with ischemic nephropathy. The question of whether there may be a renal fractional flow reserve (FFR) suggests that in contrast to the coronary circulation, renal artery circulation has afferent and efferent resistances with different response to hyperemic stimuli. Thus, a renal artery pressure gradient, P_d/P_a, at rest of less than 0.9 is associated with increased renal vein renin. Hyperemia is the highest with dobutamine infusion. Stenting for renal artery stenosis has mixed study results. The CORAL study [7] suggested no benefit despite the potential noted by observational studies. Whether physiology will guide such a study as was done in the FAME trial is yet to be determined.

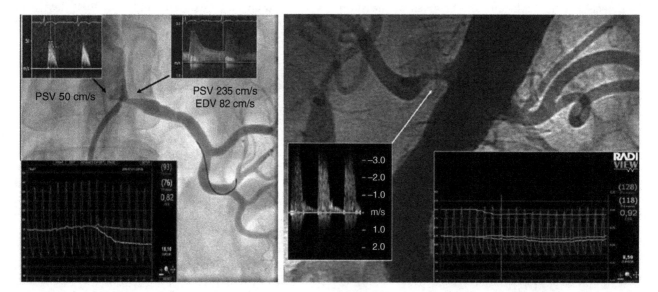

Figure 19.2 Renal artery stenosis, translesional flow velocity, and hemodynamics. (Left) Peak aortic systolic velocity (PSV) 50 cm/sec, with post-stenotic PSV of 235 cm/sec. Corresponding aortic (P_a) and distal renal artery pressure (P_d) ratio = 0.82. (Right) PSV is 300 cm/sec with P_d/P_a 0.90. EDV = end-diastolic volume. *Source:* Drieghe 2008 [3]. Reproduced with permission of Oxford University Press. (*See insert for color representation of the figure.*)

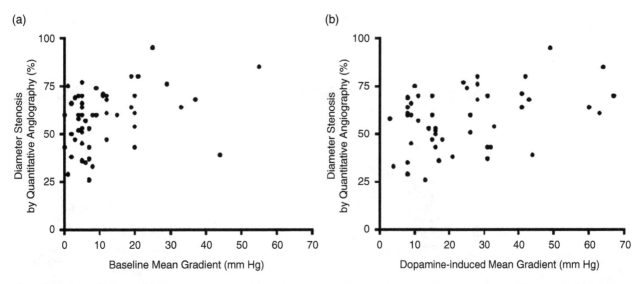

Figure 19.3 Lack of relationship between transarterial renal pressure gradient and percent diameter angiographic stenosis. (a) baseline mean gradient (mm Hg) and (b) Dopamine-induced Mean Gradient (mm Hg). *Source:* Mangiacapra 2010 [2]. Reproduced with permission of Wolters Kluwer Health, Inc.

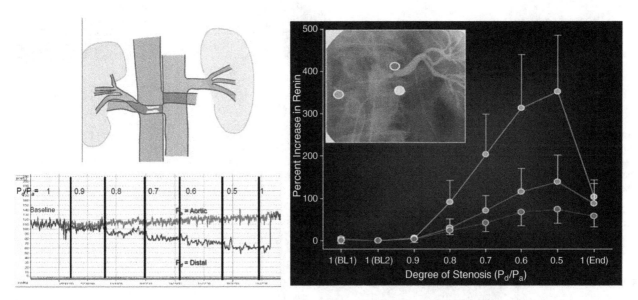

Figure 19.4 Model of renal artery stenosis created after patient receives a renal stent. (Top left) The cineangiogram frame has colored dots corresponding to the sampling locations for renal vein and artery renin. (Lower left) Pressure ratios (P_d/P_a) during partial artery occlusion created by balloon inflation. (Lower right) Renal vein begins to increase when P_d/P_a is less than 0.90. P_a = aortic pressure; P_d = distal pressure. *Source:* De Bruyne 2006 [1]. Reproduced with permission of Elsevier. *(See insert for color representation of the figure.)*

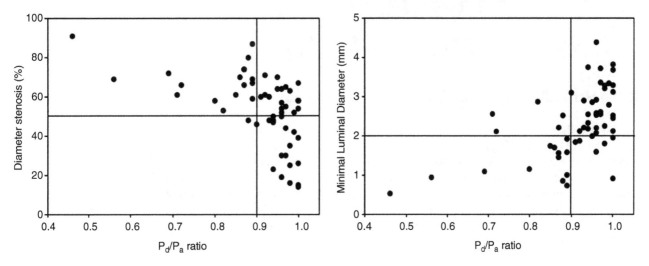

Figure 19.5 Comparison of diameter stenosis (left) and minimal luminal diameter (right) vs. renal distal (P_d) and aortic (P_a) pressure ratio. *Source:* Drieghe 2008 [3]. Reproduced with permission of Oxford University Press.

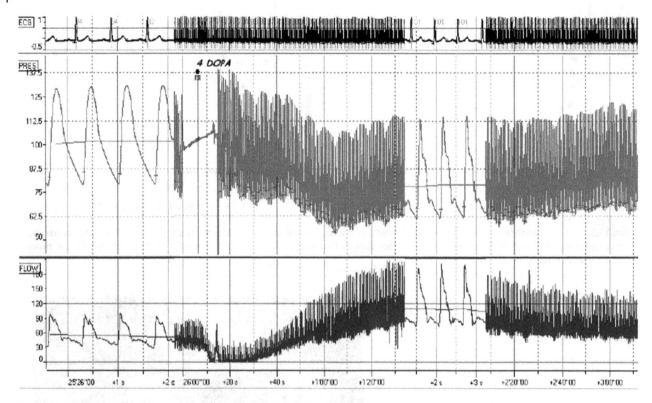

Figure 19.6 Effect of vasodilators on renal artery flow velocity. Example of simultaneous pressure and velocity pressure tracings before, during, and after intrarenal administration of a bolus of 50 μg · kg − 1 of dopamine (DOPA); immediately after administration of the bolus, a marked decrease in renal artery average peak velocity is observed, followed by an almost twofold increase in flow velocities, without changes in blood pressure nor in heart rate. *Source:* Manoharan 2006 [4]. Reproduced with permission of Elsevier. (*See insert for color representation of the figure.*)

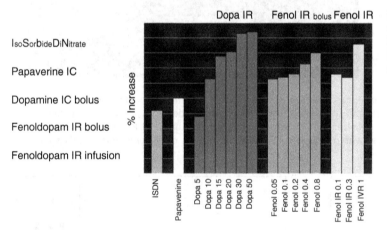

Figure 19.7 Effect of vasodilators on renal artery flow velocity. IC = intracoronary; IR = intrarenal. *Source:* Manoharan 2006 [4]. Reproduced with permission of Elsevier. (*See insert for color representation of the figure.*)

Renal Hemodynamics: Practical Tips

Dr. Tariq S. Siddiqui and colleagues from the University of Louisville, Louisville, KY performed physiologic assessment of several angiographic renal artery stenoses [8]. As noted for the assessment of coronary stenoses, angiographic assessment of RAS is often difficult and unreliable. A hyperemic systolic pressure gradient (HSPG) of over 20 mm Hg provided the highest concordance with an intravascular ultrasound (IVUS) minimal lumen cross-sectional area less than 8.6 mm^2.

Renal artery stenosis is the most common cause of secondary hypertension and is present in 0.5–5% of all hypertensive patients [9, 10]. The prevalence of atherosclerotic RAS in patients with coronary artery disease and/or peripheral vascular disease is 20–30% [11–13].

A number of studies have demonstrated that revascularization of RAS can improve blood pressure control

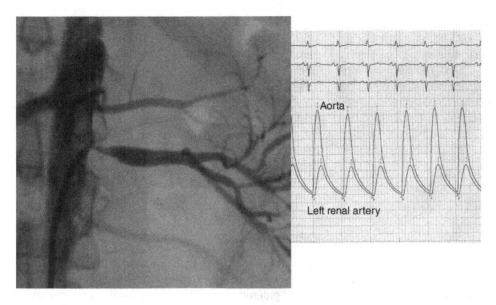

Figure 19.8 Renal artery stenosis with a peak systolic gradient between aorta and left renal artery of about 50 mm Hg. The relief of the stenosis produced symptomatic change for preservation of renal function.

and renal function [14–17]. Even though conventional angiography has been the "gold standard" to assess the severity of RAS, it does not correlate well with the physiologic severity of RAS, as determined by recent studies [18, 19]. Both intravascular ultrasound and fractional flow reserve are established modalities for the physiologic assessment of a coronary stenosis [20, 21]. Recently, the pressure gradient and FFR of the renal artery have been used for physiologic assessment of RAS [18, 19]. In this respect, a number of series [18, 19] demonstrated poor correlations comparing renal angiography with renal FFR, hyperemic mean pressure gradient (HMPG), and resting systolic pressure gradient (RSPG) [22].

Four patients who had RAS underwent pressure gradient and IVUS examination after administration of 200 mcg intrarenal nitroglycerin. The renal angiography was performed with a 5 F Cobra catheter (Boston Scientific Inc., Natick, MA). A 0.014 inch Sparta-Core guidewire (Guidant Inc., Temecula, CA) was advanced through the Cobra catheter into the renal artery and positioned distally. The Cobra catheter was removed and a 6 F Veripath guiding catheter (Guidant) was advanced over the Sparta-Core wire and engaged the renal artery. Next, the Sparta-Core wire was removed and a 0.014 inch pressure guidewire was advanced into the renal artery through the guiding catheter. In order to normalize the aortic pressure with the pressure guidewire, the pressure transducer and guiding catheter were withdrawn to the aorta, while the floppy tip of the wire remained in the renal artery. After identical pressures of the guiding catheter and pressure guidewire were confirmed at this position, the pressure transducer was advanced into the renal

artery and crossed the stenosis. After the RSPG was obtained, the guiding catheter was engaged and a 30 mg bolus dose of papaverine was injected into the renal artery to induce hyperemia. Following papaverine injection, the guiding catheter was retracted from the ostium of the renal artery to prevent dampening of pressures, and then pressure measurements were recorded. HSPG was calculated as a pressure gradient between the systolic aortic and distal renal pressures during hyperemia. The mean aortic pressure (P_a) and distal renal artery pressure (P_d) were measured continuously by the guiding catheter and the pressure guidewire, respectively. Renal FFR was calculated as FFR = P_d/P_a, where P_d and P_a were recorded simultaneously during maximal renal hyperemia. After measurements of FFR, a 2.6 F Atlantis SR Pro mechanical transducer catheter (Boston Scientific) was advanced into the renal artery and passed beyond the stenosis, then withdrawn at a speed of 0.5 mm/sec by using a motorized automatic pullback device. Online measurements of IVUS parameters were made after removal of the IVUS catheter. Images were recorded on half-inch high-resolution super-VHS videotape for offline quantitative analysis using computer planimetry, according to previously validated and published protocols [20, 23]. Following IVUS, parameters at the target lesion and reference segments were measured: (i) minimum and maximum lumen diameters (mm); (ii) minimal lumen cross-sectional area (mm^2); (iii) the reference segment, which was the normal-looking cross-section within 5 mm distal to the stenosis; (iv) plaque plus media cross-sectional area (P&M CSA, mm^2), equal to external elastic membrane (EEM) cross-sectional area minus

MLA; (v) cross-sectional narrowing (CSN, %) calculated as P&M CSA divided by EEM CSA; and (vi) area stenosis (AS, %) calculated as (reference lumen CSA – lesion MLA) × 100/(reference lumen CSA). The stenosis site was the image slice with the smallest lumen CSA. The use of an automatic pullback device enabled us to select the smallest MLA at the stenosis site.

Case Studies

Case #1

A 64-year-old man with a history of coronary artery disease, peripheral vascular disease, and hypertension underwent magnetic resonance angiography (MRA) to assess the severity of RAS. MRA demonstrated bilateral RAS: the right renal artery stenosis was greater than the left renal. Renal angiography revealed left and right RAS of 20% and 70%, respectively (Figure 19.9). The right renal artery RSPG, HSPG, and FFR were 9.0 mm Hg, 16.0 mm Hg, and 0.94, respectively (Figure 19.9). The IVUS MLA, reference lumen area, and area stenosis were 9.5 mm², 16.3 mm², and 42%, respectively (Figure 19.9). The functional, IVUS, and angiographic data are depicted in Table 19.1. Since the RAS was deemed not to be significant by both HSPG and IVUS criteria, the patient was continued on medical therapy. During the 12-month follow-up period, both the renal function and blood pressure have remained stable.

Case #2

A 71-year-old female with a history of coronary artery disease, peripheral vascular disease, diabetes mellitus, hyperlipidemia, and a status of post-bilateral renal artery

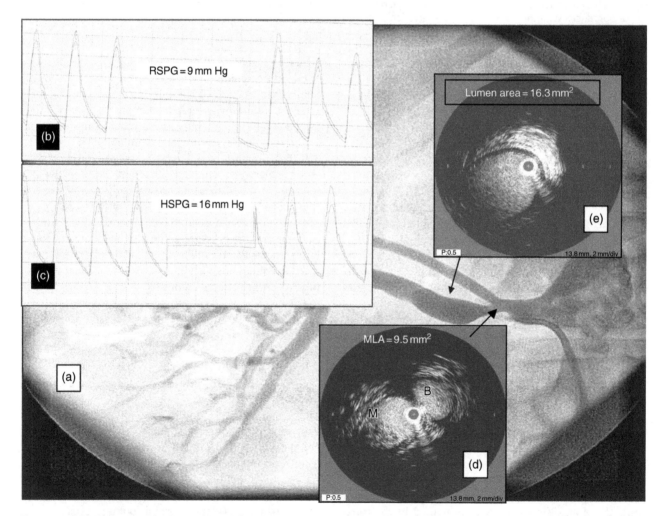

Figure 19.9 (a) Angiogram of right renal artery demonstrating a 70% stenosis of the ostial right renal artery; (b) Resting systolic pressure gradient (RSPG) after crossing the lesion with a pressure guidewire; (c) Hyperemic systolic pressure gradient (HSPG); (d) Intravascular ultrasound (IVUS) of ostial right renal artery: M indicates main branch and B indicates side branch (MLA = minimal lumen cross-sectional area); (e) IVUS of reference segment of right renal artery.

Table 19.1 Functional, intravascular ultrasound, and angiographic data.

Patient #	RSPG mm Hg	HSPG mm Hg	FFR	IVUS	Angiography RAS
1	9	16	0.94	MLA = 9.5 mm^2	70%
2	22	34	0.83	MLD = 3.0 mm AS = 42% CSN = 45% MLA = 5.1 mm^2 MLD = 1.9 mm AS = 68% CSN = 68%	50%
3	3	12	0.96	MLA = 10.6 mm^2 MLD = 3.5 mm AS = 50% CSN = 40%	70%
4	20	32	0.84	MLA = 4.9 mm^2 MLD = 2.2 mm AS = 78% CSN = 79%	50%

AS = area stenosis; CSN = cross-sectional narrowing; FFR = fractional flow reserve; HSPG = hyperemic systolic pressure gradient; IVUS = intravascular ultrasound; MLA = minimal lumen cross-sectional area; MLD = minimum lumen area; RAS = renal artery stenosis; RSPG = resting systolic pressure gradient.

stenting was admitted to the hospital with unstable angina and accelerated hypertension. The patient was referred for coronary angiography. During coronary angiography, despite taking three antihypertensive drug regimens, the patient's systolic blood pressure was over 200 mm Hg. Thus, the decision was made to perform renal angiography at the same session. Selective angiogram of the right renal artery showed minimal in-stent restenosis. However, the angiogram of the left renal artery revealed a borderline in-stent restenosis, approximately 50% by visual estimation (Figure 19.10). In view of accelerated hypertension, further assessment of the left renal stenosis by a pressure guidewire and IVUS was performed. The RSPG, HSPG, and FFR were 22 mm Hg, 34 mm Hg, and 0.83, respectively (Figure 19.10). The IVUS MLA, reference lumen area, and area stenosis were 5.1 mm^2, 16.0 mm^2, and 68%, respectively (Figure 19.10). The functional, IVUS, and angiographic data are depicted in Table 19.1. In view of a significant in-stent restenosis of the left renal artery, angioplasty and stenting of the left renal artery were performed. Repeat HSPG and IVUS assessments showed no pressure gradient and IVUS MLA increased to 15.0 mm^2. Four weeks after the stenting of the left renal artery, the blood pressure improved to 120/60 mm Hg, with only two antihypertensive medications.

Case #3

A 72-year-old man with a history of coronary artery disease, hypertension, and diabetes mellitus was referred for further evaluation of renal dysfunction and hypertension. The serum creatinine was 1.8 mg/dL and blood pressure was 152/86 mm Hg on three antihypertensive medications. MRA demonstrated a significant stenosis of the right renal artery with no stenosis of the left renal artery; both kidneys were greater than 10 cm. The renal angiogram demonstrated an approximately 70% stenosis of the right renal artery (Figure 19.11). The RSPG, HSPG, and FFR of the right renal artery were 3.0 mm Hg, 12.0 mm Hg, and 0.96, respectively (Figure 19.11). The IVUS MLA, reference lumen area, and percent area stenosis were 10.6 mm^2, 21.4 mm^2, and 50%, respectively (Figure 19.11). The functional, IVUS, and angiographic data are depicted in Table 19.1. Since the RAS was deemed not to be significant by both HSPG and IVUS criteria, the patient was continued on medical therapy. During the 12-month follow-up, both renal function and blood pressure have remained stable.

Case #4

A 68-year-old female with a history of coronary artery disease was referred because of accelerated hypertension, despite taking four antihypertensive medications.

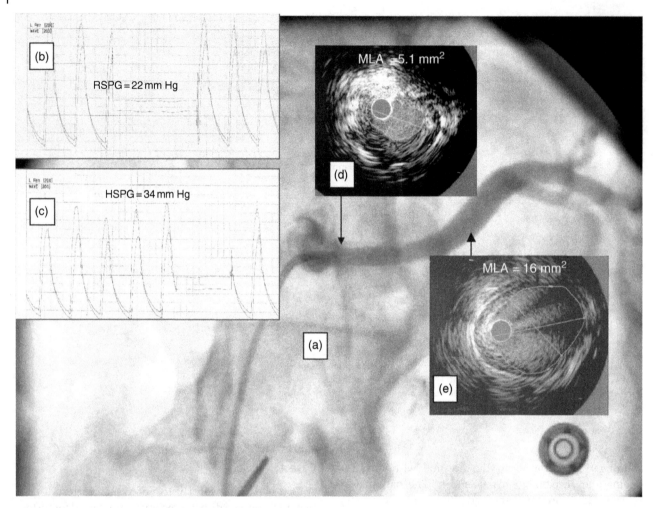

Figure 19.10 (a) Angiogram of left renal artery demonstrating a 50% in-stent restenosis of ostial left renal artery; (b) Resting systolic pressure gradient (RSPG) after crossing the lesion with a pressure guidewire; (c) Hyperemic systolic pressure gradient (HSPG); (d) Intravascular ultrasound (IVUS) of ostial left renal artery (MLA = minimal lumen cross-sectional area); (e) IVUS of reference segment of left renal artery.

MRA of the renal artery demonstrated a modest stenosis of the right renal artery, but the left renal artery had a moderate stenosis. Renal angiography demonstrated no stenosis in the right renal artery; however, there was a 50% stenosis in the left renal artery (Figure 19.12). The RSPG, HSPG, and FFR were 20 mm Hg, 32 mm Hg, and 0.84, respectively (Figure 19.12). The IVUS MLA, reference lumen area, and percent area stenosis were 4.9 mm^2, 22.0 mm^2, and 78%, respectively (Figure 19.12). In light of the presence of significant left RAS, the patient underwent stenting of the left renal artery. After stenting, IVUS MLA improved to 17 mm^2 with resolution of the pressure gradient. Four weeks after the stenting of the renal artery, the blood pressure improved to 140/82 mm Hg, with three antihypertensive medications.

Discussion

There is no established consensus with respect to the degree of RAS at which to justify stenting. The guidelines for renal artery revascularization [24] have suggested that a hemodynamically significant RAS is defined as the presence of greater than or equal to 50–70% diameter stenosis by visual estimation, a systolic pressure gradient greater than or equal to 20 mm Hg, or a mean gradient greater than or equal to 10 mm Hg, measured with a less than 5 F catheter or pressure guidewire. However, the use of a 4 F or 5 F catheter to measure the pressure gradient would overestimate the pressure gradient. In this respect, Colyer *et al.* [18] reported that a 4 F catheter significantly overestimated the severity of RAS, because a 0.014 inch pressure guidewire compared with a 4 F catheter would occupy 6% versus 24% of the renal artery, respectively.

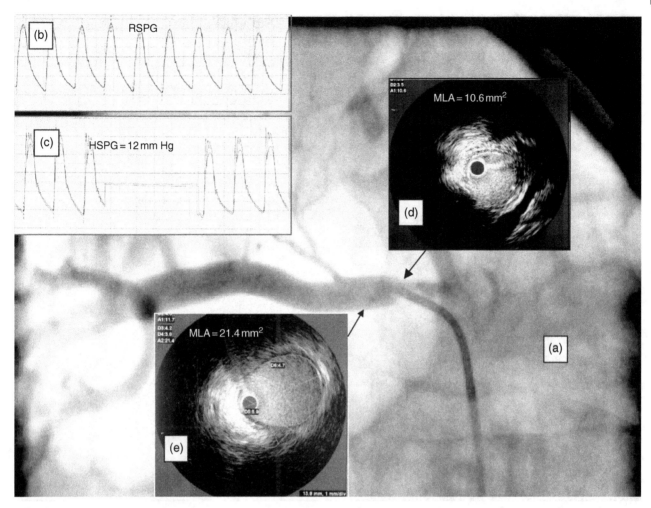

Figure 19.11 (a) Angiogram of right renal artery demonstrating a 70% stenosis of ostial right renal artery; (b) Resting systolic pressure gradient (RSPG) after crossing the lesion with a pressure guidewire; (c) Hyperemic systolic pressure gradient (HSPG); (d) Intravascular ultrasound (IVUS) of ostial right renal artery (MLA = minimal lumen cross-sectional area); (e) IVUS of reference segment of right renal artery.

A number of studies have demonstrated poor correlations comparing stenosis by angiography with renal FFR, HMPG, and RSPG [18, 19]. Subramanian *et al.* [19] reported poor correlations comparing renal FFR and HMPG with angiography. Colyer *et al.* [18] reported a poor correlation between RSPG and percent stenosis.

Leesar et al. [21] demonstrated poor concordance between HSPG and quantitative renal angiography. Thus, the renal angiogram should not be regarded as the "gold standard" for decision-making regarding revascularization in patients with RAS. HSPG can easily be performed with a pressure guidewire on the same session following renal angiography to assess the severity of RAS. On the other hand, IVUS provides detailed anatomical information, specifically in patients in whom stenting of the renal artery is being considered. IVUS helps with stent deployment. In this respect, Dangas *et al.* [25] have shown that IVUS elucidated the need for

additional intervention to achieve complete stent apposition and expansion in nearly a quarter of 153 RAS, despite an adequate angiographic result. Given dependence on acute gain and late loss, it is plausible that optimal stent deployment by IVUS may have an impact on the reduction of restenosis and event rates.

In patient #1, although the RAS appeared critical by angiography, stenting of the bifurcating ostial renal artery lesion, based on angiography, could have exposed the patient to an increased risk of side branch compromise and in-stent restenosis. An HSPG of 16 mm Hg and IVUS MLA of 9.5 mm^2, based on the recent study by Varma *et al.* [22], are not considered significant. Thus, both HSPG and IVUS provided confirmatory evidence that RAS was not significant and stenting of the RAS was deferred.

In patient #2, there was evidence for an intermediate in-stent restenosis by angiography; however, significantly

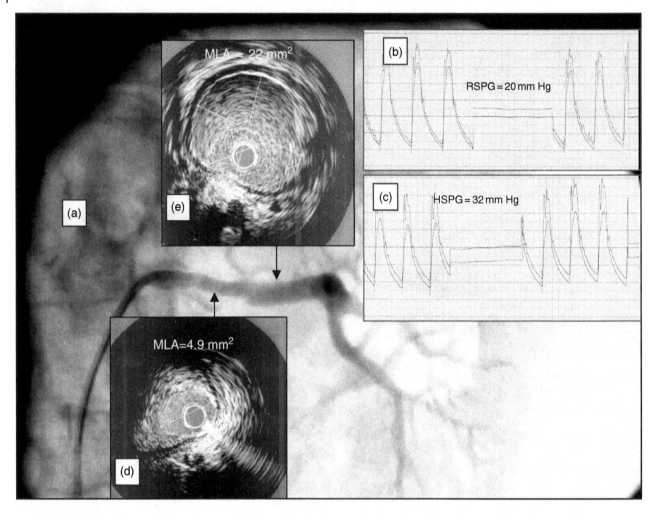

Figure 19.12 (a) Angiogram of left renal artery demonstrating a 50% stenosis of proximal left renal artery; (b) Resting systolic pressure gradient (RSPG) after crossing the lesion with a pressure guidewire; (c) Hyperemic systolic pressure gradient (HSPG); (d) Intravascular ultrasound (IVUS) of ostial left renal artery (MLA = minimal lumen cross-sectional area); (e) IVUS of reference segment of left renal artery.

increased HSPG and reduced IVUS MLA confirmed the presence of a significant RAS. In addition, the patient was highly symptomatic with accelerated hypertension, despite being on multiple antihypertensive agents. The patient responded well to angioplasty and restenting of the RAS with an improvement in blood pressure.

In patient #3, despite the fact that RAS appeared critical by angiography, HSPG and IVUS MLA were 12 mm Hg and 10.6 mm^2, respectively, indicating that RAS was not hemodynamically significant. Thus, the results of IVUS corroborated HSPG that RAS was not significantly stenosed and stenting could not have been justified. The renal size was preserved and renal dysfunction was most probably related to the presence of diabetes mellitus.

In patient #4, there was evidence for an intermediate RAS by both MRA and angiography. In contrast, both HSPG and MLA IVUS confirmed the presence of significant RAS. In addition, despite taking multiple antihypertensive agents, the patient had accelerated hypertension and responded favorably to stenting of the RAS.

Clinical Implications

These cases underscore the utility of HSPG and IVUS to further assess the significance of RAS detected during renal angiography. Because the preponderance of evidence supports the notion that a poor correlation exists between angiography and pressure gradient measured with a pressure guidewire, renal angiogram should not be regarded as the "gold standard" for decision-making regarding revascularization in patients with RAS.

Varma *et al.* [22] demonstrated that an HSPG greater than 20 mm Hg had the highest agreement with an IVUS MLA of less than 8.6 mm^2 with a predictive accuracy of 100%, and thus either an HSPG greater than 20 mm Hg or an IVUS MLA less than 8.6 mm^2 can equally predict the presence of significant RAS. HSPG can easily be performed by a pressure guidewire on the same session following renal angiography to assess the severity of RAS. On the other hand, IVUS provides detailed anatomical information, specifically in patients in whom stenting of the renal artery is being considered.

The discordance between a high procedure success rate (95%) and moderate clinical response rate (60–70%) in patients with RAS may stem from the limitations of angiography for assessing the significance of RAS. Preliminary data suggest that the use of physiological lesion assessment can enhance lesion selection and improve the clinical outcomes [26]; however, further

studies are needed to establish the role of HSPG-guided lesion assessment in clinical outcomes.

Key Points

1) Angiographic stenosis poorly correlates with transstenotic renal artery physiology.
2) A P_d/P_a of < 0.90 increases ipsilateral renal vein renin without increasing contralateral renal vein renin.
3) Treatment of renal artery stenosis in patients with hypertension who meet significant hemodynamic renal artery stenosis criteria results in reduction of hypertension.

References

1 De Bruyne B, Manoharan G, Pijls NH, Verhamme K, Madaric J, Bartunek J, *et al.* Assessment of renal artery stenosis severity by pressure gradient measurements. 48(9):1851–1855, 2006.

2 Mangiacapra F, Trana C, Sarno G, Davidavicius G, Protasiewicz M, Muller O, *et al.* Translesional pressure gradients to predict blood pressure response after renal artery stenting in patients with renovascular hypertension. *Circ Cardiovasc Interv* 3(6):537–542, 2010.

3 Drieghe B, Madaric J, Sarno G, Manoharan G, Bartunek J, Heyndrickx GR, *et al.* Assessment of renal artery stenosis: Side-by-side comparison of angiography and duplex ultrasound with pressure gradient measurements. *Eur Heart J* 29(4):517–524, 2008.

4 Manoharan G, Pijls NH, Lameire N, Verhamme K, Heyndrickx GR, Barbato E, *et al.* Assessment of renal flow and flow reserve in humans. *J Am Coll Cardiol* 47(3):620–625, 2006.

5 Parikh SA, Shishehbor MH, Gray BH, White CJ, Jaff MR. SCAI expert consensus statement for renal artery stenting appropriate use. *Catheter Cardiovasc Interv* 84(7):1163–1171, 2014.

6 Mitchell JA, Subramanian R, White CJ, Soukas PA, Almagor Y, Stewart RE, Rosenfield K. Predicting blood pressure improvement in hypertensive patients after renal artery stent placement: Renal fractional flow reserve. *Catheter Cardiovasc Interv* 69(5):685–689, 2007.

7 Murphy TP, Cooper CJ, Pencina KM, D'Agostino R, Massaro J, Cutlip DE, *et al.* Relationship of albuminuria and renal artery stent outcomes: Results from the CORAL randomized clinical trial (Cardiovascular Outcomes with Renal Artery Lesions). *Hypertension* 68(5):1145–1152, 2016.

8 Siddiqui TS, Elghoul Z, Reza ST, Leesar MA. Renal hemodynamics: Theory and practical tips. *Catheter Cardiovasc Interv* 69(6):894–901, 2007.

9 Derkx FH, Schalekamp MA. Renal artery stenosis and hypertension. *Lancet* 344:237–239, 1994.

10 Working Group on Renovascular Hypertension. Detection, evaluation, and treatment of renovascular hypertension: Final report. *Arch Intern Med* 147:820–829, 1987.

11 Simon N, Franklin SS, Bleifer KH, Maxwell MH. Clinical characteristics of renovascular hypertension. *JAMA* 220:1209–1218, 1972.

12 Rihal CS, Textor SC, Breen JF, McKusick MA, Grill DE, Hallett JW, Holmes DR Jr. Incidental renal artery stenosis among a prospective cohort of hypertensive patients undergoing coronary angiography. *Mayo Clin Proc* 77:309–316, 2002.

13 Olin JW, Melia M, Young JR, Graor RA, Risius B. Prevalence of atherosclerotic renal artery stenosis in patients with atherosclerosis elsewhere. *Am J Med* 88:46N–51N, 1990.

14 White CJ, Ramee SR, Collins TJ, Jenkins JS, Escobar A, Shaw D. Renal artery stent placement: Utility in lesions difficult to treat with balloon angioplasty. *J Am Coll Cardiol* 30:1445–1450, 1997.

15 Dorros G, Jaff M, Mathiak L, Dorros II, Lowe A, Murphy K, He T. Four- year follow-up of Palmaz-Schatz stent revascularization as a treatment for atherosclerotic renal artery stenosis. *Circulation* 98:642–647, 1998.

16 Watson PS, Hadjipetrou P, Cox SV, Piemonte TC, Eisenhauer AC. Effect of renal artery stenting on renal function and size in patients with atherosclerotic renovascular disease. *Circulation* 102:1671–1677, 2000.

17 Harden PN, MacLeod MJ, Rodger RS, Baxter GM, Connell JM, Dominiczak AF, *et al.* Effect of renal artery stenting on progression of renovascular renal failure. *Lancet* 349:1113–1136, 1997.

18 Colyer WR, Cooper CJ, Burket MW, Thomas WJ. Utility of a 0.014" pressure-sensing guidewire to assess

renal artery translesional systolic pressure gradients. *Cathet Cardiovasc Interv* 59:372–377, 2003.

19 Subramanian R, White CJ, Rosenfield K, Bashir R, Almagor Y, Meerkin D, Shalman E. Renal fractional flow reserve: A hemodynamic evaluation of moderate renal artery stenoses. *Catheter Cardiovasc Interv* 64:480–486, 2005.

20 Takagi A, Tsurumi Y, Ishii Y, Suzuki K, Kawana M, Kasanuki H. Clinical potential of intravascular ultrasound for physiological assessment of coronary stenosis: Relationship between quantitative ultrasound tomography and pressure-derived fractional flow reserve. *Circulation* 100:250–255, 1999.

21 Leesar MA, Abdul-Baki T, Akkus NI, Sharma A, Kannan T, Bolli R. Use of fractional flow reserve versus stress perfusion scintigraphy after unstable angina: Effect on duration of hospitalization, cost, procedural characteristics, and clinical outcome. *J Am Coll Cardiol* 7:1115–1121, 2003.

22 Varma J, Shapira A, Ikram S, Leesar MA. Correlations between hyperemic pressure gradient, intravascular ultrasound, Duplex ultrasound, and quantitative angiography in patients with renal artery stenosis. *J Am Coll Cardiol* 21:32B, 2006 (abstract).

23 Jasti V, Ivan E, Yalamanchili V, Wongpraparut N, Leesar MA. Correlations between fractional flow reserve and intravascular ultrasound in patients with an ambiguous left main coronary artery stenosis. *Circulation* 110:2831–2836, 2004.

24 Hirsch AT, Haskal ZJ, Hertzer NR, Bakal CW, Creager MA, Halperin JL, *et al*. ACC/AHA 2005 practice guidelines for the management of patients with peripheral arterial disease (lower extremity, renal, mesenteric and abdominal aortic). *Circulation* 113:e463–e654, 2005.

25 Dangas G, Laird JR, Mehran R, Lansky A, Mintz GS, Leon MB. Intravascular ultrasound-guided renal artery stenting. *J Endovasc Ther* 8:238–247, 2001.

26 Mitchell J, Subramanian R, Stewart R, White C. Pressure-derived renal fractional flow reserve with clinical outcomes following intervention. *Catheter Cardiovasc interv* 65:135, 2005 (abstract).

20

Adult Congenital Anomalies

Morton J. Kern, Ralf J. Holzer, and Ziyad M. Hijazi

The most common adult congenital heart lesions are ventricular septal defects, atrial septal defects, and corrected complex lesions in childhood, such as Tetralogy of Fallot [1, 2, 3]. Adult congenital cardiac abnormalities produce unusual hemodynamic tracings, often characteristic of the resultant valvular or myopathic dysfunction. A variety of right atrial pressure waveforms have been previously presented [4] reflecting tricuspid valve lesions and right ventricular dysfunction. An unusual example of one adult congenital cardiac condition can be diagnosed by simultaneous electrocardiography and right-heart hemodynamics. In conjunction with this case, we discuss ventricular septal defects. Oxygen saturation data with selected green dye curves are presented to illustrate several important aspects of intracardiac shunts.

Atrial Pressure with a Ventricular Electrogram

Patient #1 is a 29-year-old white male with a history of congenital heart disease, which included a diagnosis of an ostium secundum–type atrial septal defect, who was evaluated for palpitations. Physical examination revealed a blood pressure of 118/78 mm Hg with a heart rate of 73 beats/min and a regular rhythm. There was a loud split S_1 and fixed splitting of S_2. There was a grade II/VI systolic ejection murmur at the left sternal border. The remainder of the examination was unremarkable. An electrophysiologic study demonstrated retrograde accessory pathways on programmed stimulation. Two-dimensional and transesophageal echocardiograms demonstrated an abnormality of the tricuspid valve and the right atrium, and confirmed an ostium secundum atrial septal defect with abnormal septal motion, which was consistent with right ventricular volume overload. There was moderate tricuspid regurgitation. Using the Doppler technique, the pulmonary to systemic blood flow ratio was estimated at

1.4:1. The 12-lead electrocardiogram demonstrated right atrial and ventricular enlargement with a right bundle branch block (Figure 20.1).

Right- and left-heart cardiac catheterization was performed using a 6 F arterial sheath and an 8 F venous sheath. A 7 F balloon-tipped catheter was advanced to the right atrium. Per routine, right atrial oxygen saturations and pressures were obtained. The catheter was advanced into the right ventricle and then to the pulmonary capillary wedge position, with the balloon deflated to record the pulmonary artery pressure. Simultaneous left- and right-heart hemodynamics were obtained (Table 20.1). An oxygen saturation run was performed during right-heart catheter pullback (Table 20.2). Immediately after pullback, the atrial septal defect was crossed with the balloon-tipped catheter and pulmonary venous saturations were obtained. A minimal step-up of oxygen saturations was detected in the right-heart chambers. Systemic cardiac output was 3.1 L/min (index of 1.6 L/min/m²). Pulmonary flow was 3.4 L/min (index of 1.7 L/min/m²), resulting in a calculated Q_p/Q_s ratio of 1.1:1. Systemic and pulmonary vascular resistances were 2914 dynes*sec*cm^{-5} and 141 dynes*sec* cm^{-5}, respectively.

Left ventriculography showed normal contraction with an ejection fraction of 62%. Moderate (2+) tricuspid regurgitation was observed on the right ventriculogram, with slight right-to-left contrast shunting when injecting into the right atrial chamber.

Because of a characteristic echocardiogram, simultaneous intracavitary electrogram and hemodynamic recordings were obtained with a Zucker (pacing end-hole, woven Dacron, USCI Inc.) catheter during right ventricular catheter pullback (Figure 20.2). Examine the hemodynamic tracing and observe the right ventricular pressure as it changes to the right atrial pressure at a time when the intracavitary electrogram continues to reflect contact with right ventricular myocardium. On further pullback, the right ventricular electrogram then converts

Hemodynamic Rounds: Interpretation of Cardiac Pathophysiology from Pressure Waveform Analysis, Fourth Edition.
Edited by Morton J. Kern, Michael J. Lim, and James A. Goldstein.
© 2018 John Wiley & Sons Ltd. Published 2018 by John Wiley & Sons Ltd.

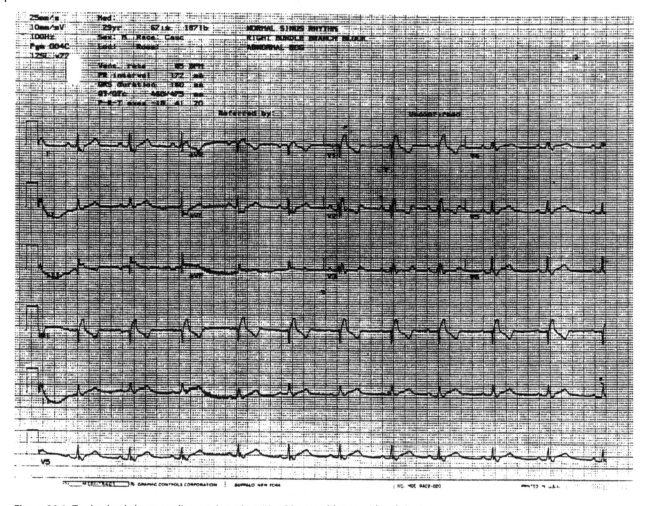

Figure 20.1 Twelve-lead electrocardiogram in patient #1, a 29-year-old man with palpitations.

Table 20.1 Hemodynamic data in patient #1.

Right atrial mean (a, v) (mm Hg)	4(6, 5)
Right ventricular (mm Hg)	23/5
Pulmonary artery (mm Hg)	23/11
Pulmonary capillary wedge mean (a, v) (mm Hg)	8(8, 6)
Left ventricular (mm Hg)	105/10
Aortic (mm Hg)	105/70
Cardiac output/cardiac index (L/min, L/min^2)	3.1/1.6
Systemic vascular resistance (dynes·sec·cm^{-5})	2195
Pulmonary vascular resistance (dynes·sec·cm^{-5})	141
$Q_p Q_s$	1.1:1

Table 20.2 Oxygen saturation data in patient #1.

Site	Saturation (%)
Inferior vena cava (low)	85
Inferior vena cava (right atrial)	70
Right atrial (low)	71
Right atrial (mid)	67
Right atrial (high)	68
Superior vena cava (right atrial)	63
Superior vena cava (high)	64
Right ventricular (tricuspid valve)	71
Right ventricular (apex)	70
Right ventricular (outflow)	73
Pulmonary artery (right)	73
Pulmonary artery (main)	73
Left atrial (pulmonary vein)	96
Left ventricular	96

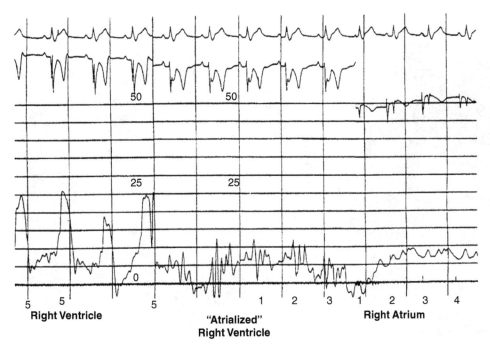

50 **50**

25 **25**

0

5   5   5   1   2   3   1   2   3   4

Right Ventricle   **"Atrialized"**   **Right Atrium**
Right Ventricle

Figure 20.2 Right-heart catheter pullback in patient #1. The lower electrocardiographic tracing is an intracavitary electrogram. See text for details.

into a normal right atrial electrogram with minor alteration of the pressure wave. The transition to the atrial pressure with a simultaneous ventricular electrogram is the classic hemodynamic finding of Ebstein's anomaly, and, although rarely seen, serves to illustrate the use of hemodynamics in documenting the histologic atrialization of the right ventricle, with pressure becoming "atrialized" during ventricular electrocardiographic activity.

Of note is that the Zucher pacing electrode catheters are obsolete and are seldom used. To obtain simultaneous right ventricular pressures and electrograms, simply place an angioplasty guidewire through a 6 F multipurpose catheter and position it in the right ventricle. Advance the angioplasty wire out of the catheter to contact the myocardium, and then flush the right ventricle lumen for pressure recordings. Next, connect the proximal end of the angioplasty wire to the V_1 electrode on the electrocardiogram. Slowly pull the catheter and wire back while recording both the pressure and the electrogram.

Ebstein's anomaly occurs in less than 1% of patients with congenital heart disease [5]. Although no family or genetic transmission of the syndrome is described, congenital cardiac anomalies in infants of mothers taking lithium have been reported. Ebstein's anomaly is characterized by a downward displacement of the tricuspid valve into the right ventricle. Anomalous attachments of the tricuspid valve leaflets are a result of dysplastic formation. The displaced tricuspid valve involves both the right atrium and the right ventricle. The tricuspid valve takes a funnel-like form leading into the right ventricle,

with the septal and inferior cusps adherent to the right ventricular wall at a variable distance from the atrioventricular junction (Figure 20.3). The anterior leaflet of the tricuspid valve is usually large and dysplastic, often with rudimentary septal and inferior leaflets connecting to the body of the right ventricle. The tricuspid valve is also variably regurgitant. The inflow region of the right ventricle is generally hypoplastic with a fibrotic and poorly contractile ventricular wall. The atrialized portion of the right ventricle may be thin-walled and dilated, or thick and fibrotic, with variations in the size and degree of tricuspid leaflet displacement.

As demonstrated in this patient, a patent foramen ovale or atrial septal defect is present in more than 75% of patients with Ebstein's anomaly [6, 7]. Left-sided Ebstein's anomaly has been reported in corrected transposition of the great vessels [8].

The clinical presentation of Ebstein's anomaly usually involves symptoms of dyspnea, fatigue, and occasionally cyanosis, usually occurring during exertion. Dyspnea and fatigue may occur in the absence of cyanosis. Chest pain resembling angina has also been reported [5]. As the patient progresses through childhood and adolescence, right-heart failure increasingly becomes the predominant cause of death. As occurred in our patient, atrial tachyarrhythmias are present in approximately 25% of patients, with 15% of patients dying suddenly. Approximately 10% of these patients have accessory pathways. Nearly 25% of patients may die before the age of 10 and 87% die before the age of 25, with few adults

(a)   (b)

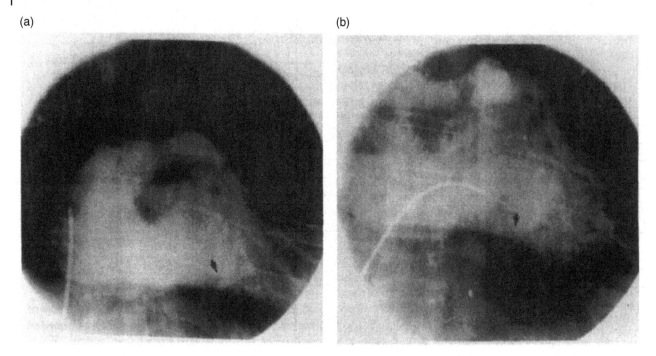

Figure 20.3 (a) Right ventriculogram of the 29-year-old man in Figure 20.1. The right ventricle is small. The tricuspid valve (arrow) is markedly displaced downward into the right ventricular cavity. (b) Right atrial angiogram emphasizing the size of the right atrium and location of the tricuspid valve.

surviving over 50 years [8–10]. Increasing heart size, cyanosis, and paradoxical embolization or other complications of right-to-left shunting are more prevalent with increasing age. Infectious endocarditis is uncommon unless other cardiac lesions are also present.

Typical findings during cardiac catheterization usually involve elevation of right atrial pressure. As shown on Figure 20.2, the magnitude of right atrial A and V waves depends on the compliance of the right atrium, amount of inter-atrial shunting, and right ventricular end-diastolic pressure. The typical atrialized hemodynamics with the right ventricular electrocardiographic complex alone do not unequivocally identify Ebstein's anomaly. However, false positives are rare. The catheter in the location of the atrialized right ventricle usually induces ventricular extra-systoles despite recording atrial pressure. Also, the catheter position in Ebstein's anomaly is left of the spine in the posterior/anterior, confirming the unusual location of pressure with the electrogram.

Cardiac catheterization in patients with Ebstein's anomaly may be associated with increased risks relative to other cardiac anomalies, since catheterization-related serious arrhythmias have been reported in as many as 28% of patients. Death in 5% of such patients has been noted [8–10]. Nonetheless, we believe that patients who have Ebstein's anomaly requiring electrophysiologic testing should have a complete catheterization to identify the extent and degree of hemodynamic abnormalities and intracardiac shunting.

Intracardiac Shunts

Intracardiac shunts may be the most common congenital anomalies encountered in adults and can be detected by five methods: oximetry, indocyanine green dye dilution curves, angiography, radionuclide angiographic techniques [11], and inhaled hydrogen arrival time [12]. Measurement of the arrival time of inhaled hydrogen gas using a platinum-tipped catheter in the venous circulation [12] permits detection and localization of left-to-right shunting. However, actual quantitation of a shunt necessitates serial oximetry or indicator dilution techniques. The oximetry findings of the intracardiac shunt in the first patient example were clinically insignificant. Sophisticated techniques for shunt detection often relegate oximetric and hemodynamic confirmation to a secondary role. However, standard oxygen saturation sampling has clinical importance in modem catheterization laboratories because of acute presentations of patients with complications of ischemic heart disease, postseptostomy assessment after mitral valvuloplasty, and unsuspected atrial or ventricular septal defects. Oxygen saturations should be collected in duplicate (1–3 cc heparinized syringes), if possible, and from the sites shown in Table 20.2.

For left-to-right shunts, oxygen saturation data are generally clinically satisfactory, with good correlation to hemodynamic findings. A brief simplified formula for rapid computation of left-to-right atrial septal defects can be obtained by computing the arterial (art) minus mixed venous oxygen (MVO_2) saturation over the pulmonary vein (PV) minus pulmonary artery (PA) oxygen saturation, providing a quick Q_p/Q_s ratio [(Art – MVO_2)/(PV – PA)]. Well-known limitations of the oximetric technique include a low sensitivity. Oximetry may fail to detect shunts smaller than a 20% shunt fraction. The Pick principle to calculate blood flow presumes a steady state during the diagnostic run and must also assume that complete mixing is achieved instantly during sampling of blood at representative locations. A high systemic flow tends to equalize arteriovenous difference across the heart. Elevated systemic blood flow thus produces mixed venous oxygen saturation that is higher than normal and intrachamber variability that is also higher than normal. When systemic blood flow is reduced, the mixed venous oxygen saturation is lower. A larger step up must be detected before significant left-to-right shunting is diagnosed. Although the more sensitive techniques such as green dye or inhaled hydrogen arrival time could be used to exclude left-to-right shunting, they are now obsolete and no longer used. For right-to-left shunts, the localization technique is more difficult. Saturation data demonstrating a "step down" on the left heart is not always diagnostic, since the saturation of arterial blood has several contributing explanations.

The quantitation of a shunt depends on accurate measurement of blood flow through the right and left heart using indicator dilution (thermodilution or green dye) and Fick or angiographic cardiac output techniques. Advantages and limitations of these methods have been described in detail elsewhere [11, 13, 14].

Consider the case of a 39-year-old woman with progressive dyspnea. Longstanding pulmonary hypertension was present, with a clinical and echocardiographic examination revealing a ventricular septal defect. She had been away from follow-up medical care for several years and now presented with markedly increasing dyspnea. Aortic pressure was 95/72 mm Hg. Right-heart pressures revealed pulmonary hypertension (Figure 20.4), with a pulmonary artery pressure of 100/50 mm Hg, a right ventricular pressure of 100/10 mm Hg, and a mean right atrial pressure of approximately 15 mm Hg with prominent A and V waves. Mean pulmonary capillary wedge pressure was also elevated to approximately 25 mm Hg with striking A and V waves (Figure 20.4). The elevation of mean pulmonary capillary wedge pressure was thought to be a predominant cause of dyspnea. Oxygen saturations on the right heart did not demonstrate a step up, with right atrial, right ventricular, and pulmonary artery saturations nearly the same at 52%. Arterial oxygen saturation was 88%. Because of the documented ventricular septal defect by noninvasive methods, green dye curves to confirm and localize the shunt were obtained.

An injection of a small bolus of green dye with sampling of arterial blood from the femoral artery normally produces a brisk upstroke with a uniform curve. Recirculation causes characteristic deflections of dye early on the curve for right-to-left shunts or late on the curve for left-to-right shunts (Figure 20.5). In our patient, when injecting into the pulmonary artery and sampling in the aorta, the dye passes through the pulmonary circuit and left heart with no evidence of recirculation of left-to-right shunting (Figure 20.6). However, on injection of green dye into the right ventricle, an early recirculation deflection can be seen, with a less prominent but similar rise in the major bolus of green dye as it passes through the left heart (Figure 20.7). On further pullback into the right atrium, the pattern of green dye traversing from right to left is duplicated, with a slightly later appearance of the recirculation deflection and a similar pattern of green dye bolus travel through the right heart, indicating the shunt to be at the ventricular level. Dye circulation curves have been used to quantitate flow by computing the area beneath the curve [14].

Ventricular septal defects may be divided into the membranous, muscular, canal type, and supracristal type. The location has prognostic importance in the presence of associated lesions. Membranous septal-type defects occur in 70% of cases and are located inferior to the crista supraventricularis. Fibrous tissue proliferation after infancy may close these defects. Rare septal aneurysms in this region have been reported to protrude into the right ventricle, sometimes becoming large and obstructive [15].

Muscular septal defects comprise 20% of ventricular septal defects and may be single or multiple, located in the supra crista area. Atrioventricular canal-type defects (also approximately 5–10% of ventricular septal defects) occur largely in patients with Down's syndrome and are commonly associated with abnormalities of the A–V valves. Supracristal infra-aortic ventricular septal defects are the least common entity, comprising under 5% of patients (in infancy). These defects are located beneath the aortic annulus, above and anterior to the crista supraventricularis, and are generally hemodynamically insignificant, unless the aortic valve becomes regurgitant.

A step up in the oxygen content of 4–6 volumes percent at the ventricular level identifies a ventricular septal defect with left-to-right shunting [11]. Ventriculography performed in the left anterior oblique view with the septum en face may also visualize the defect, with contrast opacification of the right ventricle during left ventriculography. Green dye curves are extremely sensitive to detecting very small shunts. A comparison of oximetry and indicator dilution techniques for the assessment of left-to-right intracardiac shunting in adults demonstrates a close correlation by both techniques. Hillis *et al.* [16] note that shunt volume by oximetry exceeded shunt

(a)

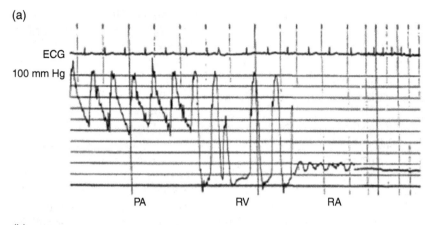

(b)

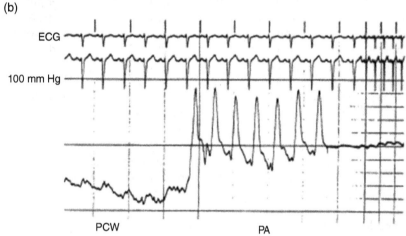

(c)

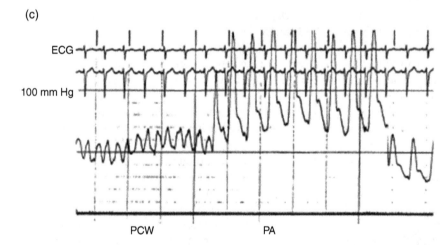

Figure 20.4 (a) Right atrial (RA), right ventricular (RV), and pulmonary artery (PA) pressures (0–100 mm Hg scale) in a patient with arterial desaturation. (b) Pulmonary artery and pulmonary capillary wedge (PCW) pressures in the same patient (0–100 mm Hg scale). (c) Pulmonary artery and pulmonary capillary wedge pressures in the same patient (0–40 mm Hg scale).

volume by indocyanine green technique by 20% in a majority of adult patients. In infants, indicator dilution technique yielded larger shunt values than did the oximetric technique.

The early appearance of an indicator in the systemic circulation in Figure 20.7 identifies a right-to-left shunt [17].

There is an early hump in the dye curve prior to the primary peak. The indocyanine green technique can detect right-to-left shunts as small as 2.5% of the systemic cardiac output [16]. Serial injection sites are used to detect shunts at the level of the atrium, ventricle, and pulmonary artery. Moving the injection site more distally further

(a)

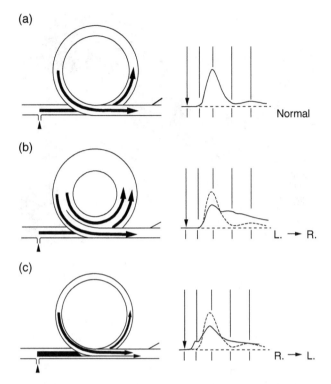

(b)

(c)

Figure 20.5 Diagram of intracardiac shunting. (a) Normal circuit through the lungs (upward circle). The dye curve on the right shows normal tracing when injecting into the pulmonary artery and sampling in the systemic artery. (b) Left-to-right shunting (L→R) shows additional flow through the pulmonary circuit (larger upward circle), with dye dilution curve showing flattened peak with later recirculation hump as the dye recirculates through the lungs and out to the systemic circulation a second time. (c) Right-to-left shunt (R→L) showing addition of flow to systemic circulation with relatively reduced pulmonary flow (smaller upward circle). Dye dilution curve shows early shoulder with flattened peak and attenuated late downstroke. Areas beneath curves are used for quantitation. *Source:* Kern 1991 [13]. Reproduced with permission of Elsevier.

localizes the shunt by noting when the early appearance of the "hump" on the primary curve is no longer evident. Right-to-left shunting across an atrial septal defect or patent foramen ovale would be best detected by injection into the inferior vena cava, because of preferential streaming of the blood [18]. The Valsalva maneuver often will accentuate shunt through a patent foramen ovale, because of the hemodynamics of right atrial pressure increasing more than left atrial pressure during phase II.

Case Studies in Congenital Cardiac Anomalies

This section is provided by Dr. Holzer and Dr. Hijazi. Hemodynamic evaluation of acquired heart disease in the adult mainly centers around the assessment of valvular

(a)

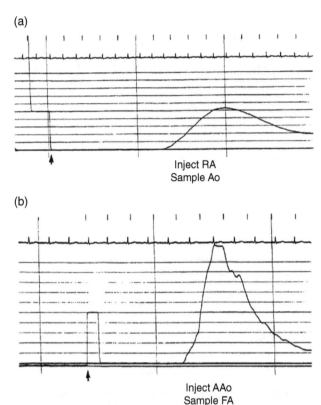

Inject RA
Sample Ao

(b)

Inject AAo
Sample FA

Figure 20.6 (a) Green dye curve injection site is the pulmonary artery (PA) and sampling in the aorta (Ao). Injection occurs at arrow. (b) Green dye curve when injecting into the proximal aorta (AAo) and sampling in the femoral artery (FA).

and ventricular function, and the number of identifiable alterations are to a degree limited in their scope. In contrast, congenital heart disease in the child and/or adult frequently presents in a larger variety and combination of hemodynamic abnormalities that are not always expected or diagnostic for a specific lesion. Hemodynamic evaluation in this population frequently delivers unusual and unexpected findings that are not considered during non-invasive assessment. Therefore, the invasive evaluation of congenital cardiac lesions requires the utmost diligence: frequently the accurately obtained and interpreted hemodynamic data is essential to decide upon the appropriate treatment strategy, be it interventional percutaneous therapy, cardiothoracic surgery, hybrid therapy, or conservative medical management. The three cases selected below will provide a flavor of the spectrum of hemodynamic abnormalities that can be found in patients with congenital heart disease.

Atrial Septal Defect and Diastolic Dysfunction of the Left Ventricle

A 56-year-old white female was evaluated for exertional dyspnea and intermittent chest pain. She had a history of

(a)

Green Dye Curve

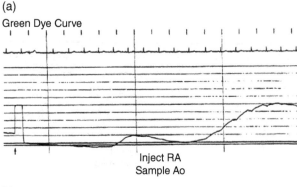

Inject RA
Sample Ao

(b)

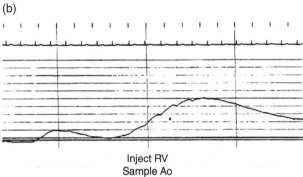

Inject RV
Sample Ao

Figure 20.7 (a) Green dye curve injection site is the right atrium (RA) and sampling in the aorta (Ao). See text for details. (b) Green dye curve injection site is the right ventricle (RV) and sampling in the aorta. See text for details.

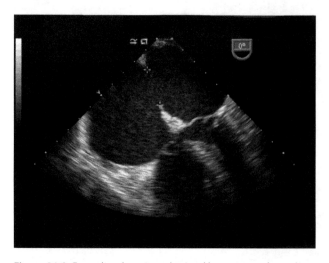

Figure 20.8 Four-chamber view obtained by transesophageal echocardiography documenting a large (25 mm) secundum atrial septal defect in a 56-year-old female patient.

systemic hypertension. Physical examination revealed wide fixed splitting of the second heart sound, with a soft II/VI mid-systolic murmur best audible at the left sternal border at the second intercostal space. A 12-lead electrocardiogram demonstrated right axis deviation with right ventricular conduction delay. The patient subsequently underwent cardiac catheterization at an adult medical center combined with transesophageal echocardiography (TEE). This documented pulmonary artery pressure to be 51/15 mm Hg, with systemic pressures of 134/64 mm Hg and an atrial-level step up in oxygen saturations, suggesting a $Q_p:Q_s$ of about 3:1. There was isolated coronary plaque disease, but no significant coronary artery stenosis that would warrant intervention. TEE documented a large secundum atrial septal defect with right atrial and right ventricular volume load. Systolic right ventricular pressure was estimated by Doppler to be 40 mm Hg above the right atrial pressure. There was also a degree of diastolic dysfunction of the left ventricle.

The patient was subsequently placed on increased diuretic therapy as well as afterload reduction using angiotensin-converting-enzyme (ACE) inhibitors, in preparation for a subsequent atrial septal defect (ASD) closure device. After an interval of three months, the patient was recatheterized at a pediatric and congenital

heart center. TEE evaluation demonstrated a large secundum atrial septal defect with a borderline inferior rim, and a nonstretched diameter on bicaval view, short-axis view, as well as four-chamber view of about 25 mm (Figure 20.8). Hemodynamic evaluation documented a $Q_p:Q_s$ of 4.1:1 with pulmonary artery pressure of 41/15 mm Hg. A 12 F Hausdorf sheath (Cook Inc., Bloomington, IN) was placed in the left upper pulmonary vein and subsequently a 32 mm Amplatzer Septal Occluder (ASO; AGA Medical Corporation, Golden Valley, MN) was deployed (but not released) in standard technique across the ASD. With the pre-existing history of systemic hypertension and documented left ventricular diastolic dysfunction, it was felt that evaluation of left pulmonary capillary wedge pressures should be performed prior to releasing the device. A second hemostatic sheath was placed in the right femoral vein and an 8 F wedge catheter manipulated into a distal left pulmonary artery (LPA) position. The mean left pulmonary capillary wedge pressure increased from 15 to 27 mm Hg after ASD (test) occlusion (Figure 20.9). This significant increase in LPA wedge pressure was reversible when recapturing the septal occluder. Interestingly, the mitral valve showed an increased amount of mitral regurgitation which was clearly not device related, as documented by the distance of the device to the mitral valve, but instead related to increased loading of a left ventricle with diastolic dysfunction, which was reflected in more prominent V waves on the wedge tracings. Again, this was completely reversible by recapturing the septal occluder. The device was left in place for about 20 minutes, but pressure tracings did not change and the patient required a slight increase in ventilatory support during that time. However, the findings were completely reversible when recapturing the device. At this point it was felt that closure of the defect could not be safely undertaken, and

(a)

(b)

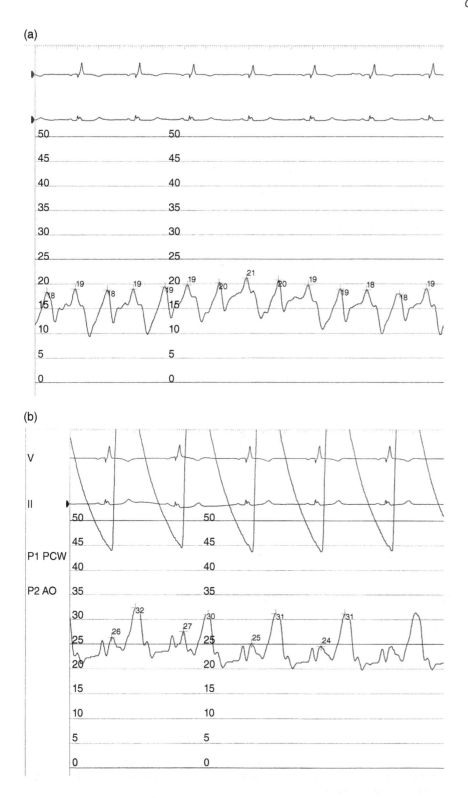

Figure 20.9 Pulmonary capillary wedge (PCW) pressure recorded in a 56-year-old female with a large secundum atrial septal defect at baseline (a) as well as during (test) occlusion of the ASD (b) using a 32 mm Amplatzer septal occluder. Note the overall increase in wedge pressure and the tall V waves (increased mitral insufficiency). AO = aortic pressure.

additional increased diuretic and afterload-reducing therapy may be of further benefit. The patient was recatheterized four months later with similar hemody-namic findings. Implantation of a fenestrated Amplatzer Septal Occluder was considered at that time, but the patient elected not to undergo any further therapy.

(a)

(b)

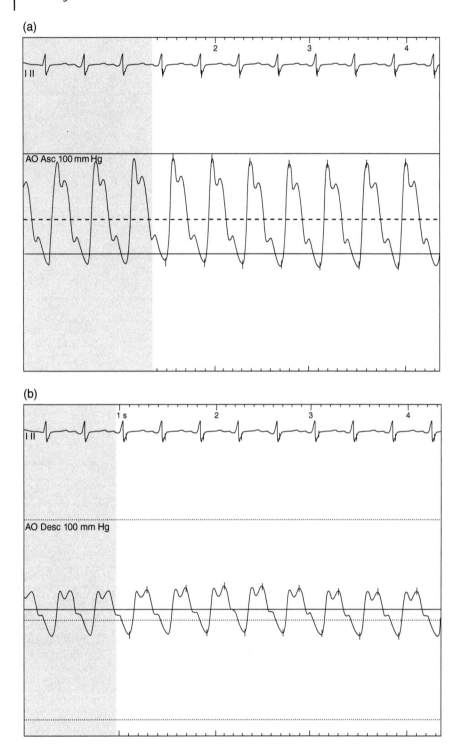

Figure 20.10 Ascending (a) and descending (b) aortic (AO) pressure in a 14-month-old male infant with a medium-sized persistent ductus arteriosus as well as juxtaductal coarctation. Note the relatively wide pulse pressure in the ascending aorta (despite coarctation), as well as the 30 mm Hg peak systolic gradient between ascending and descending aorta.

While the technical aspects of treating adults with atrial septal defects are not dissimilar to the treatment of smaller children, there are important pathophysiologic differences that may have a negative impact on how ASD closure is tolerated. This is especially the case in older patients with evidence of left ventricular diastolic dysfunction. As shown in the previous example, closure of a large inter-atrial communication in "unprepared" patient with left ventricular diastolic dysfunction can lead to a significant increase in left atrial pressure due to the loss of "pop-off" via the atrial septum, with resulting pulmonary edema and ventilator dependency [19]. Therefore, the left atrial/wedge pressure should be evaluated at baseline as well as after test occlusion of the defect. Even though a small increase in left atrial pressure may be reasonably well tolerated, an increase of left atrial pressure, for example from a mean of 15 mm Hg to a mean of 27 mm Hg as the case in the above example, is clearly prohibitive to occlusion of the septal defect. The treatment of any patient in whom these physiologic changes are expected should be optimized prior to engaging in any transcatheter procedure, and include aggressive diuretic therapy as well as afterload-reducing agents. If a patient, despite appropriate pretreatment, still develops significant left atrial hypertension after test occlusion, the placement of a fenestrated device may be beneficial [20, 21].

Persistent Arterial Duct Associated with Preductal Coarctation of the Aorta

A 14-month-old male infant was initially evaluated for a cardiac murmur. He was asymptomatic from a cardiovascular point of view and feeding well. On physical examination he did not have an upper-to-lower limb blood pressure gradient and femoral pulses were felt to be adequate without brachial-femoral delay. He had a typical grade II–III/VI continuous murmur, best audible at the lower left sternal border. The murmur was also audible at the back. An ECG demonstrated normal sinus rhythm without left or right ventricular hypertrophy. A two-dimensional echocardiographic evaluation documented a typical angiographic type A persistent ductus arteriosus (PDA), with continuous left-to-right shunt in excess of 4 m/sec across, suggesting the duct to be pressure restrictive. The pulmonary arterial end was estimated to be about 2–3 mm in diameter. The branch pulmonary arteries appeared to be of normal size with laminar flow across. The aortic arch was not very well visualized and there was a mild degree of left ventricle volume overload.

The patient was brought to the cardiac catheterization laboratory for elective PDA occlusion, which was performed under general endotracheal anesthesia. The initial hemodynamic evaluation demonstrated not only a fairly wide pulse pressure in the ascending aorta, but, even more surprisingly, a 30 mm Hg peak systolic gradient across the aortic isthmus (Figure 20.10). Oximetry data did not suggest a very large left-to-right shunt (Q_p:Q_s < 1.5:1). Angiography was obtained in the descending aorta and demonstrated a typical type A PDA measuring 2.2 mm at the pulmonary arterial end,

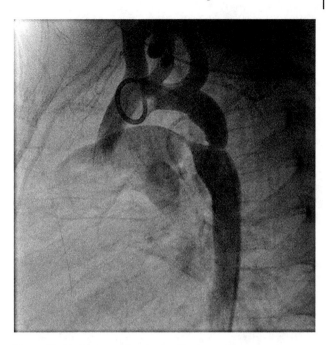

Figure 20.11 Angiography obtained in descending aorta in straight lateral projection, documenting a typical conical type A persistent ductus arteriosus of medium size with a discrete juxtaductal coarctation of the aorta.

11.5 mm at the aortic ampulla, with a total length of 11.9 mm. There was a localized juxtaductal coarctation, measuring at its narrowest 4.4–5.7 mm, the aorta distal to the left subclavian artery was 7.9 mm, and the aorta at the diaphragm was 8.2–8.6 mm (Figure 20.11). Subsequently the PDA was closed by deploying a 6/4 mm Amplatzer Duct Occluder (AGA Medical Corporation), followed by placement of a 19 mm Genesis XD stent across the coarctation using a 9 mm x 2 cm OptaPro balloon (Cordis Endovascular, Warren, NJ). Hemodynamic evaluation subsequently documented no residual gradient across the aortic arch, and a reduced pulse pressure in the aorta compared to baseline (Figure 20.12). A final angiography obtained in the descending aorta documented no residual shunt across the PDA and excellent relief of the coarctation (Figure 20.13). The patient has been followed for about 14 months without evidence of recoarctation or residual PDA shunting.

This case documents the need to pay particular attention to hemodynamic recordings even in "standard" situations. The unexpected finding of primary coarctation could easily be missed if not looked for appropriately. While the oximetry data did not suggest a significant left-to-right shunt, this data can be misleading, and the evidence of a fairly wide pulse pressure in the aorta prior to duct occlusion suggests at least a moderate run-off via the PDA in diastole, which resolved after successful PDA occlusion.

(a)

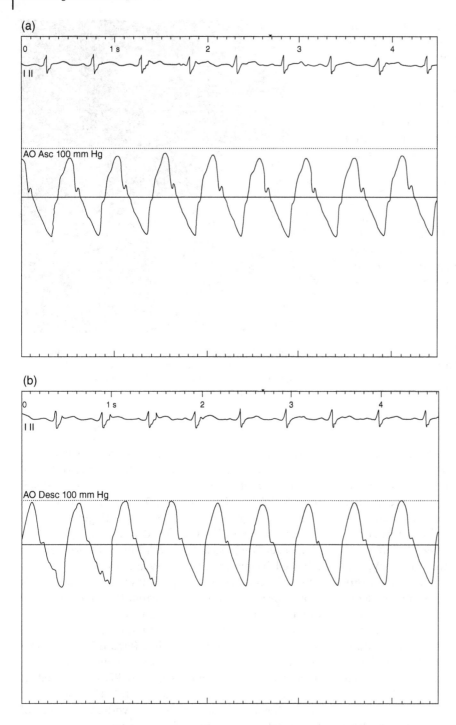

(b)

Figure 20.12 Ascending (a) and descending (b) aortic (AO) pressure after persistent ductus arteriosus occlusion as well as stenting of a discrete primary coarctation. Note the resolution of the ascending-to-descending aortic gradient as well as the decrease in pulse pressure in the ascending aorta.

Ventricular Tachycardia Arrest Nine Months after Surgical Ventricular Septal Defect Closure: Mitral Insufficiency with Subaortic Stenosis

A 22-month-old white male with trisomy 21 presented acutely with diaphoresis and vomiting. After arrival at the local emergency room, he was placed on a cardiac monitor. Within one hour of arrival the patient had a pulseless ventricular tachycardia (VT) arrest requiring full resuscitation and direct current (DC) cardioversion. He had a past history of surgical patch closure of a large inlet-type ventricular septal defect (VSD) at 5 months of age. He was also known to have a cleft left AV valve which was not repaired during initial surgery. On follow-up, there was evidence of moderate left AV valve regurgitation as well as a

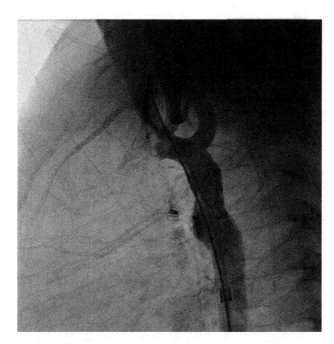

Figure 20.13 Angiography obtained in descending aorta in straight lateral projection after occluding the persistent ductus arteriosus using a 6/4 mm Amplatzer Duct Occluder, as well as subsequent placement of a 19 mm Genesis XD stent expanded to 9 mm across the juxtaductal coarctation.

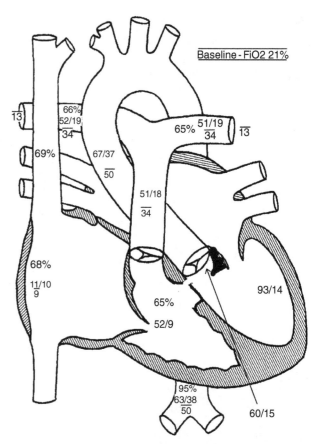

Figure 20.14 Baseline hemodynamic data in a 22-month-old male child with Trisomy 21 and subaortic stenosis, a cleft left AV valve with moderate regurgitation, and a small residual ventricular septal defect (VSD) after previous VSD closure.

degree of subaortic stenosis caused by mitral valve tissue, which created systolic gradient across the left ventricular outflow tract of 60 mm Hg peak systolic (mean 33 mm Hg). The degree of subaortic stenosis had remained unchanged since surgical repair and therefore he was followed medically to delay the possible need for mitral valve replacement. The patient also had a small residual ventricular septal defect. After the initial VT arrest the patient was transferred to a tertiary congenital center for further management. Physical examination documented a single S_2 with a grade II/VI mid-systolic murmur audible at the upper right and left sternal border, radiating to the neck. The patient also had a more prominent grade III/VI pan-systolic murmur audible at the apex and the axilla. The liver was not enlarged. Baseline toxicology screening and laboratory tests were unremarkable, and a repeat echocardiography documented unchanged findings with a moderate amount of left AV valve regurgitation and a peak systolic gradient across the left ventricular outflow tract (LVOT) of 55 mm Hg. An ECG immediately preceding the initial event documented some ST depression, but completely recovered back to baseline after the event, documenting RV conduction delay. The patient was taken to the cardiac catheterization laboratory for hemodynamic evaluation and delineation of the coronary anatomy.

The baseline hemodynamic data is depicted in Figure 20.14. This demonstrated a 33 mm Hg peak systolic

gradient across the left ventricular outflow tract (no gradient across the aortic valve), and elevated distal pulmonary artery pressures, with a transpulmonary mean gradient of 21 mm Hg in 21% O_2. Figure 20.15 demonstrates the pressure tracings obtained in left ventricle (apex), left ventricular outflow tract underneath the aortic valve, as well as ascending aorta. A pulmonary capillary wedge tracing demonstrated significantly tall V waves (Figure 20.16). The pulmonary vascular resistance index (PVR) was calculated at 5.8 Wood units. The patient was subsequently placed in 100% inspired oxygen as well as nitric oxide at 80 ppm, leading to a reduction in the transpulmonary gradient to 12 mm Hg, with an unchanged gradient across the LVOT. The PVR was calculated at 3.4 Wood units. Selective coronary angiography did not reveal any abnormality. Given the severity of the near-miss event, it was felt that surgical repair was mandatory, even though each hemodynamic lesion on its own would not necessarily be a clear indication for surgical intervention. The patient underwent successful repair of the left AV valve and resection of subaortic tissue, combined with closure of a small residual VSD and placement of an implantable cardioverter defibrillator (ICD). The procedure was well tolerated

(a)

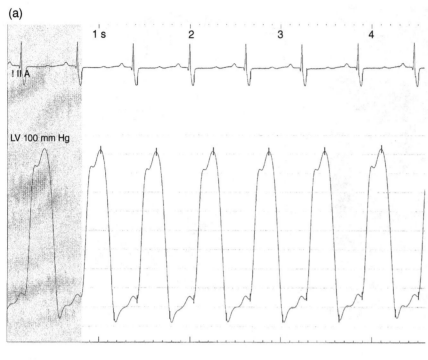

(b)

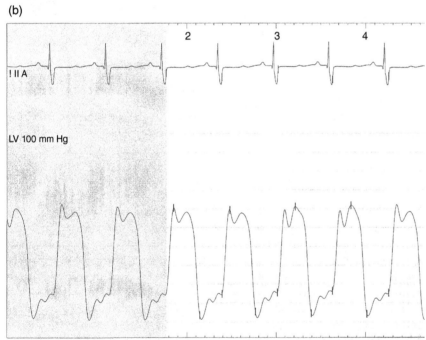

Figure 20.15 Pressure tracings obtained in left ventricle (LV, a), subaortic area (b), and ascending aorta (AO Asc, c) using an end-hole catheter in a 22-month-old child with subaortic stenosis.

with excellent hemodynamic results, and the patient made an uneventful postoperative recovery.

This case again demonstrates the necessity for accurate hemodynamic evaluation in patients with congenital heart disease. Any patient with any type of LVOT obstruction should have pressure recordings obtained using an end-hole catheter, rather than for example a pigtail catheter. Discrete subaortic stenoses can otherwise easily be missed and surgeons may then find themselves attempting to repair or replace a valve which is not the cause of the underlying hemodynamic alteration. Again, subtle changes of the pulmonary capillary wedge tracings may

(c)

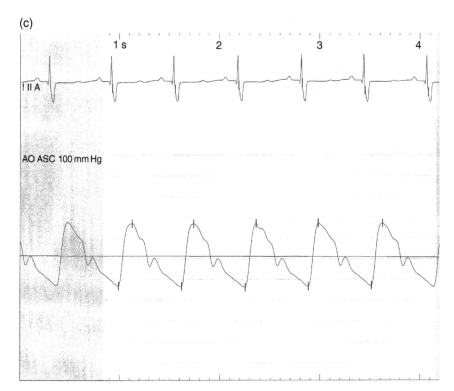

Figure 20.15 (Cont'd)

Figure 20.16 Pulmonary capillary wedge (PCW) tracing in a 22-month-old child with subaortic stenosis and cleft left AV valve with moderate insufficiency. Note the large V waves on the wedge tracing. LV = left ventricle.

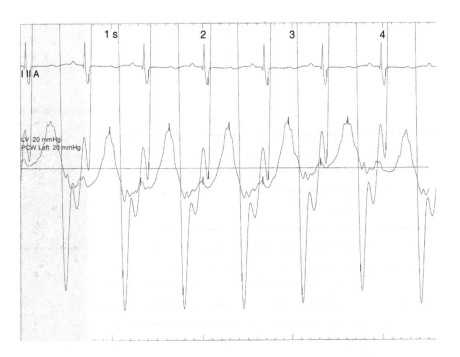

certainly complement the overall assessment, and the large V waves that were demonstrated in this patient are typical for severe mitral regurgitation. Hemodynamic evaluation of congenital cardiac lesions frequently necessitates the assessment of the pulmonary vascular bed and, as such, nitric oxide needs to be readily available to allow assessment of pulmonary vascular reactivity.

Summary

Congenital anomalies are unusual in adults, but characteristic hemodynamic data facilitate precise diagnoses (Table 20.3) [22, 23]. A complete evaluation, including assessment for intracardiac shunts, is usually indicated in patients prior to major surgical procedures or electrophysiologic interventions.

Table 20.3 Most common adult congenital anomalies.

Defect	Epidemiology	Clinical	ECG	CXR	Echo
ASD	Most common defect F > M 3:1	Asymptomatic early After fourth decade: fatigue, DOE, palpitations Wide split S₂, mid-systolic ejection murmur	Right axis deviation RBBB	Right atrial and ventricular enlargement Increased pulmonary vascular markings	Pulmonary artery dilatation Dilated RA and RV Paradoxical septal motion Increased RV end-diastolic diameter Subcostal/parasternal visualize defect Bubble study may increase sensitivity TEE helpful for sinus venosus
Ostium secundum (fossa ovalis)	75% of ASDs Associated with MVP				
Ostium primum (AV septal defect)	15% of ASDs Associated with Down's Syndrome AV valve abnormalities common	Late: cyanosis and clubbing Holosystolic murmur in ostium primum	Left axis deviation common		
Sinus venosus (high in atrial septum)	10% of ASDs Associated with anomalous connection of pulmonary vein to RA/SVC		Junctional rhythm First-degree AV block Ectopic atrial pacemaker		
VSD	Most common defect in children 90% close spontaneously in first 10 years of life F = M	Determined by size of defect and resistance of P and S systems DOE, CP, syncope, hemoptysis Late: cyanosis and clubbing Holosystolic murmur at LSB with thrill RV heave if PAH present Graham Steel murmur as PAH increases	Normal initially Large defect may show LA and LV enlargement Right axis deviation, Right atrial enlargement if PAH present	If PAH present: enlarged pulmonary arteries with rapid tapering, Oligemic lung fields	Confirms presence and location of defect Doppler studies to evaluate shunt size and direction Left atrial enlargement and LVH
Membranous	70% of VSDs				
Muscular	20% of VSDs				
Below aortic valve	5% of VSDs				
Near MV/TV junction	5% of VSDs				
PDA	10% of adult CHD Common in pregnancy due to rubella, hypoxia, premature birth Usually close immediately after birth 1/3 die by age 40, 2/3 by age 60	Machinery murmur at LUSB Palpitations, DOE, CHE, IE Nml S₁, wide pulse pressure, hyperdynamic PMI Large defects result in PAH with differential cyanosis	Usually normal May show LA and LV hypertrophy	Pulmonary plethora Prominent ascending aorta Proximal pulmonary artery dilatation	Visualize defect Doppler shows continuous flow in pulmonary trunk Retrograde color flow in PA along leftward axis
Coarctation of the aorta	7% of CHD M > F 2:1 Most common distal to left subclavian origin Associated with Turner's syndrome, VSD 70% have biscuspid aortic valve	Delayed femoral pulses HTN in UE, more developed UE Wide pulse pressure Harsh systolic murmur at LSB and back Aneursymal dilatation/rupture of circle of Willis Headache, epistaxis, cold extremities/claudication	LVH	Rib notching 3 sign (pre/post stenotic dilatation)	Location of stenosis Estimate transcoarctation pressure gradient LVH

Tetralogy of Fallot	Most common CHD surviving until adulthood 4% survive to age 15 without intervention a) Subpulmonic stenosis b) VSD c) Right deviated over-riding aorta d) RVH	TR, increased A wave, RV lift Asymptomatic in adults with prior intervention Unoperated: cyanosis/tet spells Recurrence: DOE, palpitations, right-heart failure, syncope, sudden death	Normal vascularity Right-sided aortic arch Boot-shaped heart	RVH with RBBB Ventricular arrhythmias common	Confirm lesions in parasternal and subcostal views Evaluate PI, RVH Evaluate shunt size and direction
Pulmonic Stenosis	10–12% of adult CHD 90% of RV outflow obstruction valvular usually isolated May be associated with Noonan's or William's syndrome	DOE, fatigue, right-heart failure, peripheral edema, cyanosis/clubbing Wide split S_2, RV impulse at LSB Crescendo–decrescendo systolic murmur, increased with inspiration	Post-stenotic dilatation of PA Decreased pulmonary vascular markings Chen's sign: fullness of left lung base	Right axis deviation RVH Normal until RV systolic pressure is > 60 mm HG	RVH, show PI, TR Paradoxical septal motion Localize site of obstruction, evaluate valve morphology Bubble for shunting Doppler to assess severity

Defect	Findings
ASD	Increased pulmonary to systemic blood flow (E > 1.5/1 indicates significant defect Early: left-to-right shunt, step up in oxygenation of right chambers Late: Right-to-left shunt, pulmonary hypertension → Eisenmenger's syndrome
VSD	Step up in oxygenation of right-heart chambers from left-to-right shunt Early appearance of indicator (indocyanine green) in systemic circulation suggests right-to-left shunt Surgery indicated when symptomatic with Q_p/Q_s > 1.5/1 Early: SVR > PVR (left-to-right shunt) Late: PVR > SVR (right-to-left shunt), pulmonary hypertension → Eisenmenger's syndrome
PDA	Step up in oxygenation distal to pulmonary outflow tract Early: continuous left-to-right shunt (SVR > PVR) Late: Right-to-left shunt with differential cyanosis (PVR > SVR)
Coarctation of the aorta	Surgical intervention indicated when pressure gradient > 30 mm Hg
Tetralogy of Fallot	PI pressure half-time < 100 msec VSD shunt > 1.5/1
Pulmonic stenosis	Pulmonic stenosis jet directed toward left PA → increased blood flow of left lung Increased RA pressure may result in opening of patent foramen ovale and a right-to-left shunt Normal: valve area 2.0 cm^2, pressure gradient 0 mm Hg Mild: valve area 1–2 cm^2, gradient < 50 mm Hg, peak pressure < 75 mm Hg Moderate: valve area 0.5–1 cm^2, gradient 50–80 mm Hg, peak pressure 75–100 mm Hg Severe: valve area < 0.5 cm^2, gradient > 80 mm Hg, peak pressure > 100 mm Hg

ASD = atrial septal defect; AV = aortic valve; CHD = congenital heart disease; CHF = congestive heart failure; CXR = chest X-ray; DOE = dyspnea on exertion; F = female; HTN = hypertension; LA = left atrium; LSB = left sternal border; LUSB = left upper sternal border; LV = left ventricle; LVH = left ventricular hypertrophy; M = male; MVP = mitral valve prolapse; PA = pulmonary artery; PAH = pulmonary hypertension; PDA = patent ductus arteriosus; PI = pulmonary insufficiency; PVR = pulmonary vascular resistance; Q_p/Q_s = pulmonary/systemic shunt flow; RA/SVC = right atrial/superior vena cava; RBBB = right bundle branch block; RVH = right ventricular hypertrophy; S_2 = second heart sound; SVR = system vascular resistance; TEE = transesophageal echocardiography; VSD = ventricular septal defect.

Key Points

1) Congenital anomalies are unusual in adults, but characteristic hemodynamic data facilitate precise diagnoses.

2) A complete evaluation, including assessment for intracardiac shunts, is usually indicated in patients prior to major surgical procedures or electrophysiologic interventions.

3) $Q_p/Q_s > 1.5$ indicates closure of atrial septal defect.

References

1 Kern MJ, Aguirre F, Donohue T, Bach R. Hemodynamic rounds: Interpretation of cardiac pathophysiology from pressure waveform analysis: Adult congenital anomalies. *Cathet Cardiovasc Diagn* 27:291–297, 1992.

2 Mitchell SC, Korones SB, Berendes HW. Congenital heart disease in 56,109 births: Incidence and natural history. *Circulation* 43:323, 1971.

3 Liberthson RR. Congenital heart disease in the child, adolescent and adult patients. In RA Johnson, E Haber, GE Austin (eds), *The Practice of Cardiology*. Boston, MA: Little, Brown, 1980, pp. 755–887.

4 Kern MJ, Deligonul D. Hemodynamic rounds: Interpretation of cardiac pathophysiology from pressure waveform analysis. II: The tricuspid valve. *Cathet Cardiovasc Diagn* 21:278–286, 1990.

5 Vacca JB, Bussmann DW, Mudd JG. Ebstein's anomaly: Complete review of 108 cases. *Am J Cardiol* 2:210, 1958.

6 Lev M, Liberthson RR, Joseph RH, Seten CE, Eckner FA, Kunske RD, *et al.* The pathologic anatomy of Ebstein's disease. *Arch Pathol* 90:334, 1970.

7 Nora JJ, Nora AH, Toews WH. Lithium, Ebstein's anomaly and other congenital heart defects. *Lancet* 2:594, 1974.

8 Marcelletti C, McGoon DC, Mair DC. The natural history of truncus arteriosus. *Circulation* 54:108, 1976.

9 Watson H. Natural history of Ebstein's anomaly of tricuspid valve in childhood and adolescence: An international cooperative study of 505 cases. *Br Heart J* 36:417, 1974.

10 Braunwald E, Godin R. Cooperative study on cardiac catheterization: Total population studied, procedures employed and incidence of complication. *Circulation* 37(suppl III):8–16, 1968.

11 Dalen JE, Grossman W. Shunt detection and measurement. In JE Dalen, W Grossman (eds), *Cardiac Catheterization and Angiography*, 2nd ed. Philadelphia, PA: Lea and Febiger, 1980, pp. 131–143.

12 Hugenholtz PG, Schwark T, Monroe RG, Gamble WJ, Hauck AJ, Nadas AS. The clinical usefulness of hydrogen gas as an indicator of left-to-right shunts. *Circulation* 28:542–551, 1963.

13 Kern MJ, Deligonul D, Gudipati C. Hemodynamic and ECG data. In MJ Kern, D Deligonul, C Gudipati (eds), *The Cardiac Catheterization Handbook*. St. Louis, MO: Mosby Year Book, 1991, pp. 119–177.

14 Yang SS, Bentivoglio LG, Maranhao V, Goldberg H. Assessment of cardiovascular shunts. In SS Yang, LG Bentivoglio, V Maranhao, H Goldberg (eds), *From Cardiac Catheterization Data to Hemodynamic Parameters*, 3rd ed. Philadelphia, PA: FA Davis, 1988, pp. 166–188.

15 Shumacker HB Jr, Glover J. Congenital aneurysms of the ventricular septum. *Am Heart J* 66:405–408, 1963.

16 Hillis LD, Winniford MD, Jackson JA, Firth BG. Measurement of left-to-right intracardiac shunting in adults: Oximetric versus indicator dilution techniques. *Cathet Cardiovasc Diagn* 11:467–472, 1985.

17 Castillo CA, Kyle JC, Gilson WE, Rowe GG. Simulated shunt curves. *Am J Cardiol* 17:691, 1966.

18 Swan IDC, Burchell HB, Wood EH. The presence of venoarterial shunts in patients with interatrial communications. *Circulation* 10:705–713, 1954.

19 Ewert P, Berger F, Nagdyman N, Kretschmar O, Dittrich S, Abdul-Khaliq H, *et al.* Masked left ventricular restriction in elderly patients with atrial septal defects: A contraindication for closure? *Catheter Cardiovasc Interv* 52:177–180, 2001.

20 Holzer R, Cao QL, Hijazi ZM. Closure of a moderately large atrial septal defect with a self-fabricated fenestrated Amplatzer septal occluder in an 85-year-old patient with reduced diastolic elasticity of the left ventricle. *Catheter Cardiovasc Interv* 64:513–518, 2005.

21 Cheatham JP. Now we are making a hole in a device meant to close a hole: Why? How? Is there a better answer? *Catheter Cardiovasc Interv* 64:519–521, 2005.

22 Bashore T. Adult congenital heart disease right ventricular outflow tract lesions. *Circulation* 115:1933–1947, 2007.

23 Inglessis I, Landzberg MJ. Interventional catheterization in adult congenital heart disease. *Circulation* 115;1622–1633, 2007.

21

Extra Hearts: Unusual Hemodynamics of Heterotopic Transplant and Ventricular Assist Devices

Morton J. Kern

Unusual and complex pressure waveforms present in patients with "extra" hearts, for example left ventricular (LV) assist devices or heterotopic heart transplant [1]. Most if not all of the heterotopic heart patients may never be seen again in clinical practice, since the technique has been made obsolete. Nonetheless, assisted pressure pulsation systems, either biological or mechanical, often produce confusing and interesting hemodynamic waveforms. The principles applied to interpreting hemodynamics in native hearts are even more important when examined in this context. This chapter has several of the most unusual hemodynamic tracings illustrating the concept. Review the hemodynamic tracings before reading the textual explanation. In this way, the curiosities of pressure delivery in functioning and nonfunctioning extra hearts will be even more educational.

"Extra" Arterial Pressure

A 43-year-old man with a history of mitral valve replacement for mitral stenosis developed coronary artery disease and class IV left ventricular failure due to ischemic cardiomyopathy which was refractory to medical therapy [1].

Because of longstanding pulmonary hypertension, a surgical procedure was performed (to be discussed below). Retrograde left- and right-heart catheterization was performed. Measurement of aortic pressure was obtained through an 8 F femoral side arm sheath. Simultaneous left ventricular pressure was measured with a 7 F pigtail catheter. The hemodynamic tracings are shown in Figures 21.1 and 21.2. Examine the arterial pressure wave (Figure 21.1). The electrocardiogram has an irregularly irregular rhythm. An aortic gradient is observed in Figure 21.1, beats # 1, 2 and 3. Can you explain the waveform configuration and pressure generation of beats #4, 5 and 6 on this figure? Before

moving to Figure 21.2, when can aortic pressure normally exceed left ventricular pressure?

Figure 21.2 is a continuous tracing from Figure 21.1 of the patient described above, showing deterioration of left ventricular pressure despite maintained aortic pressure. The catheter position is unchanged and aortic pressure continues around 120/70 mm Hg. What is causing the change in left ventricular pressure?

Consider another patient, a 37-year-old man having had the same procedure as the preceding patient. The "surgical" treatment for refractory idiopathic congestive heart failure was successful. The arterial pressure and electrocardiogram are shown in Figure 21.3 and demonstrate a highly irregular arterial pulse pattern with a more regular electrocardiogram. Explain the systolic arterial pressure wave in the absence of apparent high-grade atrial or ventricular ectopy.

This puzzling sequence of tracings represents unusual examples of pressure generation occurring from one or two ventricles in patients after heterotopic heart transplant (Figure 21.4). Heterotopic heart transplantation has a long experimental history and was the technique used by Christian Barnard and his colleagues in South Africa when performing the first clinical heart transplantation in 1967. Although 95% of all heart transplantations done in 1990 were orthotopic replacements, heterotopic heart transplantation is indicated in patients with pulmonary hypertension who need left ventricular assistance, but has fallen into obsolescence. Orthotopic replacement of a "new" donor heart, unaccustomed to high pulmonary artery pressures, would result in severe, potentially fatal right ventricular failure after transplantation. For historical background, the vascular communications of heterotopic transplantation are varied [2]. One common method used in the patient examples is as follows: the aorta of the accessory (donor) heart is attached end to side directly to the aorta of the native heart and the donor pulmonary artery by graft to the native pulmonary artery.

Hemodynamic Rounds: Interpretation of Cardiac Pathophysiology from Pressure Waveform Analysis, Fourth Edition.
Edited by Morton J. Kern, Michael J. Lim, and James A. Goldstein.
© 2018 John Wiley & Sons Ltd. Published 2018 by John Wiley & Sons Ltd.

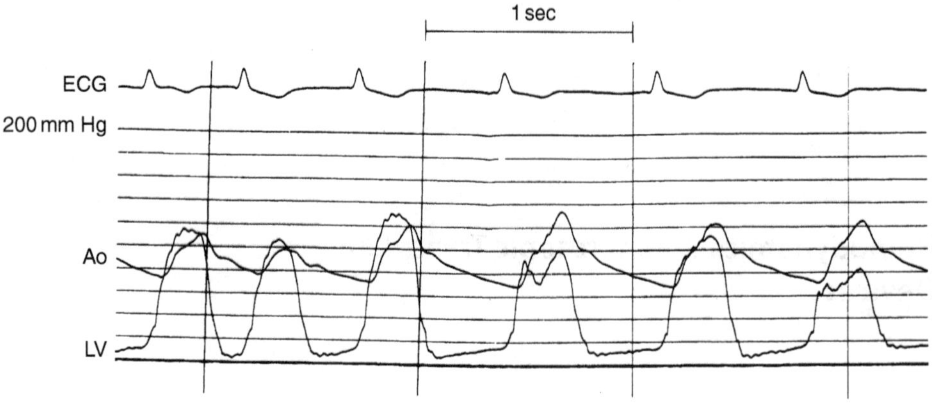

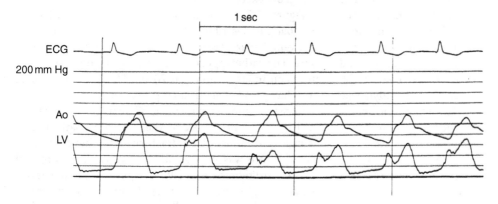

Figure 21.1 Simultaneous aortic (Ao) and left ventricular (LV) pressures (200 mm Hg scale). See text for details.

Figure 21.2 Simultaneous aortic (Ao) and left ventricular (LV) pressures (200 mm Hg scale). See text for details.

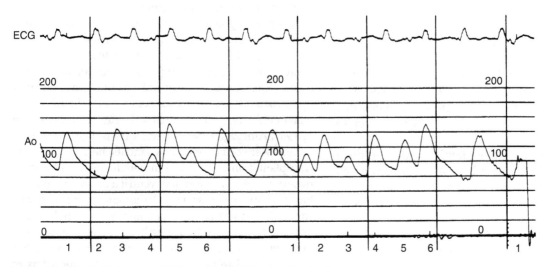

Figure 21.3 Aortic (Ao) pressure (200 mm Hg scale). See text for details.

A communication between both left atria is created (large "atrial" septal defect) to allow filling of the donor left ventricle. The donor right ventricle is filled by right atrial flow from the native heart. Since the function of the native left ventricle is generally very poor and, at times, insufficient to influence systemic pressure, the arterial pulse depends principally on the Frank–Starling mechanism of filling of the donor heart. However, the electrocardiographic complex which is most prominent may not be that of the native heart, often accounting for the disparity between electrocardiographic rhythm and pressure waves.

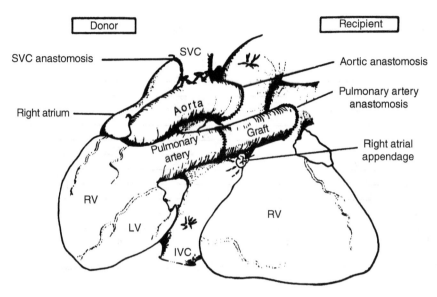

Figure 21.4 Graphic representation of heterotopic heart transplant surgical anastomoses. IVC = inferior vena cava; LV = left ventricle; RV = right ventricle; SVC = superior vena cava.

There are several advantages of heterotopic over orthotopic heart transplantation. The donor heart acts as a built-in left ventricular assist device (LVAD) and maintains the systemic circulation. Heterotopic heart transplantation allows for possible recovery of recipient heart failure after viral myocarditis, and can be performed in the presence of very high pulmonary vascular resistance, as the hypertrophied native right ventricle continues to support the pulmonary circulation. However, the transplanted heterotopic heart patient also carries a severe risk of systemic emboli from thrombus in the poorly contracting recipient left ventricle and requires long-term anti-coagulation. Moreover, the native ventricle may be subject to continuing angina related to ischemic cardiomyopathy. The risk of infection in the recipient heart is also a continuing problem.

Customary hemodynamic waveforms may be significantly affected by the dysrhythmic activity of the recipient heart, occasionally requiring high doses of anti-arrhythmic agents. Abnormal hemodynamic patterns of donor left ventricular pressure may indicate early transplant rejection. Failing function of the heterotopic transplant often appears as a significant decline in the magnitude and slowed and diminished pattern of the peripheral pressure wave. The ratio of the arterial pulse of each of the two contracting ventricles is thought to be an indicator of impending cardiac rejection [2].

In many patients, the donor heart functions as a pressure "assist" pump. The donor heart influences the systemic pressure in two ways: (i) co-pulsation, in time with the native heart; or (ii) counter-pulsation, pumping in the native heart's diastole. These coincident or counterpoint beats are evidenced by the changing waveform of aortic pressure and occasionally by the two different QRS complexes inscribed on the electrocardiographic tracing above the pressure waves. The timing of the two left ventricular pressures and influence on aortic pressure can be seen in Figures 21.5 and 21.6, which were taken from patient #2, whose arterial pressure was provided in Figure 21.3. The subtle small waves in the electrocardiogram mistakenly appearing as P waves are the electrocardiographic complexes of the donor heart, with the largest complexes being the native heart. This rhythm is more complicated because a ventricular premature complex (VPC) in the donor heart may not be detected electrocardiographically and may confuse the pressure wave interpretation. However, in patients with reduced native left ventricular function insufficient to exceed systemic pressure, the magnitude of arterial pressure is dependent on donor heart R–R interval and Frank–Starling filling force relationship.

The intrinsic cardiac rhythm for many patients may be atrial fibrillation, with the donor heart in a sinus rhythm. In Figures 21.1 and 21.2, there was coincident timing of the native and donor left ventricular pressures, explaining why native left ventricular pressures could fall under the higher aortic pressure wave. Synchrony of the two hearts was maintained for long periods of time, giving the impression that native left ventricular pressure was sufficient to generate adequate pressure in the systemic circulation. Most of the native left ventricular beats in Figure 21.2 were clearly insufficient to generate arterial pressure. The false gradient (aortic higher than left ventricular pressure) demonstrated in beat #1 (Figure 21.1)

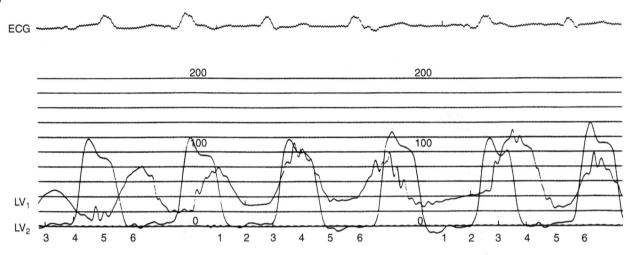

Figure 21.5 Simultaneous left ventricular (LV$_1$, LV$_2$) pressures (200 mm Hg scale). LV$_1$ = native left ventricle; LV$_2$ = donor left ventricle. See text for details

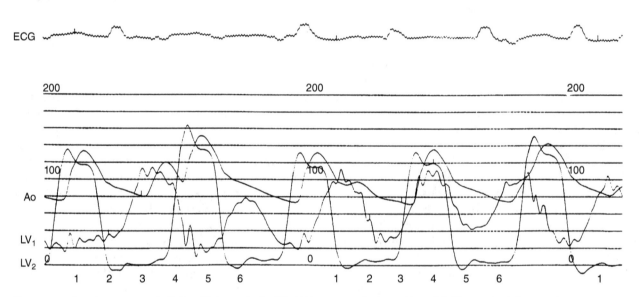

Figure 21.6 Simultaneous aortic (Ao) and left ventricular (LV$_1$, LV$_2$) pressures (200 mm Hg scale). LV$_1$ = native left ventricle; LV$_2$ = donor left ventricle. See text for details.

is a result of pressure being satisfactory in the native heart, with reduced output of the donor heart. The highest aortic pressure (beat #4, Figure 21.1, and beat #3, Figure 21.6) occurs with co-pulsation of the ventricles. The lowest arterial pressure waves (beat #2, Figure 21.1, and beat #3, Figure 21.6) occurring during dyssynchrony of ventricular contraction may be evident. The timing cycle of the co-pulsation and counter-pulsation beats is particularly evident in Figure 21.7. To determine which electrocardiographic signal and which waveform originates from the donor versus native heart, drop a vertical line from the QRS and identify the corresponding pressure upstroke. Usually the weaker pressure is the native heart.

Co-Pulsation and Counter-Pulsation

A 42-year-old man with pulmonary hypertension and class IV refractory congestive heart failure received a heterotopic heart transplant six weeks prior to evaluation (Figure 21.7). The electrocardiogram demonstrates two QRS complexes, representing the donor and native hearts. The donor left ventricular pressure (identified with the dark star) and the recipient's native left ventricular pressure (identified with the open star) show their influence on the aortic pulse pressures. Compare the synchrony of the two hearts on beats labeled X and Y. The size of the aortic pulse waves depends on the co-pulsation or counter-pulsation (i.e., synchrony) of

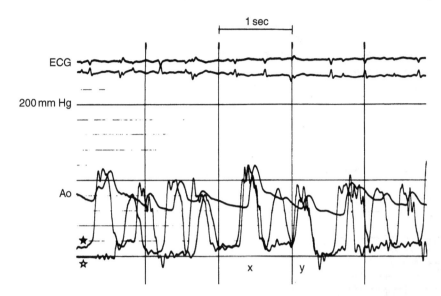

Figure 21.7 Simultaneous aortic (Ao) and left ventricular pressures (200 mm Hg scale). Dark star represents left ventricular pressures of the donor heart. Open star represents left ventricular pressure of the native heart. See text for details.

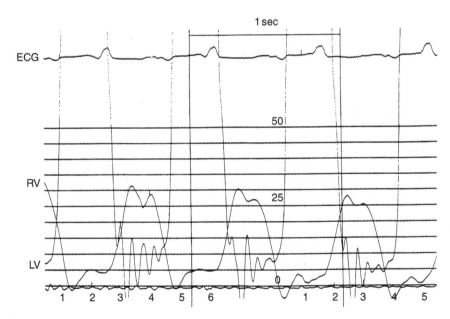

Figure 21.8 Simultaneous right ventricular (RV) and left ventricular (LV) pressures (50 mm Hg scale). Notice the small abnormal QRS complex of the native left ventricle.

native and donor left ventricular pressure augmentation. Synchrony of the two left ventricular pressures produces a large aortic pulse (X beat). The next beat barely generates a small arterial pulse wave with only the native left ventricular pressure. The following beat (Y beat) has both left ventricular pressures, but the native left ventricle is not filled adequately preceding the "premature" contraction.

Although considered artifact by the unsuspecting, the electrocardiographic rhythm consistently demonstrates the two different QRS complexes, one for each ventricle, and corresponds to the arterial pressure wave pattern. The hemodynamic responses of the two ventricles over time become clinically important when considering early allograft rejection.

As one might expect, right ventricular pressure in the donor heart is normal and is independent of native left ventricular contraction (Figure 21.8). In this example, the native QRS on the electrocardiogram is small and nearly unrecognizable relative to the large donor QRS complexes coupled to right ventricular pressure.

"Extra" Atrial Pressure

Atrial activity, at times, becomes dyssynchronous from ventricular contraction in certain orthotopic and heterotopic transplant patients. A 52-year-old man had received orthotopic transplant one year prior to study. Left ventricular and aortic pressures measured simultaneously show elevated systemic pressures (180/100 mm Hg), no aortic–left ventricular gradient, and only mild elevation of left ventricular end-diastolic pressure (Figure 21.9a).

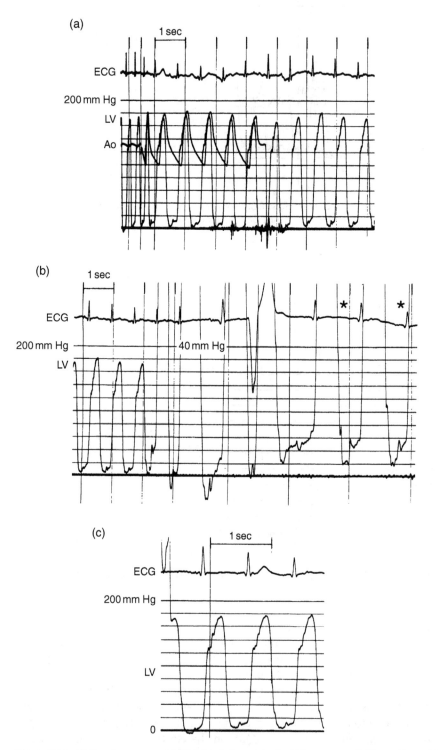

Figure 21.9 (a) Simultaneous aortic (Ao) and left ventricular (LV) pressures (200 mm Hg scale). See text for details. (b) Simultaneous aortic and left ventricular pressures (both 200 mm Hg and 40 mm Hg scales). See text for details. (c) Left ventricular pressure (G–200 mm Hg scale). See text for details.

However, the diastolic left ventricular pressure wave-form is consistently, but irregularly, deformed by "notches" in mid to late diastole (Figure 21.9b). Although uncommon, atrial contraction stimulated from the remaining native atrial tissue can produce this pressure artifact. The A wave may occur at variable times in the diastolic or systolic periods and appear separate from the electrocardiographic atrial activity of the donor heart (Figure 21.9b and 21.9b).

Consider the right-heart pressure tracings in a 53-year-old man six months after orthotopic transplantation (Figures 21.10 and 21.11). Dyssynchronous atrial

activity is also evident. Residual native atrial activity is more easily discerned on the electrocardiogram in this patient than that in Figure 21.9 and is shown by the "p'" wave relative to the "normal" P wave. The sinus (p) beats have their normal A and V waves, but when the ectopic atrial beat (P') appears, the right atrial waveform becomes distorted (see beat A'). Also note the diastolic right ventricular pressure notch (Figure 21.11, asterisk). The dyssynchronous atrial contraction superimposed on right ventricular systole may be appreciated on beat #2. Although hemodynamically interesting, atrial dyssyn-chrony does not present a serious clinical problem.

Applying the traditional hemodynamic principles to the cardiac cycle with its attendant electrical-mechani-cal events is complicated in patients with "extra" hearts. When non-physiologic events are present, investigate all possible sources of artifact along the fluid path to the transducer, catheter malposition, and congenital or "acquired" anatomic anomalies.

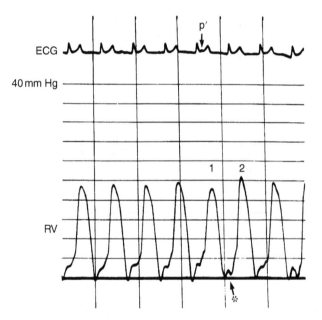

Figure 21.10 Right ventricular (RV) pressure in a patient with cardiac transplantation (40 mm Hg scale). See text for details.

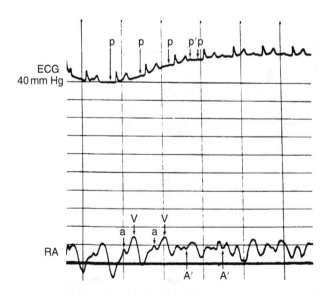

Figure 21.11 Right atrial (RA) pressure in a patient with cardiac transplantation (40 mm Hg scale). See text for details.

Left Ventricular Assist Devices

The pressure waves generated by mechanical assist device as an extra heart may be the result of two principal modes: either partial or complete support of systemic pressure. Current partial support devices would include intra-aortic balloon pumps and left atrial (LA) bypass (TandemHeart) Complete support devices generate flow through centripetal, roller-type, clam-shell, or other unique pump designs and are used as left, right, or biventricular support devices [3–6]. The total artificial heart is another of several types of these complete support devices. Pressure waves generated by these devices depend on the contribution and timing of both mechanical and intrinsic myocardial pulsatile activity.

Myocardial Ischemia and the Extra Heart

A 52-year-old man with severe coronary artery disease underwent coronary artery bypass graft surgery after a complicated myocardial infarction in 1985 [7]. Because of progressive ischemia and atherosclerosis in the saphen-ous vein grafts, a second coronary artery bypass surgery, complicated by a cardiac arrest, was performed. Successful resuscitation was accomplished with the institution of a left ventricular cardiac assist device. He was fully active with a normal exercise capacity in the hospital. Unusual serum antibodies precluded earlier donor heart matching. The patient did well for nine months after device implan-tation, while awaiting cardiac transplantation. Despite a well-functioning assist device, angina pectoris with decreasing exercise tolerance became incapacitating. A cardiac catheterization and exercise hemodynamic study was performed. Aortic and left ventricular pressures were simultaneously measured from an 8 F femoral sheath and 7 F pigtail catheter in the left ventricle (Figure 21.12). Explain the arterial pressure without a corresponding left ventricular pressure. The waveform of aortic pressure indicates that an extra heart must be performing the work to generate a systemic pulse. Note that the electrocardiogram does not correlate to the aortic pressure, but does precede each left ventricular pressure wave. Left ventricular pressure rarely exceeds minimal aortic pressure. Why are alternate left ventricular pressures higher? Which mechanical mechanisms

trigger the assist device? The extra heart in this patient was a clam-shell-type pump [8]. The Novacor® and other similar pulsatile ventricular support devices function by employing volume triggers, producing a pressure pulse when the "new" left ventricle is passively filled to a predetermined volume. "Heart rate" is then driven by filling pressures (and volume) related to systemic muscular activity. When examining simultaneous left and right ventricular pressures (Figure 21.13), a majority of beats demonstrate relatively small differences in the ventricular pressures without features of myocardial restrictive physiology.

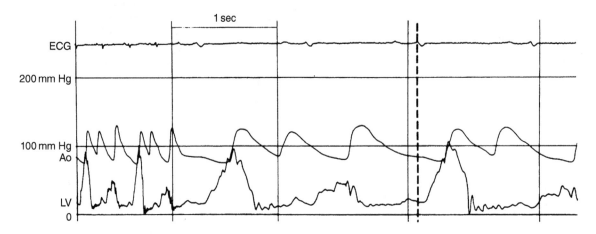

Figure 21.12 Aortic (Ao) and left ventricular (LV) pressures in a patient with an extra heart. The timing of the QRS corresponds to the left ventricular pressure (dotted line). Aortic pressure is generated in a pulsatile manner unrelated to left ventricular pressure. See text for details.

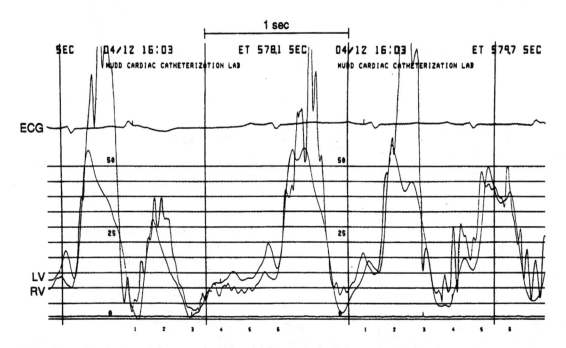

Figure 21.13 Simultaneous left ventricular (LV) and right ventricular (RV) pressures in the patient in Figure 21.12 (0–50 mm Hg scale). Note the correspondence of pressures of the left and right ventricles in most beats. There is no evidence of restrictive physiology. See text for details.

The variation of the left ventricular pressure is related to the rate of emptying through the apex conduit to the pump. As one might expect, left ventriculography is unusual, showing the volume of contrast passing through the left ventricle and exiting from the apex conduit into the assist device (Figure 21.14a). With each pump, the stroke volume is moved to the ascending aorta through the abdominally implanted conduit from the clam-shell pump (Figure 21.14b and 21.14b). Reduced left ventricular pressure occurs when the timing of pump filling exceeds the timing of the native left ventricular ejection, and thereby results in the alteration of left ventricular pressures.

To assess the etiology of cardiac dysfunction, coronary angiography was performed and showed total occlusion of the left anterior descending, right coronary, and circumflex arteries. The single saphenous vein graft to the right coronary artery had a 50% ostial narrowing with mid graft 90% lesion. Contrast opacification of the posterior descending artery and faint circumflex collaterals

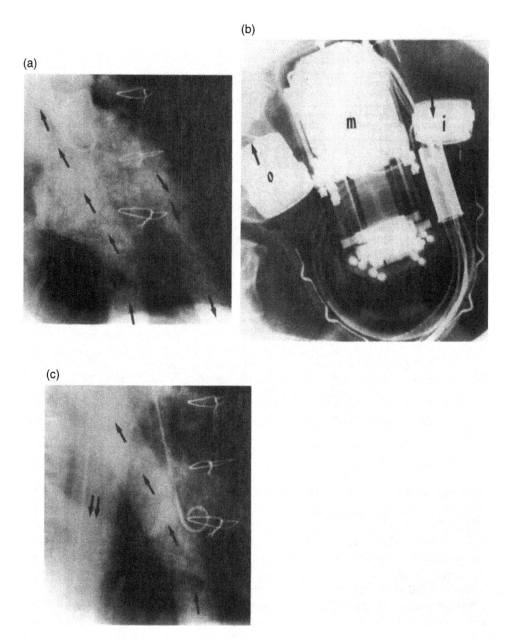

Figure 21.14 (a) Ventriculogram after injection of contrast into the mid ventricle. Contrast empties through the apex of the heart (three down arrows). (b) It enters the input port of the Novacor® pump (i with the down arrow), exits through the output port (o with the up arrow), and returns to the aorta via conduit (panel a, five up arrows). (c) Late phase of the left ventriculogram with the pump to aortic conduit filling (four up arrows) and the descending aorta filled with blood (two down arrows). The aortic valve does not open. m = motor.

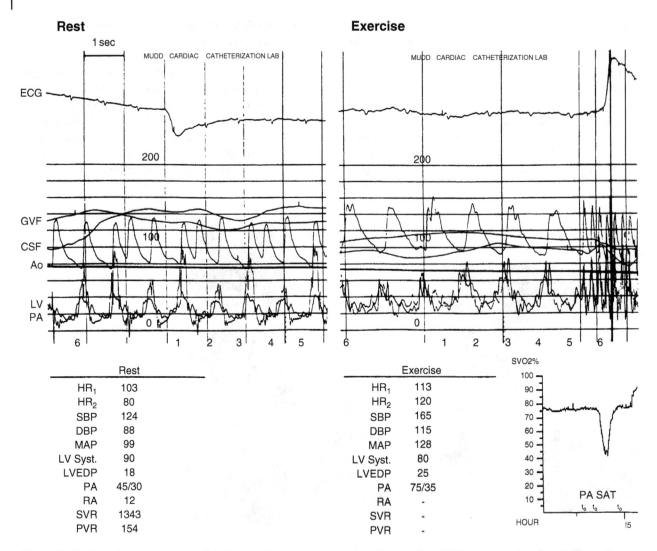

Rest   **Exercise**

	Rest
HR$_1$	103
HR$_2$	80
SBP	124
DBP	88
MAP	99
LV Syst.	90
LVEDP	18
PA	45/30
RA	12
SVR	1343
PVR	154

	Exercise
HR$_1$	113
HR$_2$	120
SBP	165
DBP	115
MAP	128
LV Syst.	80
LVEDP	25
PA	75/35
RA	-
SVR	-
PVR	-

Figure 21.15 Hemodynamics at rest and during exercise, measuring great cardiac vein flow (GVF), coronary sinus flow (CSF), aortic pressure (Ao), left ventricular pressure (LV), and pulmonary artery pressure (PA). The higher coronary blood flow is toward the bottom of the tracing. In the lower right corner is a continuous signal of pulmonary artery oxygen saturation, showing a decline at peak exercise from 78% to approximately 40%. DBP = diastolic blood pressure; HR = heart rate; LVEDP = left ventricular end-diastolic pressure; LV syst = left ventricular systolic pressure; MAP = mean arterial pressure; RA = right atrial pressure; SBP = systolic blood pressure; SVR, PVR = system and pulmonary vascular resistance.

were noted. An exercise hemodynamic study was also performed. Aortic and left ventricular pressures, coronary sinus thermodilution blood flow (catheter inserted through the left antecubital vein), continuous pulmonary artery oxygen saturation, and pressures were measured during weighted leg raising for 6 min (Figure 21.15; Table 21.1). Exercise increased the assisted heart rate (103 to 113 beats/min), mean arterial pressure (99 to 128 mm Hg), aortic diastolic pressure (88 to 115 mm Hg), left ventricular end-diastolic pressure (18 to 25 mm Hg), and pulmonary artery pressure (45/15 to 75/28 mm Hg). Cardiac output (by thermodilution and confirmed by the console values) rose minimally (5.2 to 6.5 L/min), with a marked decline in pulmonary artery oxygen saturation

(78% to 40%) and accompanying symptomatic fatigue and mild angina. Coronary blood flow (great cardiac vein) increased (43 to 56 min) with only modest lactate generation. Consider the hemodynamic results of exercise in this patient with a left ventricular assist device with regard to exercise responses in normal subjects. Exercise normally increases heart rate by more than 25%, decreases aortic diastolic pressure due to decreased systemic vascular resistance, minimally changes right ventricular and pulmonary artery pressures, and markedly increases cardiac output and coronary blood flow at least fourfold. In our patient, the blunted heart rate and the increase in diastolic aortic and mean systemic pressures indicate a failure to lower systemic vascular resistance

Table 21.1 Hemodynamic data.

	HR$_{native}$	**HR**$_{pump}$	**BP**	**MAP**	**LVP**	**PA**	**RA**
Rest	80	103	124/80	99	65/18	38/15	12
Exercise	120	113	150/98	128	65/25	65/25	—

					Oxygen Saturations (%)		
	CO$_{Td}$	**CO**$_{pump}$	**SVR**	**PVR**	**Ao**	**PA**	**CS**
Rest	5.18	6.46	1343	154	94	75	36
Exercise	5.90	6.47	—	—	97	42	41

	Lactate (mEq/L)					
	Art	**CS**	**Diff**	**GVF (mL/min)**	**MVO$_2$ (mL/dL)**	
Rest	1.3	1.1	0.2	43	273	
Exercise	6.0	4.3	2.3	96	406	

Art = arterial lactate; BP = blood pressure (mm Hg); CO$_{pump}$ = assist device pump output (L/min); CO$_{TD}$ = thermodilution cardiac output (L/min); CS = coronary sinus lactate; Diff = aorta–CS difference; GVF = great cardiac vein flow; HR = heart rate (beats/min); LVP = left ventricular pressure (mm Hg); MAP = mean arterial pressure (mm Hg); MVO$_2$ = myocardial oxygen consumption; PA = pulmonary artery pressure (mm Hg); PVR = pulmonary vascular resistance (dynes·sec·cm^{-5}); RA = right atrial pressure (mm Hg); SVR = systemic vascular resistance (dynes·see·cm^{-5}).

appropriately. The decline in pulmonary artery oxygen saturation is a markedly exaggerated response compared to a normal subject.

The increase in pulmonary artery pressures also required explanation, with a left ventricular pump which is presumed to be substituting for native left ventricular work. The limited capacity of the assist pump to empty the native left ventricle results in increased left ventricular end-diastolic pressure and also pulmonary pressures. As one might anticipate, limited coronary blood flow through this severely diseased heart might be due to arterial conduit blockage, as well as attenuated oxygen demand, with myocardial muscle performance supplemented by mechanical support. Despite mechanical ventricular assistance, myocardial oxygen demand (MVO$_2$) was increased and signs of ischemia occurred.

Can one explain the increase in left ventricular end-diastolic pressure and MVO$_2$ in a left ventricle that supposedly is *not* doing its normal share of pressure work? We speculate that the marked increase in pulmonary pressures reflects ischemia from the inferior left ventricular and right ventricular functioning zones. Right ventricular ischemia in the unassisted right ventricle might well be the cause of progressive dyspnea, with compromised function of the remaining active myocardium of the inferior and lateral walls. Progression of coronary artery disease in the right coronary artery bypass graft (the only remaining arterial blood supply) was evident. Limited blood flow to the inferior left ventricular distribution most likely affected the pressure responses to exercise.

Unfortunately, a complete answer to the questions raised cannot be provided from the hemodynamic data

alone. Several issues regarding alteration of left and right ventricular chamber dimensions, mitral and tricuspid regurgitation, and left ventricular ischemic dysfunction require combined echocardiographic imaging. This unusual hemodynamic case is illustrative of both the insights and limitations of hemodynamic data interpretation. In situations where complex questions of physiology are anticipated, explanations may be obtained with combined echocardiographic and hemodynamic techniques.

Portable Cardiopulmonary Bypass

The systemic pressure generated by the clam-shell pumping device in the previous case involved decompression of left ventricular filling and hence LV pressure [9]. This type of pump is generally associated with reduced myocardial oxygen demand and is, at times, considered to "rest" the heart [10, 11].

Cardiopulmonary bypass has been used as an emergency "extra heart" to support circulatory collapse after acute myocardial infarction or cardiac arrest in the catheterization laboratory during diagnostic or therapeutic intervention [12–15]. The hemodynamics of cardio-pulmonary support (CPS) are illustrated by the following case.

Blood Pressure with a Closed Aortic Valve

A 34-year-old woman had severe crushing chest pain with electrocardiographic evidence of extensive anterior and lateral myocardial infarctions. Because of a history of uncontrolled hypertension, thrombolytic therapy was

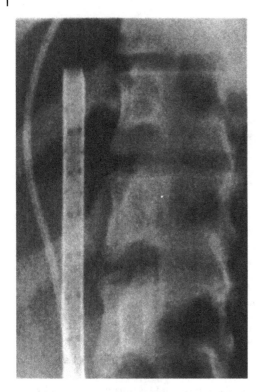

Figure 21.16 Angiogram of inferior vena cava showing the long 20F venous cannula of the cardiopulmonary bypass circuit located just beneath the inferior right atrial entrance. A pulmonary artery balloon flotation catheter can be seen traversing the inferior vena cava. The catheter was inserted from the left femoral vein.

not administered. Twelve hours after admission to a community hospital, hypotension and ventricular tachyarrhythmias occurred. Emergency helicopter transport was performed. On arrival in the intensive care unit, the patient had a cardiac arrest. Initial resuscitative efforts were successful, with subsequent intubation and placement of femoral arterial and venous sheaths. Intravenous infusions of dopamine, lidocaine, and bretylium were required to maintain a systolic blood pressure of 80 mm Hg and stable sinus tachycardia. One hour after initial resuscitation and stabilization, hypotension and ventricular arrhythmias recurred. Because of failure to maintain a systolic pressure of 60 mm Hg, emergency portable cardiopulmonary bypass was instituted, inserting an 18 F arterial cannulation into the right femoral artery and a 20 F cannulae into the inferior vena cava (Figure 21.16). Systemic blood flow using a centripetal pump system was maintained at 4.0 L/min, generating a mean blood pressure of 85 mm Hg. The patient was transferred to the cardiac catheterization laboratory for diagnostic study and possible angioplasty.

The electrocardiogram at the time of catheterization, while on cardiopulmonary bypass, showed new right bundle branch block, left axis deviation, and low anterior R wave voltage (Figure 21.17). Coronary angiography showed a normal and co-dominant right coronary artery, 90% left main stenosis, and 100% occlusion of both the left anterior descending and circumflex arteries

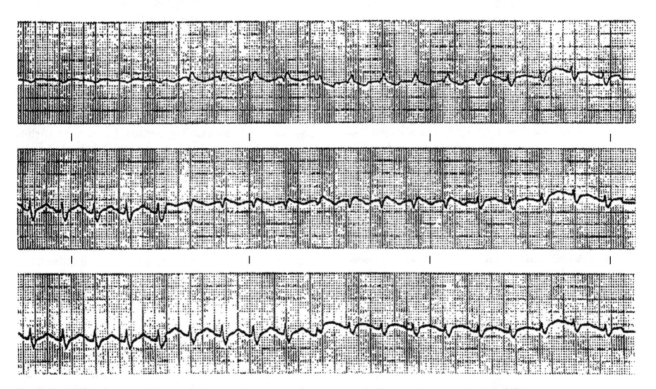

Figure 21.17 The electrocardiogram during portable cardiopulmonary bypass. Sinus tachycardia with left axis deviation, poor R wave progression, and diffuse low voltage across the anterior leads was different from the previous tracing, with marked ST elevation over leads V_1–V_4.

(a)

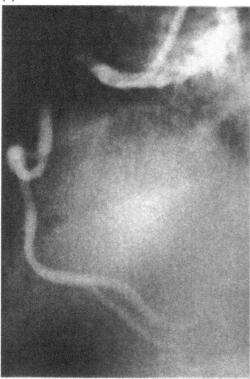

(b)

Figure 21.18 (a) Normal right coronary artery in the left anterior oblique projection. (b) Subtotal occlusion of the left coronary artery, with only an obtuse marginal branch evident. Neither the left anterior descending nor the circumflex artery was visualized. The aortic valve did not open during contrast injection.

(Figure 21.18). Left ventricular function was assessed before the cardiovascular surgeon would consider emergency coronary artery bypass grafting. Examine the hemodynamic pressure tracings measured through an 8 F pigtail catheter in the left ventricle (Figure 21.19). Left ventricular pressure is 58/20 mm Hg (Figure 21.19a, left side, beats #1–4) and is abnormal in both rate of pressure development and pattern of left ventricular relaxation, as indicated by the sharp downslope across

diastole. Continuous pressure recording during left ventricular–aortic catheter pullback is shown at the right side of the tracing after beat #4. The pressure scale is changed to 0–200 mm Hg. The phasic character of left ventricular pressure quickly changes to a mean pressure of the cardiopulmonary bypass circuit when the catheter is pulled across the aortic valve.

From the difference in left ventricular–aortic pressure, it is obvious that the aortic valve cannot open. To demonstrate the pressure at which the aortic valve did open, the flow rate of the cardiopulmonary bypass pump was turned down while continuously recording aortic pressure (Figure 21.19b). Note that the phasic arterial pressure waves do not appear until the mean aortic pressure falls below 60 mm Hg. These phasic waves reflect the left ventricular pressure opening the aortic valve. During cardiopulmonary bypass, the left ventricle is contracting against a closed aortic valve with no means of left ventricular decompression. Mitral regurgitation was not evident hemodynamically. Left ventricular strain and wan stress are certainly elevated, as is myocardial oxygen demand. However, aortic pressure is maintained sufficiently to perfuse the cerebral, renal, and coronary circulations.

The critical nature of cardiopulmonary bypass–augmented coronary perfusion was also demonstrated shortly after turning down the cardiopulmonary bypass system, reducing the mean blood pressure to below 60 mm Hg. The aortic and right atrial pressures were recorded during cardiopulmonary bypass flow at a low level, generating a mean pressure of less than 40 mm Hg (Figure 21.19c, left side). Aortic pressure is 55/40 mm Hg and right atrial pressure is 16 mm Hg (0–40 mm Hg scale). The rhythm degenerated into a wide complex tachyarrhythmia (compare to Figure 21.19b). With increasing cardiopulmonary bypass flow and restoration of an adequate systemic pressure, the phasic aortic pressure is obliterated and the right atrial pressure falls as inferior vena caval blood is returned to the cardiopulmonary bypass circuit. With maintenance of coronary perfusion pressure, the rhythm was converted into a sinus tachycardia.

Because of the critical need to assess myocardial function more than 18 hours after near total occlusion of the left coronary artery, a 15 cc contrast injection (low osmolar media, 15 cc/sec) was made into the left ventricle. The contraction pattern and regions of potential viability were measured using a digital angiographic technique. It is important to reduce the cardiopulmonary bypass flow to permit aortic valve opening during ventriculography for a realistic assessment of left ventricular contraction. A severely reduced ejection fraction would not be surprising when viewing the left ventricle trying to eject blood through a closed aortic valve. In this patient, the left ventricular ejection fraction was less than 10%, with

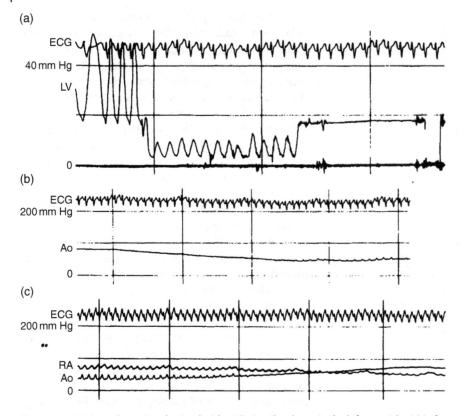

(a)

(b)

(c)

Figure 21.19 Hemodynamics obtained with a 7F pigtail catheter in the left ventricle. (a) Left ventricular (LV) pressure on a 0–40 mm Hg scale (beats #1–4, left side) and a 0–200 mm Hg scale (beats #5 and on toward the right). Left ventricular pressure demonstrated a slow increase in pressure generation and abnormal pressure decline during diastole. After beat #17, the catheter was pulled into the aorta and the mean systemic pressure of the portable cardiopulmonary bypass can be observed. (b) Alteration of pressure waveform during reduction of cardiopulmonary bypass flow volume to reduce systemic pressure below that of left ventricular pressure. Far right of the tracing shows phasic beats of aortic valve opening. Ao = aortic pressure. (c) Tight atrial (RA) and aortic (Ao) pressures during very low cardiopulmonary bypass flow rate. As flow rate is increased, the aortic pressure increases to a mean of 85 mm Hg and right atrial pressure falls from 16 to 10 mm Hg.

global hypokinesis and inferior as well as anterior akinesis. A decision for emergency coronary angioplasty was made after consultation with the cardiothoracic surgeon. Incomplete revascularization of the left main and circumflex arteries was achieved (Figure 21.20). The occluded left anterior descending artery could not be reopened. The patient expired 36 hours later because of acidosis, hypoxia, and renal failure.

Extra hearts of the cardiopulmonary bypass variety without ventricular decompression can maintain systemic perfusion, but do so at the cost of increased myocardial work. Systemic pressure support facilitates emergency resuscitation and should be employed briefly until revascularization can be performed. The hemodynamic waveforms in this patient illustrate the paradox of systemic perfusion with increased myocardial ischemia. Without restoration of coronary perfusion, myocardial salvage, and ultimately survival, is highly unlikely. An excellent review of the physiologic basis for left ventricular assist devices is provided by Naidu *et al.* [16].

Mechanical Circulatory Support Devices

Left ventricular mechanical circulatory support devices (MCS) are designed to provide hemodynamic stability with maintenance of cardiac output, mean arterial pressure, pulmonary venous pressure, and adequate oxygen perfusion.

The three most commonly used devices include the intra-aortic balloon pump (IABP), the Impella hemodynamic support system, and the Tandem Heart extracorporeal bypass system (Figures 21.21, 21.22, and 21.23 and Tables 21.2, 21.3, and 21.4). Those patients with the highest risk and usually the lowest cardiac reserve were candidates for the most powerful support (e.g., LVAD type). Recently, the development of a small catheter-based LVAD, the Impella system, permits use of more powerful hemodynamic support (relative to the IABP) which can be instituted earlier and with more facility than extracorporeal systems.

The goals of MCS are achieved through different mechanisms, producing different metrics of hemodynamic success. Among the many hemodynamic parameters, probably most strongly associated with survival in patients in cardiogenic shock is that of cardiac power output (CPO) measured in watts, defined as mean arterial pressure multiplied by the cardiac output and divided by 451 [18]. The prognostic power of CPO to predict mortality indicates that a CPO less than 0.6 watts predicts worsening heart failure in patients in a pre-shock state. CPO less than 0.53 watts demonstrated significant mortality in cardiogenic shock [19, 20]. The cardiac assist device selected should be capable of maintaining the CPO above 0.6 watts whenever possible. Additional benefit is provided through the modification of the oxygen supply and demand balance, improving myocardial ischemia. The reduction in myocardial oxygen demand can be estimated using the pressure–volume loop of cardiac function (Figures 21.24 and 21.25). The principal driving pressure of coronary blood flow is the aortic–LV pressure gradient during diastole. Devices that can favorably alter the end-diastolic and end-systolic pressure–volume relationships can decrease myocardial work and provide myocardial protection from ischemia simultaneous with increased myocardial function.

The basic mechanism of the IABP is the diastolic displacement of blood (40–50 mL) during balloon inflation, augmenting mean pressure and diastolic flow, and on balloon deflation, producing afterload reduction. The IABP is a 7 F catheter which is easily inserted using standard femoral puncture technique. IABP inflation at the onset of diastole increases diastolic pressure, which can increase coronary artery perfusion. Balloon deflation at the onset of systole decreases ventricular afterload and hence myocardial oxygen consumption (demand). Both diastolic augmentation and afterload reduction act to increase cardiac output BY approximately 0.2–0.4 L/min. A 20–30% increase in cardiac output in patients with low-output syndromes can be

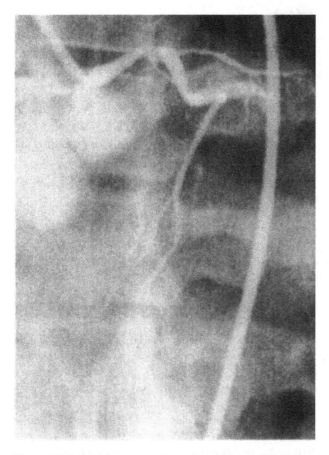

Figure 21.20 The left coronary artery after coronary angioplasty of the left main and proximal circumflex coronary lesions. The left anterior descending artery could not be recanalized.

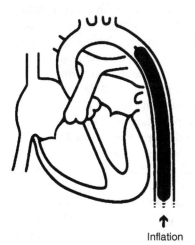

Inflation

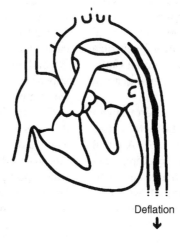

Deflation

Figure 21.21 Intra-aortic balloon pump shown inflated in diastole (left) and deflated during systole (right). *Source:* Kern 1991 [17]. Reproduced with permission of Elsevier.

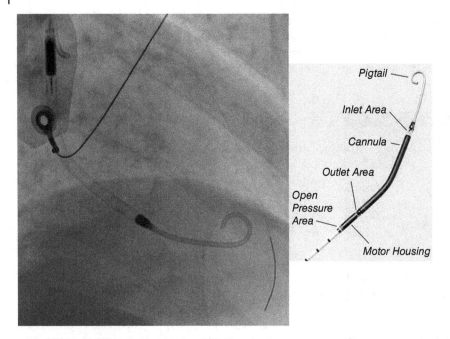

Figure 21.22 (Left) Frame from cineangiogram during percutaneous coronary intervention with the Impella device. The device consists of a single pigtail 12F catheter with inflow positioned in the left ventricle, outflow in the ascending aorta, and an incorporated intravascular axial pump (maximal rotation 51,000 rotations per minute) that can deliver up to 2.5 L/min of continuous flow. (Right) Drawing of the Impella device. *Source:* Naidu 2011 [16].

expected [21, 22]. Direct measurement of coronary blood flow during IABP demonstrates augmentation in nondiseased and patent post-angioplasty vessels, but no increase in vessels with a significant stenosis [23]. All effects are modest at best relative to the Impella and Tandem Heart devices.

The Impella LV support device is an alternative to IABP and full LV 'extra-corporeal' circulatory support (CPS or Tandem Heart). The Impella 2.5 is a 9–13 F catheter-based miniaturized "intracorporeal" LV pump that is placed across the aortic valve and directly unloads the left ventricle, reduces myocardial workload and oxygen consumption, and increases cardiac output and coronary and end-organ perfusion [24]. The micro-axial Archimedes impeller draws blood from the left ventricle through an inflow cannula and delivers nonpulsatile blood flow up to 2.5 L/min into the ascending aorta through an outflow port.

The Impella 2.5 is more complicated to insert than an IABP, but less so than a Tandem Heart. The method uses a 6 F multipurpose catheter placed in the LV. A 0.018 inch stiff guidewire is introduced and the multipurpose catheter is exchanged for the Impella catheter and positioned across the aortic valve and into the left ventricle. The Impella catheter's pigtail tip facilitates safe positioning in the left ventricle. Peripheral vascular disease and aortic valve disease are contraindications to the use of the Impella system.

The Impella simultaneously unloads the LV while increasing aortic pressure [6]. Increased aortic flow and pressure increase flow velocity and decrease coronary microvascular resistance. The Impella-induced increase in coronary flow probably results from both an increased perfusion pressure and a decreased LV pressure–volume relationship. The lower LV pressure facilitates reduced myocardial resistance to coronary flow and reduced end-organ damage.

The Impella device provides benefit through active transport of LV blood continuously into the aorta, with ventricular unloading and coronary flow augmentation well above that of the IABP. The Impella has also been shown to immediately improve overall hemodynamics in cardiogenic shock [25], including cardiac power output [9] and end-organ microcirculation [26]; both results appear to be favorable predictors of 30-day outcomes in acute myocardial infarction with shock [27].

The Tandem Heart percutaneous ventricular assist device is designed for short-term mechanical LV support. The Tandem Heart involves the placement of a 21 F catheter inserted into the left atria from the femoral vein via a transseptal puncture [28]. Blood is withdrawn from the left atrium by an external centrifugal pump and infused into the femoral artery via a 15–17 F catheter. The Tandem Heart can provide up to 4.5 L/min of cardiac support. Because of the large catheter diameter, iliac-femoral angiography must be performed prior to cannula insertion.

(a)

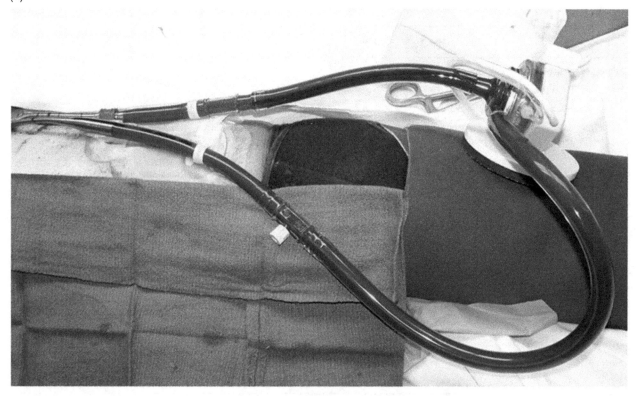

(b)

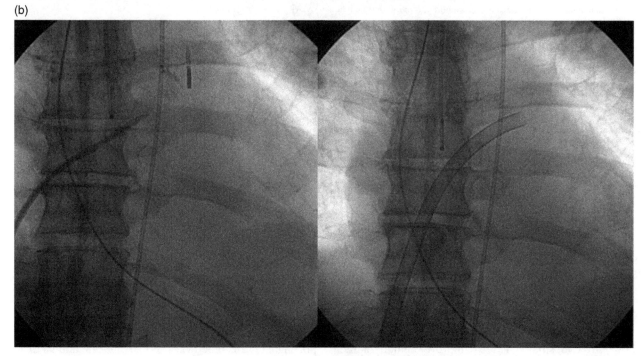

Figure 21.23 (a) Tandem Heart cannula and centripetal pump during hemodynamic support. The blue-tagged cannula draws blood from the left atrium to the pump, which returns it to the femoral artery cannula. (b) Insertion of the Tandem Heart device requires a transseptal puncture (left), dilation of the atrial septum, followed by passage of the large cannula to the left atrium (right).

Table 21.2 Technical features of hemodynamic support devices for the high-risk percutaneous coronary intervention patient.

	Tandem Heart	IABP	Impella
Vascular surgical access	Yes	No	Rarely
Arterial and venous access	Yes	No	No
Cannula/catheter size	15–17 F	7–8 F	13 F
Ease of insertion	Transeptal access required	Standard femoral technique, minimal set-up	LV guidewire exchange, console set-up needed
Ease of removal	Surgical assistance occasionally	Manual compression	Manual compression, surgical assistance occasionally
Cost	High	Low	High

IABP = intra-aortic balloon pump; LV – left ventricle.

Table 21.3 Hemodynamic parameters of cardiac support devices.

	Systolic	Diastolic	MAP	CO augmentation	LV wall stress	Oxygen demand	Coronary blood flow
IABP	–	++	+	0.5 L/min	+	–	+/–
Impella	+	+	+	2.5 L/min	–	– –	+
TH	+	+	++	3.5 L/min	++	+/–	+/–

CO = cardiac output; IABP = intra-aortic balloon pump; LV = left ventricular; MAP = mean arterial pressure; TH = Tandem Heart; + = increase; – = decrease.

Table 21.4 Comparison of IABP, Impella, and Tandem Heart for decisions in the catheterization laboratory.

	Advantages	Disadvantages
Ease of placement	IABP, IMP	TH
Rapidity of insertion	IABP > IMP	TH
Complications	IABP = IMP	TH
Hemodynamic support	IMP > > IABP	IMP < TH
Duration of support	IABP > IMP*	TH
Sheath/catheter size	IABP 7 F	IMP 9–13 F, TH 14 F
Console functions	IMP = IABP = TH	

*Several days of support have been reported.
IABP = intra-aortic balloon pump; IMP = Impella; TH = Tandem Heart device.

Compared with the IABP, the Tandem Heart has been shown in two small trials to improve hemodynamic parameters [29, 30]. However, there is a higher rate of complications with device use, including bleeding, tamponade, and vascular complications. The complexity of its insertion (>30 min in some cases) and higher complication rate compared to the Impella or IABP has limited the use of the Tandem Heart in the high-risk percutaneous coronary intervention patient.

The Tandem Heart mechanism unloads the LV by transporting left atrial blood via a transseptal LA cannula to an external centripetal pump, returning the blood to the femoral artery to maintain pressure, but compromises, to some degree, the intrinsic myocardial work of contraction in overcoming the afterload of supplemented arterial pressure. Nonetheless, as a result of the unloading mechanisms, the Impella and Tandem Heart have the greatest impact on cardiac function and hemodynamic stabilization.

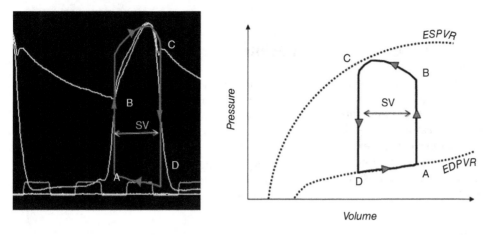

Figure 21.24 (Left) Left ventricular and aortic pressures obtained during cardiac catheterization. (Right) A pressure–volume loop is constructing moving from the initiation of systole, point A. Pressure in the left ventricle (LV) closes the mitral valve and isovolumetric contraction increases pressure, eventually exceeding aortic pressure, point B, when the aortic valve opens. LV ejection continues across systole until repolarization signals the onset of diastole and the LV ceases to eject. LV pressure falls and when below aortic pressure the aortic valve closes, point C. Isovolumetric relaxation occurs, with LV pressure falling to that below the left atrium, point D, at which time the mitral valve opens. The pressure–volume loop is bounded by the end-systolic and end-diastolic pressure–volume relationships, ESPVR and EDPVR. The pressure–volume area (PVA) is defined as the area between the ESPVR and EDPVR bounded by LV ejection (line A–B–C) and is a measure of oxygen consumption per beat. PVA is the sum of stroke work (stroke volume by heart rate, SV*HR) and potential energy (PE). Unloading occurs by reducing the PVA. (*See insert for color representation of the figure.*)

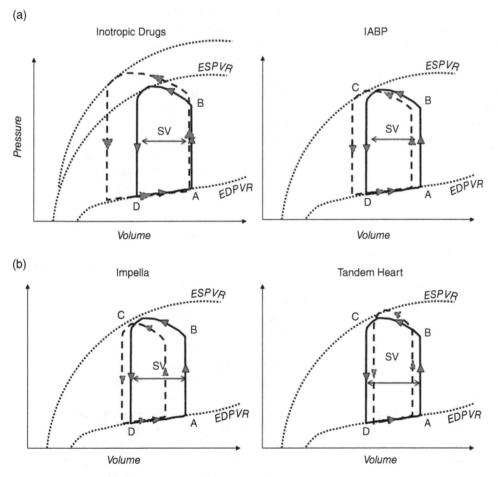

Figure 21.25 (a) Inotropic drugs shift the end-systolic pressure–volume relationship (ESPVR) upward and enlarge the stroke volume (SV) and pressure–volume area (PVA), increasing oxygen demand. The intra-aortic balloon pump (IABP) only minimally shifts the PV loop leftward by reducing afterload, resulting in a modest reduction in PVA and oxygen consumption. (b) Impella shifts the PV loop leftward, decreasing preload, PVA, and oxygen consumption. Tandem Heart decreases preload while also increasing afterload, resulting in modest changes (+/-) in the PVA. EDPVR = end-diastolic pressure–volume relationship. (*See insert for color representation of the figure.*)

Some of the advantages and disadvantages of the IABP, Impella, and Tandem Heart devices are listed in Table 21.4. From the CRISP study [31], one can conclude that if powerful hemodynamic support is needed in the acute myocardial infarction patient, even before the requirement for multiple vasopressors, the early insertion of the Impella device will permit successful completion of the procedure with a reduction of vasoconstrictors, and achieve an acceptable hospital survival rate.

Key Points

1) Heterotopic heart transplant, while now obsolete, demonstrates some of the most interesting and unique hemodynamics showing the influence of synchronous and dysynchronous systolic contraction of the donor heart.
2) Extracorporeal hemodynamic support devices provide unique hemodynamic effects specific for their mechanism of action.

References

1 Kern MJ, Deligonul U, Miller L. Hemodynamic rounds: Interpretation of cardiac pathophysiology from pressure waveform analysis. IV. Extra hearts: Part I. *Cathet Cardiovasc Diagn* 22:197–201, 1990.

2 Melvin KR, Pollick C, Hunt SA, McDougall R, Goris ML, Oyer P, *et al.* Cardiovascular physiology in a case of heterotopic cardiac transplantation. *Am J Cardiol* 49:1301–1307, 1982.

3 Pennington DG, Samuels LD, Williams G, Palmer D, Swartz MT, Codd JE, *et al.* Experience with the Pierce–Donachy ventricular assist device in postcardiotomy patients with cardiogenic shock. *World J Surg* 9:37–46, 1985.

4 Davis PK, Pae WE, Miller CA, Parascandola SA. Myocardial oxygen consumption: Comparison between left atrial pulsatile synchronous and asynchronous bypass. *Trans Am Soc Artif Intern Organs* 35:461–463, 1989.

5 Moulopoulos SD, Topaz S, Kolff WJ. Diastolic balloon pumping (with carbon dioxide) in the aorta: A mechanical assistance to the failing circulation. *Am Heart J* 63:669, 1962.

6 DeBakey ME. Left ventricular bypass pumps for cardiac assistance. *Am J Cardiol* 27:3–11, 1971.

7 Kern MJ, Deligonul U. Hemodynamic rounds: Interpretation of cardiac pathophysiology from pressure waveform analysis. IV. Extra hearts: Part II. *Cathet Cardiovasc Diagn* 22:302–306, 1990.

8 DeBakey ME. Left ventricular bypass pumps for cardiac assistance. *Am J Cardiol* 27:3–11, 1971.

9 Kern MJ, Deligonul U. Hemodynamic rounds: Interpretation of cardiac pathophysiology from pressure waveform analysis. IV. Extra hearts: Part III. *Cathet Cardiovasc Diagn* 23(1):50–53, 1991.

10 Smalling RW, Cassidy DB, Merhige M. Felli PR, Wise GM, Barrett RL, Wampler RD. Improved hemodynamic and left ventricular unloading during acute ischemia using the left ventricular assist device compared to intra-aortic balloon counterpulsation. *J Am Coll Cardiol* 13:160A, 1989 (abstract).

11 Shani J, Hollander G, Nathan I, *et al.* Percutaneous left atrial femoral artery bypass with a pulsatile pump: Initial experience in cardiogenic shock. *J Am Coll Cardiol* J3:53A, 1989 (abstract).

12 Vogel RA, Shawl F, Tommaso C, O'Neill W, Overlie P, O'Toole J, *et al.* Initial report of the National Registry of Elective Cardiopulmonary Bypass Supported Coronary Angioplasty. *J Am Coll Cardiol* 15:23–29, 1990.

13 Shawl FA, Domanski MJ, Wish MH, Davis M. Percutaneous cardiopulmonary bypass support in the catheterization laboratory: Technique and complications. *Am Heart J* 120:195–203, 1990.

14 Stack RK, Pavlides GS, Justeson G, Schreiber TL, O'Neill WW. Hemodynamic and metabolic effects of cardiopulmonary support during PTCA. J Am Col; Cardiol 15:250A, 1990 (abstract).

15 Rose EA, Gelijns AC, Moskowitz AJ, Heitjan DF, Stevenson LW, Dembitsky W, *et al.* Long-term use of left ventricular assist device for end-stage heart failure. *N Engl J Med* 345:1435–1443, 2001.

16 Naidu H. Novel percutaneous cardiac assist devices: The science of and indications for hemodynamic support. *Circulation* 123:533–543, 2011.

17 Kern MJ. *The Cardiac Catheterization Handbook*, 5th ed. Philadelphia, PA: Elsevier, 2011.

18 Mendoza DD, Cooper HA, Panza JA. Cardiac power output predicts mortality across a broad spectrum of patients with acute cardiac disease. *Am Heart J* 153(3):366–370, 2007.

19 Fincke R, Menon V, Slater JN, Webb JG, *et al.* Cardiac power is the strongest hemodynamic correlate of mortality in cardiogenic shock: A report from the SHOCK trial registry. *J Am Coll Cardiol* 44(2):340–348, 2004.

20 Torgerson C, Schmittinger CA, Wagner S, Ulmer H, Takala J, Jakob SM, Dünser MW. Hemodynamic variables and mortality in cardiogenic shock: A retrospective cohort study. *Crit Care* 13(5):R157, 2009.

21 Sjauw KD, Engström AE, Vis MM, van der Schaaf RJ, Baan J Jr, Koch KT, *et al.* A systematic review and

meta-analysis of intra aortic balloon pump therapy in ST-elevation myocardial infarction: Should we change the guidelines? *Eur Heart J* 30(4):459–468, 2009.

22 Perera D, Stables R, Thomas M, Booth J, Pitt M, Blackman D, *et al.* Elective intra-aortic balloon counterpulsation during high-risk percutaneous coronary intervention: A randomized controlled trial. *JAMA* 304:867–874, 2010.

23 Kern MJ, Aguirre F, Bach R, Donohue T, Segal J. Augmentation of coronary blood flow by intra-aortic balloon pumping in patients after coronary angioplasty. *Circulation* 87:500–511, 1993.

24 Reesink KD, Dekker AL, Van Ommen V, Soemers C, Geskes GG, van der Veen FH, Maessen JG. Miniature intracardiac assist device provides more effective cardiac unloading and circulatory support during severe left heart failure than intra-aortic balloon pumping. *Chest* 126(3):896–902, 2004.

25 Seyfarth M, Sibbing D, Bauer I, Fröhlich G, Bott-Flügel L, Byrne R, Dirschinger J, *et al.* A randomized clinical trial to evaluate the safety and efficacy of a percutaneous left ventricular assist device versus intra-aortic balloon pumping for treatment of cardiogenic shock caused by myocardial infarction. *J Am Coll Cardiol* 52(19):1584–1588, 2008.

26 Meyns B, Stolinski J, Leunens V, Verbeken E, Flameng W. Left ventricular support by catheter-mounted axial flow pump reduces infarct size. *J Am Coll Cardiol* 41(7):1087–1095, 2003.

27 Remmelink M, Sjauw KD, Henriques JP, de Winter RJ, Vis MM, Koch KT, *et al.* Effects of mechanical left ventricular unloading by Impella on left ventricular dynamics in high-risk and primary percutaneous coronary intervention patients. *Catheter Cardiovasc Interv* 75(2):187–194, 2010.

28 Vranckx P, Meliga E, De Jaegere PP, Van den Ent M, Regar ES, Serruys PW. The Tandem Heart, percutaneous transseptal left ventricular assist device: A safeguard in high-risk percutaneous coronary interventions: The six-year Rotterdam experience. *Eurointervention* 4:331–337, 2008.

29 Kovacic J, Nguyen HT, Karajgikar R, Sharma SK, Kini AS. The Impella Recover 2.5 and Tandem Heart ventricular assist devices are safe and associated with equivalent clinical outcomes in patients undergoing high-risk percutaneous coronary intervention. *Catheter Cardiovasc Interv* 82(1):E28–E37, 2011.

30 Thiele H, Sick P, Boudriot E, Diederich KW, Hambrecht R, Niebauer J, Schuler G. Randomized comparison of intra-aortic balloon support with a percutaneous left ventricular assist device in patients with revascularized acute myocardial infarction complicated by cardiogenic shock. *Eur Heart J* 26:1276–1283, 2005.

31 Patel MR, Smalling RW, Thiele H, Barnhart HX, Zhou Y, Chandra P, *et al.* Intra-aortic balloon counterpulsation and infarct size in patients with acute anterior myocardial infarction without shock: The CRISP AMI randomized trial. *JAMA* 306(12):1329–1337, 2011.

22

Invasive Hemodynamic Assessment of Shock and Use of Mechanical Support for Acute Left and Right Ventricular Failure

Ivan D. Hanson and James A. Goldstein

Shock is a life-threatening clinical condition. Rapid identification of the mechanisms contributing to hemodynamic compromise is essential because (i) if not treated expeditiously, shock often leads to death; (ii) its management varies depending on the cause; and (iii) management for one etiology may be deleterious for another.

Shock evaluation is based on the two keys of establishing the etiology and assessing the hemodynamic status, processes which proceed concurrently and immediately:

1) *Hemodynamic assessment*: Immediate bedside assessment of hemodynamic status serves as the foundation of emergency management. Physical examination stratifies the patient by hemodynamic subset (Table 22.1). Hemodynamic classification can be further refined by invasive assessment with right-heart catheterization. Whereas this is not typically necessary or appropriate in cases of clinically obvious hypovolemic or septic shock, it is critical for all cases of cardiogenic shock. Cardiogenic shock is defined as systemic tissue hypoperfusion secondary to inadequate cardiac output despite adequate circulatory volume and ventricular filling pressure. The usual diagnostic criteria include a systolic blood pressure (BP) less than 90 mm Hg for more than 30 min; a drop in mean arterial BP more than 30 mm Hg below baseline, with a cardiac index (CI) less than 1.8 L/min/m^2 without hemodynamic support or less than 2.2 L/min/m^2 with support, and elevated ventricular filling pressure (right atrial [RA], pulmonary capillary wedge [PCW], or both) [1].

2) *Etiology*: It is axiomatic that rapid steps must be taken to establish the etiology of hemodynamic instability. The etiology may in some cases be clear by careful history, physical examination, and simple noninvasive testing (electrocardiography [ECG], chest X-ray [CXR], etc.), which may confirm causes such as hypovolemic shock or acute myocardial infarction. However, further assessment is often necessary, including urgent noninvasive evaluation (e.g., ECG, computed tomography [CT], etc.) and invasive assessment (i.e., coronary angiography, invasive hemodynamics).

The following cases illustrate principles of evaluation and strategies for management of complex cardiogenic shock.

Case #1

A 62-year-old man with coronary artery disease and peripheral arterial disease presented with non-ST elevation myocardial infarction. Left ventricular (LV) ejection fraction was 30%, with multiple regional wall motion abnormalities. Coronary angiography revealed culprit severe stenosis in left anterior descending (LAD) artery, and chronic total occlusions of distal right coronary and obtuse marginal arteries. Drug-eluting stenting of LAD artery was performed, with good angiographic result. The patient was discharged against medical advice the following day. One day later, he suffered cardiac arrest. An ECG revealed anterolateral ST elevation myocardial infarction. Blood pressure was 60 mm Hg systolic, with a heart rate of 110 beats/min. BP improved to 80 mm Hg systolic after vasopressors were initiated. The patient was obtunded, but followed commands. His extremities were cold, and lung examination revealed diffuse crackles. Jugular venous pressure was elevated. He was electively intubated and mechanical ventilation was instituted. A limited echocardiogram revealed a LV ejection fraction of 10%, with normal right ventricular (RV) size and function.

The patient was immediately triaged to the catheterization laboratory. Coronary angiography revealed hazy filling defect in LAD, consistent with in-stent thrombosis. Before intervention was undertaken, mechanical support was instituted with Impella CP (Abiomed, Danvers, MA) via a 14 F introducer sheath inserted in

Hemodynamic Rounds: Interpretation of Cardiac Pathophysiology from Pressure Waveform Analysis, Fourth Edition.
Edited by Morton J. Kern, Michael J. Lim, and James A. Goldstein.
© 2018 John Wiley & Sons Ltd. Published 2018 by John Wiley & Sons Ltd.

Table 22.1 Summary of clinical and invasive hemodynamic characteristics of the various etiologies of shock.

	Extremities	JVP	Lungs	Heart	Invasive hemodynamics				
					CVP	PCW	PA	CO	SVR
Hemorrhagic or hypovolemic	Cool, no edema	↓	Clear	Flow murmur	↓	↓	↓	↑	↑
Distributive	Warm, no edema	↓	May be wet if pneumonia, ARDS, etc.	May be abnormal if IE	↓	↓	↓	↑	↓
Cardiogenic (left-heart failure)	Cool, +/− edema	↑	Wet	Abnormal	↑	↑↑	↑	↓	↑
Cardiogenic (right-heart failure)	Cool, +/− edema	↑↑	Clear	RV heave	↑↑	↔	↔	↓	↑

ARDS = acute respiratory distress syndrome; CO = cardiac output; CVP = central venous pressure; IE = infective endocarditis; JVP = jugular venous pressure; PA = pulmonary artery; PCW = pulmonary capillary wedge pressure; RV = right ventricular; SVR = systemic vascular resistance.
↑increased or augmented value, ↓decreased or diminished value, ↔ no change or unaffected.

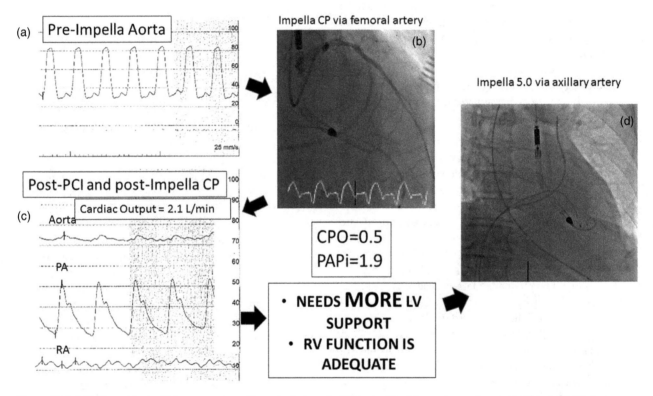

Figure 22.1 (a) Left ventricular (LV) pressure recording prior to Impella CP implant is abnormal, revealing reduced systolic pressure, blunted systolic upstroke, and elevated end-diastolic pressure. (b) After Impella CP insertion and revascularization of occluded left anterior descending artery, (c) hemodynamics were obtained. Given the inadequate cardiac power due to left ventricular failure and preserved right ventricular (RV) function, (d) the Impella CP catheter was exchanged for an Impella 5.0. CPO = cardiac power output; PA = pulmonary artery pressure; PAPi = pulmonary artery pulsatility index; RA = right atrial pressure.

the left femoral artery (somewhat difficult owing to severe peripheral arterial disease). LV pressure prior to insertion of Impella CP is shown in Figure 22.1. The reduced systolic BP, marked elevation in LV end-diastolic pressure, echocardiographic evidence of acute on chronic LV systolic dysfunction, and acute occlusion of LAD satisfied diagnostic criteria for cardiogenic shock

due to ischemic LV failure. Additional hemodynamic evaluation at that time was not necessary, particularly given the emergent need to revascularize the occluded LAD. Intravascular ultrasound revealed subtle dissection at the distal stent edge, which was treated with an overlapping drug-eluting stent. Repeat intravascular ultrasound revealed a well-expanded and well-apposed stent

Table 22.2 Hemodynamic data in patient with cardiogenic shock from acute ischemic left ventricular systolic dysfunction.

	Baseline	Impella CP	Impella 5.0
RA (mm Hg)		13	10
PA (mm Hg)		52/27	40/20
PAPi		1.9	2.0
PCWP (mm Hg)		30	25
Ao (MAP, mm Hg)	72/53 (58)	75/75 (75)	115/90 (100)
CO (L/min)		3.2	4.0
CI (L/min/m^2)		1.5	1.9
CPO (watts)		0.5	0.9

Ao = aortic pressure; CI = cardiac index; CO = cardiac output; CPO = cardiac power output (see text for definition); MAP = mean arterial pressure; PA = pulmonary artery; PAPi = pulmonary artery pulsatility index; PCWP = pulmonary capillary wedge pressure; RA = right atrium. Cardiac output and cardiac index were calculated using the Fick method.

in LAD, with improved flow in the distal vessel. Following coronary intervention, additional hemodynamic measurements were obtained (Table 22.2). At an augmented flow rate of 3.5 L/min with the Impella CP catheter, the mean aortic pressure was 75 mm Hg, with minimal pulse pressure. Cardiac power output (CPO) was 0.5 watts. Pulmonary artery pulsatility index (PAPi) was 2.0. Based on these measurements, it was elected to increase LV support with implantation of Impella 5.0 (Abiomed, Danvers, MA) (Figure 22.1).

The patient was transferred to the operating room, where the right axially artery was exposed by surgical cutdown. One end of a 10 mm Dacron graft was sewn into the axillary artery, and a 23 F sheath was affixed to the other end. The Impella 5.0 catheter was advanced into the left ventricle over a guidewire inserted via the axillary artery sheath. The Impella CP catheter was then removed. The Impella 5.0 catheter generated 4.5 L/min of forward flow. The mean aortic pressure increased from 75 to 90 mm Hg, with some return of pulsatility. The cardiac power output increased to 0.9 watts. The right atrial pressure increased from 13 to 20 mm Hg, with some decrement in PAPi. With institution of continuous veno-venous hemodialysis and fluid removal, the right atrial pressure gradually declined to 12 mm Hg. Blood pressure further improved to 110/70 mm Hg. The Impella 5.0 device was successfully weaned and explanted after two weeks.

Case #2

A 61-year-old man with chronic, severe mitral regurgitation and heart failure manifesting as progressive exertional dyspnea, orthopnea, and lower-extremity edema

presented to an outside institution for diagnosis and management. The electrocardiogram revealed atrial fibrillation with rapid ventricular response. The ECG documented severe left atrial enlargement, LV ejection fraction of 40%, severe degenerative mitral regurgitation with posterior leaflet prolapse, and mild dilation of the right-heart chambers. Coronary angiography revealed nonobstructive coronary artery disease. During heart catheterization, the patient developed cardiac arrest, hypoxic respiratory failure, and shock, requiring emergent airway intubation and institution of vasopressor support. Hemodynamics failed to recover after initiation of high-dose vasopressor support and insertion of an intra-aortic balloon pump (IABP). The patient was emergently transferred to our institution for further management. Given the available clinical information, the presumptive diagnosis was that the patient had acute mitral regurgitation (MR) leading to pulmonary edema and shock.

In our catheterization laboratory, the patient was unresponsive, cool, and clammy. Noninvasive blood pressure was unobtainable. Bilateral femoral venous and arterial access was obtained. In anticipation of Impella CP implantation, LV pressure was recorded (Figure 22.2). There was no transaortic gradient. Note the left ventricular pressure. Unlike in Case #1, LV end-diastolic pressure was relatively low. Given marked hemodynamic instability, it was elected to institute mechanical support in lieu of obtaining additional hemodynamic data at that time. After uneventful insertion of Impella CP and removal of the IABP, mean central aortic pressure declined to 40 mm Hg. Flow augmentation with the Impella catheter was minimal. Right-heart catheterization was performed via the left femoral vein. Based on the hemodynamic data in Table 22.3, it was decided to institute RV hemodynamic support. Via the right femoral vein, an Impella RP was inserted (Figure 22.2). Flow from the Impella RP was 2.7–3.2 L/min. Flow from the Impella CP was 2.4–3.3 L/min. There was a marked improvement in systemic blood pressure.

In the cardiac intensive care unit, a transesophageal echocardiogram demonstrated markedly reduced LV and RV systolic function and posterior mitral valve leaflet flail, with severe mitral regurgitation. Because of anuric renal failure, contrast computed tomography to evaluate pulmonary embolism was deferred, but a lower-extremity venous duplex revealed right leg deep vein thrombosis (DVT). Systemic heparin was initiated. The patient developed intravascular hemolysis, and the Impella CP was replaced with IABP. Eventually, the IABP was weaned and hemodynamics remained stable, with complete recovery of neurologic and renal function. The patient ultimately underwent successful

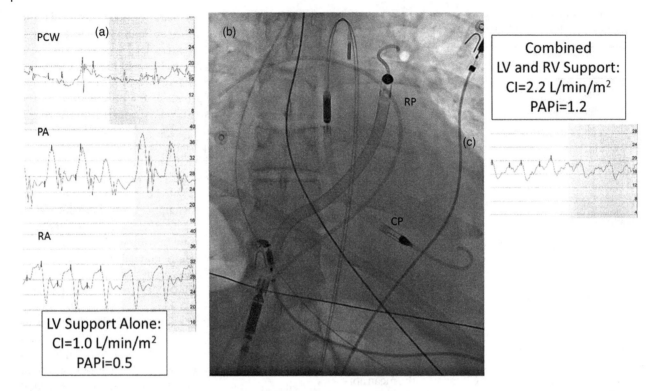

Figure 22.2 (a) Invasive hemodynamics immediately following implantation of Impella CP. (b) Given evidence of right ventricular failure, Impella RP was inserted, resulting in improved cardiac output and reduced right atrial (RA) pressure (c). CI = cardiac index; LV = left ventricular; PA = pulmonary artery pressure; PAPi = pulmonary artery pulsatility index; PCW = pulmonary capillary wedge pressure; RV = right ventricular.

Table 22.3 Hemodynamic data in patient with biventricular heart failure treated with various combinations of mechanical support.

	Immediately following LV support	Immediately following LV and RV support	IABP and Impella RP	IABP alone
RA (mm Hg)	30	14	5	4
PA (mm Hg)	40/25	35/18	40/18	44/18
PAPi	0.5	1.2	4.4	6.5
PCWP (mm Hg)	16	17	18	15
CO (L/min)	2.10	4.9	5.2	8.4
CI (L/min/m²)	1.05	2.2	2.4	3.9

CI = cardiac index; CO = cardiac output; IABP = intra-aortic balloon pump; LV = left ventricular; PA = pulmonary artery; PAPi = pulmonary artery pulsatility index; PCWP = pulmonary capillary wedge pressure; RA = right atrium; RV = right ventricular. Cardiac output and cardiac index were calculated using the Fick method.

mitral valve replacement using a tissue prosthesis and was discharged in stable condition. At the one-year follow-up visit, he had no signs or symptoms of congestive heart failure. An echocardiogram revealed moderately reduced LV ejection fraction, mildly reduced RV ejection fraction, and a normally functioning prosthetic mitral valve.

Discussion

Shock Due to Acute Left Ventricular Failure

Case #1 illustrates profound LV failure in the setting of acute myocardial infarction. The clinical examination is consistent with this diagnosis. The presence of hypotension, cold extremities, and pulmonary edema is highly suggestive. The mortality rate of cardiogenic shock in the setting of acute myocardial infarction is 50%, and has not significantly changed in recent years [2]. Cardiac power output, expressed in watts, is easily calculated by multiplying mean systemic blood pressure by cardiac output and dividing by a constant, 451: CPO = (MAP x CO)/451. A CPO of 0.53 watts was shown to most accurately predict in-hospital mortality compared to a host of other hemodynamic parameters. The probability of in-hospital mortality with a CPO less than or equal to 0.53 watts was 58%, whereas the probability of survival given a CPO greater than 0.53 watts was 71% [3]. The IABP does not substantially augment cardiac power. In contrast, the left-heart Impella catheters (2.5, CP, 5.0) both unload the LV and directly augment cardiac power [4]. The left-heart Impella is an inline axial flow pump that aspirates blood from the LV and ejects it into the aorta, thereby directly unloading the ventricle and actively generating cardiac power output. The Impella 2.5 and CP catheters are designed for femoral insertion via 13 F and 14 F peel-away sheaths, respectively. The Impella 5.0 requires a 23 F sheath for implantation, so insertion usually requires surgical cutdown in the axillary artery, but the device can also be inserted percutaneously via transcaval access [5]. Although the Impella has never been shown to improve mortality in cardiogenic shock in a randomized trial, outcomes are more favorable when support is instituted prior to, rather than after, primary percutaneous intervention in shock due to acute myocardial infarction [6]. This suggests a link between time to support and survival, but this hypothesis requires further investigation.

The patient in Case #1 developed shock due to LV pump dysfunction upon presentation with stent thrombosis in LAD, the last remaining conduit for coronary blood flow. The lack of discernible aortic pulse pressure signified markedly reduced stroke volume. Furthermore, CPO was calculated to be 0.5 watts. Right ventricular function was deemed adequate, given the preserved RV function on echocardiography and finding of PAPi greater than 1.5 (see discussion of Case #2 for the calculation and validation of PAPi). Escalation to the Impella 5.0 resulted in a dramatic improvement in systemic blood pressure and cardiac output, and this hemodynamic "bridge" likely aborted multisystem organ failure long enough for the patient to be transferred for advanced heart failure therapy with an implantable left ventricular assist device (LVAD). Unfortunately, the patient suffered embolic strokes, likely a result of plaque disruption in the aortic arch and its major branches during insertion of the large-bore Impella devices.

Shock Due to Acute Right-Heart Failure and Biventricular Failure

Shock due to predominant acute right-heart failure may be identified by the clinical findings of hypotension; low cardiac output; compensatory increase in systemic vascular resistance, often manifesting as cool, clammy extremities; clear lungs, signifying normal left ventricular filling pressure; and elevated jugular venous pressure, signifying increased RV preload. Acute RV failure is most commonly attributable to decreased contractility, as in patients with acute inferior myocardial infarction with RV involvement (RVI), post-LVAD implantation, or post-cardiotomy after any cardiac surgical procedure. Acute RV failure is often seen as a result of acute pressure overload due to pulmonary emboli. Less common is acute right-heart valve insufficiency (e.g., acute tricuspid valve regurgitation). Echocardiography provides supportive evidence of RV failure, characterized by RV dilation, depressed RV free wall motion, and diminished RV ejection fraction [7]. The RV may be larger than the LV (RV:LV end-diastolic area ratio > 0.6) and there is often reverse septal curvature. Invasive hemodynamics may further characterize the basis of RV failure. It is important to consider that RV failure often co-exists with and may be a consequence of left-heart failure, whether from primary myocardial or left-heart valve disease. Although the working diagnosis of the patient in Case #2 was acute MR leading to shock, the history of more chronic heart failure symptoms and finding of an enlarged left atrium suggested that MR was more chronic. The finding of only mildly elevated LV diastolic pressure further supports the chronic duration of MR. The cause of hemodynamic collapse refractory to the IABP is unclear, since invasive hemodynamics were not assessed during the index catheterization procedure. Perhaps the contrast load from angiography led to overwhelming biventricular failure. Alternatively, the patient may have had a pulmonary embolism (deep vein thrombosis was identified by duplex ultrasound, but never confirmed by CT angiography).

There are several interesting observations after the Impella CP was implanted. First, right-heart failure developed acutely after the institution of left-heart support. In the setting of acute RV dysfunction, the RV free wall is unable to contribute to stroke work, RV systolic performance, or maintenance of forward flow into the pulmonary artery, and ultimate delivery of stroke volume across the lungs to the left heart is dependent on LV–septal contractile contributions via systolic interactions mediated by the septum [8–10]. When the LV is decompressed, the interventricular septum shifts toward the left ventricle, which may impair its contribution to RV performance. This, combined with increased RV preload in the setting of increased venous return with the LVAD, creates the "perfect storm" of acute RV dysfunction and hemodynamic compromise.

Acute RV failure is a recognized complication of both percutaneous and implantable LVAD [11–13] and is associated with poor outcome [12]. The incidence of this complication is 20–25% [14]. The Impella RP was designed to offer temporary "active" right-heart support and its efficacy has been demonstrated in patients suffering RV shock attributable to RVI, post-cardiotomy, and post-LVAD. The RECOVER-RIGHT study included 30 patients with acute RV failure treated with the Impella RP; 18 patients had acute RV failure complicating implantable LVAD implantation [15]. In this cohort, survival to 30 days or hospital discharge was 83.3%. In contrast, in the subset of patients treated with the Impella RP for acute RV failure due to cardiotomy or acute myocardial infarction, survival was 58.3%. A ratio of central venous pressure to pulmonary capillary wedge pressure greater than 0.63, need for pre-operative mechanical ventilation, and blood urea nitrogen level greater than 39 mg/dL are recognized predictors of RV failure after LVAD implantation [12]. The pulmonary artery pulsatility index may be the most accurate predictor of RV failure after LVAD [16], and can be easily calculated using commonly collected hemodynamic parameters as follows: PAPi = (systolic pulmonary artery pressure – diastolic pulmonary artery pressure) / mean right atrial pressure.

Conclusion

In summary, most patients with cardiogenic shock should be managed with invasive hemodynamics, which provide crucial prognostic and anatomic information. Support with Impella for both left-heart failure and right-heart failure may result in dramatic hemodynamic improvement, but only if guided by appropriate invasive data.

Key Points

1) There are many potential etiologies of shock, and the astute clinician must take into account physical examination, noninvasive assessment by echocardiography, and invasive hemodynamic data to establish the precise diagnosis.
2) Invasive hemodynamics are often needed to fully characterize the presence and extent of dysfunction attributable to the left ventricle, right ventricle, or both.
3) Accurate diagnosis guides optimal hemodynamic support.

References

1 Rihal CS, Naidu SS, Givertz MM, Szeto WY, Burke JA, Kapur NK, *et al.* 2015 SCAI/ACC/HFSA/STS Clinical Expert Consensus Statement on the Use of Percutaneous Mechanical Circulatory Support Devices in Cardiovascular Care: Endorsed by the American Heart Assocation, the Cardiological Society of India, and Sociedad Latino Americana de Cardiologia Intervencion; Affirmation of Value by the Canadian Association of Interventional Cardiology-Association Canadienne de Cardiologie d'intervention. *J Am Coll Cardiol* 65(19):e7–e26, 2015.

2 Puymirat E, Fagon JY, Aegerter P, Diehl JL, Monnier A, Hauw-Berlemont C, *et al.* Cardiogenic shock in intensive care units: Evolution of prevalence, patient profile, management and outcomes, 1997–2012. *Eur J Heart Fail* 19(2):192–220, 2017.

3 Fincke R, Hochman JS, Lowe AM, Menon V, Slater JN, Webb JG, *et al.* Cardiac power is the strongest hemodynamic correlate of mortality in cardiogenic shock: A report from the SHOCK trial registry. *J Am Coll Cardiol* 44(2):340–348, 2004.

4 Seyfarth M, Sibbing D, Bauer I, Fröhlich G, Bott-Flügel L, Byrne R, *et al.* A randomized clinical trial to evaluate the safety and efficacy of a percutaneous left ventricular assist device versus intra-aortic balloon pumping for treatment of cardiogenic shock caused by myocardial infarction. *J Am Coll Cardiol* 52(19):1584–1588, 2008.

5 Frisoli TM, Guerrero M, O'Neill WW. Mechanical circulatory support with Impella to facilitate percutaneous coronary intervention for post-TAVI bilateral coronary obstruction. *Catheter Cardiovasc Interv* 88(1):E34–E37, 2016.

6 O'Neill WW, Schreiber T, Wohns DH, Rihal C, Naidu SS, Civitello AB, *et al.* The current use of Impella 2.5 in acute myocardial infarction complicated by cardiogenic shock: Results from the USpella Registry. *J Interv Cardiol* 27(1):1–11, 2014.

7 Goldstein JA. Pathophysiology and management of right heart ischemia. *J Am Coll Cardiol* 40(5):841–853, 2002.

8 Goldstein JA, Barzilai B, Rosamond TL, Eisenberg PR, Jaffe AS. Determinants of hemodynamic compromise with severe right ventricular infarction. *Circulation* 82(2):359–368, 1990.

9 Goldstein JA, Tweddell JS, Barzilai E, Yagi Y, Jaffe AS, Cox JL. Importance of left ventricular function and systolic ventricular interaction to right ventricular performance during acute right heart ischemia. *J Am Coll Cardiol* 19(3):704–711, 1992.

10 Goldstein JA, Harada A, Yagi Y, Barzilai B, Cox JL. Hemodynamic importance of systolic ventricular interaction, augmented right atrial contractility and atrioventricular synchrony in acute right ventricular dysfunction. *J Am Coll Cardiol* 16(1):181–189, 1990.

11 Kapur NK, Jumean M, Ghuloom A, Aghili N, Vassallo C, Kiernan MS, *et al.* First successful use of 2 axial flow catheters for percutaneous biventricular circulatory support as a bridge to a durable left ventricular assist device. *Circ Heart Fail* 8(5):1006–1008, 2015.

12 Kormos RL, Teuteberg JJ, Pagani FD, Russell SD, John R, Miller LW, *et al.* Right ventricular failure in patients with the HeartMate II continuous-flow left ventricular assist device: Incidence, risk factors, and effect on outcomes. *J Thorac Cardiovasc Surg* 139(5): 1316–1324, 2010.

13 Barbone A, Holmes JW, Heerdt PM, The' AH, Naka Y, Joshi N, *et al.* Comparison of right and left ventricular responses to left ventricular assist device support in patients with severe heart failure: A primary role of mechanical unloading underlying reverse remodeling. *Circulation* 104(6):670–675, 2001.

14 McIlvennan CK, Magid KH, Ambardekar AV, Thompson JS, Matlock DD, Allen LA. Clinical outcomes after continuous-flow left ventricular assist device: A systematic review. *Circ Heart Fail* 7(6):1003–1013, 2014.

15 Anderson MB, Goldstein J, Milano C, Morris LD, Kormos RL, Bhama J, *et al.* Benefits of a novel percutaneous ventricular assist device for right heart failure: The prospective RECOVER RIGHT study of the Impella RP device. *J Heart Lung Transplant* 34(12):1549–1560, 2015.

16 Morine KJ, Kiernan MS, Pham DT, Paruchuri V, Denofrio D, Kapur NK. Pulmonary artery pulsatility index is associated with right ventricular failure after left ventricular assist device surgery. *J Card Fail* 22(2):110–116, 2016.

Part Six

Clinical and Bedside Applications of Hemodynamics

23

An Anatomic-Pathophysiologic Approach to Hemodynamic Assessment

James A. Goldstein

Symptoms and physical signs reflect distinct pathophysiologic derangements of anatomic components and mechanics, a construct which serves as the foundation for clinical evaluation of the cardiovascular system. This chapter outlines an approach to the evaluation of cardiac symptoms and signs based on interrogation of a cardiac anatomic-physiologic approach to circulatory pathophysiology, employing bedside examination integrated with invasive hemodynamic assessment.

Clinical-Anatomic-Pathophysiologic Correlations to Symptom Assessment

Pathophysiologic derangements of cardiac anatomic components manifest "cardinal" cardiovascular symptoms, most of which are reflected as distinct hemodynamic disturbances. These symptomatic-hemodynamic constellations include (i) dyspnea, reflecting pulmonary venous congestion; (ii) fatigue, attributable to inadequate cardiac output; (iii) syncope, resulting from transient profound hypotension; and (iv) peripheral edema, related to systemic venous congestion. Chest pain typically suggesting ischemia does not usually result directly from primary hemodynamic derangements, and does not lend itself to this anatomic-pathophysiologic hemodynamic approach, so will not be addressed in these discussions.

It is important to emphasize that these symptom groups in isolation are nonspecific. Identical complaints reflecting disparate pathophysiologic processes can occur due to a variety of mechanisms. For example, dyspnea is an expected symptomatic manifestation of pulmonary venous hypertension attributable to a spectrum of left-heart derangements, the underlying mechanisms of which vary greatly (e.g., mitral stenosis, mitral regurgitation, left ventricular cardiomyopathy, etc.).

The treatments and prognoses also vary greatly. Dyspnea is also commonly of pulmonary origin, with circumstances in which the heart may be completely normal or impacted only as innocent bystander (e.g., cor pulmonale). Similarly, peripheral edema and ascites reflect systemic venous congestion resulting from a spectrum of right-heart failure mechanisms (e.g., tricuspid valve disease, right ventricular cardiomyopathies, pericardial disorders, etc.). However, edema may also develop under conditions with normal systemic venous pressures, as may occur in patients with cirrhotic liver disease, inferior vena caval (IVC) compression, and so on. Thus, for cardiovascular assessment, symptoms and signs must be characterized according to the underlying anatomic-pathophysiologic mechanisms, the next step to delineating the specific etiological entity.

Cardiac Anatomy, Mechanical Function, and Hemodynamics

To establish an anatomic-pathophysiologic differential diagnosis, it is essential first to consider the anatomic cardiac components (myocardium, valves, arteries, pericardium, and conduction tissue) that may be involved, and then to focus on the fundamental mechanisms that impact each anatomic component, finally asking how such anatomic-pathophysiologic derangements and hemodynamic perturbations are reflected in the symptoms, physical signs, and invasive waveforms.

The purpose of the cardiovascular system is to generate cardiac output to perfuse the body. However, although perfusion is the heart's "bottom line," the circulation is also a pressure-based system, with organ perfusion determined by arterial driving pressure modulated by vascular bed resistance. The regulation of the circulation (pressure and flow) can be understood by the application

Hemodynamic Rounds: Interpretation of Cardiac Pathophysiology from Pressure Waveform Analysis, Fourth Edition.
Edited by Morton J. Kern, Michael J. Lim, and James A. Goldstein.

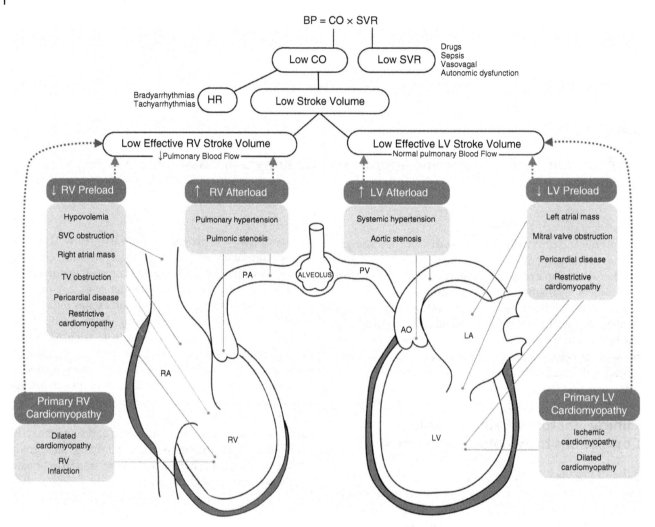

Figure 23.1 Anatomic pathophysiologic approach to evaluation of low cardiac output and hypotension. AO = aorta; BP = blood pressure; CO = cardiac output; HR = heart rate; LA = left atrium; LV = left ventricle; PA = pulmonary artery; PV = pulmonary vein; RA = right atrium; RV = right ventricle; SVR = systemic vascular resistance; TV = tricuspid valve.

of Ohm's law. In classical physics applied to an electrical circuit, Ohm's law states:

$$\Delta V = I \times R$$

where ΔV is the driving voltage potential difference across the circuit, I the current flow, and R the circuit resistance. Circuit output or current flow thus is a function of the "driving" voltage divided by circuit resistance or $I = \Delta V/R$.

Ohm's law applied to the cardiac circulation translates to Blood pressure = Cardiac output (CO) x Systemic vascular resistance (SVR) and can be applied to the systemic circulation or to individual organ beds. The key components of blood pressure can be further considered. Thus, CO = Heart rate (HR) x Stroke volume (SV). Further, SV is a function of three cardiac mechanisms: preload, afterload, and contrac-

tility. Systemic vascular resistance is determined by total blood volume and vascular tone (a function of intrinsic vessel contraction or relaxation interacting with systemic and local neuro-hormonal influences, metabolic factors, other vasomotor mediators, and so on; Figure 23.1).

Pertinent Aspects of Cardiac Mechanics

The hemodynamic evaluation of the circulation may be considered as two sides of a single coin of cardiac function: systolic function, the ability of the heart to pump and perfuse; and diastolic performance, the ability of the chambers to fill at physiologic pressures with the preload necessary to generate SV.

Systolic Performance

Systolic function reflects the ability of the ventricle to contract and generate stroke work, a function determined by its loading conditions (both preload and afterload) and the contractile state. Systolic dysfunction then develops due to primary derangements of volume overload, pressure overload, or cardiomyopathic processes. It is important to distinguish depression of systolic performance due to pressure/volume overload from primary "contractile failure" related to cardiomyopathy with damage to the contractile apparatus (e.g., ischemic or nonischemic cardiomyopathies). Systolic dysfunction reduces SV, leading to low CO, resulting in fatigue and, in the most severe stages, organ hypoperfusion and finally hypotension.

Diastolic Function and Cardiac Compliance

Diastolic function is the ability of a chamber to obtain its necessary preload at physiologic filling pressures. Functional preload is the amount of blood actually distending the cardiac chamber. This volume is reflected in filling pressure according to individual chamber compliance. Compliance is a reflection of the relationship between diastolic pressure and volume in each individual cardiac chamber. Measurement of intracardiac filling pressures (for example pressure at end-diastole) is used for two basic purposes: (i) to determine whether there is elevated pressure exerting adverse congestive effects; and (ii) to check whether preload is adequate to assist with appropriate forward ejection. With respect to assessing true preload, pressure is a convenient surrogate of chamber volume, which is exquisitely influenced by the compliance of the chamber being interrogated. Therefore, filling pressure reasonably reflects chamber volume and preload only if chamber compliance is normal. However, impaired compliance, attributable either to extrinsic influences such as pericardial disease or ventricular interaction, or intrinsic diastolic dysfunction associated with hypertrophy, infiltration, or ischemia, or primary pressure and volume overload, will influence compliance. In such cases pressure less accurately reflects true chamber volume. For example, left ventricular (LV) preload may be markedly reduced but intracardiac pressures strikingly elevated under conditions of cardiac tamponade or severe pulmonary hypertension. Conversely, chronic volume overload lesion such as aortic regurgitation may result in dramatically increased chamber volumes, but when cardiac compensation is present intracardiac pressures are relatively normal, as chamber and pericardium dilate and become more compliant.

Diastolic function is influenced by myriad factors, including the intrinsic physical properties of the chamber (thickness, ischemia, infiltration, fibrosis, etc.), as well as extrinsic factors including septal-mediated ventricular interactions, pericardial pressure, and intrapleural pressure. Diastolic dysfunction results in abnormal chamber compliance, the result of which is a stiff chamber that has a higher filling pressure for any given preload. Impaired compliance (that is, a stiff heart) leads to pulmonary and/or systemic venous congestion, depending on which side of the heart is involved. Severe diastolic dysfunction reduces filling and results in chamber preload deprivation, contributing to low cardiac output.

It is important to differentiate "primary" and "secondary" diastolic dysfunction. Primary diastolic dysfunction is designated as abnormal compliance with intact contractility (e.g., with LV hypertrophy with normal ejection fraction). Primary diastolic dysfunction may cause pulmonary venous hypertension, resulting in symptoms and signs of congestive heart failure, and in the most extreme states limits maximal LV preload impairs stroke volume and cardiac output despite normal contractility. Secondary diastolic dysfunction is that associated with ventricular systolic dysfunction. Impaired diastolic properties resulting from poor pumping performance lead to chamber dilatation, complicated by the primary myocardial insult (pressure overload, volume overload, or cardiomyopathy).

Pertinent Aspects of Normal Pressure Waveforms: Relationship of Cardiac Mechanics to Atrial Waveforms, Venous Flow Patterns, and Respiratory Physiology

An appreciation of atrial waveform hemodynamics, the physiology of the venous circulations, and the dynamic effects of intrathoracic pressure (ITP) and respiratory motion on cardiovascular physiology is critical. Analysis of the atrial waveforms yields insight into cardiac chamber and pericardial compliance. The atrial waveforms are constituted by two positive waves (A and V peaks) and two collapsing waves (X and Y descents; see Part One: Normal Waveforms). The atrial A wave is generated by atrial systole following the P wave on ECG. Atrial mechanics behave similarly to ventricular muscle. The strength of atrial contraction is reflected in the rapidity of the A wave upstroke and peak amplitude. The X descent follows the A wave and is generated by two events: the initial decline in pressure reflecting active atrial relaxation, with a latter descent component reflecting pericardial emptying during ventricular systole (also called systolic intrapericardial depressurization, a condition which is exaggerated when pericardial space is compromised). The X descent second component is affected by the pericardial space and is more pronounced when intrapericardial volume decreases when the ventricles are maximally emptied.

During ventricular systole, venous return results in atrial filling and pressure which peaks with the V wave, whose height reflects the atrial pressure–volume compliance characteristics. The subsequent diastolic Y descent represents atrial emptying and depressurization. The steepness of the Y descent is influenced by the volume and pressure in the atrium just prior to AV valve opening (height of the V wave) and resistance to atrial emptying (AV valve resistance and ventricular–pericardial compliance).

Venous return to both atria is inversely proportional to the instantaneous atrial pressure, which is itself dependent on atrial compliance. The lowest return occurs when atrial will pressure is highest. Normal intrapericardial pressure is subatmospheric, nearly equal to intrapleural pressure, and decreases during inspiration. Intrapericardial pressure also tracks right atrial (RA) pressure and shows fluctuations that are associated with cardiac cycle. In general, the intrapericardial pressure increases when cardiac volume is increased and vice versa. Under physiologic conditions, venous return to both atria is biphasic, with a systolic peak determined by atrial relaxation (corresponding to the X descent of the atrial and jugular venous pressure [JVP] waveforms) and a diastolic peak determined by tricuspid valve (TV) resistance and right ventricular (RV) compliance (corresponding to the Y descent of the atrial and JVP waveforms).

Intrapericardial pressure both approximates and varies with pleural pressure. The inspiratory decrement in pleural pressure normally reduces pericardial, RA, RV, wedge, and systemic arterial pressures slightly. However, IPP decreases somewhat more than RA pressure, thereby augmenting right-heart filling and output.

Under physiologic conditions, respiratory oscillations exert profound and complex effects on cardiac filling and dynamics. However, the effects on the right and the left heart are disparate, owing to differences in the anatomic relationships of the respective venous return systems to the intrapleural space. The entire left heart and its tributary pulmonary veins are entirely intrathoracic. In contrast, although both right-heart chambers are intrathoracic, the tributary systemic venous system is extrapleural. Normally, inspiration-induced decrements in intrathoracic pressure are transmitted through the pericardium to the cardiac chambers. On the right heart, these decrements in ITP enhance the filling gradient from the extrathoracic systemic veins to the right atrium, thereby enhancing the caval–right atrial gradient and augmenting venous return flow by 50–60%, which increases right-heart filling and output. Since pleural pressure changes are evenly distributed to the left heart and pulmonary veins, the pressure gradient from the pulmonary veins to the left ventricle shows minimal change with respiration. Early diastolic transmitral filling pressure as well as LV filling are essentially unchanged throughout the respiratory cycle. However, left-heart filling, stroke volume, and aortic systolic pressure normally decrease with inspiration (by up to 10–12 mm Hg), a phenomenon termed (normal) pulsus paradoxus or paradoxical pulse. The mechanisms responsible for this normal inspiratory oscillation in aortic pressure include variable ventricular volumes as each ventricle competes for intrapericardial volume. This competition leads to leftward septal displacement due to augmented right-heart filling, increased LV "afterload," and inspiratory delay of augmented RV output through the lungs.

Pertinent Aspects of Ventricular and Arterial Waveforms

Ventricular waveforms reflect systolic and diastolic function. The ventricular pressure upstrokes (dP/dt) approximately reflect contractility. A brisk upstroke suggests reasonable function versus a sluggish or delayed pressure rise indicating depressed performance. The peak amplitude reflects both contractility and afterload. The pressure wave of the downstroke relaxation phase is an active adenosine triphosphate (ATP)-requiring process and closely mirrors systolic function. The downstroke can also be used to assess cardiac dysfunction. A slurred negative dP/dt may indicate cardiomyopathy and adversely influenced diastolic properties. Arterial waveforms reflect the input from the corresponding ventricle (and therefore its preload, contractility, and afterload), together with the intrinsic resistance and compliance of that circuit.

Anatomic-Pathophysiologic Approach to Differential Diagnosis

To assess each patient hemodynamically, it is essential to think of each cardiac structure, consider the disease processes that may affect each, and then compile a differential diagnostic list of pathophysiologic syndromes that may manifest in symptoms. From a simple anatomic perspective, the components of the heart from "outside in" include pericardium, myocardium, valves, coronary arteries, conduction system, and great vessels. Each of these structures may undergo various pathophysiologic alterations that result in a spectrum of specific hemodynamic derangements and subsequent symptoms related to those abnormalities.

Pericardial Abnormalities

Elevated intrapericardial pressure exerts deleterious effects on cardiac compliance and filling. This is most commonly attributed to (i) primary pericardial disease (constriction or tamponade); or (ii) abrupt chamber dilatation, as may occur with acute right ventricular infarction. The dilated right ventricle acutely crowds the interpericardial space and may also increase interpericardial pressure. Regardless of the etiology, increased pericardial resistance impairs chamber compliance, resulting in increased filling pressures. Abnormal cardiac compliance also limits ventricular filling, with reduced preload resulting in limited cardiac output.

Myocardial Abnormalities

The anatomic-pathophysiologic approach to myocardial dysfunction for any given chamber is based on consideration of the three primary determinants of myocardial performance: preload, contractility, and afterload (in aggregate the determinants of SV). All abnormalities of cardiac performance must be related to (i) primary volume overload, associated with valve regurgitation, shunts, or high-output states; (ii) primary pressure overload, due to outflow obstruction or excess vascular resistance; or (iii) primary derangements of contractility due to ischemic or nonischemic cardiomyopathy. A dilated and depressed ventricle must result from either intrinsic cardiomyopathy or decompensation attributable to primary volume or pressure overload. A dilated ventricle with intact contractility may result from primary volume overload (valve leaks and shunts) or high-output states.

Myocardial diastolic dysfunction—that is, contractility intact—may be categorized as due to intrinsic and extrinsic abnormalities. Intrinsic diastolic dysfunction may result from primary chamber volume overload (dilation and hypertrophy), pressure overload (hypertrophy and later dilation), or cardiomyopathic processes (ischemic, infiltrative, inflammatory, fibrotic, etc.). Extrinsic factors leading to diastolic dysfunction include those mediated by pericardial restraint, septal-mediated ventricular interactions, or intrapleural influences.

Valvular Pathophysiology

The hemodynamic manifestations of valvular heart disease can be simplified into two obstructive categories: pressure overload and regurgitant (volume-overload) lesions. Obstructive lesions exert dual adverse effects, imposing increased afterload on the "upstream chamber" delivering flow through the narrowed orifice and limiting preload or blood flow into the "downstream chamber"; they also limit the outflow into the downstream chamber and therefore reduce the preload or perfusion volume, depending on the position of the valve to the downstream conduit. The effect of excess afterload on the "upstream chamber" is hypertrophy and ultimately dilatation and pump failure, resulting in higher filling pressures and lesser forward flow. Obstructions limit preload and therefore maximal stroke volume and cardiac output (preload deprivation).

Regurgitant valvular lesions result in primary volume overload of the chambers impacted by the leak. In the case of semilunar valve regurgitation, the ventricle bears the predominant load. However, atrio-ventricular valve insufficiency impacts not only the atria suffering the direct brunt of the regurgitant leak, but the ventricle itself, which must receive both the normal forward venous return as well as the excess recirculated volume. Regurgitant lesions result in chamber volume overload predisposing to diastolic dysfunction; prolonged severe overload leads to systolic dysfunction. Even when ventricular performance is intact, regurgitant leaks may limit forward cardiac output by compromising maximum effective forward stroke work.

Basics of the General Approach to Cardiovascular Examination

Clinical hemodynamic assessment should be based on interrogation of cardiac (imaging) anatomy with the focus on pathophysiology and differential diagnosis. The primary goal is establishment of the pathophysiologic differential diagnosis of the patient's symptoms in concert with the history, physical examination, and/or noninvasive or invasive assessments.

Bedside Hemodynamics

The fundamental purpose of the circulation is to perfuse the body. Therefore, the initial step in hemodynamic assessment is the determination of whether forward cardiac output and perfusion are adequate. According to Ohm's law, pressure drives flow. Consequently, when CO is limited (regardless of the reason), neuro-hormonal compensatory mechanisms (reflex vasoconstriction, sinus tachycardia, increased contractility) are activated to maintain BP and priority perfusion to the most critical organ, the brain.

The bedside assessment of perfusion status starts with evaluation of whether cerebral perfusion is adequate. If the patient is awake, alert, mentating well, and able to communicate in lucid sentences, overall cerebral perfusion must at least be adequate to maintain flow to the brain. Bedside analysis of peripheral perfusion focuses on the presence of reflex compensatory mechanisms, reflecting response to adequacy of cardiac output: when CO is low, compensatory systemic vasoconstriction is elicited to augment blood pressure. Those organ beds that are preferentially constricted are those that can most successfully withstand periods of hypoperfusion, specifically the skin, skeletal muscle, and bowel. Thus, if the patient is awake and alert, mentating well, and the skin is warm and pink with brisk capillary refill, overall cardiac output and perfusion are reasonable; conversely, the patient may be awake, alert, and mentating well, indicating intact cerebral perfusion, but if the extremities are cool, clammy, mottled, and there is poor capillary refill, indicating severe vasoconstriction, then cerebral perfusion may only be maintained by intense vasoconstriction, indicating severely low output.

A key component to appreciating systolic function and perfusion at the bedside is the arterial pulse, including both the rate and contour of the pulse wave. When cardiac output is low (not attributable to primary arrhythmias), the expected compensatory response is sinus tachycardia. Therefore, the presence of a compensatory sinus tachycardia is an important sign of a compensatory hemodynamic mechanism attempting to stem the effect of low CO. It should be kept in mind that patients with chronotropic incompetence due to primary electrical disturbances, drugs, or other metabolic abnormalities may not be able to elicit a sinus tachycardia despite neuro-hormonal stimulation to achieve that desired effect. Examination of the arterial pulse waveform, particularly the carotid artery, provides important insights into cardiac function. The carotid pulse components (upstroke, peak amplitude, and downstroke) provide a physical examination window into cardiac performance, which correlates with invasive aortic waveform interrogation. The carotid pulse waveform reflects the stroke volume ejected by the LV, modulated by the aortic valve and intrinsic compliance of the aorta–carotid vessels. Accordingly, the carotid reflects LV preload, contractility, and afterload. Therefore, in a patient with adequate perfusion where cardiac output is an issue, interrogation of the carotid pulse may provide the critical information as to whether cardiac output is contributing to this problem.

Evaluation of cardiac diastolic function may also be approached at the bedside. Diastolic dysfunction on the left side of the heart results in pulmonary venous congestion, manifest symptomatically as dyspnea, initially during exertion and later at rest. At the bedside, if the patient is awake and alert and breathing comfortably, with a normal respiratory rate and the lungs are absolutely clear, the patient will not be suffering significant pulmonary venous congestion at that time. Caution must be applied to patients with chronic LA pressure elevation due to mitral valve disease or cardiomyopathy, in whom adaptive changes of the pulmonary circulation and lymphatics may allow a resting elevated wedge pressure to be tolerated without resting dyspnea. However, such patients will typically develop dyspnea on exertion, as the increased preload from augmented venous return during exercises causes the cardiac chambers to ascend their pressure–volume curve, resulting in dramatic increases in diastolic pressure and culminating in shortness of breath. Conversely, if the patient is short of breath at rest and the lung examination reveals rales and/or rhonchi, dyspnea is likely cardiac in nature. This will be considered in detail in the next section on evaluation of dyspnea.

Hemodynamic Evaluation of Dyspnea

Dyspnea can only be ascribed to cardiac origin if the pulmonary capillary wedge (PCW) pressure is elevated, typically over 15–20 mm Hg. If the PCW pressure is normal, then dyspnea must either be of primary pulmonary origin (upper airway, lower airway, alveolar processes, parenchymal disease, pulmonary arterial problems, etc.) or related to a metabolic condition such as anemia.

The differentiation of "cardiac" versus "noncardiac" dyspnea is based on evidence of conditions that induce elevated PCW. This approach simplifies the evaluation of dyspnea interactive interrogation by physical examination (Figure 23.2) or by invasive catheterization, focused on whether there are cardiac abnormalities that could lead to pathophysiologic perturbations resulting in elevated PCW pressure. It is important to note that chronic resting elevations of PCW pressure, even over 25 mm Hg, may be tolerated without resting dyspnea, due to thickening of the pulmonary capillaries, development of pulmonary hypertension, and increased capillary lymphatic drainage of the lung.

Dyspnea with Elevated Pulmonary Capillary Wedge Pressure (Over 15–20 mm Hg)

Whether an elevated PCW is responsible for dyspnea is based on interrogation of the anatomic course of the circulation from the pulmonary capillaries through the entire left heart. Accordingly, proceeding along the course of blood flow, if PCW is elevated then cardiac dyspnea must reflect pulmonary venous hypertension. A simple anatomic approach reveals a very limited number of anatomic mechanisms responsible for an elevated back pressure, a finding which may be found at the bedside and by invasive evaluation. Excepting the rare instances of pulmonary

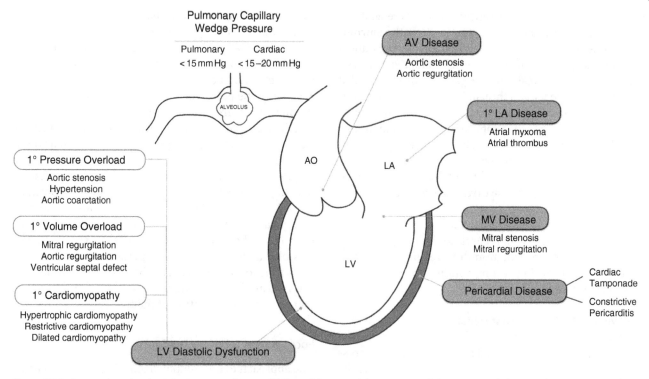

Figure 23.2 Anatomic pathophysiologic approach to evaluation of dyspnea. AO = aorta; LA = left atrium; LV = left ventricle; MV = mitral valve.

veno-occlusive disease, pulmonary venous hypertension equates to left atrial hypertension due to one of several mechanisms, including (i) space-occupying lesions (e.g., myxoma) of the LA; (ii) pressure overload from mitral valve obstruction or left ventricle compliance abnormalities; (iii) volume overload due to mitral regurgitation or increased pulmonary blood flow from ventricular-level shunts or high-output states; or (iv) intrinsic atrial cardiomyopathies, which may be ischemic or nonischemic.

In the absence of an atrial mass, the next anatomic site to interrogate is the mitral valve, which if primarily to blame for dyspnea must be either obstructed or regurgitant. If the mitral valve is normal, then dyspnea due to LA hypertension can only be explained by LV diastolic dysfunction imposing increased afterload on the left atrium. LV compliance abnormalities may reflect either intrinsic chamber processes (e.g., primary LV pressure overload, volume overload, or cardiomyopathic processes) or extrinsic abnormalities related to abnormalities of the pericardium. LV pressure overload may result from fixed-outflow obstructions (aortic stenosis, coarctation), dynamic (hypertrophic cardiomyopathy) obstructions, or increased systemic vascular resistance due to hypertension (± coarctation). Primary LV volume overload is induced by aortic insufficiency, mitral regurgitation, or ventricular-level shunts (ventricular septal defect, VSD, and patent ductus arteriosus, PDA).

Keys of Physical Examination

Primary Left Atrial Disease

LA mass obstruction presents with dyspnea, intact carotid upstrokes, and quiet LV or precordial examination. Unfortunately, assessment of LA size and pressure is not feasible by physical examination. Other than rare instances when prolapsing atrial mass lesions are indicated by a "plop" and flow rumble that may change with position, echocardiography is necessary to confirm the presence of an LA mass.

Primary Mitral Valve Disease

Bedside interrogation should easily establish whether the mitral valve is normal, regurgitation, or obstructed. A normal S_1 intensity and the absence of murmurs are sufficient clues to exclude mitral valve disease.

Mitral stenosis is associated with a loud S_1, and an opening snap (if the valve leaflets are still compliant), together with diastolic flow rumble, a loud P_2, and right ventricle (RV) heave indicate longstanding severe obstruction and secondary pulmonary hypertension.

Mitral regurgitation of magnitude sufficient to induce dyspnea is associated with a holosystolic blowing murmur radiating from apex to axilla and intensified by handgrip exercise. The intensity and length of the murmur as well as the presence of LV enlargement by palpation help grade the severity of mitral regurgitation.

It should be noted that in patients with severe acute or chronic decompensated mitral regurgitation, the murmur may be less than holosystolic and quieter, as pressure is rapidly equilibrated between the LV and the LA. The precordial exam reveals an enlarged, volume-overloaded LV and the presence of a thrill indicates severe regurgitation. Severe mitral regurgitation (MR) results in a peripheral pulse characterized by rapid upstroke and amplitude, but diminished pulse volume. The physical examination stigmata of mitral regurgitation are virtually indistinguishable from acute post-infarction VSD; in such cases, echocardiography or invasive oximetry differentiates the two entities.

One must also remember that in patients with dynamic ischemic mitral regurgitation or hypertrophic cardiomyopathy in whom mitral regurgitation may not be present during resting conditions, auscultation during exercise may be necessary.

Left Ventricular Diastolic Dysfunction

Elevated LV diastolic pressure can be transmitted and thereby lead to increased LA and pulmonary pressures. LV diastolic and systolic function can be assessed at the bedside. A pronounced point of maximal impulse (PMI) together with S_3 and S_4 gallops is an indicator of ventricular enlargement and diastolic dysfunction that may contribute to dyspnea. Ventricular systolic function can be evaluated through assessment of the carotid upstroke and amplitude. If the LV is quiet and the carotid (upstroke, amplitude, and volume) is normal, then LV systolic function and stoke volume are usually reasonable. Conversely, a depressed carotid waveform and enlarged LV suggest either primary LV cardiomyopathy (ischemic or nonischemic) or outflow obstruction. Interrogation of the LV outflow tract and aortic valve is straightforward. If the carotid upstroke and volume are intact and there is no systolic murmur in the LV outflow or aortic region, including during Valsalva's maneuver, there is no obstruction. Conversely, aortic stenosis is indicated by loud and late-peaking systolic murmur together with diminished upstroke and amplitude of the carotid waveform (pulsus parvus et tardus), reversed split S_2, and LV enlargement by precordial examination. It is important to search for dynamic LV outflow tract obstruction. Obstructive hypertrophic cardiomyopathy typically results in a bisfiriens carotid pulse and a brisk upstroke with reduced volume and a notched bifid waveform, together with a loud left sternal border–apical murmur that intensifies with Valsalva.

Aortic insufficiency is established by presence of a diastolic decrescendo murmur along the left sternal border. Chronic aortic insufficiency results in LV volume overload, evident on precordial examination by cardiac enlargement and displacement of the PMI. The carotid waveform reflects the volume-overloaded LV generating a brisk, large-volume bounding pulse, whereas regurgitation back into the LV results in a dramatic diastolic collapse of the pulse, together producing a widened aortic pulse pressure. Aortic insufficiency may be subtle, paradoxically quiet when the lesion is acute, and severe with hemodynamic decompensation. Under such conditions, the murmur may shorten or disappear as the aorta empties rapidly into the left ventricle early in diastole, resulting in abrupt early diastolic equilibration between the LV and aorta. The intensity of S_1 softens and may disappear, emphasizing the importance of timing the murmur to the carotid to differentiate its systolic versus diastolic nature. Acute aortic regurgitation (AR) may not allow time for the LV to dilate, thus patients may develop severe heart failure but do not manifest volume overload on precordial examination of the LV.

Focus on the Carotid Waveform

The approach to differential diagnosis of dyspnea can be simplified and keyed to assessment of the carotid pulse waveform.

Dyspnea and Depressed Carotid Waveform

If the patient is short of breath and the carotid upstroke is depressed, dyspnea is likely related either to aortic stenosis or LV cardiomyopathy (except in those instances in which the carotid arteries are themselves diseased). Examination can differentiate these two entities. Aortic stenosis has a slow-rising, delayed, diminished-amplitude carotid pulse (parvus et tardus) together with late-peaking systolic murmur, reversed split S_2, and sustained LV apical impulse. LV cardiomyopathy is characterized by a depressed carotid pulse, diffuse LV impulse with gallops, and often a murmur of secondary mitral insufficiency. Importantly, end-stage aortic stenosis may result in a dilated depressed LV, leading to a mixed picture.

Dyspnea and Brisk Carotid Waveform

If the carotid upstroke is brisk with a large volume and collapsing character, the differential diagnosis includes aortic insufficiency, mitral regurgitation, or high-output states. A bounding pulse with large volume and collapse suggests AR, whereas a brisk upstroke with a modest volume should stimulate consideration of MR. Aortic and mitral regurgitation is readily detected by auscultation. These murmurs must be searched for, particularly AR, which may be missed when increasing regurgitation severity causes the murmur to shorten as aortic and LV pressures rapidly equilibrate.

Dyspnea and Normal Carotid Waveform

If the patient is short of breath and the carotid is normal, then the only cardiac entities that are likely to lead to pulmonary venous hypertension are mitral valve obstruction (stenosis or myoxoma), or more commonly severe LV diastolic dysfunction related to LV hypertrophy, infiltrative-restrictive processes, or acute ischemia (prominent LV apical impulse and loud S_4). Diastolic dysfunction may also be a manifestation of pericardial disease, which should be suspected by the JVP pressure and waveform.

One important caveat to emphasize is that cardiac symptoms and their physical stigmata may be evident only with exercise. Under conditions of exercise and stress, venous return is augmented, contractility increases, heart rate is elevated, and systemic vascular resistances may vary dramatically. Therefore, normal examination (and invasive hemodynamics) at rest does not imply the *absence* of significant abnormalities that may be develop during dynamic provocations.

Invasive Hemodynamic Evaluation of Dyspnea

Invasive interrogation of patients with dyspnea can be approached by the anatomic-pathophysiologic processes already described. Analogous to the bedside examination, the key to determining whether dyspnea is due to a cardiac condition is whether the PCW pressure is elevated (>15–20 mm Hg).

Dyspnea with Normal Pulmonary Capillary Wedge Pressure

If the PCW is less than 15 mm Hg, then dyspnea is not attributable to a cardiac condition but is more likely of primary pulmonary origin. However, two important caveats must be emphasized. First, PCW may be normal at rest but increase dramatically during exercise or stress. Thus in the dyspneic patient, if the resting PCW is normal, hemodynamics should be measured during leg lifts, volume challenge, or following contrast administration. Secondly, it is important to note that dyspnea may be also be an "angina equivalent," a condition of myocardial ischemia which should be established by coronary arteriography.

Dyspnea with Elevated Pulmonary Capillary Wedge Pressure

If the PCW is elevated, greater than 15–20 mm Hg, it is highly likely that left-heart failure is the major contributor to dyspnea. Evaluation of the PCW and simultaneous LV pressure measurements together with ventriculography fully delineates the causes of left-heart failure. The rare conditions of pulmonary veno-occlusive disease or LA hypertension due to space-occupying lesions are best established by noninvasive imaging studies.

If PCW is elevated, specific waveform abnormalities may indicate underlying pathophysiology, including the following:

1) Augmented A wave and X descent reflect augmented atrial contraction/relaxation due either to mitral valve obstruction or stiff noncompliant LV. The PCW in a patient with mitral stenosis is characterized by a prominent A/X and blunted Y descent. Simultaneous LV–PCW pressure measurements demonstrate a pan-diastolic gradient. LV diastolic dysfunction results in a prominent A wave/X descent, but there is no end-diastolic gradient on simultaneous LV–PCW tracings.

2) A prominent V wave suggests either mitral regurgitation or a VSD (particularly acquired post-infarction VSD). The height of the V wave reflects the degree of volume overload and LA compliance; if either lesion is acute, the V wave may be particularly large, as the LA has not had the opportunity to stretch and accommodate to the volume overload. A prominent V wave may be reflected in the pulmonary artery pressure trace, resulting in a "rabbit ears" morphology. In patients with VSD, the V timing of the wave peak may be delayed, but the V waveform pattern may be indistinguishable from severe mitral regurgitation. With a right-heart catheter in place, oximetry across the right heart establishes the presence of a VSD with left-to-right shunts. LV cineangiography can also assist in distinguishing MR from VSD.

When LA and PCW pressures are chronically elevated, over 25 mm Hg, pulmonary hypertension is an expected response, due both to the back pressure from the elevated left-heart filling pressures as well as to the compensatory responses by the lung to protect itself from the overload. The magnitude of pulmonary hypertension reflects the severity of the LA hypertension, its chronicity, and intrinsic lung predisposition to developing a hypertensive response.

Careful interrogation of simultaneous LV and PCW pressures and the LV gradient across the aortic valve, with LV cineangiography, further defines the cardiac pathology that could result in dyspnea. LV diastolic pressure may show elevated mid- and end-diastolic pressure with a prominent A wave ("atrial kick"), reflecting LV noncompliance of hypertrophy, fibrosis, infiltration, or external pericardial restraint. If LV and RV diastolic filling pressures are elevated and equalized, differential considerations include increased intrapericardial pressure (tamponade, constriction, or due to acute RV infarction), restrictive cardiomyopathy, or massive acute pulmonary embolus. Hemodynamic differentiation of these conditions is discussed in detail in Part Three: Constriction and Tamponade.

Dynamic and fixed obstructions in the LV outflow tract and the level of the aortic valve may also result in LV diastolic and systolic dysfunction, and are easily revealed by measurement of LV–aortic systolic gradients during catheter pullback, including with provocative maneuvers to elicit dynamic obstructions. Finally, LV cineangiography documents underlying LV dilatation and systolic dysfunction, as well as the presence of mitral regurgitation or VSD.

Bedside Evaluation of Low Output/Hypotension

Investigation of hypotension can be focused on Ohm's law as applied to the circulation: Blood pressure (BP) = Cardiac output (CO) x Systemic vascular resistance (SVR). Accordingly, low output/hypotension must be explained either by diminished CO, low SVR, or both. Specific contributing mechanisms involve the determinants of CO and SVR. Recall that CO is a function of heart rate and stroke volume, the latter determined by ventricular preload, contractility, and afterload. SVR is determined by total blood volume and vascular tone (e.g., autonomic influences, drugs, sepsis, neuropathies, etc.; Figure 23.1).

Low Output/Hypotension Due to Arrhythmias

The first step is assessment of the physiologic cardiac rhythm. Under conditions of low output due to depressed SV, reflex sinus tachycardia is the expected compensatory rhythm; lack thereof suggests chronotropic incompetence, which contributes to hemodynamic compromise. If the patient has a first-degree arrhythmia and/or chronotropic incompetence, restoration of physiologic rhythm is the first therapeutic intervention (e.g., cardioversion or bolus antiarrhythmic drugs).

Low Output/Hypotension Due to Low Systemic Vascular Resistance

In patients with low output/hypotension and physiologic rhythm, the next step is to assess SVR. SVR, determined by total blood volume and vascular tone, is gauged clinically by peripheral perfusion. Low SVR is suggested by distal extremities that are warm and pink with brisk capillary refill. In such cases, hypotension likely reflects factors associated with vasodilatory stimulation such as sepsis, autonomic dysfunction, overdose of vasodilating drugs, or peripheral neuropathies (e.g., diabetes) and other neurological disorders.

However, if the extremities are cool, clammy, and mottled with poor peripheral capillary refill, low output is associated with reflex vasoconstriction as the primary problem. In patients with chronic congestive heart failure (CHF), low output and reflex vasoconstriction may not manifest these peripheral stigmata. In such cases, invasive evaluation of cardiac output and systemic vascular resistance are confirmatory.

Low Output/Hypotension due to Diminished Stroke Volume

In patients with low output/hypotension and a physiologic cardiac rhythm, low CO can only be explained by diminished SV. An inadequate SV can only be explained by inadequate preload, poor contractility, or excess afterload. Analysis of SV should be approached according to anatomic-pathophysiologic principles, with a step-wise focus on each cardiac chamber, as well as for the heart as a whole.

Compliance Properties Pertinent to Preload Assessment

Cardiac preload is the amount of blood distending the cardiac chamber. In assessment of preload, measured the chamber filling pressure is a convenient surrogate for chamber volume. The compliance characteristics of the chamber being interrogated have a striking effect on the pressure–volume relationship. Therefore, filling pressure reasonably reflects chamber volume and preload only if chamber compliance is normal. Since chamber compliance is influenced by numerous intrinsic (e.g., hypertrophy, ischemia, infiltration, inflammation, etc.) and extrinsic factors (e.g., pericardial pressure elevations or intraventricular or intra-arterial interactions), it follows that there are numerous conditions in which filling pressure may be elevated but preload limited. For example, LV preload may be markedly *reduced* but intracardiac pressures strikingly *elevated* under conditions of cardiac tamponade or severe pulmonary hypertension. Conversely, chronic volume overload lesion such as aortic regurgitation may result in dramatically increased chamber volumes but relatively normal intracardiac pressures as chamber and pericardium dilate, become compliant, and compensate for the pathophysiology.

Finally, LV filling is the final common preload pathway that generates effective forward SV and thus CO. However, it is not uncommon for the LV to be preload deprived but other chambers to be overloaded. Thus, preload assessment must consider all cardiac chambers and conduits and be interrogated according to the course of venous blood returning to and ultimately delivered to the LV cardio-pulmonary circulation.

Reduced Cardiac Preload Due to Decreased Total Blood Volume

Low output due to systemic hypovolemia is detected clinically by low jugular venous pressure, orthostatic blood pressure changes, sinus tachycardia, and clear lungs. Invasive hemodynamics document diminished RA, PCW, and LV diastolic filling pressures. If LV function is intact, the carotid and aortic waveforms reveal intact upstrokes with a small pulse volume. Volume administration will restore filling pressures, increase cardiac output, normalize blood pressure, and ultimately resolve the compensatory sinus tachycardia (lower HR). If volume challenge results in dramatic increases in filling pressures without the expected increase in CO and blood pressure, then preload was not the predominant factor, although it certainly may have been contributory.

Decreased Cardiac Preload Despite Increased Total Blood Volume

Right-Heart Inflow Obstruction

Elevated JVP exceeding RA pressure with a demonstrable JVP–RA gradient indicates inflow obstruction at the level of the superior or inferior vena cavae; central venous waveforms proximal to the obstruction are typically blunted. Noninvasive imaging confirms the site and nature of the obstruction. Elevated RA pressure exceeding RV diastolic pressure with an end-diastolic RA–RV gradient indicates either a space-occupying RA mass lesion or tricuspid valve obstruction. RA mass lesions manifest an overall blunted RA waveform. Tricuspid valve obstruction results in a prominent A wave with a sharp X descent resulting from enhanced atrial contraction/relaxation against the stenotic valve, with a blunted Y descent reflecting impaired RV inflow. Matched and elevated RA and RV filling pressures may indicate primary RV diastolic dysfunction. The differential diagnosis includes primary RV derangements (pressure overload, volume overload, or cardiomyopathy) or pericardial disease. Elevated equalized diastolic pressures throughout the cardiac chambers with an RV "dip and plateau" configuration suggest either constriction, restriction, or acute RV infarction. The differentiation of these entities is discussed in detail in Chapter 14: Hemodynamic Manifestations of Ischemic Right-Heart Dysfunction.

Decreased Right Ventricular Outflow

Elevated right-heart filling pressures with normal or low PCW pressure indicate impaired delivery of preload from right heart to left heart, attributable to (i) RV systolic dysfunction (e.g., RV infarction), (ii) excess RV afterload due to outflow obstruction (at the level of the outflow tract or pulmonary valve), or (iii) pulmonary arterial hypertension. Diminished effective RV stroke volume limits LV preload due not only to reduced transpulmonary blood flow, but also to the effects of RV pressure/volume overload. RV overload can induce septal-mediated diastolic ventricular interactions, which adversely influence LV compliance and filling. Severe RV infarction depresses RV stroke work, leading to depressed transpulmonary delivery of LV preload. Thus RV infarction with decreased LV preload results in a syndrome of hypotension, low output with clear lungs, and elevated right-heart filling pressures. The clinical and invasive hemodynamic patterns for RV infarction are discussed in Part Three: Constriction and Tamponade.

Excess RV afterload is delineated by elevated RV systolic pressure: RV outflow obstructions are evident by elevated JVP with RV heave and loud late-peaking ejection murmur along the left sternal border. Invasively, right ventricle systolic pressure (RVSP) greater than pulmonary arterial systolic pressure (PASP) suggests either subvalvular RV outflow obstruction or pulmonary valve stenosis. Clinical evaluation delineates pulmonary hypertension, characterized by an RV heave and loud P_2. Invasive assessment documents elevated RV systolic pressure equal to PA systolic pressure. The magnitude of the PA diastolic pressure increase is dependent on the mechanism of pulmonary hypertension. Calculated pulmonary resistance is elevated and reflects the magnitude of obstruction in the pulmonary bed. If attributable to left-heart etiology, pulmonary hypertension will be associated with elevated PCW.

Left Heart Inflow Obstruction

Under conditions of left-heart inflow obstruction, reduced LV preload results in low output/hypotension despite expanded total blood volume, elevated right-heart preload, and increased PCW pressure. Inflow obstruction may occur at the level of the pulmonary veins, LA, or mitral valve. LV preload is reflected by LV diastolic pressure, which must be interpreted within the context of LV compliance. Elevated PCW pressure with an end-diastolic gradient across the mitral valve suggests either a space-occupying lesion in the left atrium or mitral valvular obstruction. The lack of opening snap and diastolic flow rumble on examination excludes mitral stenosis, and should lead to suspicion of an atrial mass or pulmonary veno-occlusive disease. Noninvasive imaging is confirmatory. Elevated and equal PCW and LV filling pressures indicate LV diastolic dysfunction, which may be primary (with intact LV contractility) or secondary (associated with depressed LV systolic function). Primary LV diastolic dysfunction reflects intrinsic LV abnormalities (primary pressure overload/outflow obstruction, volume overload, or cardiomyopathic processes) or extrinsic constraint (pericardial disease or intense ventricular interactions from the

RV). Occasionally, acute LV ischemia with global paralysis of LV function may result in abrupt diastolic dysfunction with "flash pulmonary edema" and low output/hypotension. LV contractility may be intact or depressed depending on the duration of the ischemia. Severe LV diastolic dysfunction may result from a hypertrophic noncompliant cavity (e.g., severe hypertensive LV hypertrophy, aortic stenosis, or hypertrophic obstructive cardiomyopathy), with elevated filling pressures but reduced LV preload and stroke volume, further limiting cardiac output.

Low Output Due to Diminished Left Ventricular Outflow: Depressed Left Ventricular Contractility

Reduced LV stroke volume may be attributable to (i) impaired systolic performance, (ii) decompensated primary pressure overload (hypertension or outflow resistance), (iii) volume overload (mitral insufficiency, aortic regurgitation, or ventricular level shunts), or (iv) primary cardiomyopathies (either ischemic or nonischemic). It is important to differentiate "contractile failure" resulting from ischemic or nonischemic myocardial depression from "pump failure" attributable to chronic excess afterload conditions such as severe aortic stenosis. Regardless of the cause, systolic dysfunction reduces stroke volume and cardiac output. The LV systolic pressure waveform may reflect the severity of depression of contractility, as indicated by diminished upstroke, reduced peak, and delayed relaxation. These derangements are similarly reflected in the aortic pressure waveform as diminished carotid aortic upstroke, amplitude, and overall small stroke volume. End-stage LV pump failure may result in pulsus alternans. LV systolic dysfunction results in dilatation and secondary diastolic dysfunction, leading to elevated diastolic filling pressures.

LV dilatation and depressed systolic dysfunction by cineangiography indicate either decompensated primary volume overload, a primary afterload lesion, or intrinsic cardiomyopathy (ischemic or nonischemic). Volume overload due to aortic insufficiency is indicated by the expected characteristic murmur and pulse amplitude on physical examination, invasively by elevated LV filling pressure with widened aortic pressure, and contrast aortography is confirmatory.

Severe mitral regurgitation is evident by the physical examination findings and invasively by elevated PCW pressure and a prominent V wave, also with LV cineangiography confirming the regurgitant mitral leak.

Ventricular septal defect has a characteristic physical examination, but otherwise appears similar to MR (especially acquired post infarction). The diagnosis is easily established by oximetry and LV cineangiography.

Transient acute ischemic LV dysfunction is excluded by coronary angiography. If present, severe left main or multivessel equivalents are noted and occasionally result in episodic low output/hypotension, often with "flash" pulmonary edema; more commonly LV contractility is depressed due to ischemic cardiomyopathy.

Depressed Cardiac Output Due to Increased Left Ventricular Afterload

Increased LV afterload impairs stroke volume and cardiac output, either with intact LV contractility or LV systolic dysfunction. Increased LV afterload can be categorized mechanically and anatomically as (i) dynamic LV outflow tract due to hypertrophic obstructive cardiomyopathy, (ii) fixed obstructions due to subvalvular (membranes) or valvular stenosis, or (iii) post-valve-level resistance attributable to systemic hypertension or aortic coarctation.

Valvular aortic stenosis is evident invasively by fixed gradient across the aortic valve and a dramatic difference in aortic and LV waveform morphologies. The LV upstroke and amplitude are brisk, whereas in the carotid and aortic waveforms there is a depressed upstroke and delayed and diminished peak, often with shudder findings, associated with low cardiac output. The aortic waveforms will be characteristic, with aortic stenosis revealing a slow-rising and diminished amplitude, pulsus parvus et tardus. In contrast, hypertrophic obstructive cardiomyopathy demonstrates a bifid or bisfiriens pulse waveform. The severity of the obstruction will be reflected in the mean and peak gradients and cardiac output.

Hypertrophic obstructive cardiomyopathy results in an LV–aortic dynamic gradient that may be present at rest and is demonstrated by a pressure pullback from the LV apex through the body and LV outflow tract into the aorta. An intraventricular gradient is located by carefully watching the slow catheter pullback under fluoroscopy, showing that the gradient occurs within the ventricle before it is pulled across the aortic valve. The arterial pressure waveform pattern often demonstrates a unique morphology, a "spike and dome" or bisfiriens waveform with an intact upstroke, mid-systolic delay, or notch, reflecting the obstruction and an overall very small stroke volume.

Algorithm Focused on the Carotid Waveform

Hypotension/Low Output and Normal Carotid Waveform

A normal carotid upstroke and amplitude, together with absence of LV enlargement or murmurs indicating left-heart valve disease, effectively narrow the differential considerations of low output. If the carotid pulse is normal, the next critical determinant of stroke volume to assess is "preload." Evaluation of the lung fields and the JVP will serve to establish evidence of pulmonary congestion which, if present, suggests pulmonary venous hypertension related to mitral valve obstruction, LV diastolic dysfunction, or primary lung disease. Two-dimensional echocardiography is usually effective in establishing the underlying etiology in such patients. In patients with hypotension/low output, a physiologic rhythm and normal carotid exam with evidence of predominant right-heart failure (elevated by JVP elevation or clear lung fields), the algorithm will proceed as described for differentiation of right-heart failure (JVP algorithm). If the carotid pulse is normal with clear lung fields and flat neck veins, such patients should be assumed to be relatively volume depleted and should receive a fluid challenge. Persistent hypotension in such patients suggests sepsis.

Hypotension/Low Output and Depressed Carotid Waveform

If the patient has low output/hypotension, a diminished carotid waveform indicates either LV outflow obstruction (fixed valvular aortic stenosis with depressed delayed parvus et tardus pulse or dynamic obstruction resulting in bisfiriens pulse) or depressed LV contractility due to cardiomyopathy.

Hemodynamic Evaluation of Right-Heart Failure

Right-heart failure (RHF) results in systemic venous congestion, manifest initially as peripheral edema. More advanced stages of RHF lead to hepatomegaly and ascites. Importantly, there are numerous cardiac conditions with disparate pathophysiologic mechanisms that manifest systemic venous congestion. Furthermore, edema and ascites often result from liver disease or peripheral venous derangements unrelated to the right heart. Accordingly, peripheral edema and ascites can only be attributed to right-heart failure under conditions of RA hypertension. Figure 23.3 summarizes the bedside hemodynamic evaluation of right-heart failure.

Physical Examination of the Jugular Venous Pressure and Right Atrial Waveform

The JVP and RA waveform pressures reflect right-heart anatomy and mechanics, as well as total blood volume. To interpret abnormalities of the JVP, it is essential to appreciate the normal waveform components and their relationship to anatomic and mechanical events, including intrapericardial pressure and intrathoracic pressure oscillations.

Abnormalities of the JVP and RA waveforms are categorized according to pathophysiologic considerations, including (i) augmented A wave/X descent, reflecting enhanced atrial contraction/relaxation attributable either to increased outflow resistance imposed by tricuspid valve obstruction or to RV noncompliance resulting from intrinsic RV hypertrophy, infiltration, ischemia, or extrinsic pericardial constraint; (ii) depressed A wave/X descent, reflecting diminished atrial contractility due to ischemic and nonischemic cardiomyopathies—the A wave may be completely absent owing to loss of electrical activation, e.g., atrial fibrillation; (iii) augmented V wave, resulting from tricuspid valve regurgitation; (iv) sharp Y descent, reflecting rapid early atrial emptying as in severe tricuspid regurgitation or constrictive pericarditis; and (v) blunted Y descent attributable to impaired atrial emptying caused by tricuspid valve obstruction or RV noncompliance, reflecting intrinsic RV disease or extrinsic constraint due to cardiac tamponade.

Algorithmic Evaluation of Right-Heart Failure: Focus on the Jugular Venous Pressure

To ascribe peripheral congestive symptoms and signs to right-heart failure, there must be evidence of elevated JVP. Thus, patients with clinical right-heart failure can be evaluated by employing an anatomic-pathophysiologic algorithm based on the JVP, together with precordial examination of the right ventricle and auscultatory examination of the tricuspid and pulmonary valves.

Elevated Jugular Venous Pressure without Right Ventricular Enlargement

When the JVP is elevated, the key to differential diagnosis is physical examination. The presence of RV enlargement is indicated by an RV heave (or "lift") along the left sternal border. If the JVP is elevated and the RV is quiet, then move along the anatomic route from the distended neck veins toward the heart. Is the elevated JVP due to superior vena cava (SVC) obstruction? The JVP is characterized by elevated mean pressure but an overall blunted waveform, particularly the Y descent, which reflects poor flow from the great veins through the SVC obstruction into the heart. Respiratory oscillations are blunted. Thus the inspiratory reduction in the JVP will be attenuated. Physical examination often reveals distention and engorgement of upper thoracic systemic venous channels, whereas chest X-ray and other imaging studies reveal the obstructive mass.

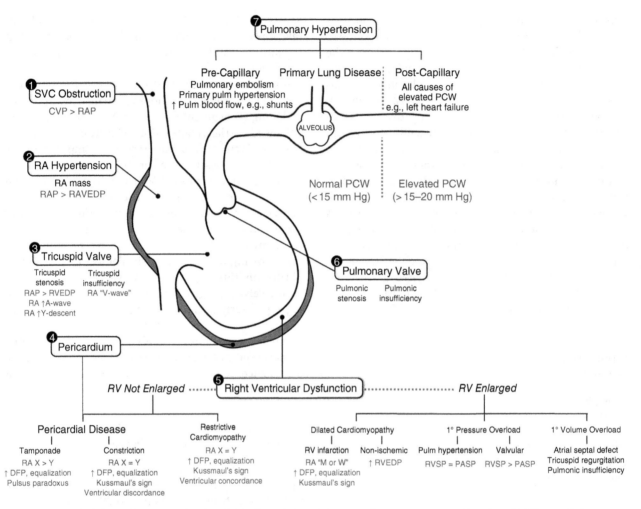

Figure 23.3 Bedside hemodynamic evaluation of right-heart failure. CVP = central venous pressure; DFP = diastolic filling period; PASP = pulmonary artery systolic pressure; PCW = pulmonary capillary wedge; RA = right atrium; RAP = right atrial pressure; RAVEDP = right atrial end-diastolic pressure; RV = right ventricle; RVEDP = right ventricular end-diastolic pressure; RVSP = right ventricular systolic pressure; SVC = superior vena cava.

Next, excluding SVC obstruction, an elevated JVP directly reflects RA hypertension. Entities resulting in RA pressure elevation without RV enlargement include RA space-occupying lesions (tumor masses, thrombi, and vegetations). The elevated RA–JVP pressure has a blunted waveform, especially the Y descent, reflecting poor transit of blood through the obstructive mass, one consequence of which is blunted inspiratory augmentation of right-heart filling, producing Kussmaul's sign. Auscultation may reveal a tumor plop and diastolic flow rumble. Tricuspid valve obstruction due to rheumatic heart disease results in elevated mean RA pressure with a prominent A wave/X descent, reflecting augmented atrial contraction boosting flow through the obstructed orifice. The sharp X descent reflects accelerated atrial relaxation coincident with augmented atrial contraction. The blunted Y descent reflects poor inflow resulting in impaired emptying of the RA. Auscultation reveals

diastolic flow rumble and an opening snap. Primary RV diastolic dysfunction without RV enlargement related to infiltrative processes (e.g., amyloid) produces an RA waveform with an "M" shape, with relatively blunted components due to impaired atrial contraction and delayed RV inflow. Pericardial disease can also elevate RA pressure. In cardiac tamponade, the magnitude of JVP elevation directly reflects elevated RA pressure and intrapericardial pressures. The waveform is characterized by a prominent A wave and sharp X descent, reflecting enhanced atrial contraction into the RV made stiff by pericardial fluid. The Y descent is blunted, reflecting pan-diastolic resistance to RV filling. In tamponade, inspiratory augmentation of venous return to the compressed right heart is intact. The resulting inspiratory competition between the ventricles for preload within the crowded pericardium is responsible for pulsus paradoxus, the magnitude of which reflects the severity of tamponade. In constrictive pericarditis, the JVP is elevated, with augmented atrial contraction and relaxation reflected in a prominent A wave and X descent. However, in constrictive pericarditis, in contrast to tamponade, the first third of diastole is resistance free and thus the Y descent is sharp. In constriction, the heart is isolated from the lungs, resulting in a lack of transmission of intrathoracic pressure changes to the encased cardiac chambers. The lack of respiratory augmentation of right-heart filling precludes forming pulsus paradoxus. Instead, since inspiration does increase venous return toward the chest but not into the heart, JVP pressure increases, resulting in Kussmaul's sign (the hemodynamic obverse of paradoxical pulse).

Infiltrative restrictive processes cause severe RV diastolic dysfunction without RV dilatation. The resultant syndrome is pathophysiologically and hemodynamically similar to and often indistinguishable from constriction. The elevated RA pressure with Kussmaul's sign indicates poor inspiratory augmentation of venous return into the stiff right heart.

Acute Right Ventricular Infarction

Acute RV infarction (see Part Three: Constriction and Tamponade) results in elevated RA pressure with RV dilation, but the acutely noncompliant pericardium limits the appreciation of an RV heave by physical examination. The clinical presentation is hemodynamically similar to tamponade, but the diagnosis is suspected by its association with acute transmural inferior myocardial infarction. The differentiation from tamponade is made obvious by ECG and echocardiography.

Elevated Jugular Venous Pressure with Right Ventricular Enlargement

If RA–JVP pressure is elevated and there is a palpable RV heave, the differential diagnosis now includes (i) primary RV pressure overload, (ii) primary volume overload, and (iii) intrinsic cardiomyopathy (usually nonischemic, as discussed above). The key to the differentiation of these abnormalities is based on the presence of increased RV afterload, most commonly due to pulmonary hypertension (or rarely in adults pulmonary stenosis). On physical examination, pulmonary hypertension is denoted by the presence of a loud P_2. The components of S_2 are best judged by comparing its loudness to that of S_1. The louder and more "booming" the S_2, the higher the PA pressure. S_2 is further analyzed by comparing the intensity to S_1 at the left upper sternal border pulmonary region, where P_2 is normally more prominent. Over the mitral position, S_1 is normally louder than S_2. When pulmonary pressure is elevated, P_2 becomes louder with a snapping sound, particularly in the mitral region, where S_2 will appear louder than S_1.

Elevated Jugular Venous Pressure–Right Atrial Pressure and Right Ventricular Enlargement without Pulmonary Hypertension

If JVP is elevated with an RV heave and soft P_2, then RV dilatation and right-heart failure are related to (i) primary volume overload, (ii) pressure overload proximal to the pulmonary artery, or (iii) intrinsic RV cardiomyopathy. Volume overload lesions include primary tricuspid regurgitation, pulmonary insufficiency, or an atrial septal defect (ASD), all of which are easily differentiated by physical examination. Tricuspid regurgitation is indicated by a holosystolic murmur along the left sternal border that augments with inspiration (Carvullo's sign). The elevated JVP has a prominent V wave and sharp Y descent. Pulmonary insufficiency is evident by a diastolic decrescendo murmur similar to aortic insufficiency, but without the collapsing wide arterial pulse. Atrial septal defect results in JVP elevation with a nonspecific waveform pattern. Auscultation reveals a characteristic wide split S_2, a diastolic flow rumble, and a mid-peaking systolic flow murmur across the RV–PA outflow tract. Increased RV afterload without pulmonary hypertension may result from pulmonary outflow obstruction at the subvalvular, valvular, or postvalvular level. Pulmonary outflow obstruction is indicated by a loud, late-peaking systolic murmur over the RV outflow tract region. RV cardiomyopathy manifests enlarged RV and elevated JVP, and is often associated with secondary functional tricuspid regurgitation (TR).

Elevated Jugular Venous Pressure–Right Atrial Pressure and Right Ventricular Enlargement with Pulmonary Hypertension

Right-heart failure due to pulmonary hypertension is evident by an elevated JVP, an RV heave, and a loud P_2. Right-heart failure attributable to RV pressure overload often results in RV systolic "pump" failure with secondary RV volume overload. It is important to emphasize that under conditions of RV dilatation, the tricuspid valve is vulnerable to functional incompetence, as the dilated RV tends to tether the tricuspid mural (septal) leaflet, rendering the valve prone to functional leakage. Secondary TR is common when the RV fails and enlarges as a consequence of pulmonary hypertension, the increased afterload forcing the RV to preferentially regurgitate backward across the lower-resistance tricuspid valve, thereby perpetuating a vicious cycle of right-heart dilation and low output.

Differential Diagnosis of Pulmonary Hypertension

Right-heart failure due to pulmonary hypertension may be differentiated based on anatomic-pathophysiologic hemodynamic considerations as to whether pulmonary hypertension is pre-capillary, intra-pulmonary, or post-capillary (Figure 22.3). Pre-capillary pulmonary hypertension reflects primary abnormalities of the pulmonary arterial bed, resulting from thromboembolic disease, primary pulmonary hypertension, or occasionally extrinsic mass obstruction of the major pulmonary arteries from mediastinal tumors. Primary intrapulmonary processes include the broad range of primary obstructive or restrictive lung diseases. Post-capillary pulmonary hypertension is attributable to increased pulmonary capillary wedge pressure. Therefore, post-capillary pulmonary hypertension resulting in right-heart pressure failure can be determined through the same approach used for the evaluation of dyspnea, an algorithm based on why and how LA pressure is elevated, as previously described.

Invasive Hemodynamic Assessment of Right-Heart Failure

Invasive evaluation of right-heart failure follows from the anatomic-pathophysiologic approach described based on physical examination.

Employing standard right-heart catheterization techniques, in those patients with elevated central venous pressure, a gradient between the cavae and right atrium indicates obstruction (e.g., mass), in which case the central venous pressure proximal to the obstruction will be elevated. Pressure distal to the obstruction will more closely reflect a normal RA pressure. Even a small gradient across the obstructive mass can produce significant clinical problems.

If RA mean pressure is elevated, RA waveform perturbations provide insights into the pathophysiologic differential diagnosis. A prominent RA A wave/X descent indicates enhanced atrial contraction/relaxation, reflected in increased upstroke and amplitude of the A wave and a sharp initial component of the X descent. Augmented atrial contraction may occur with (i) tricuspid obstruction, associated with a blunted Y descent reflecting impaired atrial emptying and diastolic gradient across the tricuspid valve; (ii) RV diastolic dysfunction, with a lesser blunted Y descent, without a gradient; or (iii) cardiac tamponade, indicated by elevated equalized diastolic filling pressures, a prominent RA A wave/X descent with a blunted Y descent, reflecting pan-diastolic resistance to RV filling and arterial paradoxical pulse, the magnitude of which reflects the severity of tamponade.

Pericardial constriction is also associated with elevated and equalized diastolic filling pressures. The RA waveform manifests an augmented A wave and X descent, but a prominent Y descent, reflecting a pattern of late pericardial resistance. The initial third of diastole is resistance free and

the RV waveform reveals a diastolic "dip and plateau," followed by resistance to filling with a pressure plateau. Constriction results in distinct respiratory oscillations in hemodynamics, with inspiration eliciting a pattern of systolic ventricular pressure discordance and Kussmaul's sign of RA pressure. RV dilated cardiomyopathies also result in marked elevation of right-heart filling pressures. RV infarct results in a marked elevation of right-heart filling pressures. An "M" or "W" pattern in the RA waveform reflects a depressed atrial contraction due to ischemia, a blunted Y descent due to impaired RV filling, and elevated intrapericardial pressure attributable to acute RV dilatation and elevated equalized filling pressures throughout the right and left heart. Restrictive cardiomyopathy and constrictive pericardial disease present nearly identically with regard to hemodynamics. Dynamic respiratory systolic pressure ventricular concordance occurs with restrictive cardiomyopathy. Ventricular systolic pressure discordance is helpful, but not sufficiently diagnostic alone to refer patients for surgery. Pericardial thickening by imaging studies clarifies whether the hemodynamic findings are pericardial or myocardial in nature. The RV pressure waveforms express diastolic abnormalities, as described above. RV systolic pressure reflects RV contractility and afterload. Severely depressed RV contractility (e.g., RV infarction) results in a depressed, sluggish waveform with diminished upstroke and amplitude, as well as delayed relaxation. Increased RV afterload leads to elevated RV systolic pressure. RV outflow obstruction at the subvalvular and valvular levels is identified by a gradient between RV and PA systolic peak and mean pressures. Pulmonary hypertension is indicated by equivalent elevations of RV and PA systolic pressures. Post-capillary pulmonary hypertension due to LA hypertension is suspected whenever PCW pressure is greater than 20–25 mm Hg.

Key Points

This chapter articulates a bedside approach to hemodynamic assessment based on fundamentals of anatomy and pathophysiology.

1) Dyspnea is evaluated based on the delineation of overt left heart derangements based on the carotid waveform, the presence of precordial LV heave and auscultation to elucidate left heart valve abnormalities.
2) Peripheral edema is evaluated based on the delineation of Jugular venous pressure elevation and its waveform, the presence of precordial RLV heave and auscultation to elucidate right heart valve abnormalities.
3) Low Output-Hypotension is evaluated based on blood pressure, the carotid, precordial LV and RV heaves and auscultation of the valves, together with assessment of pulmonary congestion by lung exam.

Appendix

Hemodynamic Rounds, Fourth Edition, 2018

The following citations have been used in the chapters identified by chapter number from the 3rd edition of *Hemodynamic Rounds*. Most of these chapters were originally published in *Catheterization and Cardiovascular Diagnosis* and continue to comprise the basis for most of the chapters in *Hemodynamic Rounds*, 4th edition.

Chapter 1   Kern MJ, Aguirre FV, Donohue TJ. Hemodynamic rounds: Interpretation of cardiac pathophysiology from pressure waveform analysis: Pressure wave artifacts. *Cathet Cardiovasc Diagn* 27:147–154, 1992.

Chapter 2   Kern MJ. Pitfalls of right heart hemodynamics. *Cathet Cardiovasc Diagn* 43:90–94, 1998.

Chapter 3   Kern MJ, Deligonul U. Hemodynamic rounds: Interpretation of cardiac pathophysiology from pressure waveform analysis. II. The tricuspid valve. *Cathet Cardiovasc Diagn* 21:278–286, 1990.

Chapter 4   Kern MJ. Hemodynamic rounds: Interpretation of cardiac pathophysiology from pressure waveform analysis: The left-side V wave. *Cathet Cardiovasc Diagn* 23:211–218, 1991.

Chapter 5   Kern MJ. The LVEDP. *Cathet Cardiovasc Diagn* 44:70–74, 1998.

Chapter 6   Kern MJ, Donohue TJ, Bach R, Aguirre FV. Hemodynamic rounds: Interpretation of cardiac pathophysiology from pressure waveform analysis: Simultaneous left and right ventricular pressure measurements. *Cathet Cardiovasc Diagn* 28:51–55, 1992.

Chapter 7   Kern MJ, Aguirre FV, Hilton TC. Hemodynamic rounds: Interpretation of cardiac pathophysiology from pressure waveform analysis: The effects of nitroglycerin. *Cathet Cardiovasc Diagn* 25:241–248, 1992.

Chapter 8   Schoen WJ, Talley JD, Kern MJ. Hemodynamic rounds: Interpretation of cardiac pathophysiology from pressure waveform analysis: Pulsus alternans. *Cathet Cardiovasc Diagn* 24:315–319, 1991.

Chapter 9   Kern MJ. Editorial comments for hemodynamic rounds: Interpretation of cardiac pathophysiology from pressure waveform analysis: Acute aortic insufficiency. *Cathet Cardiovasc Diagn* 28:244–249, 1993.

Chapter 10   Kern MJ, Aguirre FV. Hemodynamic rounds: Interpretation of cardiac pathophysiology from pressure waveform analysis: Aortic regurgitation. *Cathet Cardiovasc Diagn* 26:232–240, 1992.

Chapter 11   Kern MJ, Aguirre FV. Hemodynamic rounds: Interpretation of cardiac pathophysiology from pressure waveform analysis: Aortic regurgitation. *Cathet Cardiovasc Diagn* 26:232–240, 1992.

Chapter 12   Kern MJ, Aguirre FV, Guerrero M. Abnormal hemodynamics after prosthetic aortic root reconstruction: Aortic stenosis or insufficiency? *Cathet Cardiovasc Diagn* 44:336–340, 1998.

Chapter 13   Godlewski KJ, Talley JD, Morris GT. Interpretation of cardiac pathophysiology from pressure waveform analysis: Acute aortic insufficiency. *Cathet Cardiovasc Diagn* 28:244–248, 1993.

Hemodynamic Rounds: Interpretation of Cardiac Pathophysiology from Pressure Waveform Analysis, Fourth Edition.
Edited by Morton J. Kern, Michael J. Lim, and James A. Goldstein.
© 2018 John Wiley & Sons Ltd. Published 2018 by John Wiley & Sons Ltd.

Chapter 14 Kern MJ, Aguirre FV, Donohue TJ, Bach RG. Hemodynamic rounds: Interpretation of cardiac pathophysiology from pressure waveform analysis: Multivalvular regurgitant lesions. *Cathet Cardiovasc Diagn* 28:167–172, 1993.

Chapter 15 Suh WM, Kern MJ. Addressing the hemodynamic dilemma of combined mitral and aortic stenosis. *Cathet Cardiovasc Interv* 71: 944–949, 2008.

Chapter 17 Kern MJ, Aguirre FV. Hemodynamic rounds: Interpretation of cardiac pathophysiology from pressure waveform analysis: Mitral valve gradients, part I. *Cathet Cardiovasc Diagn* 26:308–315, 1992.

Chapter 18 Kern MJ. Mitral stenosis and pulsus alternans. *Cathet Cardiovasc Diagn* 43:313–317, 1998.

Chapter 19 Azrak E, Kern MJ, Bach RG, Donohue TJ. Hemodynamic evaluation of a stenotic bioprosthetic mitral valve. *Cathet Cardiovasc Diagn* 45:70–75, 1998.

Chapter 20 Kern MJ. Left ventricular puncture for hemodynamic evaluation of double prosthetic valve stenosis. *Cathet Cardiovasc Diagn* 43:466–471, 1998.

Chapter 22 Freihage JH, Joyal D, Arab D, Dieter RS, Loeb HS, Steen L, *et al.* Invasive assessment of mitral regurgitation: Comparison of hemodynamic parameters. *Cathet Cardiovasc Interv* 69:303–312, 2007.

Chapter 23 Kern MJ. Hemodynamic rounds: Interpretation of cardiac pathophysiology from pressure waveform analysis: The pulmonary valve. *Cathet Cardiovasc Diagn* 24:209–213, 1991.

Chapter 24 Kern MJ, Bach RG. Pulmonic balloon valvuloplasty. *Cathet Cardiovasc Diagn* 44:227–234, 1998.

Chapter 25 Kern MJ, Aguirre FV. Hemodynamic rounds: Interpretation of cardiac pathophysiology from pressure waveform analysis: Mitral valve gradients, part II. *Cathet Cardiovasc Diagn* 27:52–56, 1992.

Chapter 29 Kosmicki D, Michaels AD. Hemodynamic rounds: Left heart catheterization and mitral balloon valvuloplasty in a patient with a mechanical aortic valve. *Cathet Cardiovasc Interv* 71(3):429–433, 2008.

Chapter 30 Higano ST, Azrak E, Tahirkheli NK, Kern MJ. Hemodynamics of constrictive physiology: Influence of respiratory dynamics on ventricular pressures. *Cathet Cardiovasc Interv* 46:473–486, 1999.

Chapter 32 Kern MJ, Aguirre FV. Hemodynamic rounds: Interpretation of cardiac pathophysiology from pressure waveform analysis: Pericardial compressive hemodynamics, part II, *Cathet Cardiovasc Diagn* 26:34–40, 1992.

Chapter 33 Kern MJ, Aguirre FV. Hemodynamic rounds: Interpretation of cardiac pathophysiology from pressure waveform analysis: Pericardial compressive hemodynamics, part III. *Cathet Cardiovasc Diagn* 26:152–158, 1992.

Chapter 34 Kern MJ, Aguirre FV. Hemodynamic rounds: Interpretation of cardiac pathophysiology from pressure waveform analysis: Pericardial compressive hemodynamics, part I. *Cathet Cardiovasc Diagn* 25:336–342, 1992.

Chapter 35 Azrak EC, Kern MJ, Bach RG. Hemodynamics of cardiac tamponade in a patient with AIDS-related non-Hodgkin's lymphoma. *Cathet Cardiovasc Diagn* 45:287–291, 1998.

Chapter 36 Strote JA, Dean LS, Goldberg SL, Krieger EV, Stewart DK. A novel assessment for a constrictive pericarditis. Personal communication, 2008.

Chapter 38 Kern MJ, Donohue TJ, Bach RG, Aguirre FV. Hemodynamic rounds: Interpretation of cardiac pathophysiology from pressure waveform analysis: Cardiac arrhythmias. *Cathet Cardiovasc Diagn* 27:223–227, 1992.

Chapter 39 Kern MJ, Deligonul U. Hemodynamic rounds: Interpretation of cardiac pathophysiology from pressure waveform analysis: Pacemaker hemodynamics. *Cathet Cardiovasc Diagn* 24:22–27, 1991.

Chapter 40 Kern MJ, Puri S, Donohue TJ, Bach RG. Hemodynamics of dual-chamber pacing and Valsalva maneuver in a patient with hypertrophic obstructive cardiomyopathy. *Cathet Cardiovasc Diagn* 44:438–442, 1998. Kern MJ, H, Bach RG. Hemodynamics effects of alcohol-induced septal infarction for hypertrophic obstructive cardiomyopathy. *Cathet Cardiovasc Interv* 47:221–228, 1999.

Chapter 41   Kern MJ. Hemodynamic rounds: Interpretation of cardiac pathophysiology from pressure waveform analysis. Coronary hemodynamics: I. Coronary catheter pressures. *Cathet Cardiovasc Diagn* 25:57–60, 1992.Kern MJ. Hemodynamic rounds: Interpretation of cardiac pathophysiology from pressure waveform analysis. Coronary hemodynamics: II. Patterns of coronary flow velocity. *Cathet Cardiovasc Diagn* 25:154–160, 1992.Kern MJ, Aguirre FV, Donohue TJ, Bach RG. Hemodynamic rounds: Interpretation of cardiac pathophysiology from pressure waveform analysis. Coronary hemodynamics III: Coronary hyperemia. *Cathet Cardiovasc Diagn* 26:204–211, 1992.Kern MJ, Puri S, Craig WR, Bach RG, Donohue TJ. Coronary hemodynamics for angioplasty and stenting after myocardial infarction: Use of absolute, relative coronary velocity and fractional flow reserve. *Cathet Cardiovasc Diagn* 45:174–182, 1998.

Chapter 44   Kern MJ, Aguirre FV, Donohue TJ, Bach RG. Hemodynamic rounds: Interpretation of cardiac pathophysiology from pressure waveform analysis: Adult congenital anomalies. *Cathet Cardiovasc Diagn* 27:291–297, 1992.

Chapter 46   Kern MJ, Deligonul U, Miller L. Hemodynamic rounds: Interpretation of cardiac pathophysiology from pressure waveform analysis. IV. Extra hearts: Part I. *Cathet Cardiovasc Diagn* 22:197–201, 1990.Kern MJ, Deligonul U. Hemodynamic rounds: Interpretation of cardiac pathophysiology from pressure waveform analysis. IV. Extra hearts: Part II. *Cathet Cardiovasc Diagn* 22:302–306, 1990.Kern MJ, Deligonul U. Hemodynamic rounds: Interpretation of cardiac pathophysiology from pressure waveform analysis. IV. Extra hearts: Part III. *Cathet Cardiovasc Diagn.* 23:50–53, 1991.

Index

Hemodynamic Rounds: Interpretation of Cardiac Pathophysiology from Pressure Waveform Analysis, Fourth Edition.
Edited by Morton J. Kern, Michael J. Lim, and James A. Goldstein.
© 2018 John Wiley & Sons Ltd. Published 2018 by John Wiley & Sons Ltd.